The Veterinary Medical Team Handbook

The Team Approach to Veterinary Medicine

The Veterinary Medical Team Handbook
The Team Approach to Veterinary Medicine

Andrew J. Rosenfeld DVM

Diplomate, American Board of Veterinary Practitioners
Canine and Feline

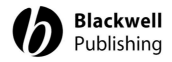
Blackwell Publishing

Andrew J. Rosenfeld, DVM, Diplomate ABVP, is the founder and president of Veterinary Team Education Course. He lectures frequently on topics in emergency medicine, small animal anatomy and physiology, and cardiology. He has practiced small animal critical care and emergency medicine for 16 years and served as hospital director of Paradise Valley Emergency Animal Clinic in Scottsdale, Arizona, for 3 years. Previously, Dr. Rosenfeld was director of technical education for the Pet's Choice family of veterinary hospitals and specialty practices and an adjunct professor at Mesa Community College and Arizona State University.

Blackwell Publishing Professional
2121 State Avenue, Ames, Iowa 50014, USA

Orders: 1-800-862-6657
Office: 1-515-292-0140
Fax: 1-515-292-3348
Web site: www.blackwellprofessional.com

Blackwell Publishing Ltd
9600 Garsington Road, Oxford OX4 2DQ, UK
Tel.: +44 (0)1865 776868

Blackwell Publishing Asia
550 Swanston Street, Carlton, Victoria 3053, Australia
Tel.: +61 (0)3 8359 1011

Authorization to photocopy items for internal or personal use, or the internal or personal use of specific clients, is granted by Blackwell Publishing, provided that the base fee is paid directly to the Copyright Clearance Center, 222 Rosewood Drive, Danvers, MA 01923. For those organizations that have been granted a photocopy license by CCC, a separate system of payments has been arranged. The fee codes for users of the Transactional Reporting Service is ISBN-13: 978-0-7817-5759-1/2007.

First edition, 2007

Library of Congress Cataloging-in-Publication Data

Rosenfeld, Andrew J.
  The veterinary medical team handbook: the team approach to veterinary medicine/Andrew J. Rosenfeld.—1st ed.
      p.   ; cm.
  Includes bibliographical references and index.
  ISBN-13: 978-0-7817-5759-1 (alk. paper)
  ISBN-10: 0-7817-5759-2 (alk. paper)
  1. Veterinary medicine—Handbooks, manuals, etc. I. Title.
  [DNLM: 1. Veterinary Medicine—Handbooks. 2. Animal Diseases—nursing—Handbooks. 3. Animal Technicians—Handbooks. SF 748 R813v 2007]

  SF748.R67 2007
  636.089—dc22
                                                                                          2006036123

The last digit is the print number: 9 8 7 6 5 4 3 2 1

Dedicated to Lisa, Lauren, and Jillian, who act as my center, my practicality, my imagination, and my world

Contents

Preface

Veterinary medicine is a dynamic field, allowing all team members growth in every aspect of the science and profession. It is the only medical profession that allows a medical team member to be part of surgical, radiological, emergency medicine, internal medicine, and surgery teams all in one day. With increasing expectations of quality care and technology, a team member's knowledge and responsibilities are growing at an exponential rate.

This book is dedicated to that veterinary team that works as one unit to

- focus the doctor's attention where the hospital needs him or her most,
- utilize the staff to their fullest potential,
- increase staff satisfaction and loyalty as well as decrease employee turnover,
- increase revenue by becoming more effective communicators and increasing their ability to sense health problems and deal with upset clients, and
- turn the veterinary technician field into a profession that can be financially and professionally rewarding.

This book is intended to be used as a training and interactive resource to help train the medical team to be a resource for the veterinarian, the patient, and the client.

How to Use This Book

Each section of this book is divided into sections. The sections are broken down into the following: The First Two Days on the Job, Anatomy and Physiology—The Science behind the Diseases, Clinical Diagnostics—The Science behind the Diagnostics, Understanding the Concepts of Disease and Treatment, and the Appendix. The overall goal of this book is to

- give the paraprofessional the education and tools to discuss and understand the different disease, diagnostic, and treatment processes that may be required;
- serve as a quick reference source for the paraprofessional on general practice subjects; and
- reinforce the concepts of each section with interactive clinical cases in a PowerPoint format.

Using this book either as a simple resource or as a part of a formal training program will help refine the skills of the staff and make them greater resources within the hospital team.

Acknowledgments

Thanks to the following professionals who reviewed the book: Dr. Curt Coffman, Fellow of the Academy of Veterinary Dentistry, Aid Animal Dental Clinic, Scottsdale, Arizona; Dr. Kimberly Coyner, DVM ACVD, Dermatology Clinic for Animals, Phoenix, Arizona; Dr. Sharon Dial, DVM ACVP (Clinical and Anatomic Pathology), associate research scientist, Department of Veterinary Science and Microbiology at University of Arizona, Tucson, Arizona; Victoria M. Lukasik, DVM, Diplomate ACVA, Southwest Veterinary Anesthesiology, and assistant research scientist, Radiology, University of Arizona College of Medicine, Phoenix, Arizona.

Thanks also to Stephen Bistner, DVM DACVO, Plymouth, Minnesota, and Jeffrey Bowersox, DVM ACVO, Wilmington, Delaware, for editing support and images.

Special thanks to Caron Cann, who has been my professional sounding board and a compass for me while I finished this project.

Veterinary Medical Team Handbook Interactive CD-ROM

The goal of the interactive CD-ROMs is to practice the key concepts of each section of the book. The CD-ROM is split into two programs.

The first CD-ROM is meant for practice with the first two sections of the book with special focus on:

- **Auscultation Trainer**—Reviews basic concepts of auscultation and allows team members to practice ausculting hearts with different murmurs in case formats.
- **Section I Cases**—Helps the team member apply basic concepts of nomenclature, lesion position, and obtaining a medical history and understanding the concepts of surgery, vaccination, and heartworm prevention.
- **Section II Cases**—A slightly more advanced program outlining and testing concepts of basic anatomy and physiology, diseases, clinical diagnostics, and communication with clients about the cardiac, renal, liver, and pancreatic organs.

The second CD-ROM contains advanced rounds for the medical team focusing on physical examination, clinical diagnostics, and treatment concepts. Topics contained on the CD-ROM are:

- **EKG Trainer and Case Rounds**—This section reviews the basic concepts of the electrical rhythm of the heart, step-by-step protocols on how to evaluate an EKG, and how recognize basic arrhythmias.
- **Emergency Triage Trainer**—The program takes the medical team through two emergency cases that enter the hospital at the same time; the team has to evaluate which animal is more of an emergency at each step of the evaluation.
- **Toxin Rounds**—This program takes the medical team through toxin and poison ingestion cases and focuses on common physical symptoms and clinical diagnostics associated with common poison ingestion.
- **Complete Blood Count Rounds**—This program shows the medical team how to evaluate a complete blood count focusing on red blood cell morphology, white blood cell changes, and platelet estimation on the blood film.
- **Fluid Rounds**—This section takes the medical team through how to evaluate the patient for dehydration, determine fluid need, and practice fluid calculation.

To Load the CD

Both CD-ROMs contain self-loading narrated PowerPoint based programs that work on any computer (PC or Macintosh). Both contain large files and will take 3 to 5 minutes to load. Simply place the CD-ROM into your CD-ROM drive and allow the program to load. The program will then instruct you on how to navigate through each program.

To Navigate in the PowerPoint Environment

Once in the PowerPoint environment, you will be able to navigate through each slide by clicking on selected tabs to move forward, answer a question, evaluate a heart rhythm, or make choices where to go in the program. To fully enjoy this process, please follow these guidelines to navigate in this environment.

1. **When the program begins, you get a Macro Warning.** These programs contain commands called "macros" that allow the participant to move throughout the environment, listen to sound files, and view image files contained on these CDs. These are not meant to affect your computer or its ability to function. In order to use the CD-ROMS you will need to select to activate the macros in this presentation.

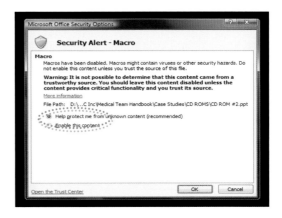

In order to view this program properly, please select Enable Macro and click Okay. The program will then load and run normally.

2. **When selecting a tab, make sure that the mouse arrow has changed to a small hand before left clicking the mouse button**. This will select the proper tab, and will not move you one slide forward in the program.

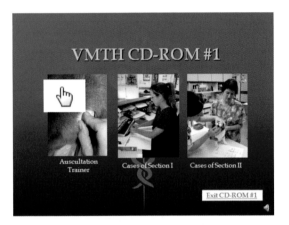

Correct way—The mouse has gone from arrow to hand, showing you are selecting the proper tab.

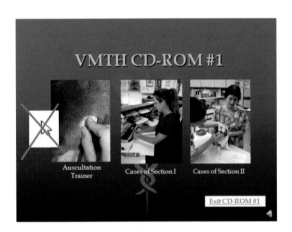

Incorrect Way—In this image the arrow has not changed into the hand, and clicking the mouse will move the program forward one slide only.

3. **When using the mouse, you inadvertently click or use the dial to move one slide forward.** If you do inadvertently move to the next slide and are out of place, simply right click the mouse, which will bring up the following options:

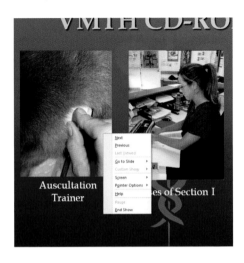

By right clicking the mouse, the following options become available, please highlight Previous and click with the left mouse button. This will move you back one slide space.

4. **There is no narration for the slide.** On occasion, PowerPoint may not initiate the narrative sequence. To restart the narration process, simply click the left mouse button once.

Finally—The programs are meant as fun exercises to reinforce the concepts of the book. At no time does the program, the book, or the author suggest that the medical team is responsible for diagnosis, prognosis, or treatment of the patient.

Section 1

The First Two Days on the Job

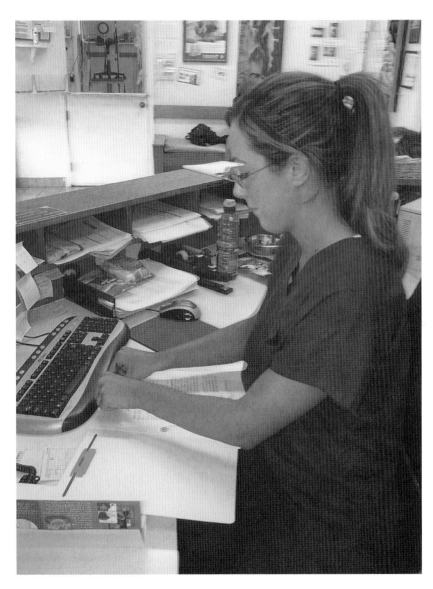

This section is for the new employee who has an active interest in learning the fundamentals of being a part of the veterinary team. It is a training manual that outlines what all team members should know on the first 2 days on the job.

Chapter 1

Basic Terminology

Introduction

As with the study of any science or profession, there is a language and terminology unique to this knowledge; veterinary medicine is no different. Understanding the basics of veterinary terminology is a critical aspect of becoming an excellent team member and will better serve your clients and patients. Many clients will use terminology that they pick up from other hospitals, the Internet, or human medicine, and if a team member does not fully understand what the client is asking for, miscommunication and poor client service can occur. For example, consider the following situations.

- A client calls and informs you that their pet needs to come in for "an allergy injection." This could refer to a steroid injection for allergies or an allergen vaccine for a pet that has been skin tested for allergies.
- A client comes in and requests that "their pet needs to be put to sleep." In most cases this suggests that their pet is to be euthanized, but clients use this terminology to ask for sedation for a pet that may need to be groomed or that is going on a car trip.
- A client brings their male cat in for a "spay." If the sex of the animal is not quickly determined, the cat may be prepped and possibly surgically set up for an ovariohysterectomy.

All these situations sound amusing, but they have occurred in everyday clinical settings. Therefore, it becomes the veterinary professional's responsibility to understand and educate the clients so that they can make an informed choice.

Directional Terminology

To properly describe a lesion, injury, or other problem, the first thing that must be mastered is the directional terminology that helps locate the problem on the pet's body (Figure 1.1). To systematically do this, we create a series of planes that split the pet into sections. The most important plane we deal with is the **median plane** that splits the pet into two symmetrical halves.

Once this plane is established, we compare where a body part or injury falls in relation to the proximity of the median plane. For example, the forelimb of a dog is illustrated in Figure 1.2. Each toe or finger is closely related to our fingers and toes. The first digit, which represents our thumb, is the dog and cat's dewclaw, a small digit that does not directly have a function in weight bearing and is often removed when the animal is young (3–4 days old).

The first digit is closest to the medial plane of the animal and hence we say that the first digit is the most **medial**. The other digits are farther away from the medial plane from the first digits and hence we refer to these digits as being **lateral** to the first digit.

Therefore, the third digit is medial to the fifth digit and lateral to the first and second digits, and the fourth digit is medial to the fifth digit and lateral to the first, second, and third digits.

Also, we must be able to inform the medical team where a region, mass, or injury lies in relation to its position on the limb. Hence the closer the area of concern lies to the body, the more **proximal** it is. The farther away the injury or area lies from the body the more **distal** it is said to be. In the illustration in Figure 1.2, the wrist is proximal to the toes, or the toes are said to be distal to the wrist. This directional terminology refers only to limbs.

When discussing the main torso of the animal's body, we define areas closer to the spine as having a **dorsal** position to regions that are closer to the pet's sternum and belly, which have a **ventral** position. Hence a dog's ears are generally dorsal to their eyes, or the eyes sit more ventral to the canine's ears.

Further directional terminology occurs when we explain where the body part lies in its relation to the head or tail. Body parts that lie closer to the head of the pet are **cranial** in their position, whereas body parts that are closer to the tail are **caudal** in their location. Thus a pet's ears are cranial to their shoulders, or their shoulders are caudal to the ears.

For a review, see Figures 1.3 and 1.4.

History Terminology

Taking a good medical history is one of the chief focuses of this book and will be discussed in detail in Chapter 5. However, there are certain abbreviations that are used in taking an accurate history and relaying this information to the medical team. Some abbreviations used in taking the animal's history are as follows:

DESCRIPTIVE TERMS – PLANES – SECTIONS

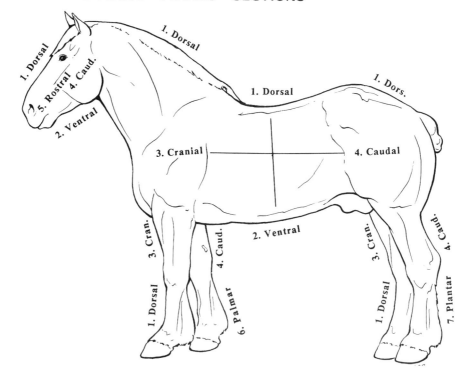

Figure 1.1. Descriptive terms. (Courtesy of *Anatomy of Domestic Animals,* 7th Edition. Pasquini, Chris, and Pasquini, Susan. Sudz Publishing, Pilot Point, Tx 1989. Used with permission from Sudz Publishing.)

- C: coughing
- S: sneezing
- V: vomiting
- D: diarrhea
- PD: polydipsia (increased thirst)
- PU: polyuria (increased urination)
- BM: bowel movement
- Anorexia: not eating
- Lethargy: depressed/decreased energy and activity

Terminology of the Physical Exam

There is specific nomenclature that is also used in discussing the pet and aspects of the pet's body system based on the physical exam. To properly communicate with the medical team, the team member must have an understanding of this terminology. Although we will discuss the physical exam in detail in Chapter 5, there are medical abbreviations that are commonly used to describe an animal properly.

Cat description abbreviations include

- DLH: domestic long hair,
- DMH: domestic medium hair, and
- DSH: domestic short hair.

There are many abbreviations for physical examination nomenclature, as well. For **mentation** (how the pet presents mentally), the abbreviations are as follows:

- BAR: bright, alert, and responsive
- QAR: quiet, alert, and responsive
- Depressed: animal is not active or normally responsive to stimuli
- Comatose/obtund: animal is not responding to any stimuli, severe depression without consciousness

For the baseline parameters of overall health the terms used are as follows:

- T: temperature
- P: pulse
- R: respiration
- MM: mucous membrane
- CRT: capillary refill time
- Hydration

Abbreviations for the body systems are as follows:

- CV: cardiovascular system (heart and vascular system)
- Resp: respiratory system (trachea, bronchi, and lungs)
- Abd: abdomen
- LN: lymph nodes
- MS: musculoskeletal system
- E-E-N-T: eyes, ears, nose, and throat
- Neuro: neurologic system
- Int: integumentary system (skin)
- Uro: urogenital system (reproductive organs)

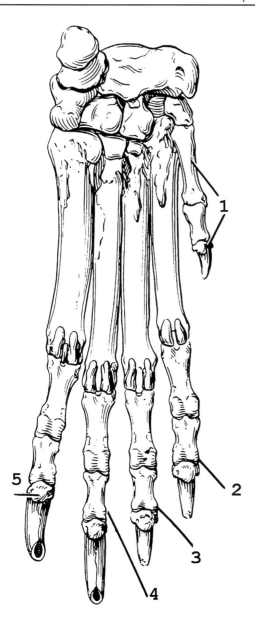

Figure 1.2. The forelimb of a dog. (Courtesy of *Anatomy of Domestic Animals,* 7th Edition. Pasquini, Chris, and Pasquini, Susan. Sudz Publishing, Pilot Point, Tx 1989. Used with permission from Sudz Publishing.)

Disease Terminology

When obtaining a thorough history and understanding the concerns of the client, it is important to define the onset and progression of the pet's disease. In these cases, the following terms are used to help define these parameters.

- **Acute** onset of disease refers to a disease entity that has affected the patient rapidly as the patient went from good health to illness in a short period of time.
- **Chronic** onset of disease refers to a disease entity that a patient has been dealing with over longer periods of time. Symptoms can worsen or stay the same during the duration of the illness, but the patient is still affected over the long term.

- **Progressive** disease refers to disease entities that have worsening symptoms over time. Both acute and chronic disease can have progressive symptoms.

Pharmacological Terminology

When dispensing medication to an animal there are specific abbreviations and terms that apply to the route by which the drug is given, how often it is given, and to what part of the anatomy it is applied. Understanding these terms is extremely important because a mistake can produce serious side effects.

Dosing

The abbreviations used for dosing, particularly the frequency of administration of medication per day, are as follows:

- EOD: every other day
- SID: once per day
- BID: twice per day
- TID: three times per day
- QID: four times per day
- PRN: as needed
- ETD: every third day
- q: normally written in lowercase case, *q* translates to *every* (i.e., q 8 hrs means every 8 hours).

See examples of using this terminology in clinical settings next.

> Example 1: You are a part of a busy medical team. Your doctor has talked with Mr. Doe about his dog Rufus at length. Rufus is on phenobarbital. Mr. Doe left a message for the doctor that Rufus is still seizing and asks what he should do about the medication. The doctor leaves you the following message: "Please call John Doe about Rufus. Instruct him to increase Rufus's phenobarbital from 1–25 mg tablet SID to 1–25 mg tablet BID by mouth (PO). If the seizing continues, I will need to see Rufus." This message indicates that you need to instruct Ms. Doe to increase Rufus's phenobarbital from 1–25 mg tablet 1×/day to 1–25 mg tablet 2×/day by mouth.

> Example 2: Your veterinarian asks you to assist her in filling a prescription for 500 mg aspirin. The chart indicates the following instructions: Give one (1) tablet q 12 hours PRN. This translates to "Give one tablet every 12 hours as needed" (for pain, limping, or for whatever the disorder indicated).

Anatomical Abbreviations for Ears and Eyes

When dealing with the eyes and ears, specialized abbreviations allow us to determine which ear or eye is to be treated.

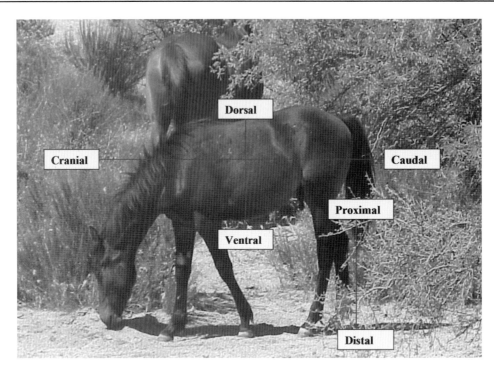

Figure 1.3. Cranial/caudal and dorsal/ventral nomenclature.

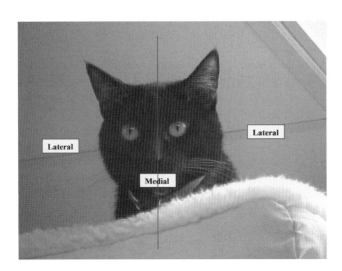

Figure 1.4. Lateral/medial nomenclature.

The following abbreviations are used for eyes:

- OD: right eye
- OS: left eye
- OU: both eyes

The following abbreviations are used for ears:

- AD: right ear
- AS: left ear
- AU: each ear

A good way to remember the letter combination is that it was once thought that people who shook hands with their left hand were thought to be "sinister." Hence *s* means left.

Administration Routes
The way a drug is administered to the animal also has its own abbreviations.

- IV: intravenous–in the vein (typically done through an intravenous catheter)
- IM: intramuscular–in the muscle
- IN: intranasal–in the nose
- IC: intracardiac–in the heart (rarely done)
- IT: intratracheal–in the throat (or intratracheal tube)
- PO: per os–by mouth
- SQ: subcutaneous–under the skin

It is very important to never fill a prescription or give a medication without full knowledge of the drug, the drug's function, and any potential side effects or drug interactions. If there is ever a question on a prescription or concern regarding the route or the dosing of a medication, the prescription should not be filled until all questions are discussed with a veterinarian. Pharmacology will be discussed comprehensively in Chapter 26.

CD-ROM 1 reviews material presented in this chapter. Please try the cases for Section 1 (The First Two Days on the Job) to help reinforce the information presented here.

Chapter 2

Vaccines, Heartworms, and Their Terminology

Although many diseases will be discussed in depth in subsequent chapters, all members of a medical team will need to have knowledge of specific diseases, vaccines, and heartworm prevention from the first day on the job. Every practice and medical team has a slightly different approach to their vaccine recommendations, how often the vaccines should be administered, and how to discuss the vaccines with the client. It is important to get an understanding of how your medical team approaches this topic; however, this section will help provide a basic overview of vaccination principles and nomenclature.

Canine Vaccines

There are generally two schedules of vaccines given to canines in a general practice, the schedule for the puppy and the schedule for the adult. The puppy is generally vaccinated three to four times over the first 6–16 weeks of life to help boost long-term immunity for many juvenile and adult diseases. The adult vaccine is generally an annual booster to help maintain the animal's immunity to specific diseases

throughout its life. The types of vaccines given can vary but in general they are as discussed next.

DHPP
Also known as DA$_2$P, the DHPP vaccine is generally given subcutaneously three to four times in the juvenile phase (6–16 weeks) every 2–4 weeks and is then repeated annually. It can be given in conjunction with other vaccines (corona virus/leptospirosis). The diseases that are vaccinated for are canine distemper, hepatitis, parainfluenza, and parvo virus.

Canine Distemper Virus
Canine distemper virus(CDV; see Chapter 11), the *D* in DHPP, is a highly infectious upper respiratory virus that can cause

- severe high body temperature (fever),
- anorexia,
- depression,
- lethargy,
- coughing,
- sneezing,
- sinusitis, and
- neurologic signs.

Fifty percent of the time CDV enters the central nervous system, causing seizures, coma, and death.

There are some basic points to raise when discussing vaccines with clients.

- Vaccines are killed or weakened bacteria or viruses that are injected into a healthy animal to help it develop immunity to a specific disease.
- In order for vaccines to be effective, the pet must be in good health with a normal immune system.
- No vaccine is 100% effective, and if the animal is exposed to enough of the infectious agent, they can still become ill. However, in some cases, the vaccines generally can help reduce the capacity of a microorganism to cause disease (**virulence**).
- Vaccines will not prevent the disease in an already infected animal.
- Although rare, any vaccine can produce an allergic reaction, and there is no way to tell if an animal will have a reaction to a vaccine until the vaccine is given.
- Vaccine reactions can occur in the first minutes to hours after inoculation.

Key Points in Discussing Distemper Virus with Clients
- Distemper virus is an upper respiratory illness that is commonly found in large kennel facilities with young animals, such as a pound or animal control facility.
- The infection will start as a severe upper respiratory infection causing loss of appetite, depression, runny purulent (pus) ocular and nasal discharge, and fever.
- Fifty percent of the time the virus will infect the central nervous system producing seizures, muscular tremors, coma, and death.
- If the animal begins to exhibit neurologic symptoms, the animal's prognosis is generally poor.
- A full set of vaccinations as a puppy and regular adult vaccines is very protective against the virus.

Canine Hepatitis Virus

Canine hepatitis virus, the *H* (or *A* in DA₂P) in DHPP, is an adenovirus that produces a life-threatening infection of the liver, causing

- depression,
- anorexia,
- yellowing of the gums, whites of the eyes and skin (jaundice),
- vomiting, and
- diarrhea.

Parainfluenza

Parainfluenza, the first *P* in DHPP**,** is a flu virus causing upper respiratory and or pneumonia.

Parvo Virus

Parvo virus (CPV; see Chapter 10), the second *P* in DHPP, is a severe viral disease of juveniles (8 weeks–18 months of age) that lives in the environment through exceptional cold and heat for years. The virus attacks the cells of the intestine that absorb water and food. The animal is unable to properly absorb food and water causing the following

- Massive diarrhea and vomiting (often bloody).
- Anorexia.
- Severe life-threatening dehydration.
- Massive whole body infection (sepsis). The virus temporarily decreases the white blood cell population in the pet. The animal is then open to massive infections from any bacterial source.

Key Points in Discussing Parvo Virus with Clients

- Parvo virus is an illness of the gastrointestinal system that is found in large numbers in the environment. The virus is very hardy and able to live through temperature extremes for years.
- The infection temporarily destroys the cells that absorb food and water, so the pet cannot properly digest and absorb it. This produces severe vomiting and diarrhea, often with blood.
- The virus also temporarily decreases the pet's white blood cell population making them very susceptible to infection.
- These pets dehydrate and become severely infected leading to a life-threatening state.
- Although the vaccine does not always prevent a pet from contracting parvo, the more vaccinations the pet has received usually decreases the virulence of the disease.

Corona Virus

Corona virus (CV) is a weak gastrointestinal virus that causes mild vomiting and diarrhea. The vaccine can be given subcutaneously with DHPP or by itself.

Leptospirosis

Leptospirosis is a spiral bacteria (spirochete) that can cause an acute kidney or liver disease and can affect blood cell populations. As the infection occurs, the animal's ability to remove toxins from the body is impaired producing signs of

- depression,
- anorexia,
- vomiting,
- diarrhea,
- profound dehydration,
- yellowing of the gums, whites of the eyes, skin (**jaundice**),
- vomiting blood (**hematemesis**),
- frank blood in the stool (**hematochezia**), and
- nose bleeds (**epistaxis**).

This vaccine can be given subcutaneously by itself or with the DHPP vaccine. This is one of the most common vaccines to produce an allergic reaction in the pet.

Canine Rabies

Rabies is a debilitating and lethal viral infection of the central nervous system that is spread through the saliva and bite of an infected animal. Rabies can be spread by wildlife (skunks, raccoons, bats, foxes, coyotes, etc.). All dogs in the United States are required to be vaccinated. Generally, the juvenile vaccine is given subcutaneously or intramuscularly. The adult vaccine is then boosted after 1 year and then repeated every 1–3 years depending on how prevalent rabies is in the geographic region (**endemic**). Rabies is also infectious to humans (zoonotic).

Bordetella

The Bordetella vaccine protects against infectious tracheobronchitis (kennel cough; see Chapter 11). *Bordetella* causes a mild upper respiratory/sore throat complex for which vaccine is administered two to four times per year through an intranasal vaccine or once a year through a subcutaneous vaccine.

Lyme Disease

Lyme disease is an intracellular parasite (*Borrelia burgdorferi*) that is spread by a tick bite and occurs in specific geographic regions of the United States (New England and other regions). It produces acute lameness, fever, anorexia, and occasionally heart disease. This vaccine is given intramuscularly in endemic regions of the country.

Feline Vaccinations

As with the canine, there are two set schedules for vaccination: one for the kitten and one for the adult. However, vaccine recommendations are currently undergoing a dramatic reexamination due to potential long-term reactions to specific vaccines (see below), and many hospitals and medical teams have very different recommendations for their vaccine schedule. However, the general vaccines for cats are discussed below.

FVRCP

The FVRCP vaccine is generally given subcutaneously three times in the juvenile phase (6–16 weeks) every 2–4 weeks and is then repeated every 1–3 years. The diseases that are vaccinated for are feline viral rhinotracheitis, feline calici virus, and feline panleukopenia virus.

Feline Viral Rhinotracheitis

Feline viral rhinotracheitis (the FVR in FVRCP) is a feline herpes virus that produces a mild to moderate upper respiratory infection generally in young kittens. As with other herpes virus in all species, the animal can overcome the infection and then be reinfected with the virus at other points in the pet's life related to stress, the animal's health status, and other factors. The signs of the disease are

- coughing,
- sneezing,
- watery ocular discharge,
- squinting,
- fever,
- anorexia, and
- corneal ulceration.

Feline Calici Virus (FCV)

Feline calici virus (FCV), the *C* in FVRCP, is an upper respiratory virus generally of the young cat or adopted cat. It produces signs of

- coughing,
- sneezing,
- watery ocular discharge,
- drooling from the mouth,
- anorexia, and
- ulcers of the tongue.

Feline Panleukopenia Virus

Feline panleukopenia virus (or feline parvo virus; FPV), the *P* in FVRCP, is often called feline distemper. However, feline panleukopenia is a parvo virus. As with the canine form of the disease, it produces a severe viral juvenile disease (8 weeks–18 months of age) that attacks the cells of the intestine that absorb water and food. The pet is unable to properly absorb food, causing massive diarrhea and vomiting (often bloody), anorexia, and severe life-threatening dehydration. The disease has a high mortality rate in cats.

Feline Rabies

Just as with the canine form, feline rabies is a debilitating and lethal viral infection of the central nervous system spread through the saliva and bite of an infected animal. Rabies vaccination and licensing in cats can be required depending on state law. Generally, the juvenile vaccine is given subcutaneously or intramuscularly. The adult vaccine is then boosted after 1 year and then repeated every 1–3 years depending on how endemic rabies is in the state. Rabies is also infectious to humans (zoonotic).

Feline Leukemia Virus

Feline leukemia virus (Felv) is an incurable, potentially lethal, viral disease that infects the cat's white blood cells, causing an inability of the white blood cells to reproduce and protect the body from infection. Cats can carry the disease for years without showing infection and can spread the disease over long-term exposure to other cats through cat fights, grooming, eating from the same food bowls, or sexual intercourse. Signs and onset of the disease can be extremely variable depending on where the viral disease begins to show itself.

Acute Felv Disease (Disease of Sudden Onset)

Respiratory disease causes an acute precipitation of white blood cells and fluid of the body building up within the chest cavity producing signs of

- shortness of breath,
- open mouth breathing,
- bluing of the gums, whites of the eyes, tongue,
- abdominal breathing, and
- death

Feline leukemia virus can invade the central nervous system producing (although rarely)

- seizures,
- fever,

Key Points in Discussing Feline Leukemia with Clients
- There is no link between human leukemia and the feline leukemia virus.
- Outside or inside/outside cats are the most at risk.
- Cats spread the disease from cat fights/bites, chronic exposure (over months to years) to infected cats through grooming and eating out of the same food bowl, sexual coitus.
- Cats can carry the disease and be infectious for years without any physical symptoms.
- Most vaccines are about 70% effective, and cats that do roam outside should be tested annually.
- Vaccines will not prevent the disease in an already infected animal, so if there is a concern with Felv, that cat should be tested prior to initial vaccination.
- Although rare, the vaccine can make the cat depressed, lethargic, and grumpy for a few days after the vaccination, similar to our reaction to a human flu shot.
- Feline leukemia vaccine does have some potential long-term side effects of concern (see below).

- depression,
- coma, and
- death.

Chronic Felv Disease (Disease of Slow Onset)

With chronic disease, signs can be dependent on which body systems the virus infects; however, general signs are

- weight loss,
- anorexia,
- severe dental disease,
- diarrhea/vomiting (if the intestinal system is affected),
- poor abilities to heal,
- muscle wasting, and
- poor hair coat.

Feline Infectious Peritonitis

Feline infectious peritonitis (FIP) vaccine protects against a viral disease of the corona virus family that produces a fatal inflammatory disease of the abdomen and chest. The virus interacts with white blood cells of the body, producing microscopic clumps of white blood cells and virus on tissue. These nests of inflammatory cells cause organ damage and disease on the tissue level. The disease is most common in young and stray cats. The disease produces signs of

- anorexia,
- lethargy,
- weight loss,
- depression,
- fever,
- accumulation of fluid in the abdomen (ascites),
- accumulation of fluid in the chest (pleural fluid), which presents as
  — shortness of breath,
  — open mouth breathing,
  — bluing of the gums, whites of the eyes, tongue,
  — abdominal breathing, and
  — death.

Key Points in Discussing FIP with Clients
- Outside or stray cats are the most at risk.
- Currently it is unknown exactly how the disease is spread.
- The virus belongs to a large family of viruses; the exact virus type within the family is so far unknown. Therefore there is no absolute test for FIP.
- FIP vaccine is given through an intranasal vaccine, typically for animals that are at risk.

Feline Immunodeficiency Virus

Feline immunodeficiency virus (FIV) is an incurable viral disease that can attack any system in the cat's body, causing a chronic wasting disease or an acute life-threatening epi-

sode. The disease usually affects the cat's immune system and then secondarily will affect other body systems. The virus can cause a wide variety of signs.

Respiratory disease presents with

- chronic nasal discharge,
- chronic ocular discharge (eyes),
- trouble breathing,
- increased respiratory rate,
- open mouth breathing, and
- collapse.

Gastrointestinal disease presents with

- severe gingivitis,
- ulcers in the mouth and tongue,
- chronic vomiting,
- chronic diarrhea,
- weight loss, and
- nonresponsiveness to medication.

Neurologic disease presents with

- seizure,
- aggression, and
- fever of unknown origin.

Key Points in Discussing FIV with Clients
- FIV is in the same family of viruses as HIV.
- There has never been a reported case of humans contracting FIV from a cat.
- Cats can carry the disease and be infectious for years without any physical symptoms.
- Outside or inside/outside cats are the most at risk.
- Cats spread the disease from cat fights/bites, chronic exposure (over months to years) to infected cats through grooming and eating out of the same food bowl, and coitus.
- There is a vaccine available, however at this time, its ability to promote protection is still under investigation.
- Any cat that has been vaccinated for FIV will show positive on the FIV screening test, making it impossible to differentiate a cat that has been vaccinated from one that has been infected.

Potential Side Effects of Vaccination

Short-Term Reactions: Allergic and Anaphylactic Reactions

There are a few basic concepts that must be understood when discussing and monitoring allergic reactions in pets.

- Any medication, whether vaccine or medicine, whether injectable or oral, can produce an allergic reaction in an animal.

There are some very basic points to raise when discussing an allergic reaction with the client. With young animals that have not been exposed to a specific vaccine before,

- inform them that allergic reactions are very rare and usually mild problems, but they can occasionally occur;
- review symptoms of a possible allergic reaction and stress to the client that they should be aware of what to look for in the next 12–24 hours;
- make sure the owner has emergency contact numbers for your hospital or a local emergency clinic if any signs are noted;
- if signs are noticed, the animal should be seen immediately to prevent a mild allergic reaction from getting worse; and
- inform the client that if a pet shows sensitivity to a specific vaccine, steps can be taken in the future to prevent the pet from having repeat incidence on their next vaccination.

With older animals that have been repeatedly exposed to the same type of vaccinations

- always check the chart and with the client to ensure that there has been no previous history of vaccine reaction; and
- check to see if there has been any concern regarding even mild changes in the pet's health prior to vaccination. If so, inform the veterinarian immediately.

- There is no way to tell if any pet given a medication for the first time will have a reaction.
- The allergic reactions in the dog and the cat manifest themselves with completely different symptoms.
- Allergic reactions are uncommon.
- Allergic reactions are generally mild; however, mild allergic reactions can precipitate into more severe reactions if the pet is not treated in a timely fashion.
- The allergic reaction can take place in the first few minutes after injection or several hours after exposure.
- Although unlikely, animals may show a first-time allergic reaction to a medication or a vaccine they have never been exposed to previously. It is not impossible for a dog to start to show a mild allergic reaction on its first rabies vaccination.
- Typically, patients produce allergic reactions after being exposed to a vaccine or medication for a second or third time. This is not usually due to a change in the manufacturer of the vaccine (see below) but can be because the pet has built up a small allergic response to the vaccine over time.

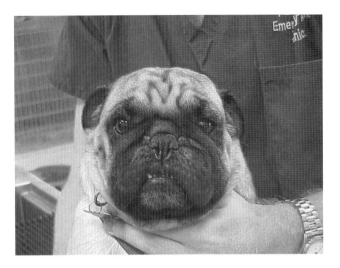

Figure 2.1.   Image of a canine allergic reaction. Note the swollen lip and skin around the nose. This type of reaction can occur minutes to hours after vaccination.

Canine Allergic Reaction

When administering puppy vaccines, remember that the pup has had very limited or no exposure to previous vaccinations, so allergic reactions to vaccinations are always possible and should be discussed with the client prior to the vaccine being given. The reaction is caused by the body responding to the chemical or metal components of the vaccine that are responsible for stimulating an immune reaction in the body. These chemicals or portions of microscopic metal that produce an immune response are called an **adjuvant**. This immune response stimulates the white blood cells of the body to capture the deactivated or killed infectious agents and produce immunity against the specific disease. With an allergic reaction, the body is overreacting to the adjuvant with a release of a substance called **histamine,** which regulates the allergic response. The most common vaccine to produce an allergic reaction is the leptospirosis vaccine; however, any vaccine may stimulate a reaction in a given animal. Common symptoms of a mild allergic reaction (see Figure 2.1) are

- swollen face,
- swollen eyes,
- itchy muzzle,
- hives, and
- red ears, abdomen, armpits.

There are rare occasions when severe reactions, called **anaphylactic** reactions, can occur. Anaphylactic reactions can be an acute problem where an oversensitized animal will go through a massive allergic reaction. However, it is important to know that a mild allergic reaction can lead into a severe anaphylactic reaction if not properly treated or recognized. Signs of an anaphylactic reaction are

- respiratory noise when breathing,
- breathing (rasps breathing pattern),

- shortness of breath,
- vomiting,
- slow heart rate,
- poor pulse quality,
- weak to nonresponsive, and
- cold.

Anaphylactic reactions are life-threatening emergencies that must be dealt with immediately or the pet may die. Since some anaphylactic reactions can precipitate from mild allergic reactions, all clients must be informed of what to do if they are concerned their pet is having a reaction to medication (see below).

Feline Allergic Reactions
As with most situations, cats react very differently from dogs when responding to an allergic reaction. Although cats will occasionally have mild to severe reactions to vaccines and medication, their symptoms can be quite different. Cats can show any of the following symptoms.

- depression
- lethargy
- reddening of the ears and mucus membranes
- profuse vomiting
- dehydration
- weak pulse
- collapse

The most common vaccine to produce mild symptoms of depression and lethargy is the feline leukemia vaccine, which can produce mild flu-like symptoms of soreness, lethargy, and change in attitude (grumpiness) in some cats.

What To Do When a Vaccine Reaction Occurs
Vaccine reactions are generally mild and reported by the owner usually in the first 12–24 hours after the vaccination. **Since the animal is not in the hospital, there is no way to assess the patient's stability over the phone.** Therefore, it is recommended that the client be rechecked immediately either by the hospital or the emergency clinic.

If the client is hesitant to have their pet seen, it is important to inform them that even a mild allergic reaction can precipitate into a more severe problem if the pet is not checked and the reaction is not halted. If the client is still hesitant to have their pet seen,

- the doctor should be consulted immediately;
- at no time should over-the-counter medication ever be suggested to a client without a veterinarian's recommendation;
- the chart should be documented with the highlights of the phone conversation and that an allergic reaction to a vaccine has occurred; and
- the folder or the top sheet of a chart (usually a patient's medical problem log) should be labeled with a bright

sticker or highlighter to indicate that the patient has a history of allergic reactions to a specific medication or vaccine.

If a Pet Had a Vaccine Reaction in the Past
Every hospital team handles patients with a history of vaccine reactions differently; however, some basic tenets of treatment are that the pet receive a dose of antihistamine 30–120 minutes prior to the vaccination. The antihistamine helps to block the release of the histamine producing the allergic reaction. The medication can be given orally by the owner or in an injection at the hospital.

The pet is then vaccinated and then must be monitored for a few hours after the vaccination for any signs of an allergic reaction. Often the pet can be hospitalized for the day; however, if owners are reluctant to leave the pet, a recommendation should be made that the pet and owner stay with the pet in the hospital for 30–60 minutes after the vaccination should be made. This allows the veterinarian the ability to assess that there is no obvious reactions in that time and discharge the pet. The owners must also be aware that these animals still need to be closely monitored with owner supervision for the next 12–24 hours and any changes reported immediately to the hospital.

Long-Term Reactions
There can be some long-term concerns from vaccinations that are also tied to the animal's response to the adjuvant. As with allergic reactions, there is no way to determine if an animal will have a long-term reaction until the vaccine is given. Overall, the owner should be aware that these reactions are extremely rare and the probability that these reactions would occur is very small in comparison with a much larger probability of a pet getting a disease if the animal is not properly vaccinated.

A sterile abcessation at the vaccine site (vaccine knot) appears as a small knot that is noticeable over the vaccination site, especially after rabies vaccination. Most of these knots are a small, nonpainful mass or nodule of chronically inflamed tissue (**granuloma**) that occurs and disappears in 14–28 days. On a few occasions, these knots can develop a clear or purulent (pus) fluid accumulation and become larger. These are extremely rare, but if noted, the abscesses may need to be lanced and drained.

Injection site sarcoma is a malignant destructive cancer that has been associated in response to exposure to the adjuvant of feline leukemia and, more rarely, feline rabies vaccine. It occurs in less than 0.1% of all cats vaccinated. However, without advanced diagnostics or surgical excision, an injection site–induced fibrosarcoma and a vaccine knot are impossible to distinguish. Therefore, all swellings or lumps in cats should be carefully monitored, especially around vaccine sites.

In some practices, the vaccines are given in different anatomical locations so that the medical team can monitor any reactions to each specific vaccine. For example, FVRCP vaccine will be given subcutaneously over the right shoulder, avoiding the midline, and as distal as possible. Felv will be given subcutaneously in the left hind leg. Rabies vaccine will be given subcutaneously in the right rear leg. Thus the medical team can be able to monitor each specific site and know what vaccine was administered there.

Vaccine Side Effect Concerns

The concerns with long-term side effects from vaccines are radically changing the recommendations of what vaccinations should be given and how often they should be administered. It is very important to discuss with the medical team what the hospital's recommendations are for vaccines, and their time table, before discussing any vaccinations with clients. Constructing a simple vaccine schedule for dogs and cats can become a useful resource for new employees. An example of a vaccine schedule is seen in Table 2.1.

Key Points in Discussing Potential Long-Term Vaccine Side Effects with Clients

- Just as with allergic reactions, there is no way to tell if a vaccine will produce a long-term side effect until the vaccination is given.
- The possibility of formation of a vaccine-induced sarcoma occurring is less them 0.1%.
- The vaccine's protection for exposed or at-risk animals far outweighs the possibilities of long-term side effects.
- The owners should monitor the vaccine sites for the next 2–4 weeks and report any changes or concerns that they note immediately.

Heartworm Disease

Note that a complete discussion of heartworm disease is covered in Chapter 12. Heartworm disease is a parasitic infection of a bloodborne parasite, *Dirofilaria immitis* (see Figure 2.2). The disease is spread by mosquitoes, which feed on infected dogs and cats. The mosquitoes pick up larval heartworms (microfilaria), which they in turn inject into an uninfected animal the next time they feed.

- The parasite is injected into the tissue, and over the next 3–6 months it migrates through the tissue to the blood supply and to the right heart.
- There the worms mature and reproduce, causing an obstructive heart disease in the right heart and lung fields (see Figure 2.2).
- The disease can be asymptotic initially (especially in felines), but as the infection worsens, the right side of the heart begins to obstruct and potentially fail.
- The infection affects dogs and cats (rarely) in mosquito-endemic regions, along the Atlantic and Gulf coasts, and

Table 2.1 Feline vaccination schedule.

Vaccines	Kittens	Adults	Recommendations
Felv	Vaccinated at 12 and 16 weeks of age	Vaccinated every 3 years	Given in left hind leg. Recommended for inside and outside or outside cats only. Cats should be tested for FELV annually.
Rabies	Vaccinated at 16 weeks of age	Vaccinated at 1 year and then every 3 years	Given in right hind leg. Per state law, all cats must be vaccinated and licensed.
FVCRP	Vaccinated at 8, 12, and 16 weeks	Vaccinated every 3 years	Given over the shoulder blades.
FIP	Not recommended at this time.	Not recommended at this time.	Only given on request of owner.
FIV	Not recommended at this time.	Not recommended at this time.	

FVCRP, Feline viral rhinotracheitis, calici virus, panleukopenia virus; FIP, feline infectious peritonitis; FIV, feline immunodeficiency virus.

other parts of the United States. Outside, unprotected animals are at the highest risk.

Common Signs in Medical History

In canines the disease produces a chronic progressive disease. In felines, the disease can be asymptotic until the pet enters acute cardiac failure. Common medical complaints can be

- sudden death (cats),
- weakness/lethargy/collapse,
- decreased ability to exercise,
- coughing (rare in cats),
- shortness of breath,
- weight loss, and
- fluid buildup in the abdomen (ascites) with formation of obstructive right heart disease in severely affected animals.

Common Points in Physical Examination

Physical signs depend on heartworm burden, length of disease, age of the pet, and other underlying disease conditions. Signs are species dependent.

In canines, patients may present with a mild to worsening cough. In severe cases animals may be unable to exercise properly. There may be evidence of a right tricuspid murmur with increased lung sounds. The pet may be coughing up blood.

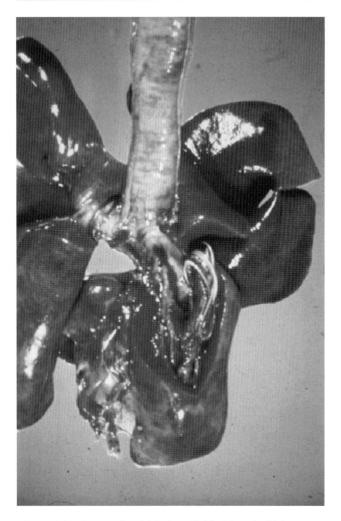

Figure 2.2. Image of multiple lung fields. Note the high number of adult heartworms in the incised lobe. These worms become obstructive to the heart and lungs, producing a severe cardiac and respiratory disease.

In felines, pets may not show any physical signs until the pet is in cardiovascular failure or death.

Diagnosis

Diagnosis is largely based on screening patient blood for antibodies against the adult heartworm. In canines, there are many excellent in-hospital tests to determine potential exposure. In feline patients, there are tests available through many of the outside animal health laboratories.

Prevention

Annual to biannual heartworm testing and routine heartworm prevention (every month to every 6 months dependent on the product) can greatly reduce the chance of heartworm infection for pets living in endemic regions.

There are some basic points to raise when discussing heartworms with the client.

Disease

- Heartworm disease is a bloodborne parasite infection that is spread by mosquito bites.
- The disease is endemic in warm climates where there are active mosquito populations.
- However, specific geographic regions are more endemic for the disease (i.e., northeast and southeast coastal states, Texas, and parts of the Midwest).
- The disease is transmitted by the mosquito that feeds on a currently infected animal and then bites an unaffected pet.
- The mosquito injects a small larval form of the parasite into the tissue, which over 4–6 months migrates into the right heart and lung fields.
- There the parasite begins to reproduce and become obstructive to the heart and lungs.

Physical Signs

- In the canine, pets generally develop a persistent worsening cough that can develop into weakness, inability to exercise, and collapse in severe cases.
- In feline heartworm disease, the worm loads can be much less, with infections having only a few worms evident. Physical symptoms are mild to nonexistent until the feline enters a cardiovascular shock/crisis.

Clinical Diagnostics

Although there are many diagnostic tests used to diagnose and confirm the extent of heartworm disease, the initial clinical test is a simple blood test that evaluates the pet's blood for the presence of antibodies against the adult heartworm. Many of these tests can be run in a few minutes within the hospital setting.

Control

Through annual to biannual heartworm testing and placing the pet on heartworm prevention, the pet is highly unlikely to develop the disease. The preventatives are monthly tablets that kill any of the larval parasites that the pet comes in contact with.

CD-ROM 1 reviews material presented in this chapter. Please try the cases for Section 1 (The First Two Days on the Job) to help reinforce the information presented here.

Chapter 3

Elective Procedures

This chapter will focus on discussing basic elective procedures with the client. Although approaches and types of elective surgical procedures vary from hospital to hospital, the basic concepts of each will be covered along with some key points regarding how to approach discussing surgery with the client.

As with all components of veterinary medicine, surgery also has its own terminology and special terms. An overview of these surgical terms follows.

- **Ovariohysterectomy (OVH),** or **spay,** refers to a complete removal of the ovaries and uterus from a female patient. After the procedure, the female is unable to reproduce or have heat cycles and has a much lower chance of developing infections of the uterus (**pyometra**) or having mammary tumors in later life.
- **Orchidectomy/castration,** or **neuter,** refers to a complete removal of both testicles of a male animal, rendering the pet unable to reproduce and decreasing secondary sex characteristics (i.e., aggression, voice change, territory marking, etc.).
- **Feline onchyectomy,** or **declawing,** refers to the removal of the claws and fingertips (**third phalanx**) in a feline. These procedures are typically done on the forelimbs or done on all four legs to prevent the pet from scratching and damaging its environment.
- **Feline tendonectomy** refers to an alternative surgical procedure to declawing where a small section of tendons that flex and exteriorize the claws is removed. This procedure prevents cats from extending their claws, but leaves the nail and fingertip intact.
- **Dental prophylaxis** is a thorough dental cleaning, oral examination, gingival examination, and polishing of the patient's mouth. With severe disease, dental x-rays can be taken and tooth extractions or advanced procedures (i.e., root canal) can be performed.

When discussing surgery with the client, there are two main topic groups. The first is what the client should know about anesthesia and surgery before the procedure. How to discuss anesthetic procedures with the client will be covered later. The discussion of surgery should focus on

- the goals of the procedure,
- how the procedure is physically done, and

- any contingencies that would make the procedure more complicated.

The second part of the discussion outlines what the client needs to monitor after surgery. This is usually discussed at the time of discharge and should be done both verbally and with written instructions for the client to take home so the client may reread the information at a later time.

Besides specific concerns that need to be discussed with each procedure, general comments about monitoring incisions and incision care should always be reviewed with the client at the time of discharge.

> **Discussing Monitoring the Incision Site with the Client**
> - The incision site should be checked daily for swelling, draining, heat, or any evidence of incision line breakdown. If there are any changes noted, the hospital should be notified immediately.
> - The incision site may have some mild, firm swelling after the first week, which is usually localized over where the last suture knot was placed. This swelling will disappear as the sutures are absorbed over the next 4–6 weeks.
> - The animal should not be bathed and the incision should not be allowed to get wet.
> - If absorbable suture is used to close the skin, the client should be informed that the suture will dissolve on its own, but the incision should be checked 10–14 days after the procedure.
> - If nonabsorbable suture is used, the incision should be checked between postoperative days 10 and 14 and the sutures removed when the incision has healed.
> - If the pet is bothering or licking the incision at any time, the hospital should be contacted and a Buster or Elizabethan collar placed on the pet to keep the animal away from the incision.

The Ovariohysterectomy

An ovariohysterectomy (OHE), or spay, is a complete removal of both ovaries and the uterus to the cervix. Once the

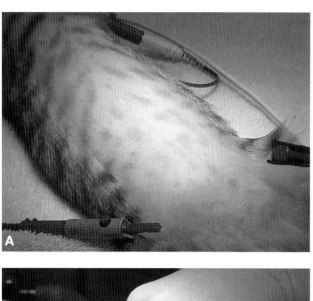
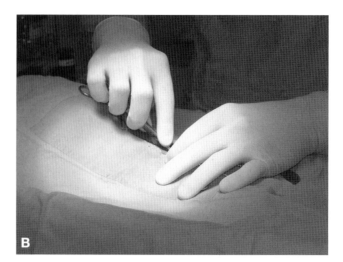
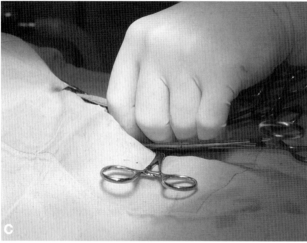
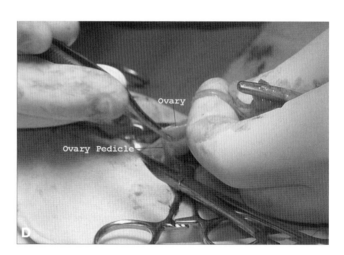

Figure 3.1.   Image of the ventral abdomen (belly) shaved and cleaned in preparation for surgery (a). An incision is made in the middle of the abdomen (b). The abdomen is then explored (c), isolating the uterine horns and exteriorizing the ovaries and ovarian pedicle (d). The pedicle is then double-ligated (tied) with absorbable suture and the ovary and uterine horn exteriorized.

pet is placed under anesthesia, the abdomen (belly) is shaved and surgically prepped with an antiseptic/antibacterial soap and then rinsed with alcohol to reduce hair and bacterial load. The surgical boundaries are then covered with sterile towels (**draped**), and an incision is made into the abdominal wall. The ovaries are first located and exteriorized; their blood and nerve supplies are tied off with an absorbable suture (**ligated**). The procedure is repeated with the other ovary (see Figure 3.1).

With both ovaries freed from their blood supply, the uterus is exteriorized and ligated just above the cervix. The uterus with its ovaries is then completely removed from the abdomen (Figure 3.2).

The abdominal wall is closed with three separate suture layers: first the muscle wall is closed with absorbable suture, then the subcutaneous tissue is closed with absorbable su-

ture, and lastly the edges of the skin are brought together. The incision is then cleaned, and animal is moved into the recovery area (see Figure 3.3).

If the female animal is in heat or pregnant at the time of surgery, the procedure will be more complicated because the uterus is larger and has an increased vascular supply. **Animals that are in heat can still be attractive to males and must be kept separated from any male animal until signs of heat disappear. If the patient is accidentally bred, the internal sutures could break down and the pet could begin to bleed internally.**

After this procedure, the patient will not be able to reproduce or go into heat. An animal is spayed to prevent heat and pregnancy but also to reduce the risk of mammary tumors and disease of the reproductive tract in middle-aged to older females (see Chapter 18).

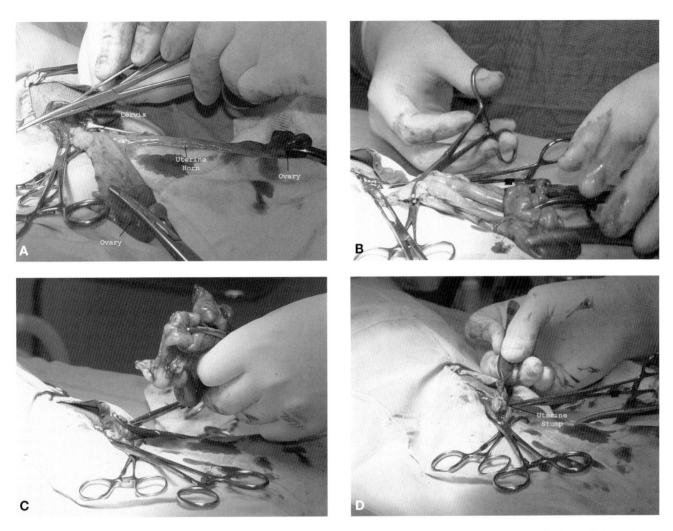

Figure 3.2. With both ovaries ligated, the entire uterine body is exteriorized to the cervix (a). Here the uterus is clamped above the cervix, and the region is double-ligated (b). The uterus, uterine horns, and ovaries are then removed (c). The cervix and uterine stump are then examined to make sure there is no obvious bleeding (d).

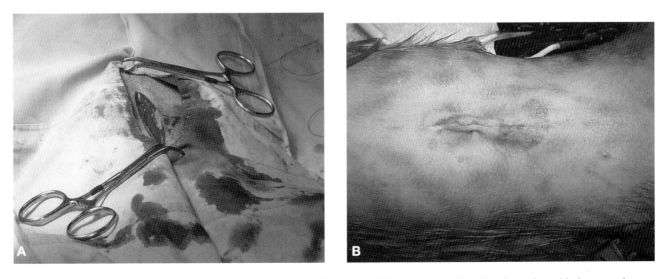

Figure 3.3. Image of the incision with all three tissue layers still open (a). These layers are then closed, starting with the muscular layer, then the subcutaneous layer, and lastly the skin is brought together (b).

Discussing an Ovariohysterectomy with a Client Before Surgery

- An ovariohysterectomy is a surgical procedure to completely remove both ovaries and the uterus of the animal to prevent the pet from going into heat, spreading sexually transmitted diseases, or being able to reproduce.
- Furthermore, a spay helps reduce the chance of mammary cancer and severe life-threatening diseases of the reproductive tract that are often seen in middle-aged to older pets (usually more than 4 years of age).
- If the pet is in heat or pregnant, the procedure can be more complicated, because the uterus is larger and has an increased blood supply.

Discussing an Ovariohysterectomy with a Client After Surgery

- The pet has been through a major abdominal surgery and may seem sore, depressed, and may not eat well for the first 24 hours.
- If the pet was in heat, she can still be attractive to males for days after the surgery and should never be left alone with a male until the sutures are removed. If she is accidentally bred, the internal sutures could break down and the pet could begin to bleed internally.
- Incision care should be discussed as previously outlined in this chapter.
- The pet should be closely monitored for the first 10–14 days after surgery, and the hospital should be contacted if
  —the pet is trying to produce urine but cannot;
  —the pet stops eating, drinking, or begins to vomit;
  —the pet's abdomen seems tense or painful;
  —there is any other change in the pet's health.

Orchidectomy/Castration

Canine Neuter

A canine neuter (castration) is a complete removal of both testicles from the scrotum. Once the pet is placed under anesthesia, an area in front of the scrotum is shaved and surgically prepped with an antiseptic soap. The boundaries of the area are then draped with sterile towels. An incision is made into the skin in front of the scrotum. The testicles are then pushed forward into the incision area and exteriorized. The blood and nerve supplies are ligated with sutures and the testicle removed. The same procedure is completed with the other testicle, and then the subcutaneous and skin tissues are brought together with suture. The area is then cleaned and the animal is moved into the anesthetic recovery area (see Figure 3.4).

In normal testicular development, the fetal testicles orig-

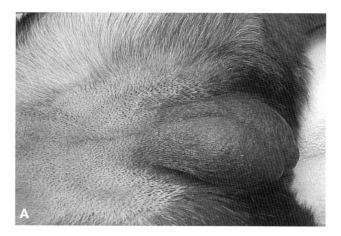

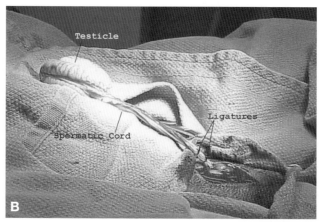

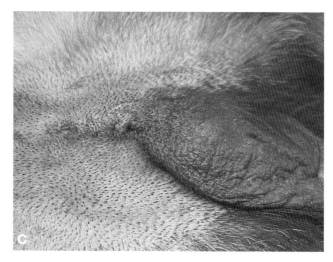

Figure 3.4. Image of the shaved region in front of the scrotum (a). Through a small prescrotal incision, each testicle is exteriorized, ligated, and then removed (b). After the excision, the subcutaneous and skin layers are closed (c).

inate behind the kidneys and descend through the abdomen into the scrotum through a slit in the abdominal muscles **(inguinal canal)** that allows the abdomen to communicate with the subcutaneous tissue and scrotum. This process is complete by birth or within the first few months of life. Some

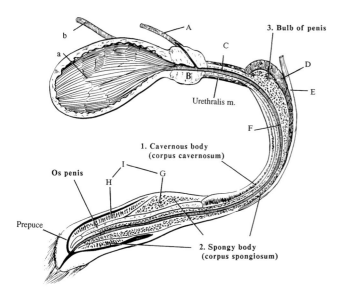

3. Bulb of penis

Urethralis m.

1. Cavernous body
(corpus cavernosum)

Os penis

Prepuce

2. Spongy body
(corpus spongiosum)

Figure 3.5. Illustration of normal testicular and penile anatomy. (Courtesy of *Anatomy of Domestic Animals*, 7th Edition. Pasquini, Chris, and Pasquini, Susan. Sudz Publishing, Pilot Point, Tx 1989. Used with permission from Sudz Publishing.)

male patients do not have their testicles descend normally and the organs may sit within the inguinal canal or anywhere within the abdominal cavity (see Figure 3.5). These animals are referred to as being **cryptorchid.** Neutering an animal with retained testicles can make the surgery a much more lengthy and complicated procedure.

Animals that are cryptorchid should be neutered young for the following reasons.

- Cryptochidism is a congenital syndrome that can be passed to males in future litters.
- The patient can still potentially breed and has all male behavioral characteristics.
- Over long periods of time, the increased body temperature can make the retained testicles more likely to become cancerous in later life. These testicular tumors can produce large quantities of sex hormones (testosterone, estrogen) that can have life-threatening effects on the patient's blood cell populations.

Feline Neuter

A feline neuter (castration) is a complete removal of both testicles from the scrotum. Once the pet is placed under anesthesia, the scrotal area is surgically prepped with an antiseptic/antibacterial soap. The boundaries of the area are then draped with sterile towels. An incision is made into the scrotum. The testicles are exteriorized; their blood and nerve supplies are ligated with sutures, surgical clips, or tied off with a section of their own blood supply; and the testicle is removed. The same procedure is done with the other testicle (see Figure 3.6). The scrotum heals together without the need for suture. After the testicles are removed, the area is cleaned.

After a castration, the pet will not be able to reproduce and is less likely to mark his territory. Male dogs neutered late in life will stiffly lift their leg and may also be able to produce an erection. Male pets are neutered to prevent accidental pregnancy, transmission of sexually transmitted diseases, and decrease the risk of prostate disease and cancer in later life.

Discussing a Castration with a Client Before Surgery
- A neuter is a surgical procedure to completely remove both testicles from the animal to prevent the pet from being able to reproduce.
- A neuter helps reduce male aggressive behavior, dogfights, marking of territory, sexually transmitted diseases, and prostatic disease and cancer.
- If the pet has retained testicles, testicles that are not evident within the scrotum of the pet, the procedure can be more complicated because the testicles must be located and removed from the inguinal canal or the abdomen.

Discussing a Castration with a Client After Surgery
- The pet has been through a surgical procedure and may seem sore, depressed, and not eat well for the first 24 hours.
- Incision care should be discussed as previously outlined in this chapter.
- The pet should be closely monitored for the first 10–14 days after surgery, and the hospital should be contacted if
  —the pet is trying to produce urine but cannot;
  —the pet stops eating, drinking, or begins to vomit;
  —the pet's abdominal, inguinal, or scrotal region seems tense or painful;
  —there is any other change in the pet's health.

Onchyectomy

The onchyectomy (feline declawing) is a highly controversial procedure. Many animal rights groups suggest this procedure is inhumane and unfair to the cat. However, for many, the procedure allows the cat to live in the household and prevents damage to the furniture and destruction to the home. Arguments of morality aside, the feline declaw is still very much apart of the general practice and a very important surgery about which to properly educate the clients.

The onchyectomy is the surgical removal of the fingertip and nail bed of the pet's digits. This prevents the animal from being able to scratch or destroy things within the home. Once the pet is placed under anesthesia, the nails and fingertips are surgically prepped with an antiseptic wash solution. A tourniquet is placed above the paw to minimize bleeding

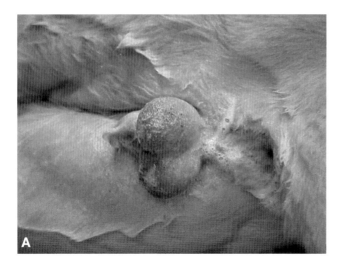

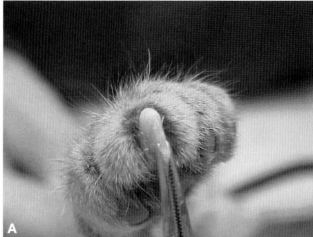

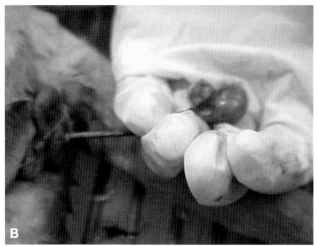

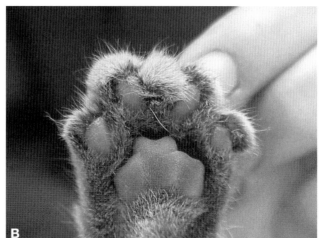

Figure 3.6. Illustration of a prepared surgical site for feline castration (a). An image of the exteriorization of the testicle and spermatic cord before ligation (b). Once ligated the testicle is removed, and the incision heals without sutures.

during the procedure. Using either a scalpel blade, sterilized nail clippers, or a surgical laser, the fingernails and fingertips are dissected away from the rest of the paw. The skin incision is closed with suture or a special glue resin and the paw bandaged to prevent postoperative bleeding (see Figure 3.7). The same procedure is repeated for the other paw. The declawing is usually done on the front paws only; however, in some circumstances all four paws are declawed.

The declaw procedure has an increased chance of mild postsurgical complications. Once the bandage comes off the feet and the cat goes home, the cat will be walking on and using the paws in litter directly on the incision sites, which greatly increases the chance for infection and breakdown of the incision line in the first 10 days after surgery. Often these patients are required to use a special paper litter for 10–14 days after surgery to prevent small particulates of normal litter from embedding themselves within the incision, increasing the chance of infection. In some cases, the

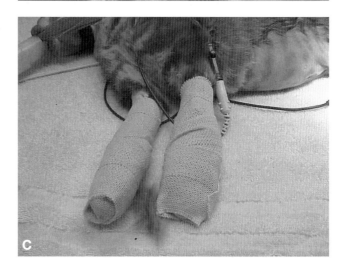

Figure 3.7. The nail is exteriorized and, with a special blade, excised from the paw (a). Once the nails have been removed, the skin margins are closed (b). Once both paws are declawed, bandages are placed on the legs to prevent oozing from the incision (c).

Discussing a Declawing with a Client Before Surgery

- A declaw is a surgical procedure in which the tips of the toes and the nails are surgically removed from the pet.
- Once declawed, the pet's abilities to defend itself and climb are greatly reduced, so the animal should remain indoors for life.
- After surgery, the pet may be feeling moderate pain, and the use of pain medications may be required.
- The cat may also have an altered or changed gait for 4–6 weeks after surgery as it adjusts to the change in dexterity.

Discussing a Declawing with a Client After Surgery

- The pet has been through a surgical procedure and may seem sore, depressed, and not eat well for the first 24 hours.
- Incision care should be discussed as previously outlined in this chapter.
- The procedure is moderately painful, and if the pet seems to still be favoring the legs or in pain even with medication, please contact the hospital immediately.
- The pet should be closely monitored for the first 10–14 days after surgery, and the hospital should be contacted if
  —the pet stops eating, drinking, or begins to vomit;
  —the pet's paws continue to be painful;
  —the pet excessively licks, chews, or bothers the incisions or there is a breakdown of the incision lines;
  —there is any other change in the pet's health.

patient may also be placed on antibiotics to further reduce the chance of infection.

The procedure can also produce a period of postoperative pain where the cat may not walk on the limbs or may hop to avoid the pain. This sensitivity can last for a day to several days after surgery. Since the tips of the digits have been surgically removed, there is a change of dexterity the pet must adjust to, so these animals can appear to have an altered or abnormal gait for up to 4–6 weeks after surgery. Finally, and most important after the procedure, the cat's ability to protect itself and climb are severely diminished; it is recommended that your cat remain indoors after having this procedure.

Not all (or any) of these complications will occur after surgery, but the client should be aware of all these concerns before the surgery is performed.

Feline Tendonectomy

A feline tendonectomy is an alternative procedure that is used in place of declawing to help control household dam-

age produced by the cat's claws. The procedure removes a small section of tendon in each toe to prevent the extension of the animal's claws. The nails and the tip of the toe still remain intact, and there is no overall change in dexterity and less postoperative pain.

Once the pet is placed under anesthesia, the interdigital regions are surgically prepped with an antiseptic wash solution. A tourniquet is placed above the paw to minimize bleeding during the procedure. With a scalpel blade, a small incision is made behind the small metacarpal pads of each digit. A small hemostat dissects and elevates the deep digital flexor tendon. A small section of the tendon is then incised. The skin incision is left open, and a bandage is placed to prevent bleeding until the skin margins begin to heal in 12–24 hours. The same procedure is repeated for the other paw.

Discussing a Tendonectomy with a Client Before Surgery

- A tendonectomy is a surgical procedure in which tendons that aid in extension of the claws of the paw are cut so that the animal cannot extend the nails normally.
- Once the tendons have been cut, the pet's ability to defend itself and climb are greatly reduced, so the animal should remain indoors for life.
- The pet's nails will continue to grow and will need regular nail trims every 2–4 weeks to prevent nail overgrowth and injury to the pads.
- Rarely, the cut tendons can repair themselves and the pet may be able to extend one or more claws. If this occurs, the procedure would have to be repeated on that digit.

Discussing a Tendonectomy with a Client After Surgery

- The pet has been through a surgical procedure and may seem sore, depressed, and not eat well for the first 24 hours.
- Incision care should be discussed as previously outlined in this chapter.
- The procedure is mildly painful, and if the pet seems to still be favoring the legs or in pain even with medication, please contact the hospital immediately.
- The pet should be closely monitored for the first 10–14 days after surgery, and the hospital should be contacted if
  —the pet stops eating, drinking, or begins to vomit;
  —the pet's paws continue to be painful;
  —the pet excessively licks, chews, or bothers the incisions or there is a breakdown of the incision lines;
  —there is any other change in the pet's health.

The tendonectomy has an increased incidence of postsurgical complications that the owner should be aware of prior to surgery. Just as with declawing, the incisions are very susceptible to postoperative infections as the pet walks, cleans its paws, and uses the litter. The patient will need to use a special paper litter to reduce grit and debris that can infect the incision sites. Secondly, the nail is still intact and growing, so regular biweekly to monthly nail trims are a necessity to prevent the nails from growing into the paws. Furthermore, since the nails do not extend and are not regularly cleaned by the cat, they are more brittle and harder to clip. Cats that are not easy to restrain in order to clip the nails regularly are not good candidates for this procedure. Lastly, on occasion the tendons of one or more digits can repair itself so that pet may be able to extend one or more claws over time.

Dental Prophylaxis

We will be discussing dental anatomy, physiology, dental diseases, and the components of a dental health program in Chapter 9. However, a dental cleaning is a routine procedure for a general veterinary practice, and a brief discussion of a dental surgery protocol is necessary.

In as little as 2–3 years, a pet's teeth begin to wear down, and the gums can become irritated. Dental tartar and plaque, which is rich in bacteria, can build up and cause moderate to severe swelling and infections of the gums **(gingivitis).** As the gums weaken, bacteria can migrate down into the tooth root, causing pain, infection, and loosening of the tooth. Owners may notice the following signs at home:

- Bad breath
- Salivating
- Inability to eat hard food or snacks or inability to eat at all
- Eating on only one side of the mouth

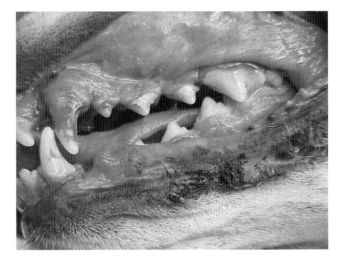

Figure 3.8. Image of teeth showing moderate dental tartar and some recession of the gums, especially over the canine teeth.

- Rolling food from one part of the mouth to the other
- Pain on palpation of tooth

Over many years chronic bacterial infection of the teeth can lead to more serious health concerns such as kidney, liver, and heart disease.

To help prevent long-term concerns and keep teeth healthy, routine dental cleanings are recommended every 6–12 months. Pets should have a thorough oral examination when presented for their annual health and vaccination visit. If there is evidence of dental tartar, recession of the gums, or broken teeth, then the medical team will discuss the need for a dental prophylaxis (see Figure 3.8).

The dental prophylaxis is a surgical procedure in which the oral cavity is examined for broken teeth, pockets in the gum line around the tooth root, exposed roots, and lesions

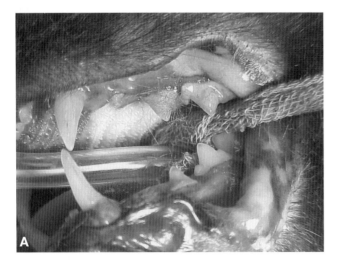
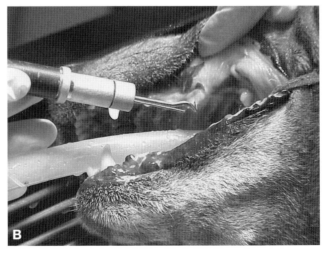

Figure 3.9. Image of a canine mouth with mild to moderate dental tarter (a). Once under anesthesia, the gum lines (gingiva) are probed and explored for deep pockets around the teeth, suggestive of dental disease (b).

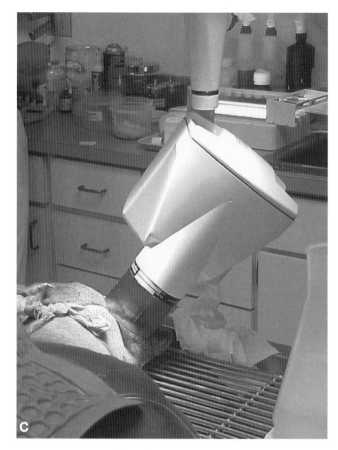

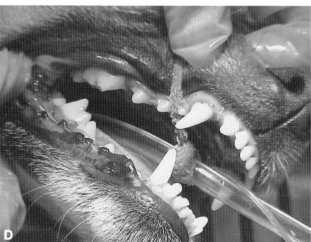

Discussing a Dental Cleaning with a Client Before Surgery

• A dental cleaning is a surgical procedure in which the teeth and gums are examined for disease and infection, the teeth are cleaned and polished, dental x-rays are taken if there is a concern regarding an infected tooth, and the gums and teeth can be medically and surgically treated.

• It is often impossible to detect serious dental disease with the pet awake. Furthermore, full proper dental cleanings and other procedures such as extractions, dental radiographs, or root canals and crowns can only be completed with the patient under anesthesia.

• After surgery, the pet may be placed on antibiotics or pain medication, depending on the procedures completed.

• Dental care is a lifetime concern, and recommendations for brushing the teeth, applying special oral rinses, and using special treats to reduce dental tartar may also be suggested after surgery.

Discussing a Dental Cleaning with a Client After Surgery

• The pet has been through a minor surgical procedure and may have some minor oral pain, act depressed, and not eat well for the first 24 hours.

• If teeth were extracted, the owner may notice a small amount of blood in the patient's food or water bowl. Furthermore, the client may notice sutures in the mouth that will dissolve in the next 2–3 weeks.

• The pet should be closely monitored for the first 10–14 days after surgery, and the hospital should be contacted if
—the pet stops eating, drinking, or begins to vomit;
—the pet acts as if it is feeling pain while eating, drools excessively, or if its mouth seems sensitive;
—there is any swelling, heat, pain, or discharge in the mouth or around the face;
—there is any other change in the pet's health.

Figure 3.9. (*continued*) In many cases, the patient will have dental x-rays performed to check questionable teeth for pathology, abcessation, and disease (c). Finally, the teeth are polished and the animal is recovered (d).

that may need medical or surgical treatment (see Figure 3.9). Once the mouth is examined, the teeth are cleaned using an ultrasonic cleaner to remove the dental tartar and bacteria. The teeth are then polished to remove any microscopic scratches that could be a site for dental plaque to reform. Dental x-rays can be also taken at this time to assess the

health of the tooth root and check for dental abcessation or disease. If a tooth root is exposed and sensitive and the tooth is weakened, a dental extraction or an advanced dental procedure (i.e., root canal and crown) may need to be completed. After the procedure, the pet may need to be placed on antibiotics and/or pain medication.

CD-ROM 1 reviews material presented in this chapter. Please try the cases for Section 1 (The First Two Days on the Job) to help reinforce the information presented here.

Chapter 4

Safety and Restraint

Within any veterinary environment, there is risk taken with one's health and well-being on a day-to-day basis. Whether the risks are from an animal bite or scratch, handling medication or cleaning supplies, or lifting a large heavy object, every hospital or clinic should have a set protocol in the handling of various health hazards and conditions. Every hospital or clinic should have an **OSHA** (Occupational Safety and Health Administration Requirements) handbook, which covers how to handle potential risks and accidents that occur within the workplace. It is the responsibility of the veterinary hospital to provide the necessary OSHA information for reference in an emergency and to provide the necessary protective equipment. Every staff member should be familiar with this information and refer to it whenever a potential exposure or danger occurs.

For example, an animal is being put to sleep with an injection of euthanasia solution. As the injection is being given, the syringe separates from the needle and euthanasia solution is sprayed into the air, landing on the technician who is restraining the pet. The solution penetrates the eyes and mouth of the team member. Although this is a scary scenario, it has occurred in many hospitals at different times. What would be the correct protocol for handling this situation? How dangerous is the drug, especially to the eyes and if received orally? What is the first thing to do? The veterinary hospital team must know the emergency protocols and first steps in handling exposure to dangerous chemicals in order to minimize trauma and injury. This is how one clinic responded to the above scenario.

- The contaminated technician immediately went to the eye-wash station and began rinsing out her eyes and washing out her mouth with cold water.
- Another team member retrieved the OSHA notebook, found the Material Data Safety Sheet for the drug, and read the information on drug contact for the eyes and what to do following oral ingestion.
- Furthermore, the technician contacted the local poison control that was listed in the OSHA notebook and discussed the concerns of exposure with a toxicologist.
- The exposed technician continued to rinse her eyes for another 15 minutes, and because there was concern regarding irritation to the eyes, the team member was taken to the hospital.

- All workers' compensation forms needed for the emergency room were in folders located with the OSHA notebook.
- Later, the appointed safety team member had an incident report filled out and filed with the veterinary hospital manager and medical director.

Although these steps sound rather formal and rigid, it is extremely important to know what to do in an emergency situation.

Personal Safety

In every veterinary hospital there are general guidelines for personal safety that should always be followed.

The first and foremost rule is that if a team member feels uncomfortable performing a specific task or assisting in a procedure they are unsure of, the team member should ask for help. It is better to make sure that the team member completely understands the assignment rather than do something that could place the patient or a team member in danger.

Anyone who is pregnant or may be pregnant should never take part in taking x-rays or assisting with gas anesthesia. The team member should notify the hospital of the health concern and should not participate in those procedures, even if there has to be a change in team member responsibilities. With the same concern, clients who may be pregnant and small children should stay away from the areas in which these procedures take place.

Proper handling of chemicals and prescription medication is everyone's responsibility within the hospital. Certain drugs and chemicals can penetrate the skin and have systemic effects on the body. For example, chemotherapeutics (i.e., cisplatin, cyclophosphamide, vincristine), if absorbed into the skin, can cause massive side effects and decreases in the white blood cell population. Other drugs (i.e., Cytotec, etc.), if handled by a pregnant employee, could produce an abortion if some of the drug were introduced into the body through a cut or irritation in the skin. The team member should always be aware of drugs that have special handling or disposal concerns.

All needles and syringes should be disposed of in an OSHA-approved container. When full, the container should be disposed of appropriately by an approved process (i.e., incinerated). Any diagnostic blood work going out to a lab should never contain needles, and all glass should be disposed of in an OSHA-approved sharps container.

There will be times when team members may be faced with an injury stemming from an animal attack or a trauma. Unless there is a certified EMT or human medical personnel on site, it is extremely important to follow the following protocols.

If the injuries seem life threatening or the person seems shocky, nonresponsive, and weak, contact 911 immediately.

Minimize Contact with Blood

If a client or another person is bleeding, the team member should not touch or handle the wounds or injuries.

If the person is able to clean up his or her own injuries, the team member should do the following:

- Take the injured person to a bathroom or sink and offer water and antiseptic solution.
- Never directly handle the wound.
- Never clean and bandage a wound. If the person wants to bandage his or her injury to stop the bleeding, give him some light bandaging material. A team member without human medical training should never attempt to dress the wound.
- Refer the injured person to a medical facility immediately. Document all incidences in written format (OSHA-approved injury report for hospital use).

If the person is unable to clean up his or her own injuries,

- contact 911 immediately,
- use gloves to separate yourself from the blood,
- refer the person to a medical facility immediately, and
- document all incidences in written format (OSHA-approved injury report for hospital use).

Bite Wounds

If an animal bites a human, rabies information on the animal should be obtained immediately, the incident should be documented, and a state bite report may need to be filed.

If the owner is bitten by her own animal, the owner may elect not to report her own animal to rabies animal control. The client should still be advised to seek medical assistance immediately.

An incident report should be filed outlining the incident, the client's refusal to contact rabies animal control against hospital advice, and the documentation for the hospital's recommendation that the client seek medical attention immediately. No matter how the incident occurred, this bite wound could still be the veterinary hospital's liability and responsibility, therefore documentation is extremely important.

If someone else is bitten by an owned or stray animal, the state animal control must be contacted immediately and the rabies status of the pet reported. These bite wounds can

occur as a team member approaches the pet for the first time, tries to get a pet out of a cage, or simply restrains a pet. There is a constant risk of any animal biting in fear, self-defense, or aggression in a new environment. An owner must accept that risk when bringing the pet into a veterinary hospital.

If an animal has a history of possible aggression or exhibits questionable behavior, the animal should be muzzled or chemically restrained. (See how to discuss restraint with the owner below.) Animals with a history of aggression should have their chart marked with a caution, and the owner should already know what precautions must be taken before the pet comes into the hospital. For example,

- some owners will already have their pet muzzled prior to the examination,
- some pets will be on sedatives provided by the hospital, and
- some pets will be placed in carriers and taken to an anesthetic chamber for sedation so that the pet can be examined.

Pet Safety

Just as we are advocates for the safety of our team members and our own safety, team members must also be primary advocates for pet safety. Animals must be protected against injury and harm from other animals, exposure to infectious disease, possible escape, or other dangerous and life-threatening scenarios. To help maintain these safety standards, the following guidelines are suggested.

Restraint in the Lobby

All animals that enter the hospital should be on a leash or in a carrier so that they may be restrained to ensure there is no contact with other animals.

- There should be a sign emphasizing hospital policy on leash restraint on all hospital entry doors.
- If an owner does not have a leash for a pet, extra leashes should be made available.
- If an owner has a small, pocket pet (rat, hamster, ferret) or cat that is not able to be restrained by a leash, and no carrier is available, the client should be moved into a room or the patient be placed in a kennel in the back until an exam room is available.
- When walking hospitalized or boarded animals use two leashes; thus if one leash breaks, there is a backup restraint.

Infectious Diseases

If based on the history there is a concern the animal may have an infectious disease, upon entering the hospital the animal and owner should be moved into isolation or a low-traffic exam room. Animals with the following complaints may fall into this category.

- **Vomiting/diarrhea**: These symptoms in a young dog or cat (usually less than 12–18 months of age) can suggest canine parvo virus or feline panleukopenia. Even if upon entry the pet appears bright and alert, these animals should be moved away from the general population.
- **Sneezing and coughing**: These symptoms in younger animals or animals that have recently been boarded, groomed, or adopted may have contagious upper respiratory disease or canine distemper virus.
- **Skin conditions:** If a pet comes in with concerns about hair loss; red, irritated skin and/or severe itchiness (pruritis); or fleas or ticks, the pet may have an infectious skin condition (i.e., ring worm, fleas, or sarcoptic mange; see Chapter 19). These patients should be isolated and human contact with the pet minimized.

Once the exam has been completed and the animal moved on to treatment, the room should be thoroughly disinfected and cleaned.

Identification of the Animal

All animals admitted to the hospital for procedures or treatment should have a breakaway paper collar that identifies the animal and gives the reason the patient has been admitted, the name of the hospital, and a contact phone number. All regular collars, tags, or halters should be removed prior to the animal being placed in its kennel. Normal tags and collars can catch on grates and kennel doors, sometimes trapping or even choking the pet.

Approaching and Handling an Animal

It is hard to always anticipate how an animal will respond to a stranger in a different environment. Many dogs may seem shy and wag their tails but will growl and try to bite without much provocation. Whether it is fear, protecting its owners, or pain, a pet's fractious behavior can be magnified. Dogs defend themselves by biting. Cats may scratch and/or bite. Horses tend to kick and bite. Rabbits also bite. In any case, even the most docile animal may render harm to the handler.

With certain neurological conditions, patients may show very abnormal behavior and then attack the team member aggressively. Patients that have ingested toxins (e.g., antifreeze), that are suffering from infectious diseases (e.g., rabies, distemper), and that have central nervous system disease (e.g., spinal meningitis) may all act abnormally with fits of aggression. Any patient that demonstrates strange behavior should be treated with caution, and client and personnel contact should be minimized. The veterinarian should be informed immediately, and if there are any concerns about exposure to rabies, the patient should be safely and quickly isolated.

It is also important to recognize a pet's body language and behavior that suggest what actions the patient may take (see Figure 4.1). Dogs will show a variety of behaviors while under stress. Some of the most common are as discussed next.

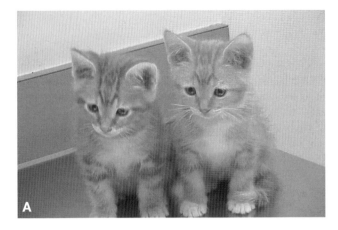

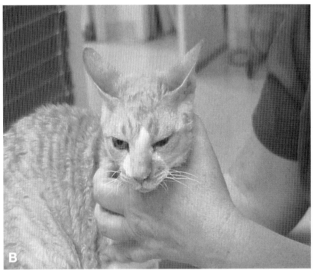

Figure 4.1. What behaviors might these animals show? Figure A. These kittens appear interested and curious in their environment and not quick to anger. However, in Figure B, the cat with its ears down and expression of angst may be a more cautious and possibly aggressive patient.

Dog Behavior under Stress
Avoidance Behavior
Avoidance behaviors are exhibited as the animal tries to relieve the tension or its concern about the situation. The pet may bite or scratch at a body part during a time of pain, fear, or dominance. The animal may also appear to be wagging its tail while baring all teeth as a team member enters the exam room. An important distinction to help identify these animals is that the animal does not generally try to make eye contact with the person but glances at them from the side of its eye, making no attempt to approach the team member.

Fight or Flight
Fear biters become so stressed or nervous due to a new or dangerous situation the pet functions on pure adrenaline. The patient acts purely on stimulus and response (fight or flight), producing a large amount of adrenaline. Physical symptoms that help us recognize possible fear biters are

bounding heart rate, dilated pupils, and tense muscles that are prepared for high energy bursts.

Aggressive Behaviors

Aggression is a form of antagonistic or conflict behavior that leads to physical signs of aggression and fighting. Aggression is dependent on the type of stimuli. Physical signs of aggressive behavior are direct eye contact, raised scruffs, and curled lips.

When approaching an unknown dog, there are a few guidelines to use to help minimize injury.

- If the pet is showing any signs of possible unfriendly behavior, ask the owner if the pet typically allows their temperature and initial exam be done without some form of restraint. Some owners already know the pet may need to be muzzled, taken to the back, or even tranquilized.
- Allow the pet to come to you. Do not approach the pet, especially if the patient is hiding in a corner or behind the owner.
- If the pet is not coming over and its behavior is questionable, ask the client to move the pet into the center of the room.
- If the patient continues to demonstrate escape or aggressive behaviors, ask the owner if they would be comfortable placing a muzzle on the pet. If at any point, the animal starts becoming aggressive with the owner, have them stop immediately and notify the veterinarian.
- In some cases, the pet can be taken to the back to be muzzled and examined; **some animals are protective of their owners and show less aggressive behavior if the owner is not present.**

Cat Behavior under Stress

Felines can show all of the previously discussed behaviors; however, cats tend to show aggressive behavior differently. Felines manifest signs of aggression as tail flipping, hissing, and spitting, and they defend themselves by biting and scratching. A dog bite or wound can be very serious and need medical attention, but a cat bite almost always results in some degree of infection. Cat bites should receive medical attention immediately; this may entail thorough cleaning of the wound and administration of antibiotics. Furthermore, when handling potential fractious cats, all doors and windows should be closed so that if the patient escapes, it has a limited area to hide in. If the team member is not careful, cats can hide for days in small unreachable areas under a cage or within a wall.

Restraining and Handling Animals

In an effort to work effectively, it is necessary to restrain the animals for treatment. The levels of restraint vary according to how the animal responds to being handled or the amount of pain the patient may be in. In some situations, it is easier to sedate or anesthetize an animal in order to perform an examination or carry out a procedure, if the patient is a safe anesthetic risk (see Chapter 29).

All team members should have a working knowledge of the handling and restraint of all pets seen by the hospital. To begin, it may be best to approach an animal with minimal restraint, and then based on its response, the veterinary technician may add more or less restraint as needed.

It is advantageous to the handler or examiner to approach the animal with caution, making slow movements so that the animal does not feel threatened or imposed upon. In the exam room, avoid cornering the animal; try to do any procedure in the middle of room or on the table. If the animal becomes uncooperative or aggressive, separate the pet from the owner. Also, when dealing with a female and her new litter, puppies and kittens should be examined in another room away from the mother.

Restraint takes practice and control. It may take many weeks to months for a team member to be able to adequately control a pet in most situations. New team members should start with animals that are easy to restrain and increase their abilities with time and experience. If the team member ever feels that the pet is too hard to restrain or the team member is becoming frustrated with the pet, the animal should be confined until more help is available.

Canine Restraint Methods

Vice Grip Restraint

The most common type of restraint for the dog is called the vice grip, where the restrainer's strong hand comes under the neck of the pet and the restrainer's body is behind and over the head of the animal. The other hand can help extend a leg and hold off a vein (see Figure 4.2). In the room, the owners can stand in front where animal can see them and they may comfort their pet; however, do not let owners touch or hold the patient's face.

Side Restraint

Another common form of restraint is to have the dog lie down on its side in lateral recumbency. To do this, the owner or another person helps to position the pet on its side and a team member grabs the pet's lower front paw while placing light pressure on the pet's neck with the elbow. The lower hind paw is similarly restrained while the team member places light pressure on the pet's hips. This prevents the pet from being able to roll or get up.

Removing an Animal from a Kennel

When trying to remove a dog from a kennel, do not make loud or quick movements into the cage or at the animal. Do not just reach in and grab the animal, let it come to you. If the animal is backing into the corner of the cage and avoiding the handler, do not lunge or attempt to grab the patient. If possible, try to lasso it with a leash. If the pet is still acting aggressively, charging, or resisting restraint, then give the pet time to calm down and relax. Discuss the concerns with the doctor.

Canine Restraint Devices

A muzzle is used by placing it over the nose and securing it behind the animal's ears. The technician's hand tightens the latch so that the animal cannot bite.

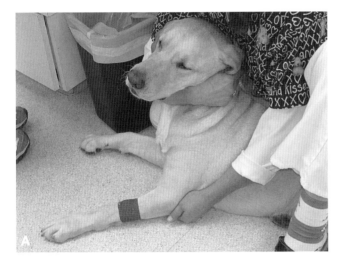

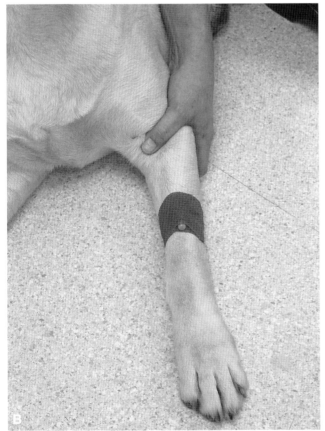

Figure 4.2. The figure demonstrates the proper approach to applying the vice grip restraint on a canine. Here the team member is placing one forearm around the patient's neck while extending the patient's limb forward for venipuncture (a). The team member can then also place the pointer finger on top of the animal's elbow to hold off the large cephalic vein to aid in blood draw (b).

A leash is placed with the looped end over the head and used accordingly.

The rabies pole is a long, rigid pole with a thick wire cable running throughout its hilt. The end of the cable is looped so that it can be secured around the animal's neck and pulled. This is used as a last resort for restraint for very aggressive animals. Usually, the rabies pole helps restrain animals while they are being sedated or anesthetized. These animals will fight back aggressively as they are being forced to the floor to be given an injection. The owner must understand the concerns and what will happen to these pets while they are being restrained. This is the last option in restraint.

Feline Restraint Methods

Cats are much more flexible and acrobatic than dogs. An aggressive cat can lunge, bite, and claw before a hand is placed on it. Caution must be taken, as well, since cats that are restrained can become severely stressed to the point of shock. Just as with dogs, restraining cats must be practiced. Types of restraint for the cat are discussed next.

Scruffing the Neck

Using the strong hand, the team member grabs and holds the top of the neck, being sure to grab skin and hair. The other hand can help hold the hind legs to prevent the cat from escaping. This does not harm the animal but is similar to how a mother cat carries her kittens. This hold is very helpful in restraining the animal for a physical examination or vaccination (see Figure 4.3).

Stretching and Scruffing

This restraint is used when simple scruffing is not sufficient and the cat is still potentially aggressive. The restrainer scruffs the cat with one hand, while the other hand grabs and holds the rear legs, stretching the cat into a straight line. Generally, this holds a cat in a secure position. It also allows

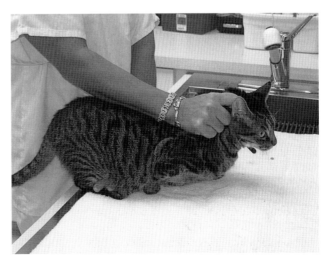

Figure 4.3. Image of the proper approach to scruffing the cat.

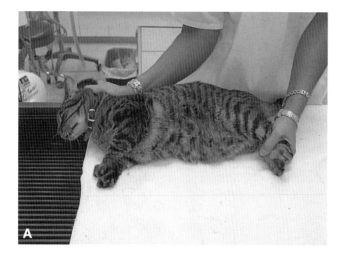

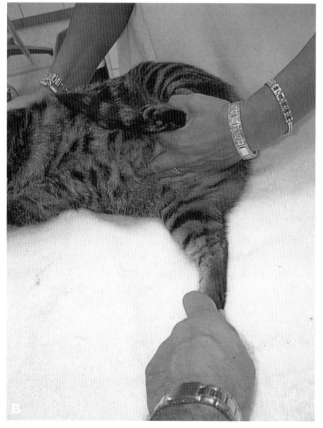

Figure 4.4. Image of the proper approach to scruffing and stretching a cat. Generally, with this restraint the cat can be held and manipulated for proper examination and blood draw (a). The hind leg can then be extended by an assistant while the medial saphenous vein is held off for blood draw with the bottom of the restrainer's hand (b).

another person to have access to a hind limb to draw blood, administer medication, or treat a region (see Figure 4.4).

Restraint for Jugular Venipuncture
The animal is placed farther forward on the table; its front legs are extended outward and the technician holds the

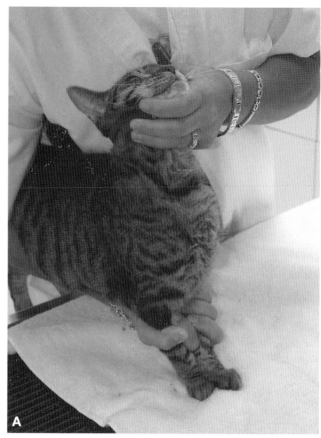

Figure 4.5. Image of the proper approach to extending the neck for a jugular blood draw (a).

wrists. The technician's other hand extends the neck dorsally by lifting the head upward by the muzzle. If need be, the cat can be placed on the end of a table to help the team member get better access to the neck (see Figure 4.5).

Feline Restraint Devices
Towel or Blanket Technique
Wrapping the cat in a towel or blanket like a "burrito" can greatly help in the physical exam and treatment of a fractious animal. A thick towel is generally placed over the animal, and using the towel to help restrain the pet, the cat is wrapped up with its head exposed. This can allow the cat to be confined while the towel is lifted in specific regions to examine or treat the pet (see Figure 4.6).

Cat Bag
A similar device is a cat bag, which allows the cat to be wrapped in a large nylon bag, leaving only the head exposed. There are zipper regions that allow a leg to be exteriorized for blood draw or treatment. Both the towel and cat bag can also be used in combination with a muzzle to further prevent the cat from biting (see Figure 4.7).

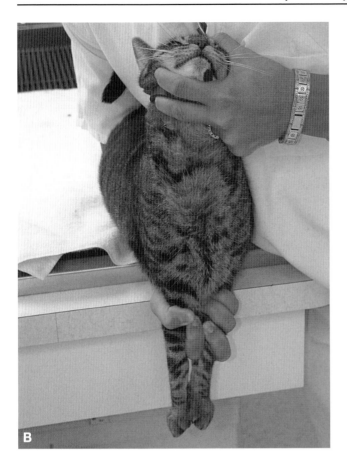

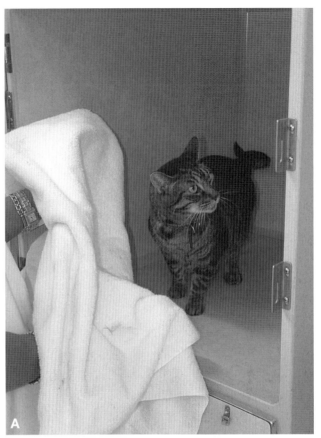

Figure 4.5. (*continued*) In some cases, extending the neck and pulling the forelimbs downward over the table edge may give some team members a better approach to the jugular vein (b).

Anesthetic Chamber

In some cases, the cat is so aggressive that no form of restraint will be sufficient. These pets need to be placed into an **induction chamber**, which is a large glass or plastic aquarium-like structure with a locking air-tight lid. Once in the chamber, anesthetic gas can be filtered to place the pet under light anesthesia. There is some moderate risk in anesthetizing animals that cannot first be examined; however, in many cases it is a safer option for the medical team, owner, and even the animal (see Figure 4.8).

Discussing and Rationalizing Restraint with the Client

The goal of restraint is using just enough to complete the examination or procedure without endangering the animal or the restrainer. The hospital and its trained technical personnel are liable for injuries and damage done by an animal

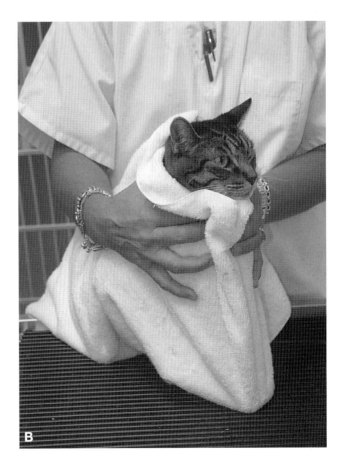

Figure 4.6. Image of cat being approached with a towel, allowing the team member to restrain the cat without risking a scratch or bite (a). Image of a towel restraint, which allows the cat to be isolated and restrained with decreased stress (b).

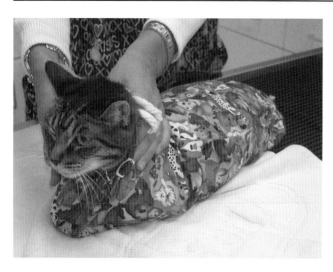

Figure 4.7. Image of cat being restrained in a cat bag. Many bags will have multiple openings that allow a patient's leg to be exteriorized while still restraining the patient.

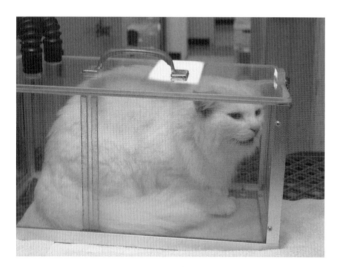

Figure 4.8. Image of cat being anesthetized in a chamber so that an examination, diagnostics, and possible treatments can be completed.

attack. It is extremely important that proper restraint is always performed or overseen by a team member (this involves transport, pain management, etc.). The owner can be helpful under proper direction but should never be allowed to be the sole restrainer of the animal without supervision.

Owners tend to under-restrain or let go when the pet becomes fractious in the new environment. The owner is under the assumption the pet will never attack them or a family member, and they do not understand that when a pet is threatened, adrenaline takes over. Even the gentlest animal can become aggressive in the right circumstance. **The team member's primary job as a restrainer is to protect the animal and the owner from injury and harm.**

Discussing Restraint with the Client
- The goal is to restrain the pet just enough to accomplish the procedure and protect the team members and the owner.
- Before attempting restraint, describe how the patient will be restrained.
- An animal in a new environment may react aggressively or defensively because it is unsure of what is going to happen. These actions can be driven largely by adrenaline and fear, and the pet may even attack the owner unknowingly.
- A muzzle is a temporary measure to help restrain the pet. It is placed on tightly so the pet cannot remove it. A muzzle does not suggest a pet is an aggressive or dangerous animal, just that the pet is in a new environment and may react unexpectedly.
- The owner can help place a muzzle on the pet, but if the animal becomes aggressive toward the owner, another means of restraint may be need to be employed.
- In some cases, the pet may become protective of the owner and will attack if the owner is present. If this occurs, it is best to take the patient in another area to be worked on.
- Some patients become so stressed that sedation is the only option. Stress can be a life-threatening concern, and in these cases sedation or anesthesia may be used to protect the pet.

CD-ROM 1 reviews material presented in this chapter. Please try the cases for Section 1 (The First Two Days on the Job) to help reinforce the information presented here.

Chapter 5

Obtaining an Adequate and Precise History

In most medical and surgical cases, obtaining an accurate medical history can be a large percentage of the diagnostic process. Because the receptionist, kennel assistant, and technical staff are the team members to make first contact with the client by phone or in person, it becomes extremely important that all personnel be able to obtain a brief but thorough history. When presented with a life-threatening emergency, it often becomes the responsibility of the technician or receptionist to take a thorough, precise history, because all other members of the medical team are treating the emergency patient. It is just as important to be able to complete a thorough physical examination, it is important to establish a set protocol of questions that covers most situations. The team member must also be able to discern if there is more going on than what the client can perceive. For example, consider the following.

> A client calls a clinic late in the day just prior to closing. The client informs the receptionist that their cat Whiskers has been acting constipated for the last 1–2 days. Whiskers is straining to defecate and is vocalizing, and now seems more and more depressed. The owner wants to know what they should do; can they give it a children's suppository? Is there some over-the-counter medication that can help? Or should the pet be seen, and can it wait to the morning?

What questions should the receptionist ask to assess if the pet is truly in need? The team member could hand the information over to a technician or take the message for a doctor to return, but what if the message does not get answered tonight? Will the pet be okay?

As many experienced medical teams know, constipated male tom cats are more often suffering from a urinary obstruction than actual constipation. If the male is not seen quickly, the inability of the pet to urinate and the buildup of toxins could put the pet in a life-threatening state. It is not up to the receptionist to decide over the phone if the pet's life is threatened. If the team member asks the right questions and reports to the doctor that a male tom cat is straining and vocalizing and acting constipated, the veterinarian will be

able to more accurately make recommendations and help the pet as quickly as possible.

Getting an Adequate History from a Client's Phone Call

Just as with the example above, there are many clients who ask questions about their pet's health that may never reach the doctor's attention unless a proper history is taken. When handling a client on the phone, a team member should not hesitate to take time to get a file and ask some basic information about the pet so that the medical team has sufficient information to make a decision. Some basic questions are as follows.

Basic Questions
What Is the Signalment of the Patient?
The signalment of the patient is the physical description, age, sex, reproductive status, and weight of the animal. This certainly can be taken from a client's file if the pet has been seen; however, reconfirming the information with the client is always helpful. On many occasions, the signalment of a patient can sometimes help the medical team prepare for a sick patient.

> For example, a client calls with a 4-month-old, male, 35-pound, gold and tan rotteweiler with vomiting and diarrhea. A well-informed medical team will already be suspicious of possible parvo virus, will have the pet immediately placed in an isolation exam room, and possibly even have the diagnostic tests pulled out and warming up to room temperature.

What is the Chief Complaint?
Although this sounds like a straightforward question, the team member must always realize the emotionally attached client does not have the same level of medical training. It is very important to discover what the client perceives as the main concern. Frequently a client may only pick up on a small symptom that may be hiding a much more serious problem (see Figure 5.1).

the team member may have to incorporate some questions from a full history (see below) to help the client distinguish if the pet is showing other specific symptoms such as

- vomiting,
- diarrhea,
- coughing,
- sneezing,
- increased thirst,
- increased urination, and
- weight loss.

These symptoms can suggest profound systemic disease and should never be ignored, whether you are dealing with an ill patient or an animal that is brought in for vaccinations.

These four basic and simple questions can set the tone for how seriously ill the patient is and what steps the hospital team may need to take in order to make sure the pet is diagnosed and treated. Clients will often expect serious decisions to be made based on the information that they give the medical team over the phone. **It is important to be very precise and get a history but not give out medical information or even suggest a diagnosis over the phone.**

Taking an Adequate History Prior to Physical Examination

As important as taking a history from clients over the phone, a full medical history prior to or during a medical examination is paramount to a proper medical diagnosis. The history

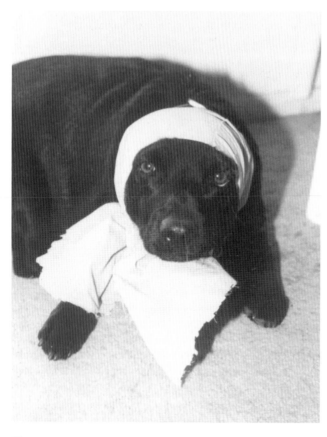

Figure 5.1. What is the signalment on this pet? (Answer): A 40- to 50-pound lab mix.

For example, a client calls to inform you that their 8-year-old, male, neutered, gray Himalayan cat is shedding and has a poor hair coat. When the pet arrives at the clinic, you discover that the pet has lost 4 pounds in 1 month and its ears, whites of the eyes, and gums are yellow. Obviously there is more going on than just a mild skin problem, but if a proper history is not taken, this pet may wait days to be seen at a busy general practice.

How Long Has This Been Happening?

Many clients take "the wait and see approach" with their own health and their pet's health. However, determining the duration of an illness can certainly help the medical team understand how serious the problem may be. Clients can vary tremendously in what they feel is the appropriate time for a condition to last until they seek medical attention. Some clients will immediately bring their pet in at the first sign of illness; some clients may wait days to weeks from the initiation of physical illness.

Is the Pet Showing Any Other Signs of Illness?

The goal of a team member is to be extremely specific in discussion with the client. When asking this last question,

A 2.5-year-old, male, neutered, 15-pound bichon frise came into an emergency hospital for acute onset of inability to balance, lack of coordination, collapse, and weakness. A technician and doctor went through the medical history thoroughly, and the client assured the team that the pet was in perfect health and had no exposure to toxins or poisons. The veterinarian informed that the pet certainly could have a serious neurologic problem, and although the pet could be started on fluids and routine blood work, a neurologic consultation be needed in the morning. The clients were willing to anything for their pet and agreed to begin treatment. The pet was admitted, started on intravenous fluids, and routine blood work was sent to the lab. The clients came to the back to say goodnight to their pet, escorted by a hospital team member. As the clients were leaving, one client looked at the other client and said, "You know I don't think he liked the vodka as much as his normal bourbon." On further questioning, it was discovered that the dog shared evening cocktails with the client and recently began drinking martinis rather than just bourbon on the rocks. The clients had no idea that a little vodka could be toxic to their pet.

When discussing health concerns with clients on the phone, there are some common questions a client may ask.

Do You Think the Pet Should Be Seen Immediately?
- **The most important concept to explain to a client is that there is no way to diagnose a patient over the phone.**
- A good rule of thumb is that if the client is worried enough to call and feels that it is an emergency, the animal should probably should be seen.
- The medical team should then be consulted using the proper history and the pet scheduled or brought in immediately per the recommendation of the veterinarian.

Is There Anything I Can Give the Pet Over the Counter?
- At no time should anyone on the medical team (except the veterinarian) recommend any medications (holistic or other) be given a pet without the veterinarian's recommendations or a physical examination.
- Even something as benign as aspirin or an aspirin-like drug can have serious to life-threatening side effects.
- As with all other examples, the medical team should be consulted and a return call made to the client.

Is There Anything I Can Do at Home for Him?
- Just as with the previous example, no recommendations of home therapy should be made without a veterinarian's advice or physical exam.
- Even discussion of placing a pet on a bland food diet should first be discussed with the doctor on staff once an adequate history is given and the veterinarian has had time to review the medical record.
- Any medical advice given to a client makes the entire hospital liable for the information. If the pet has a severe reaction or is not seen promptly and dies, the client could hold the hospital responsible for the incident.

After the conversation with client, the most important thing to do is to document the call in the client's record, including the hospital team's recommendation and the client's response. Through proper documentation, the hospital can keep track of a pet's medical history at the same time protecting itself from liability issues. The following is an example of documentation.

9/12/03 Ms. Schadler called (Owner). Buffy is vomiting for 3 days, recommended exam immediately, owner declined and will feed bland food diet for 12–24 hours, will recheck if worse. Scheduled a call back for 9/13.

should be taken initially by the admitting team member checking in the patient. The doctor can then come into the room with a clear idea of what additional questions need to be asked. This sometimes makes the client go through some aspects of the medical history twice; however, very often the client will start thinking of certain problems or concerns during the first set of questions and may expand the information to the doctor.

The history should be thorough and precise. When asking questions, the team member should be very specific in what they ask the client. A very common question to ask a client with a sick animal is, Could the pet have gotten into any poisons or toxins? The concept of a toxin or poison can sometimes mean very different things to a client.

The moral of this story is to be precise and specific when talking with clients.

A team member should develop a routine for medical questions and ask them in the same format and order each time. Medical history questions can change depending on why the pet is being seen, in what part of the country the animal hospital is located, and the living conditions of the animal. There is no set number or type of questions that should be used, but the medical team should discuss what types of

questions should be asked for pets being seen for wellness exams, admitted for surgery, or checked because of illness. Below are some basic medical questions that can be used for pets being admitted for medical concerns.

Medical History Questions
What Is the Chief Complaint?
It is very important to define what the owner is concerned about in relation to the pet's health.

How Long Has This Been Happening?
The duration of the illness can help suggest if the disease is acute or chronic in nature.

Could the Pet Have Gotten into Any Poisons, Medications (Human or Animal), or Toxins?
As illustrated by the example above, being very specific can help delineate if there has been any exposure to a possible toxic element. Remember that some pets can get into drugs that family members take, and even though these are bitter tasting, the medication will be eaten by certain animals (i.e., Labrador retrievers).

Over-the-counter products, especially aspirin-like drugs

(non-steroidal anti-inflammatory drugs) such as Aleve, ibu-profen, Tylenol, and aspirin-free medications can produce se-rious or life-threatening complications, especially in cats.

Common basic poisons/insecticides include

- rodent poison (Warfarin and others),
- gopher bait (strychnine),
- rose feed/bone meal (organophosphate),
- antifreeze (ethylene glycol),
- snail bait (metaldehyde), and
- ant/roach spray (pyrethrins).

Plants also can have toxic side effects and are specific to particular regions. Some examples of toxic plants include

- oleanders (cardiac toxin),
- mushrooms (death cap),
- algae (algae poisoning), and
- Other regional plants.

Toxic animals are also regionally specific. Some examples of these are

- scorpions,
- snakes, and
- spiders.

There are some drugs that may not be prescription, but still may be dangerous to the animal, such as marijuana, crack, etc. Remember that concerns of illegal drug con-sumption should be handled delicately and possibly may need to be handled by the veterinarian.

Any Chance of Trauma?
Be specific when asking about possible trauma (e.g., fall, hit by car, animal attack). Also, some owners do not realize that cats that climb up to 14-foot ledges could easily fall and sus-tain damage.

Is There a History of Previous Disease?
When confronted with a pet in a life-threatening emergency, owners will sometimes forget that their pet has a long his-tory of disease. Some owners will forget that their pet once had a disease if the last symptoms were seen months or years before. Also, some owners will not understand that a pet may be suffering from a serious disease if the pet was diag-nosed with a disease but never treated for the problem. For example, a client may inform you that their pet had seizures, but that the last one was many years ago. A client may say that their pet was diagnosed with Cushing's disease, for in-stance, but they never treated it.

Diseases of concern are

- heart disease,
- seizure/epilepsy,
- organ disease: kidney, liver, pancreas,

- hormonal disease: diabetes, hyperadrenocorticism, hy-poadrenocorticism, and
- hypertension.

Are There Changes in Appetite?
Changes in appetite can range from normal intake of food to complete anorexia and can certainly suggest severe disease. Long-term anorexia can produce its own life-threatening con-cerns, especially in the cat (see Chapter 14; hepatic lipidosis).

Any Evidence of C/S/V/D/PU/PD?
The acronym C/S/V/D/PU/PD stands for coughing, sneez-ing, vomiting, diarrhea, increased thirst, and increased uri-nation. Changes in these parameters can suggest diseases of major body systems.

Respiratory/Cardiovascular System
Coughing and sneezing can suggest changes in the heart and lungs. Coughing can be associated with upper respiratory, pulmonary, and cardiac disease.

Sneezing is generally associated with upper respiratory or pulmonary problems. When coughing and sneezing is combined with nasal or ocular discharge, the possibility of infectious disease is a concern, and the pet should be placed in an exam room or isolation area away from other pets.

Gastrointestinal System
Vomiting and diarrhea are common signs of many potential gastrointestinal problems. Possible categories of diseases that produce these signs can be

- dietary indiscretion,
- gastrointestinal parasites,
- infectious diseases: parvo virus,
- intestinal obstruction/foreign bodies (i.e., clothing, rocks, dog toys), and
- inflammatory disease.

Other systemic disease can also produce vomiting and di-arrhea. These are diseases where there is a buildup of toxins in the body (i.e., kidney disease, liver disease, severe dia-betes, other hormonal diseases) producing gastrointestinal signs due to the nausea and toxins the pet must deal with.

If young animals (under 12–18 months of age) with a his-tory of vomiting or diarrhea are brought in, these pets should be placed into an isolated exam room away from other waiting pets.

Polyuria/Polydipsia
Polyuria (PU) refers to a pet that has a sharp increase in urinating. **Polydipsia** (PD) is defined as an increase in water consumption.

These increases can start subtly over days to weeks and be the first indicators of chronic serious disease.

Animals tend to drink a great deal of water to help try to flush toxins out of their system when there is chronic disease increasing the amount of toxins in the body. Along with increased water consumption, animals urinate more often.

PU/PD can be the first indicator of many chronic older-age diseases.

- Kidney disease
- Diabetes mellitus
- Hyperthyroidism (cats)
- Hyperadrenocorticism (Cushing's disease)
- Liver disease
- Other systemic diseases

When asking if the dog is PU/PD, it should be noted if these symptoms have been occurring over weeks to months rather than being an acute situation.

Clients whose pets are being seen for preventative care (i.e., vaccinations) should also be questioned about changes in thirst and urination since chronic increase can be more suggestive of an underlying systemic disease.

Has There Been Any History of Fainting, Decreased Ability to Exercise (Exercise Intolerance), or Collapse?

These signs can be very serious and can suggest serious cardiac or systemic disease. Animals with inability to handle normal activity or animals that faint or collapse are potentially in a life-threatening condition and need to be handled as a critical care emergency.

These animals cannot keep up with simple demands of activity or normal stress that can be placed upon them and collapse or are unable to complete the task. Some of these animals can become so challenged that they simply collapse and die.

Some diseases that can produce these symptoms include heart disease or systemic disease causing weakness, such as

- infectious disease,
- metabolic disease,
- tumor,
- blood loss/anemia,
- bleeding abdominal tumor, and
- clotting problems.

If a pet comes in with a history of collapsing or fainting, these pets should be treated as an emergency and brought to the medical team's attention immediately (see Chapter 30).

Has the Pet Shown Any Change in Neurologic Behavior?

Changes in neurologic behavior, such as seizures, nystagmus (uncontrolled rapid eye movements), or general changes in behavior (aggression, changes in appetite, forgetfulness, sudden blindness) can suggest central nervous system disease or systemic illness. Owners will bring animals in suggesting that they have a change in attitude or behavior, suddenly or over time as the pet ages. It is very important to have the owner specifically describe the changes and when the behaviors occur because there are

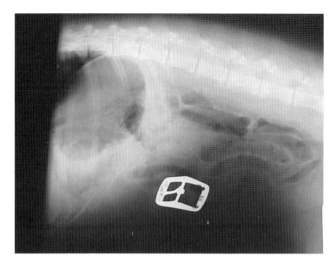

Figure 5.2. Image of an abdominal radiograph that shows that the canine ate a belt buckle.

many types of disease that can manifest themselves in how the animal acts.

Does the Pet Eat Abnormal Things?

Especially with pets being seen with complaints of vomiting and diarrhea, questions of what the pet could have gotten into need to be addressed. The team member should ask extremely specific questions because owners will sometimes assume that their pet would never eat anything that tastes bad or is abnormal (see Figure 5.2).

Some possible foreign bodies can be

- electric cords,
- toys,
- bones,
- rocks,
- clothing, and
- trash (i.e., corn cobs, feminine products, plastic).

Has the Pet Traveled?

A very important question can be if the pet has a travel history or if it has just moved from another location. These pets could have contracted a regional disease that may not show physical symptoms for weeks to months. These diseases may be uncommon or nonexistent in the current location. Some regional geographic diseases are

- heart worm,
- valley fever,
- histoplasmosis,
- leptospirosis,
- blastomycosis,
- Lyme's disease,
- Rocky Mountain spotted fever, and
- salmon poisoning.

Are There Other Animals in the Household, and How Is Their Health?

It is important to determine if there are any other pets in the household that could be showing signs suggesting an intoxication or infectious disease affecting more than one pet. Are there other pets that could potentially succumb to an infectious disease that has just been diagnosed in another animal. For example, if a new 4-month-old puppy has been tested and diagnosed with parvo viral infection, it is important to determine if there are other pets in the household that could be at risk.

In the later sections of this book that deal with specific organ systems and their diseases, each chapter will have a focused discussion on how to get a good history for pets showing specific organ disease. Just like all aspects of veterinary medicine, the entire medical team should practice and be able to routinely take an excellent history from the client.

CD-ROM 1 reviews material presented in this chapter. Please try the cases for Section 1 (The First Two Days on the Job) to help reinforce the information presented here.

Chapter 6

The Medical Record and the 30-Second Triage Examination

This chapter will review the legality of the medical record, the proper way to evaluate the stability of an incoming patient (**triage**), and basic knowledge of diseases that are infectious to both animals and humans (**zoonotic diseases**).

Although understanding the importance of the physical exam and knowing how to do a proper triage examination is important, many medical teams feel that this is the veterinarian's responsibility. However, although the ultimate liability rests squarely on the veterinarian's shoulders, all members of the team must be able to assess if a pet is getting into trouble. For example, consider the following.

- A technician monitoring a pet on fluids begins to notice that the pet is gaining weight, has increased lung sounds, and a moist cough.
- A kennel assistant notices the large-breed canine boarder is acting weak and in pain and has a large, bloated abdomen. This team member may be the only one observing this pet 90% of the time.
- A groomer notices a severe ear infection and skin rash and can help the medical team catch important medical concerns for the health of the pet.
- A receptionist that checks in a cat for an eye problem notices that the pet is severely dehydrated, icteric, and has its third eyelids elevated. This pet may need immediate attention.

It is impossible for the veterinarian to evaluate and monitor all of these patients, initiate diagnostics, and begin treatment without the help of a well-educated medical team. Building and educating the team members so they can identify abnormality is the most important tool of the hospital team. When an employee goes up to another team member and says, **"Could you please check Herman, I think there is something abnormal going on," the medical team is beginning to properly use all it resources.**

Medical Records

A medical record is the compilation of pertinent facts about the individual animal's life and health history. The medical record is the property of the hospital and should be maintained on site for at least 1–3 years, depending on state law. In some states, medical records may need to be kept in storage for up to 7 years. Radiographs, ultrasound images, and other diagnostic test reports are also part of the medical record and must be kept in conjunction with state laws. Clients are allowed to request copies of medical records as needed for veterinary specialty consultations, personal records, or other needs. Radiographs can be loaned out to the client as needed but remain the property of the hospital. Most hospitals will have a radiograph sign-out form to track the location and the responsible party for the x-rays. If a client wants to have a copy of radiographs made, there are human medical radiography offices that can duplicate the films for a set fee.

The hospital maintains a client–patient relationship with the owner who presented the pet for treatment. The client–patient relationship does not allow disclosure of pet information without the verbal or written consent of the owner. Permission to disclose medical information to another person should be documented in the chart with the date of the permission, who in the family gave the permission, and to whom the information is allowed to be given. Although rare, there can be incidences of dispute between family members, an owner and breeder, or individuals where client–patient confidentiality may need to be maintained.

There are many possible medical record formats available to a hospital. Whether written records, computer records, or records on a PDA, the basic medical record may follow many possible outlines.

- **Conventional:** This is a source-oriented file that follows chronological order of what the pet presented for each visit. Some source files will have a master problem list as a top sheet of the record. This page lists all dates of all major diseases and diagnosis and serves as a diagnostic index for the pet.
- **Problem oriented:** This file follows full documentation of a pet per problem situation. Every time the pet comes in for a continuing problem (for instance, pancreatitis), there is a specific section in the pet's file for this diagnosis, and the workup is listed chronologically.

Whatever format and medium is used, a thorough medical record should contain the following.

- Owner's information
  — Name
  — Address

- — Employment
- — Phone number
- — Financial information
- Animal information
  - — Case number
  - — Signalment
- Record
  - — Symptoms
  - — History
  - — Vaccination history
  - — Consultations
  - — Diagnosis
  - — Discharge summaries
  - — Prognosis
  - — Continuing education for aftercare
  - — Biopsy/necropsy findings
  - — Client communication

It is extremely important, from a liability perspective, that all team members understand, be able to interpret, and notate on the medical record any contact with the client and information about the pet or changes in the pet's medical status. If ever there is a dispute regarding the patient care or communication with the client, the medical record and its entries become the first document examined.

The 30-Second Triage Examination

The difference between a true emergency and a perceived emergency is derived by physical exam and history (see Chapter 5). The focus of this exam is to assess the overall status of the patient in a brief 30-second examination. The goal of this examination is not to make a nonveterinarian team member able to diagnose or give a prognosis for a patient but rather to make sure the borderline or shocky patient is seen immediately.

Each employee should have a basic understanding of what a true emergency is so the team member can communicate her concerns to the client and veterinarian. Triage examination is something that must mastered by all employees and be constantly practiced in order to perfect. If there is ever a concern regarding stability of a patient, always err on the side of caution—remember the words *"I think this is abnormal, could you please check this,"* can save lives.

The physical examination is broken into steps of observation. A patient does not need to meet a specific number of criteria for the team member to feel that the patient is of increased concern. If the medical team member is uncertain if the pet may be borderline on one aspect of the triage exam, the rest of the medical team should be informed immediately.

Point I: General Review of the Animal (Mentation)— Conscious or Unconscious?

Mentation is defined as the mental status or attitude of the pet. Very few pets come into a medical facility and calmly

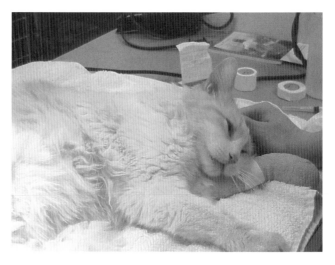

Figure 6.1. Even the friendliest cat will not often lie on its side, not moving or exploring a new environment. This pet is in trouble.

lie down on their sternum or side and relax as if they are at home. The friendliest dog often stands up and explores the environment, especially when someone new enters the room. Animals that are carried in, lie on their sides (lateral recumbency), or even on their chest (sternal recumbency) should already raise the concern level (see Figure 6.1). When encountering a potentially sick pet that seems severely lethargic or depressed and is not up and moving around, you must consider that these pets may need immediate attention where a few minutes may make the difference between life and death.

Point II: A Review of the Respiratory System—Is the Pet Breathing?

A quick visual review of how the pet is breathing can quickly differentiate an animal that is life threatened from a stable pet. Of course, if there is no respiration, the caution level is automatically critical; however, the pet's body position, its respiratory rate, and how it is breathing can tell the medical team a great deal.

Normal respiration rates are 8–30 breaths per minute (sometimes getting up to 80 breaths per minute in stressed animals).

A panting pet should not be confused with a pet in respiratory distress, and there are both dogs and cats that will pant in a stressful environment. If a cat comes in panting and is acting as if it is in respiratory distress, often asking the owner if the cat typically stresses and open mouth breathes every time it comes in may help clarify whether the cat is an emergency or just nervous. Even with a cat with a known history of panting, a team member should still evaluate the pet to make sure that this open mouth breathing is not a manifestation of a new problem.

Normal breathing patterns in a relaxed animal are slow

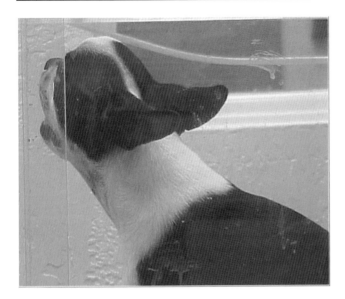

Figure 6.2. In this image the pet is in an oxygen cage. This dog is having severe respiratory difficulty. Note the following: extended head and neck, ears back, open mouth breathing. A video of this pet breathing is not needed to detect that this pet is having respiratory problems.

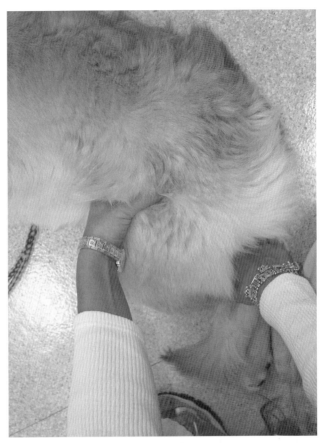

Figure 6.3. Image of a team member taking the femoral pulse. This is accomplished by placing the flat of the hand on the inside hind limb just distal to the inguinal fold. A strong pulse should be observed.

chest expansion and depression. The animal should not be extending the neck and head as it tries to breathe (see Figure 6.2). There is no component of normal breathing that includes abdominal movement or open mouth breathing. Signs of concerns are an abdominal push with breathing, open mouth breathing, or severely increased respiratory rate.

Point III: A Review of the Cardiovascular System— Is the Heart Beating?

Pulses are a reflection of cardiac output. There are times when there may be a strong heart rate, but weak pulses (i.e., shock). Pulse rates are more important than heart rates as long as the pet has an observable heart rhythm. Changes in pulse quality can suggest serious disease of the heart and lungs, massive dehydration, trauma, internal bleeding, and many other problems. Any concerns or changes in the pulse rate should be discussed immediately with the medical team and veterinarian.

All members should be able to evaluate a pulse. Whether it is necessary to evaluate a potential emergency, check a patient prior to surgery, or simply check a boarder, it is important that all team members are able to evaluate and get a pulse rate. This is mastered with practice and patience. If a team member has problems isolating a pulse, a heart rate can be observed by placing a hand at the left side of the chest at the left elbow level. Remember, the key is to feel an abnormal heart or pulse rate, so the team members should practice on large healthy dogs and work their way up to smaller pets. A quick note of caution is to make sure the pet is not aggressive or a fear biter before attempting a pulse rate.

To get a pulse, the team member should place the fingers over a large artery. A team member's thumb should not be used because the pulse of the individual can also be felt while trying to take a patient's pulse, and this could falsely increase the pet's pulse rate. There are a number of locations in which to find a strong pulse.

- **Femoral artery**: This is the most common location to take a good pulse. By placing your hand inside the inguinal fold on the medial aspect of the hind leg, where the hind leg meets the skin, the femoral pulse can be felt (see Figure 6.3).
- **Axillary pulse:** In some animals, especially in larger dogs, a pulse can be picked up behind the forearm in the armpit region. By placing your fingers against the medial aspect of the forelimb in the armpit region, a good pulse may be picked up against the fingers (see Figure 6.4).
- **Metacarpal pulse:** As with humans, a pulse can be found in some pets over the wrist below or above the metacarpal pad of the front limb (see Figure 6.5).
- **Digital pulse:** In some pets a strong pulse can be picked up in the interdigital region between the toes (see Figure 6.6).

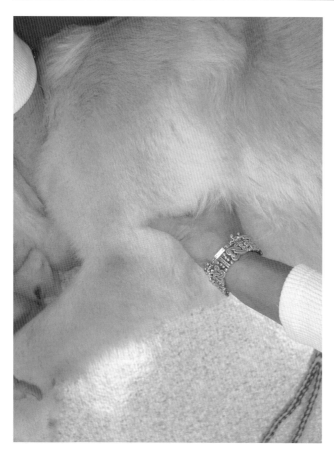

Figure 6.4. Image of a team member taking an axillary pulse. This is accomplished by placing the flat of the hand on the inside arm just dorsal to the elbow. A strong pulse can often be observed.

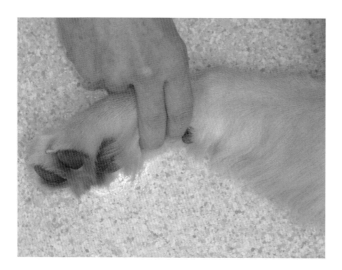

Figure 6.5. Image of a team member taking a metacarpal pulse. This is accomplished by placing the pointer and middle finger just dorsal to the larger metacarpal/metatarsal pad on the caudal aspect of the limb. A strong pulse can often be observed.

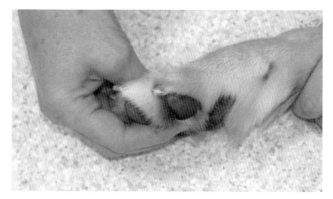

Figure 6.6. Image of a team member taking an interdigital pulse. This is accomplished by placing the pointer and middle finger in the interdigital space on the ventral aspect of the foot. A strong pulse can often be observed.

Once a pulse is identified, the following criteria should be evaluated.

Evaluating the Pulse

For the **pulse rate**, count the number of pulses in a 15-second time frame and multiply by four; this gives you pulse per minute.

- A normal pulse rate is 80–120 (canine) and 100–140 (feline).
- A pulse rate >160–180 (**tachycardia**) should be pointed out to the medical team.
- A pulse rate <80 (**bradycardia**) should also be noted and discussed with the medical team.

As important as pulse rate is the quality of the pulse—its overall strength or weakness. As the team members become more practiced in determining a normal pulse quality, they will be able to point out abnormality. Pulse quality should be evaluated as follows.

- **Yes versus no:** If no pulse is evident, with or without a heart rate, it is an absolute emergency, and the doctor and medical team should be notified immediately.
- **Weak pulse:** Pulses that seem weak or are nonexistent could suggest that an animal is in serious shock or in respiratory or cardiac arrest. Animals with weakened pulses should be brought to the attention of the medical team immediately.
- **Hyperdynamic:** This pulse type is defined as rapid, hard pulses that lift your finger off the limb. This change can suggest the body trying to keep up with an increased need, and it may soon be unable to maintain this demand. Although this can be normal in happy, excited, or even scared pets, animals that come in sick and depressed may be in early shock. Hyperdynamic pulses in depressed or ill patients should be pointed out to the medical team immediately.

Point IV: Mucus Membrane (Gums)—What is the Gum Color?

The **mucus membranes** refer to the nonhaired regions of the body where the normal color of the skin can be seen. The mucus membrane regions of the body are the gums, whites of the eyes, inside ear flaps (pinna), rectum, penis, or vulva. Caution should be taken when assessing gum color or capillary refill rate to make sure the animal is not fearful or aggressive and will not try to bite.

Normal healthy gum color is a light to moderate pink, and this color reflects proper oxygenation of tissue. Abnormal coloration of this tissue can suggest different disease entities.

- **Purple, blue, and gray** reflects an inability of the body to properly oxygenate the tissue, usually suggesting heart or respiratory disease. These colorations suggest severe life-threatening concern. The pet should be placed in an oxygen-rich environment and the doctor and medical team notified immediately.
- **Pale pink to white** suggests that the body is unable to maintain the demands placed upon it due to shock, dehydration, or blood loss. The animal must alter the blood flow to small peripheral capillaries in the gums and other mucus membranes, causing a paling or lack of color in these regions. This change should also be noted and the medical team informed.
- **Yellow** pigmentation usually suggests a buildup of toxins within the tissue that are normally detoxified and eliminated by the liver. A buildup of these toxins in the body causes a yellowing of the gums, whites of the eyes (**conjunctiva**), and skin (**icterus or jaundice**) (see Figure 6.7). Early jaundice can be detected initially by examining the roof of the mouth (**hard palate**) with a light source and observing a yellow coloration. Care must be

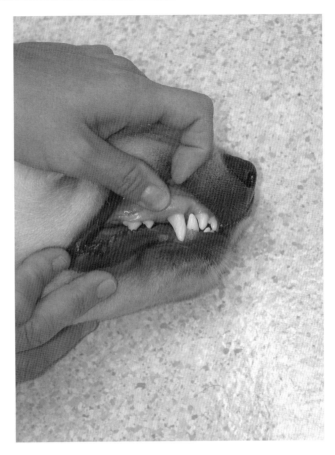

Figure 6.8. Image of evaluating the capillary refill time. Being cautious of aggressive animals, the lip is lifted and the gum color evaluated. A finger then presses on the gums with enough pressure to blanch the membrane. The finger is then removed, and the time it takes for gums to return to normal color is measured.

taken with fearful or aggressive animals when evaluating the hard palate. Icterus can suggest a serious liver disease or other disease entity.

Point V: Capillary Refill Time—Does the Gum Color Return Quickly?

The capillary refill time (CRT) refers to the time it takes for the gums to return to normal color after the mucus membranes are pressed with a light pressure. **Normally the process should take less the 2 seconds (see Figure 6.8)**.

Abnormality suggests the body is unable to refill the smallest capillaries of the body in an adequate time frame. This can be a very important factor in assessing for early shock. When the body is challenged and cannot keep up with the demands placed upon it, the CRT slows. Some causes that change the CRT are dehydration, shock, allergic reaction, toxins, and other diseases. Please note that it is not possible to get an accurate CRT on an already pale or icteric animal. The fact the animal is pale or jaundiced is enough reason to have it evaluated.

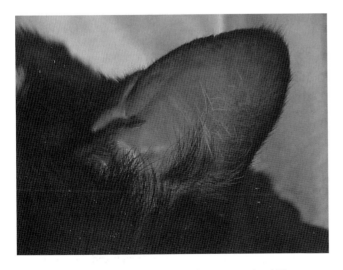

Figure 6.7. Image of a ear pinna. These areas should be checked for yellowing of the skin suggestive of jaundice or icterus.

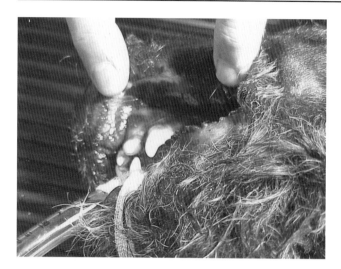

Figure 6.9. Evaluating the gums and skin for abnormal bruising is key to picking up early bleeding problems. In this image, the patient has massive bruising of the gums secondary to a rattlesnake bite.

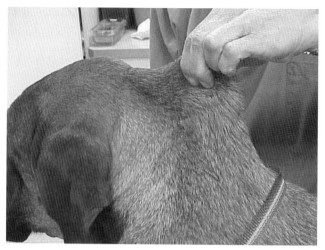

Figure 6.10. Image of a medical team member evaluating skin turgor for dehydration. In this patient the skin does not bounce back quickly, suggesting moderate to severe dehydration.

Point VI: Brusing—Is There Bruising of the Mucus Membrane?

Spontaneous bruising of the gums without evidence or history of trauma can suggest an inability of the body to clot blood normally (**coagulopathy**). This is of special concern if a sick pet begins to spontaneously bruise while in the hospital. Improper clotting of blood can be caused by a low platelet count that makes the pet more susceptible to bleeding, certain infectious diseases, rat poison or other toxin ingestion, heat stroke, and other disease entities. Spontaneous bruising or bruising in general should be pointed out to the medical team immediately (see Figure 6.9).

Point VII: Temperature—What Is the Pet's Temperature?

Both extremes of temperature can suggest serious disease.

Normal rectal temperature is 100–102.5° Fahrenheit for the dog and cat.

Hypothermia, or less than normal body temperature, can suggest the animal is severely weakened and sick, or it can suggest that the animal is in cold shock after exposure to cold or falling into icy waters. Hypothermia is life threatening and needs to be reported to the medical team at once.

Higher than normal body temperature, which is called **fever** or **hyperthermia,** can also be a strong concern, and if severely elevated (>106° Fahrenheit) can be life threatening. Fever is generally a response to internal substances and occurs secondary to infection, inflammation, or **neoplasia** (cancer). Life-threatening hyperthermia results from massive infection, inflammation, or heat stroke, which occurs when the temperature increases above 106°. Heat stroke can produce damage to the organs, the body's ability to clot blood, and central nervous system. High fevers are life threatening, and the pet must be brought to the attention of the medical team immediately and cooled down (see Chapter 30).

Point VIII: Dehydration—Is the Pet Losing or Unable to Maintain Normal Hydration?

Dehydration is a measurement of how severely a pet is fluid compromised on presentation. It is measured by observation in the physical exam through a number of parameters.

- **Skin turgor** is the overall elasticity of the skin or how quickly the skin bounces back after being lifted or tented. The more dehydrated the pet, the less the skin's ability to bounce back quickly (see Figure 6.10). Common locations to check for dehydration are the skin over the shoulders, on the forehead, and over the eyelids (typically the most sensitive).

   One exception to this rule is that animals with severe weight loss can have poor elasticity and could seem severely dehydrated.
- **Gums** are generally moist and slippery in well-hydrated animals. The gums become drier and tackier as the animal becomes more dehydrated.
- **Eyes** have fat pads behind them that help keep the eyes protruded. As an animal dehydrates, these fat pads decrease in size as moisture is removed to help rehydrate the animal. Thus the more the animal is dehydrated, the greater is the sunken appearance of the eyes. Also, as the eye sinks in, the third eyelids or lower eyelids begin to protrude over the eye, giving the appearance of a red swollen eye.

Measuring Dehydration

Dehydration is a measurement based on the physical examination of the pet (i.e., skin turgor, mucus membrane, and appearance of the eyes). Severe dehydration can be a life-threatening concern that could push a sick or injured animal into a worsening state of shock. Levels of dehydration are as follows.

- **Early dehydration**: In this stage the pet is usually not detectably dehydrated, but the history of severe fluid losses (i.e., vomiting and diarrhea) may suggest the pet's hydration status is being challenged. Although early dehydration is not a life-threatening emergency, the medical team may need to explain to the client the need to treat the patient with some form of fluid therapy before the condition worsens.
- **Mild dehydration:** In this level of dehydration, the animal is beginning to show initial dehydration; the skin turgor is slowed (slightly), gums are moist to dry, and eyes may be less shiny and slightly sunken in. Animals may be slightly depressed.
- **Moderate dehydration:** With moderate dehydration skin turgor is more severely slowed, gums are dry, eyes are sunken, and the pet tends to be more depressed.
- **Severe dehydration**: This is a life-threatening dehydration; there is no skin elasticity, gums are bone dry, eyes are severely sunken, and the animal is usually lifeless, lying on its sternum or its side. These pets require immediate medical attention.

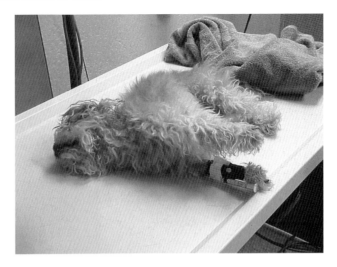

Figure 6.11. Image of a patient with Shift-Sherrington syndrome. This canine has been hit by a car and presents rigid and fixed in the front limbs and neck but is relaxed and flaccid in the hind limbs. This type of presentation after a trauma suggests a broken back.

Point IX: Changes in Body Conformation—Does the Pet's Body Look Abnormal?

There are a few changes in the pet's body conformation that may suggest an emergency condition and a need for immediate care. These changes are apparent in an initial inspection of the animal and should be dealt with as soon as possible.

Bloated Abdomen

When a dog, usually a large to giant breed, presents with a large distended abdomen with a history of gagging and trying to vomit, this suggests a true emergency in veterinary medicine. This condition, called bloat or **gastro-distention volvulus** (see Chapter 10), is a life-threatening condition in which the patient's stomach has rotated around its own axis, cutting off the blood supply to the stomach and spleen. This disease is much like a horse colic and if not treated quickly may lead to a life-threatening state and potential death.

Shift-Sherrington Syndrome

When a canine comes in after a trauma (usually from being hit by a car) and presents with a rigid unmovable forelegs and neck and a hind end that is completely relaxed, this usually suggests that there has been a fracture in the lower back and the spinal cord may be damaged or severed (see Figure 6.11). This syndrome typically carries a poor prognosis, and the pet needs to be treated with the utmost care.

Point X: Lesser Concerns: Body Conditions— Lacerations, Eye Injuries

Although very disconcerting, lacerations and superficial injuries must come second to shock and stabilization of an animal (see Figure 6.12). However, to the owner, these injuries may seem like a life and death emergency. If the nine steps

of stability discussed above are within normal limits, the team member must explain that the patient may need to wait until the medical team is able to handle the case. Or if the pet is unstable with superficial injuries, the pet may need to be stabilized before the less serious injuries are addressed.

Flowchart of Triage

Figure 6.13 is a flowchart used to evaluate the stability of a patient. There is no one right way, and any system that adequately evaluates the patient and can be repeated in a systematic way is acceptable (see Table 6.1).

Zoonotic Disease

When approaching or triaging pets, the team member should always keep in mind that there are some diseases that the animal may be infected with that can also be transmitted to humans (**zoonotic disease**). Transmission of the disease can occur via ingestion, inhalation, or direct contact. It is very easy to come into contact with blood, urine, or other specimens, especially if the team member does not wear protective gloves. Those in the human health-care field have very specific protocols to follow when handling human specimens and the patients themselves. It is important to recognize and adhere to the rules and regulations of your hospital or clinic when handling specimens and patients. Precautions include the following.

- Know specific zoonotic diseases in your geographic region that are present and potentially of high risk to humans. For example, in the Arizona mountains, bubonic plaque is endemic. This lethal disease, spread by fleas, can also infect cats. Cats will come in with severe upper

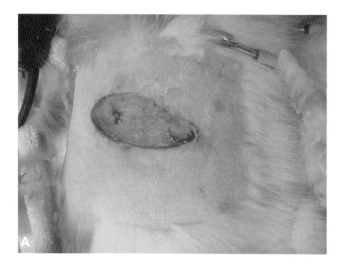 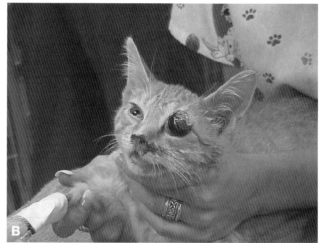

Figure 6.12. With a patient in shock, although very disconcerting to the owner, a laceration (a) or a proptosed eye (b) are non-life-threatening secondary injuries.

respiratory signs of nasal discharge, sneezing, and coughing. The animals will all have high fevers, rashes, and are usually covered in fleas. This pet is a human health hazard and must be moved into isolation immediately.

- When dealing with pets with undiagnosed skin conditions, always wear gloves and wash thoroughly when done. Many stray and owned animals may be exposed to skin diseases such as sarcoptic mange or ringworm. These diseases can cause mild to moderate discomfort to humans that come in contact with the pet.
- With dogfights, being hit by car, and other trauma accidents, it is impossible to determine whether one might come into contact with animal or human body fluids. When dealing with animal attacks or trauma, it is impossible for the inspecting team members to avoid getting blood and fluids on themselves. Some owners or concerned citizens that bring pets in may have also been injured or bitten. Although the risk of blood contamination is low, team members should always be concerned about direct contact with human or animal blood without protective clothing.

Documentation

Although discussed in the next chapter, all team members should be able to document the findings of a basic triage examination. Often the initial findings are the first real physical prior to a true emergency, and another physical examination may not be recorded until after the pet is stabilized. Therefore, it is important for the team member to be able to properly document observations for the medical record.

There is no absolute system for how to do this; however, using components of the SOAP (subjective, objective, assessment, plan) method is probably the most accepted (see Chapter 7). This method follows the following criteria.

Signalment
As discussed previously, all facts describing the animal should be listed so the medical team has a complete picture of what the animal is upon first observation.

Subjective Statement(S)
The subjective statement is a personal observation of the physical appearance, mentation, and attitude of the patient. Some common statements in this category are listed here.

- Dog is bright, alert, and responsive (BAR).
- Dog is quiet, alert, and responsive (QAR).
- Dog is depressed.
- Dog is comatose.
- Dog is aggressive.
- Dog is emaciated.

Objective Statement (O)
The objective statement is a discussion of all physical data evaluated for the patient. The temperature, pulse, respiration, mucus membrane color, CRT, and hydration are evaluated. As well, each body system is evaluated and commented on. All team members should be able to evaluate the first six parameters of the objective part of the SOAP.

Assessment (A)
The assessment part of the SOAP is done by the veterinarian to outline potential disease entities that may be producing symptoms in the patient.

Plan (P)
The plan part of the SOAP is completed by the veterinarian to outline a diagnostic and treatment plan for the patient.

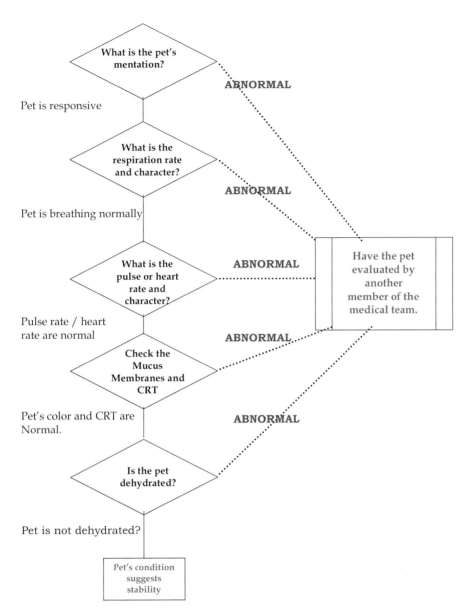

Figure 6.13. Algorithm of stability.

Table 6.1. You know you are in trouble based on physical exam when . . .

System Examined	Canine	Feline
Disposition	Nonresponsive	Nonresponsive
	Comatose	Comatose
	Lateral recumbent	Lateral recumbent
Breathing	Increased rate >45	Increased rate >45–60
	Abdominal breathing	Abdominal breathing
		Open mouth breathing (panting)
Pulses/heart beating	Increased rate >150	Increased rate >200
	Pulse quality:	Pulse quality:
	None	None
	Hyperdynamic	Hyperdynamic
	Weak	Weak
Gum color	White	White
	Purple/gray	Purple/gray
	Yellow	Yellow
Capillary refill time	CRT >2 seconds	CRT >2 seconds
Bruising	Any bruising should be monitored	Any bruising should be monitored
	Increased bruising	Increased bruising
Body temperature	Temp <98° or Temp >106°	Temp <98° or Temp >106°
Body confirmation	Bloated in abdomen	Bloated in abdomen
	Bloated in chest	Bloated in chest
	Shift-Sherrington	Shift-Sherrington

A pet is brought into your hospital. A team member completes the following triage exam.

- **Signalment**: A 40- to 50-pound black female, spayed Lab mix.
- **Subjective statement**: Dog is depressed.
- **Objective statements:**
  —Temperature: 98.7°
  —Pulse: 100 (weak)
  —Respiration: 80 (abdominal)
  —Mucus membrane: pale pink
  —CRT: >3 seconds
  —Hydration: severe

Based on this triage exam, this pet would need the immediate attention of the medical team and should be taken into a treatment area.

CD-ROM 1 reviews material presented in this chapter. Please try the cases for Section 1 (The First Two Days on the Job) to help reinforce the information presented here.

Section 2

Anatomy and Physiology—
The Science behind the Diseases

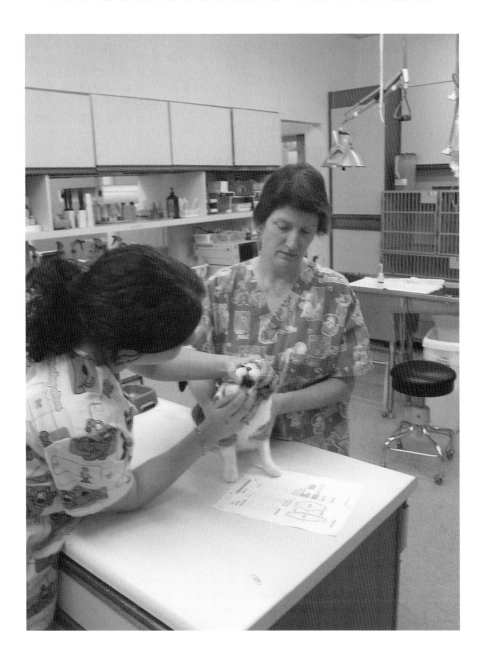

This section is an overview of the anatomical systems of the canine and feline. The goal of this section is to gain a practical understanding of the anatomy of each body system, be able to obtain a medical history from the client, look for key physical symptoms suggesting disease, understand the clinical diagnostics and diseases of each system, and be able to discuss these aspects with the client.

Chapter 7

Physical Exam

This chapter will focus on proper documentation and the full physical examination of the patient. It is a necessity that the technical team be able to document and perform a thorough physical examination. Even though the liability of the pet's health is the doctor's responsibility, the medical team must have members that can auscult, examine, and palpate hospitalized and ill pets to assist the doctor in determining the health and medical status of the animal.

SOAP Method

Documentation of the veterinary exam is achieved through the **SOAP method** (as discussed in Chapter 6). SOAP stands for

S: subjective,
O: objective,
A: assessment, and
P: plan.

Although the medical team does not typically have direct input in the assessment and plan stages of the SOAP, all team members should be aware of proper documentation styles so that they may accurately review a record to determine the health concerns of the pet and recommendations of the veterinarian.

As discussed previously, the beginning of each medical record should start with the **signalment** of the pet and the **chief complaint (cc)**. The signalment is the legal description of the pet's breed, weight, sex, hair color, species, and if the pet is altered. The chief complaint is the owner's primary concern, or why the pet is brought into the hospital. In many circumstances, the signalment itself can sometimes start the medical team preparing for the potential cases.

For example, the following might be entered in a medical record.

- **Signalment**: 3.5- month-old, 25-pound, male intact black and gold rotteweiler puppy
- **CC**: Vomiting and bloody diarrhea
- **Concern**: This could suggest an infectious disease (parvo), parasites, or other causes. Often the medical team will separate the pup into an isolation exam room to prevent possible contamination to the environment.

- **Signalment:** 1.5-year-old, male, 10-pound, black DSH cat
- **CC:** Constipation
- **Concern:** Often the owner will mistake a male tom's inability to urinate as an attempt to defecate. Blocked male cats are a life-threatening concern that should be evaluated by the medical team as soon as possible.

The subjective part of the SOAP is the evaluator's subjective opinion of the behavior or mentation of the pet and the physical disposition of the animal. Changes in the subjective evaluation of a hospitalized pet can sometimes suggest a significant change in the overall health of the animal.

For example, a pet is hospitalized for a general gastroenteritis or possible foreign body of the intestine; the pet is monitored by the medical team at 2 pm and is bright, alert, and responsive. At 6 pm the pet is reevaluated and shows signs of depression; this may be a red flag of a change in the pet's status.

Common descriptors for mentation are as follows.

- BAR: Bright, alert, and responsive
- QAR: Quiet, alert, and responsive
- Depressed
- Lethargic
- Obtund/comatose
- Aggressive
- Fearful
- Other: Seizuring, neurologic

Other common descriptors of physical body condition can be

- normal,
- thin,
- **emaciated** (the animal is skeletally thin), and
- obese.

The **objective** part of the SOAP is all of the veterinarian's or medical team's observations regarding the patient. This objective is split into two categories.

Tenets of Stability

These elements were covered in Chapter 6's discussion of the 30-second triage exam. These parameters allow the medical team member to assess stability. The brief overview of the parameters is discussed next.

Temperature

What is the pet's temperature?

> Normal temperature for canines/felines is 100–102.5° Fahrenheit.

Hypothermia, a temperature colder than normal, can be caused by environmental exposure, metabolic disease, or shock. **Fever** or **hyperthermia** can be secondary to infection, inflammation, or neoplasia (cancer).

Heat stroke, temperatures of >106°, can produce heat damage to the organs, central nervous system, and blood supply. It can occur secondary to

- extreme fever/infection,
- environmental exposure,
- prolonged seizure activity,
- toxins, and
- other causes.

Pulse

> Normal pulses (canine/feline) are 80–120 beats per minute.

Pulses are a reflection of cardiac output. There are times when there may be a strong heart rate but weak pulses.

Pulses should be monitored for both rate and quality. Slow heart rates are termed **bradycardia,** and rapid heart rates are termed **tachycardia**. Pulse weakness is indicated by those pulses that have decreased pressure and volume as compared with a normal pulse. A **hyperdynamic pulse** is one that is rapid and lifts your fingers off the artery with each pulse.

When ausculting the heart, for each heartbeat there should be a pulse. If there is not, this is called a **pulse deficit**. It can suggest abnormal contractions of the heart (premature ventricular contraction, or PVC) or shock.

A **paradoxical pulse** refers to a change in the pulse strength, from strong to weak, as the animal breaths in and out. This can suggest an accumulation of fluid around the heart (**pericardial effusion**) and can be a great concern.

Respiration

> Normal rate for the canine/feline is 20–50 breathes per minute.

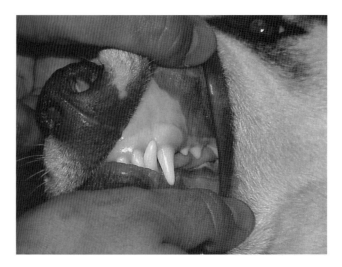

Figure 7.1.   Checking mucus membrane color.

Breathing rate should be monitored for slow respiratory rate, rapid respiratory rate (tachypnea), and breathing patterns: abdominal versus normal, open mouth versus normal, shallow.

Mucus Membrane (Gums)

- Normal gum color is light pink (see Figure 7.1).
- Abnormal gum color is white and suggests the following:
  — **Anemia:** Low red blood cell volume
  — **Dehydration:** Low blood fluid volume
  — **Bleeding:** Loss of both cells and fluid
  — **Pain**
  — **Hypotension:** Decreased peripheral blood pressure
- Red gum color suggests ingestion of toxin or hyperthermia.
- Yellow suggests
  — liver disease,
  — autoimmune disease, and
  — gall bladder obstruction.
- Purple to blue to gray suggests
  — cardiovascular disease,
  — respiratory disease, and
  — Tylenol intoxication (cats).

Bruising of the Gums

Spontaneous bruising of the gums can suggest problems with the body's ability to clot blood (**coagulopathy**). Any evidence of bruising should be reported to the medical team immediately because the pet may be beginning to bleed spontaneously.

Capillary Refill Time

Capillary refill time (CRT) is the amount of the time it takes for the gum color to return to normal when pressure is applied (see Figure 7.2).

> Normal CRT is less than 2 seconds.

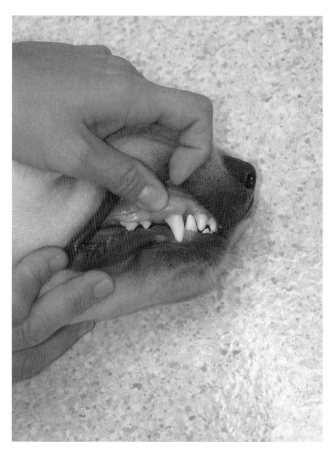

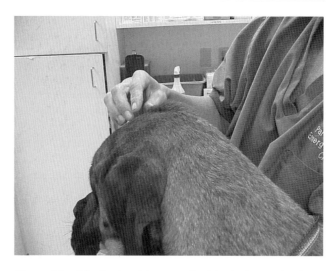

Figure 7.3. Monitoring skin turgor for dehydration can be done over the shoulder, on the forehead, or over the eyelid.

Figure 7.2. When evaluating CRT, caution should always be exercised with potentially aggressive or fearful patients.

Abnormality suggests an inability of the body to maintain normal blood flow to the tissue (**perfusion**) and to the smallest peripheral arterioles and venules, that is, blood is not moving adequately through the body.

Examples of disease that can affect the CRT are

- heart disease,
- shock,
- severe dehydration, and
- acute blood loss.

Remember that an animal must have normal gum color in order to assess the CRT properly.

Dehydration

In general, dehydration is a measurement of how severely a pet is fluid compromised (see Figure 7.3). Dehydration is never a normal finding.

Dehydration is measured qualitatively on the physical exam by a number of parameters.

- Skin turgor
- Gums
- Eyes

Measuring Dehydration

Overall, on physical examination, dehydration is measured as a percentage of the total dehydration of the animal. It is generally stated as a percentage from 0 to 12%.

- **0–5% dehydration—undetectable dehydration:** The animal may have significant losses of fluid (i.e., vomiting/diarrhea), but there are no physical symptoms at this level of dehydration.
- **5–7% dehydration—mild initial dehydration:** Physically, the patient will begin showing signs of dehydration.
  — Slowed skin turgor
  — Slightly dry gums
  — Eyes less glossy or sunken in
  — Normal mentation to mild depression
- **7–9% dehydration—moderate dehydration:** Physically, the patient is showing more severe physical signs of dehydration.
  — Significantly decreased skin turgor
  — Dry gums
  — Eyes less glossy and sunken in
  — Depressed
- **9–12% dehydration—life-threatening dehydration.** Physically, the patient will show severe symptoms that can also start to affect other body systems.
  — No skin turgor—the skin does not return to normal after tenting.
  — Severely dry gums.
  — Eyes are dull and sunken in, and third eyelids are elevated.
  — Animal is depressed and in sternal or lateral recumbency.
  — Heart rate can be variable from bradycardia to tachycardia.
  — Respiratory rate may be shallow and increased.

Systems

The next part of the objective SOAP is an evaluation of body systems by the medical team member. This requires the ability to palpate, auscult, and observe the patient system by system. It requires practice to develop the concept of what is normal for each body system and a systematic approach of how the physical is done. There is no correct step-by-step system of a proper physical exam. It is important that the team member perform the same process in every exam and not overlook a body system. The systems examined are as follows.

Cardiac System (Heart)

The best way to evaluate the cardiovascular system is by auscultation with a good stethoscope. The only way to become proficient in auscultation is to listen and practice on healthy animals. The overall goal is to identify what sound may be abnormal and then discuss those concerns with the doctor.

The steps for proper auscultation are as follows.

- Begin ausculting the heart where the left forelimb is attached to the chest, caudal to the left elbow (see Figure 7.4). This is typically the ventral third intercostal space.
- Move the stethoscope to the middle of the fourth intercostal space and again distally to the low fifth intercostal space. This will cover most of the valves of the heart.
- Repeat the same pattern on the right side of the heart.
- Then auscult the heart through the sternum.

Can You Hear the Heartbeat?

At this location a strong heart beat should be auscultable. If there is no sound, there may be a disease process present that

is obscuring the normal heart sounds. Pathology that can obscure the heart sounds are

- increased lung sounds,
- mass between the chest wall and the heart,
- mass in the lung fields (see Figure 7.5),
- mass in the chest cavity itself, and
- fluid in the chest, lungs, or pericardial cavities (see Figure 7.6)

Is There a Murmur?

A **murmur** is an alteration in the normal heart sounds from turbulent or abnormal flow of the blood through the valves, heart wall, or an abnormal blood vessel. Although a complete discussion of murmurs and cardiac pathology will be discussed in Chapter 12, it is important for the medical team to distinguish if there is a murmur present. With time and

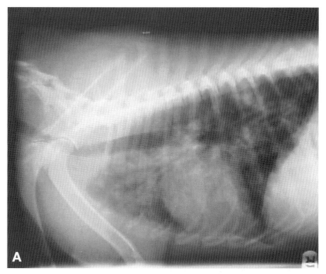

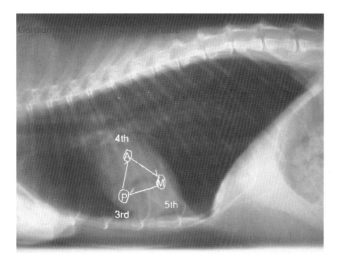

Figure 7.4. Image of how to auscult the left chest to appreciate the different valves. (P) = pulmonary, third lower intercostal space (left); (A)= aortic valve, fourth middle intercostal space (left); (M)= mitral valve, fifth ventral intercostal space. The tricuspid valve is on the lower third of the intercostal space on the right side of the pet.

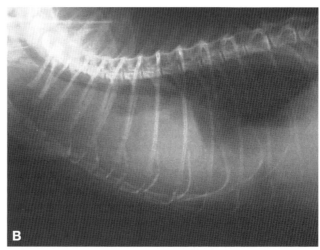

Figure 7.5. Diseases in the lungs, such as this fungal pneumonia, can produce severe lung sounds that may hide or diminish the normal cardiac sounds (a). Fluid within the chest, around the heart and lung (pleural effusion), can make the heart very hard to auscult (b).

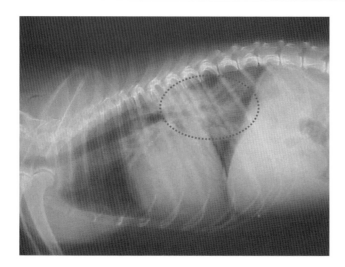

Figure 7.6. Fluid accumulation in the lungs from pneumonia, heart disease (pulmonary edema), or pulmonary injury (i.e., drowning) can produce crackles where the lung pathology exists.

experience, the team may be able to identify the location of the murmur and if the murmur is valvular or constant. Initially, it becomes important to distinguish if a murmur exists.

Are There Irregular Rhythms or a Pulse Deficit?

Lastly, and most importantly, does the rhythm seem abnormal, or does the rhythm not match the pulse? Any aberration in heart rate or pulse deficit should be brought to the attention of the veterinarian immediately.

Respiration

Appreciation of normal lung sounds comes with practice. The quiet movement of air through normal bronchi produces a slight perceivable sound of air movement. Abnormal lung sounds can sometimes aid in detection of the underlying primary disease process. Abnormal lung sounds are as follows.

- **Crackles:** The sound is best represented as the crumpling of cellophane paper. Here the normal airways and alveoli are filled with cells and fluid. The crackle sounds are produced as air passes through the cramped region (see Figure 7.6).
- **Rasps:** This sound is best represented as air flows through narrowed or constricted airways, which produces a musical whistle. Diseases that produce fibrosis or narrowing of the bronchi (e.g., feline asthma, allergic reaction, chronic obstructive pulmonary disease), produce the whistle.
- **Referred sound from the upper airway:** These sounds are produced from the trachea and the upper airway as a result of obstruction from debris, masses, or fluid. The sounds are heard with slightly decreased volume deeper in the chest. In some short-nosed breeds (pugs, English bulldogs, shar-peis) these sounds can be normal due to the narrowed, shortened airway.

Abdomen

When palpating the abdomen, a light, practiced, gentle touch to distinguish abnormality is important. Knowledge of the abdominal architecture is helpful; the overall evaluation should include the following points.

- **Abdominal Pain/abdominal tenderness**: With light palpation, if the pet begins to audibly groan, pushes the palpator's hands outward, or tenses so severely as to resist palpation, this suggests an acute abdomen. Although there are many causes of an acute abdomen (i.e., pancreatitis, intestinal foreign body, peritonitis), the evidence of abdominal pain and its severity should be noted.
- **Large, distended, painful bladder:** With light palpation, a large, distended bladder in the caudal abdomen can be detected with practice. Heavy palpation has been noted to rupture a bladder, but careful, light hands can easily detect a full, painful bladder as seen with blocked male cats, and male and female dogs.
- **Fluid in the abdomen**: With practice, a team member can detect large amounts of fluid in the abdomen. The team member can gently place their hand on one side of the dilated abdomen and gently apply an on again/off again pressure. This force will produce a wave that can be perceived by the other hand. This feeling of fluid rushing toward the other side of the abdomen is called a **fluid wave**. It suggests the evidence of blood, urine, or other fluids building up.

Musculoskeletal System

When doing an initial assessment of the musculoskeletal system, the team member is basically evaluating and documenting whether the pet seems to be **favoring** (not using) the limb, or if there is a section of the limb that has swelling, pain, or heat evident. Light palpation and pressure of the limb can sometimes be applied to evaluate pain, but caution should be used because animals can react aggressively to pain. Simply documenting the limb affected and the possible location of the physical pain or swelling is sufficient (see Figure 7.7).

Neurologic System

With the neurologic system, the focus of the evaluation is the neurologic status of the animal and the ability of the animal to stand and bear weight. Neurologic status of the animal reflects any physical symptoms that may suggest the animal's central nervous system is affected. Some possible symptoms follow.

- **Seizuring**: Animal comes in with petite to grand mal seizures. The pet can be unaware of its surroundings and be lateral recumbent, having its head extended and front legs rigid (**opisthotonus**), and losing its urine and evacuating its bowels (see Figure 7.8).
- **Depression/coma/decreased pain perception**: Animals that have suffered a severe trauma or have severe meta-

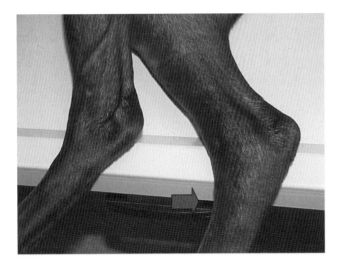

Figure 7.7. Observing the physical swelling at and distal to the hock is sufficient for the initial documentation of the patient's musculoskeletal system.

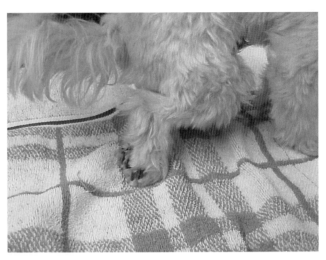

Figure 7.9. The patient does not know where his limbs are in space, so it cannot place its paws properly and cannot stand due to lack of proper innervation to the muscle groups.

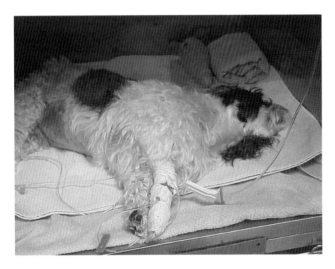

Figure 7.8. Dogs can present in constant seizures (status epilepticus) suggesting central nervous system or metabolic disease.

bolic disease can have a lack of normal neurologic response or stimulus. After a trauma event (i.e., hit by car, fall, animal attack), the lack of response does not always suggest permanent damage but may be secondary to shock or injury.

- **Inability to perceive normal position of limbs or bear weight on leg:** If there has been a spinal cord injury or peripheral nerve injury, the pet may lose the ability to bear weight or sense pain and/or position of the limb. In pets with neurologic disease, the limbs are relaxed (**flaccid**), and the pet cannot properly place them or stand normally on the limb. This is usually due to injury of the peripheral nerve of the leg, with the result that the body does not know where the limb is in space (see Figure 7.9).

Eyes/Ears/Nose/Mouth

Assessing for abnormalities in eyes, ears, nose, and mouth E-E-N-M) systems can vary tremendously depending on the diseases affecting the animals. It is important to have an idea of what the normal anatomy and physiology looks like, so abnormality and its cause can be assessed thoroughly.

Eyes

Normally, the eyes are shiny and responsive. The white of the eyes (sclera) are white with small blood vessels evident. The pupils are equal sized and responsive to light, and the cornea is clear. Changes to normal coloration of the eye can suggest systemic or ocular disease. Some noted changes can be as follows.

- **Bruising:** Spontaneous bruising or hemorrhage of the eye can suggest a severe local trauma or a systemic problem, such as clotting blood. Any spontaneous hemorrhage should be documented and reported immediately.
- **Jaundice:** A yellow tinge or color to the whites of the eyes can suggest liver or blood disorders where there is increased level of body toxins building up.
- **Anemia (lack of color):** When the animal has a low red blood cell count, the normal small vessels usually visible on the sclera disappear as the body shuts down smaller peripheral capillaries.
- **Red/swollen/irritated eye:** Red, irritated, swollen sclera can suggest specific diseases of the eyes (see Figure 7.10; see also Chapter 20).

Changes in the cornea, pupil, and internal architecture of the eye can also suggest central nervous system, ocular, or systemic disease.

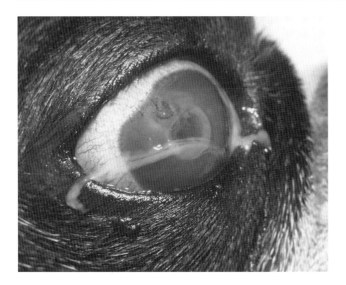

Figure 7.10. Changes in the sclera and cornea of this eye suggest severe corneal disease.

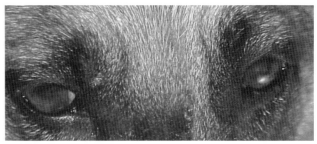

Figure 7.11. Pupils with different iris sizes (anisicoria) can suggest a concussion or CNS damage, especially after a severe trauma. Pupils should be regularly evaluated when assessing and monitoring traumas.

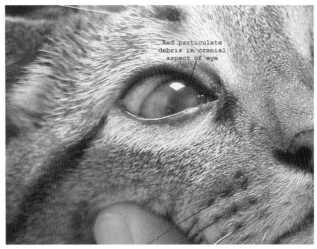

Figure 7.12. Blood in the eyes can suggest a serious possible life-threatening condition for the pet.

- **Is there squinting, excessive blinking, increased tearing or sensitivity to light**? Painful eyes can show increased sensitivity to bright light, increased tearing, squinting, and holding the eye closed.
- **Are the pupils fixed, abnormal, or an uneven size (anisicoria)?** Abnormalities can suggest central nervous system disease, concussion, or ocular damage. Pupils should be checked regularly after any life-threatening trauma for symmetry (see Figure 7.11).
- **Is there a normal pupillary light response?** The eye responds to the amount of light present in the environment (see Chapter 20). The light level is analyzed and the iris of the eye is opened or closed by a reflex pathway of the optic nerve. If there is low light or darkness, the iris opens up, increasing the amount of light coming in. If the environment is bright, the iris constricts, decreasing the level of light reaching the retina. This is called the **pupillary light response (PLR)**. Both irises will respond to a bright light perceived by one iris. If a light shines into one iris and it constricts, we call this a **direct PLR**. If a light shines into one iris and the opposite pupil constricts as well, it is called an **indirect PLR**. If a direct or indirect PLR is absent in a pet, it can suggest disease of the eye, optic nerve, or a part of the central nervous system.
- **Rapid irregular eye movements:** Rapid irregular eye movements from side to side, up and down, or in a circular motion (**nystagmus**) can suggest a balance problem caused by an ear infection or central nervous system disease. The eyes are moving rapidly from side to side because the body is having a hard time establishing normal balance.
- **Blood inside the eye**: The presence of blood inside the eye (**hyphema**) can suggest trauma or an inability of the pet to clot blood normally (see Figure 7.12).

Ears
Generally, the ear canal and ear flap (**pinna**) should be light pink and free of discharge. Changes in the ear itself can suggest local infection or inflammation. The pinna should also be monitored for changes suggestive of whole body disease.

In the ear canal, debris, swelling, and odor can suggest mild to severe infections. Serious inner ear infections can also produce balance and coordination problems for the pet (see Figure 7.13).

Just as with the sclera of the eye, the pinna can suggest systemic disease by changes in its appearance. Bruising in the ear pinna suggests an inability of the blood to clot normally and could indicate a serious, possibly life-threatening, disease. Icteric or jaundiced pinna, a yellow tinge or coloration to the ear flap, can suggest liver or blood disorders in the pet (see Figure 7.14).

Nose
Changes in discharge in the nose can suggest local or systemic respiratory diseases. When nasal discharge is en-

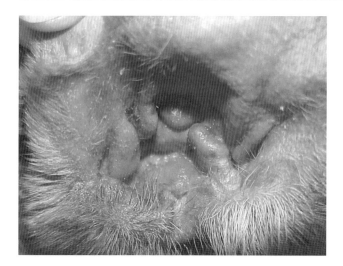

Figure 7.13. A red, swollen ear can suggest a serious ear problem.

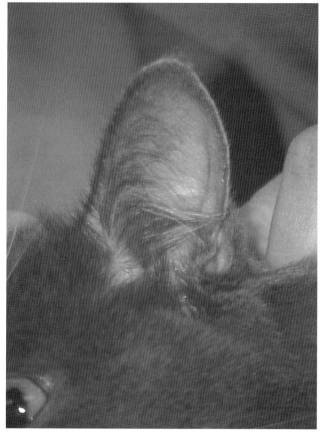

Figure 7.14. Check the ear flap for yellow pigmentation. It may be the first hint that there is a serious disease in the pet.

countered, several points should be evaluated and documented.

The team member should note if the discharge is coming from one or both nostrils (unilateral or bilateral discharge). A unilateral discharge usually suggests disease localized to that nostril from infection, a foreign body, mass, or trauma.

A bilateral discharge usually suggests that a systemic or respiratory disease process is occurring. Especially with purulent debris, the material will come up from the lungs and fill both nostrils.

Discharge can consist of blood or pus. Unilateral blood can suggest bleeding from a trauma, a mass, or a foreign body. Bilateral bleeding can suggest a problem with the body's ability to clot blood. Purulence (pus) found in a unilateral discharge suggests a localized upper respiratory infection, tooth root abscess, or reaction to a foreign body or mass (see Figure 7.15). Bilateral discharge suggests purulence and infection evident from the lower respiratory tract and the lungs.

Mouth

The mouth refers to the gums, teeth, and oral cavity. The mucus membrane color and CRT should have already been assessed. The team member should be evaluating the mouth for changes that are suggestive of disease.

- **Is there halitosis?** Although bad breath can simply be linked with diet and dietary indiscretions, severe halitosis can suggest underlying disease, especially if the halitosis comes on acutely in a sick pet. Such disease states could include
  — kidney disease,
  — liver disease,
  — severe diabetes (ketoacidotic diabetic),
  — severe periodontal disease,
  — tooth root abscess,

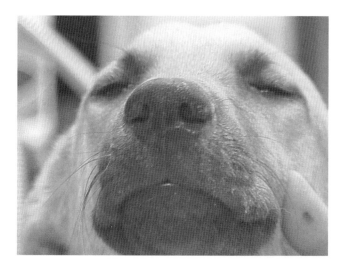

Figure 7.15. Unilateral nasal discharge can suggest localized infection, foreign body, or mass.

  — oral tumor, and
  — oral foreign body.
- **Are there lacerations or ulcers of the gums?** Ulcerations of the gums can sometimes suggest acute severe

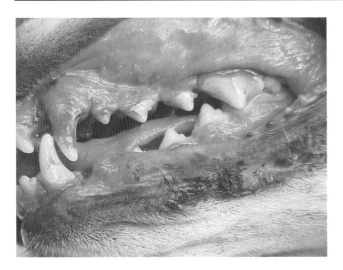

Figure 7.16. Severe dental disease can set up other serious diseases of the older pet, such as liver, kidney, or heart disease.

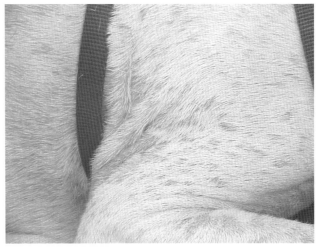

Figure 7.17. These localized regions of hair loss in this animal suggest a primary mite infection (demodex).

disease where toxins are building up so quickly within the body, they are burning the skin lining inside the mouth lateral to the teeth (**buccal mucosa**). Diseases such as acute renal and liver disease or antifreeze intoxication can produce acute ulcers. Some upper respiratory virus (i.e., **calici virus**) can also produce marked ulceration of the gums and tongue.

- **Is there dental disease?:** Dental disease can suggest a primary disease of middle-aged to older animals, and if not monitored and treated, chronically infected teeth and gums could produce severe secondary disease (see Figure 7.16; see also Chapter 9).

Lymph Nodes

The lymph nodes of the body are part of the immune system of the animal. They produce white blood cells and filter the white blood cell system and lymph systems for infection or debris. There are numerous locations of lymph nodes throughout the body. They enlarge secondary to infection or cancer. Common locations are

- submandibular,
- popliteal,
- inguinal,
- prescapulary, and
- axillary.

Skin (Integument)

The skin is a great reflection of the overall health of the pet. Subtle chronic diseases may first manifest themselves with physical changes to the hair coat. A thick, normal, healthy, shiny hair coat that begins to thin or look unkempt may suggest the pet is beginning to suffer from a chronic disease, nutritional deficiency, hormonal disease, or primary skin problem (i.e., allergies, ringworm, skin mites, etc.) There are changes that should be monitored and documented.

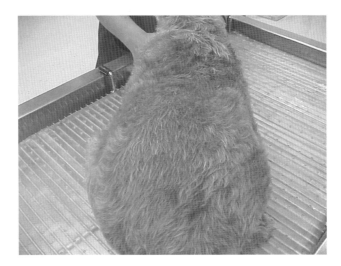

Figure 7.18. Chronic symmetrical hair loss, thin fragile skin, and increased pigmentation can suggest underlying systemic disease.

- **Is there hair loss?** Hair loss can suggest either primary skin disease or be secondary to an underlying chronic disease (see Figure 7.17). Localized asymmetrical hair loss can suggest primary skin disease (i.e., ringworm, **mange** [skin mites], allergies). Symmetrical hair loss over the entire body or over the flank could suggest a chronic systemic or hormonal disease. Also, increased pigmentation of the skin, fragile thin skin, or even chronically infected skin can suggest an underlying systemic disease (see Figure 7.18).
- **Is the skin red and inflamed?** Red and inflamed skin usually suggests localized infection or allergies. However, it is important for the team member to note the location and extent of the inflammation because this can sometimes suggest systemic allergic reaction, insect bite

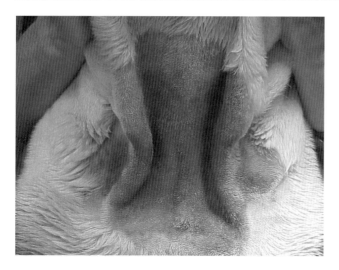

Figure 7.19. Red inflamed areas can be secondary to allergies (hot spots), infections, bites, or stings, or even chemical or physical burns.

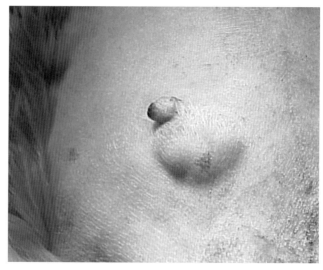

Figure 7.20. Nodules and masses within the mammary chain can suggest a serious possible malignancy.

or sting, snake bite, and other localized trauma (see Figure 7.19).

- **Is there severe itchiness?** Severe itchiness (**pruritus**) is usually linked to primary skin disease caused by allergies, infection, or inflammation.

Genitourinary Systems

The genitourinary system refers to the reproductive and urinary system of the body. Although more attention will be focused on these systems in Chapter 18, a team member should note any changes in the following reproductive organs.

In the female, the mammary chain should be monitored for irregularities and abnormalities. The following changes should be monitored and documented.

- **Masses or tumors in the mammary tract:** Potential masses of the mammary tract can suggest serious malignancy in spayed and intact females (see Figure 7.20).
- **Generalized swelling, heat, and pain:** Focal or generalized swelling and pain in an intact, usually lactating female can suggest infection or inflammation within the mammary chain (see Figure 7.21).

The vulva should be checked for the following.

- **Discharge:** Bloody and purulent (pus) discharges can suggest infection or a mass and is evident within the reproductive tract or bladder.
- **Mass:** There are some vaginal/vulva masses that can be evident and extend outside the vulva.

In the male, both the penis and testicles should be monitored and documented for abnormalities.

- **Testicles:** Testicles should be lightly palpated for normal size and shape. Any difference in one testicle in compar-

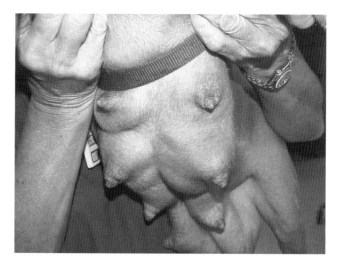

Figure 7.21. Generalized swelling of the mammary chain can suggest a massive infection or inflammation.

ison with the other should be documented as well (see Figure 7.22).
- **Penis:** Abnormal swelling or discoloration of the penis could suggest entrapment or injury. Any purulent or bloody discharge should be documented as well because it can suggest a urinary or prostatic disease (see Figure 7.23).

Assessment

The assessment is performed by the veterinarian and lists the overall medical concerns that are challenging the animal. The assessment of problems should be directly linked to the observations noted on the physical exam. See the following example.

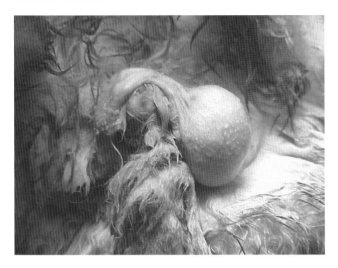

Figure 7.22. Abnormal testicular size and shape could suggest a testicular tumor or infectious disease; in this image note one enlarged testicle and one small or **atrophied** testicle.

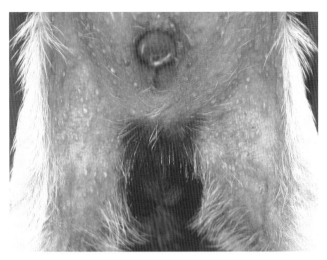

Figure 7.24. Image of severe pustular rash on inguinal canal of male dog.

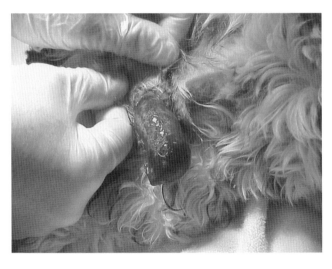

Figure 7.23. Entrapment of the penis in the young dog can be severely painful and damaging to the animal.

- **Objective—INT**: Severe rash and pustules on inguinal region and abdomen (see Figure 7.24).
- **Assessment—skin**:
  —Bacterial infection
  —Mites (demodex, sarcoptes)
  —Fungal infection (i.e., ringworm)

Plan

The plan is produced by the veterinarian and lists the diagnostic and treatment plans that are recommended by the doctor. For example, with the case above, the doctor may recommend the following.

- Skin scrape
- Fungal culture
- Antibiotic trial

Prognosis

The prognosis is also completed by the veterinarian and outlines the overall prognosis for the pet given the information available. Common descriptors for the prognosis are

- excellent,
- good,
- fair,
- poor,
- guarded, and
- grave.

Documentation of the Physical Exam

Although the responsibility of the physical examination is the veterinarian's, the technical team should be able to perform and document a cursory full physical exam. All hospitalized animals should have a full physical examination done at least one to two times per 24-hour period to reassess the animal's hydration, weight, overall health, and/or changes from initial physical presentation. Furthermore, with critical care patients, a brief triage exam should be conducted and documented every 3–4 hours minimum. Parameters that should be assessed are

- temperature,
- pulse,
- respiration,
- hydration,
- capillary refill time,

- mucus membranes,
- mentation,
- fluid input/urinary output,
- food intake,
- fecal output, and
- fluid loses (vomiting/diarrhea).

Example of SOAP

Signalment: A 40–50 pound, black, female, spayed Lab mix (see Figure 7.25).

- CC: Owners found dog down and suddenly weak.
- S (subjective): Dog is depressed to obtund.
- O (objective): Tenets of stability.
  - Temperature: 98.7°.
  - Pulse: 80 (weak)
  - Resp: 80 (abdominal)
  - MM: pale pink
  - CRT >3 seconds
  - Hydration: severely dehydrated

System

- Cardiovascular (CV): Bradycardia ± mild murmur, unsure of where murmur is loudest.
- Respiration (Resp): Increased lung sounds ± crackles in upper airway.
- Musculoskeletal (MS): Within normal limits (WNL)
- Neurologic (Neuro): Dog is depressed
- Lymph node (LN): Increased popliteal lymph node
- Abdomen (Abd): Pain on abdominal palpation.
- Eyes, Ears, Nose, and Throat (E-E-N-T): WNL
- Genitourinary (Genit): WNL

Assessment (done by the veterinarian)

- Congestive heart disease
- Pneumonia
- Cancer (neoplasia)

Plan (done by the veterinarian)

Recommend IV fluids, complete blood work, x-ray, urinalysis. Depending on outcome, hospitalization and fluid care may be required.

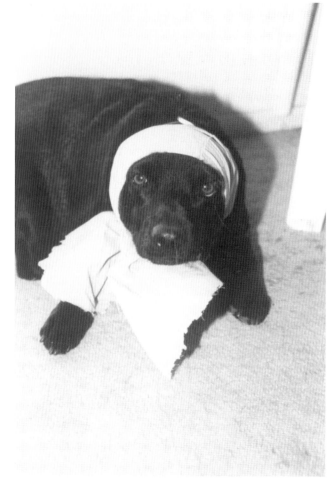

Figure 7.25. Signalment of the patient.

CD-ROM 1 reviews material presented in this chapter. Please try the cases for Section 2 (Anatomy and Physiology—The Science behind the Diseases) to help reinforce the information presented here.

Chapter 8

Skeletal System

Bone is a living, constantly changing organ that supplies stability, flexibility, and movement to the animal. Bone is composed of rapidly changing, actively metabolizing tissue that may be altered in size, shape, and position by mechanical and biochemical demands. It responds in a variety of ways to vitamin, mineral, and hormone deficiencies and excesses. The inner aspect of the bone, the **bone marrow**, is a location of blood precursor cells responsible for the production of much of the body's red and white blood cells and platelets. Without a careful understanding of bone and cartilage, common serious and potentially life-threatening disease could not be diagnosed and treated. Overall, bone functions to

- support and protect the body and its organs,
- act as a protective outer defense for internal organs,
- work as a lever for muscular action,
- serve as a storehouse for minerals, and
- be a site for blood cell formation.

Classification of Skeletal Elements

Bone is classified according to shape and size. There are five basic divisions.

Short Bones
These bones are confined to the carpus (wrist) and the tarsus (ankle). Each joint contains seven short bones. The bones have variable size and shape. Their surfaces can either be interlinked with a joint where bone is on bone (**articular**) or not associated with a joint (**nonarticular**). The bone surfaces provide locations for placement of ligaments, arteries, and veins (see Figure 8.1).

Sesamoids
These small bones formed in muscle tendons function to protect tendons at the points of greatest friction. They increase the ability of the tendons to pull and move. The sesamoid tends to be articular, with its surface in contact with the bone (see Figure 8.2).

Flat Bones
Typically, flat bones are found in the limb girdles (pelvis) to serve as muscular attachments. Also, flat bones are present in the head where they surround and protect the sense organs and the brain (see Figure 8.3).

Irregular Bones
Irregular bones are commonly found in the spinal column, making up the bone of the vertebral body (see Figure 8.4).

Long Bones
The long bones (e.g., femur, radius, or ulna) are generally used to provide movement and stability (bone shaft), as well as red, white, and platelet cell precursors (bone marrow). The anatomy of a long bone has very similar architecture (see Figure 8.5).

Epiphysis (Growth Plate)
In young animals, the epiphysis is an active area of bone growth where soft spongy bone (**cancellous bone**) is produced. There can be multiple growth plates in a bone. They are usually only visible in young, growing animals (see Figure 8.6).

Metaphysis
The metaphysis is the area of primary (**trabecular**) soft bone located on the farthest ends of the bone. This area of bone flares out to increase the articular surface of the joint, providing a larger surface area to more evenly balance weight distribution.

Diaphysis
Diaphysis is the area of dense **cortical bone** in the middle of the bone shaft, also called the bone shaft. The thickened strong bone is used for support of the axial skeleton.

Medullary Canal
The medullary canal lies inside the column of bone. This is where the blood precursor cells (red blood cells, white blood cells, and platelets) develop in the bone marrow.

Perisoteum
The perisoteum is a thick, connective tissue membrane covering the bone. It is responsible for protection and nutrition of the bone.

Joints
Joints are the intersections of bones or other articulations that serve to unite the bones firmly or allow free movement. The first category of joints is the **fibrous joint (synartho-**

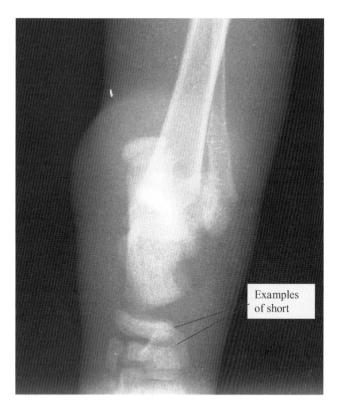

Figure 8.1. Bones in the wrist (carpus) and in the ankle (tarsus) are examples of short bones. This is a radiograph of the hock.

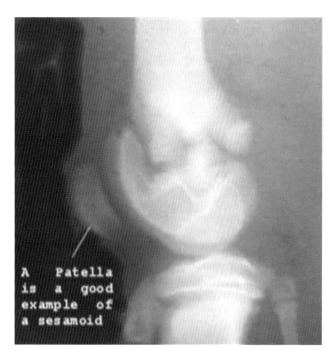

Figure 8.2. The most common sesamoid is the patella.

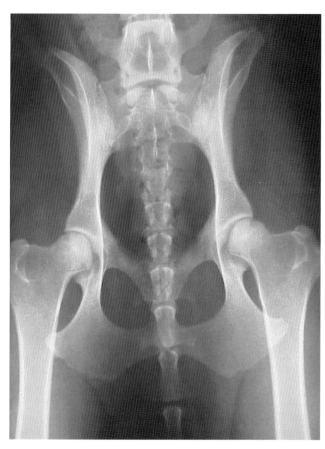

Figure 8.3. Flat bones are located in the pelvis and head for protection and attachment of ligaments and tendons.

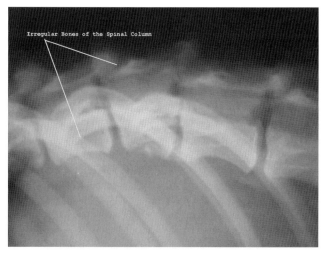

Figure 8.4. Image of irregular bones that make up the vertebral column. These bones grow around and protect the spinal cord and spinal nerves.

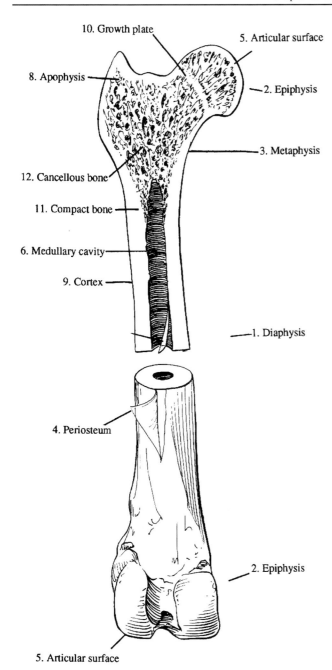

Figure 8.5. Illustration of long bone. (Courtesy of *Anatomy of Domestic Animals*, 7th Edition. Pasquini, Chris, and Pasquini, Susan. Sudz Publishing, Pilot Point, Tx 1989. Used with permission from Sudz Publishing.)

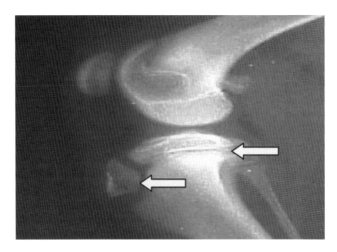

Figure 8.6. Image of a young proximal tibia (distal to the stifle). The radiolucent lines within the long bones show the growth plate. These areas will calcify as the animal ages.

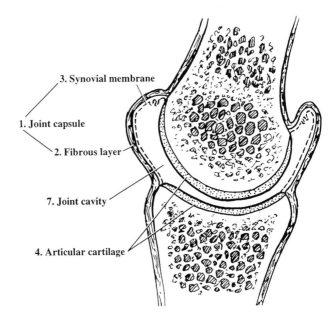

Figure 8.7. Example of a synovial joint—the stifle. (Courtesy of *Anatomy of Domestic Animals*, 7th Edition. Pasquini, Chris, and Pasquini, Susan. Sudz Publishing, Pilot Point, Tx 1989. Used with permission from Sudz Publishing.)

sis); these bones are connected by dense connective tissue. These mostly occur in the skull, also called **sutures.** Sutures allow the developing skull to grow as the animal ages.

The second type of joints are **cartilaginous joints;** these are bones connected by dense cartilage. These types of joints are called **synchondrosis;** this includes the joints formed between the epiphysis and diaphysis of young animal long bones.

The most common form of the joint is the **synovial joints**

(diarthrosis). These joints are freely movable and are united by a fluid-filled cavity (see Figure 8.7). The joint consists of the following.

Joint Capsule and Joint Cavity
The joint capsule is a thick connective band of fibrous tissue that surrounds the joint and keeps the bone aligned. The joint capsule is innervated. The area within the joint capsule filled with the lubricating synovial fluid is the joint cavity.

Articular Surface

The articular surface refers to the region within the joints where bones contact and move with other bones. These bony regions are covered with articular cartilage, typically hyaline cartilage. This tissue conforms to the underlying bone to help cushion and support the joint. The articular cartilage has variable thickness depending upon the location within the joint. The cartilage has no vascular or nerve supply.

Synovial Membrane

The synovial membrane is the thin layer of connective tissue that stretches out over the entire articular surface (where bone interdigitates with bone). The overlying joint capsule strengthens the membrane that serves to produce the **synovial fluid**. The synovial fluid helps to lubricate and aid in the nutrition of the joint. When the joint is inflamed from injury or disease, the joint capsule begins to swell outward as joint fluid production increases secondary to inflammation. The presence of these swollen palpable regions, called a **joint effusion,** helps to diagnose joint inflammation.

Menisci or Discs

The menisci structures are formed from hyaline cartilage, fibrocartilage, and fibrous tissue. They sit within the joint surface to add stability and shock absorption to the joint.

Ligaments

Thick cartilaginous ligaments help maintain normal movement of bones within the joint as the limb moves. A good example of this type of structure is the **cranial (anterior) cruciate ligament**. This ligament attaches to the femur and the tibia to prevent abnormal movement (cranial or medial) as the joint moves (see Figure 8.8).

Nomenclature of the Fracture

When discussing and documenting a fracture with the medical team, there are a number of factors that must be considered.

- Name of bone or joint affected (Figure 8.9 shows the skeleton of the dog and outlines the nomenclature for each bony structure of the skeleton.)
- The location of the fracture on the bone
- The type of fracture
- If the fracture is communicative with the outside of the skin
- How many bone fragments occur with the fracture.

Location of the Fracture in the Bone

The location of the fracture in the bone helps the veterinarian evaluate the type of fracture and the type of fixation that may be needed. The location of the fracture could be

- diaphyseal,
- metaphyseal, or
- epiphyseal.

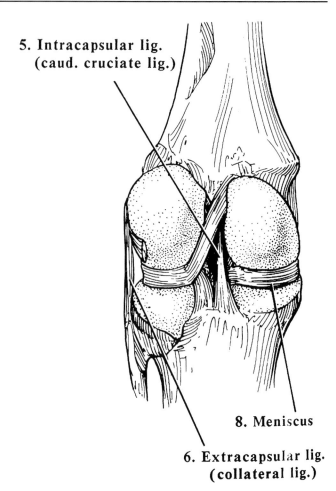

5. Intracapsular lig. (caud. cruciate lig.)

8. Meniscus

6. Extracapsular lig. (collateral lig.)

Figure 8.8. The anterior cruciate ligament (cranial) helps prevent forward or medial movement of the femur on the tibia. If the ligament is ruptured, the pet is unable to stand, and if the patient bears weight, the movement of the femur on the tibia causes pain and joint swelling. (Courtesy of *Anatomy of Domestic Animals,* 7th Edition. Pasquini, Chris, and Pasquini, Susan. Sudz Publishing, Pilot Point, Tx 1989. Used with permission from Sudz Publishing.)

Furthermore, the fracture can also be categorized as a proximal or distal fracture depending on its position within the bone.

Type of Fracture

The type of fracture refers to how the bone is broken and can suggest to the medical team the level of fixation needed. The types of fracture are discussed below.

- **Greenstick fracture:** A greenstick fracture is generally a mild fracture of one side of the bone column, but it is not a complete fracture of the bone. These fractures are not severe and can generally be repaired with simple fixation (i.e., cast/splint; see Figure 8.10).
- **Transverse fracture:** A transverse fracture is a complete fracture of the bone straight across the bone column (see Figure 8.11).

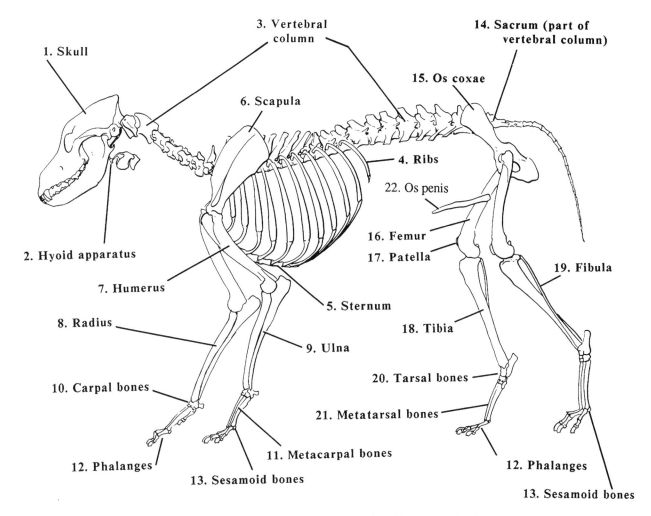

1. Skull
3. Vertebral column
14. Sacrum (part of vertebral column)
15. Os coxae
6. Scapula
4. Ribs
22. Os penis
2. Hyoid apparatus
16. Femur
17. Patella
19. Fibula
7. Humerus
5. Sternum
18. Tibia
8. Radius
9. Ulna
20. Tarsal bones
10. Carpal bones
21. Metatarsal bones
11. Metacarpal bones
12. Phalanges
13. Sesamoid bones
12. Phalanges
13. Sesamoid bones

Figure 8.9. Canine skeleton. (Courtesy of *Anatomy of Domestic Animals,* 7th Edition. Pasquini, Chris, and Pasquini, Susan. Sudz Publishing, Pilot Point, Tx 1989. Used with permission from Sudz Publishing.)

- **Oblique fracture:** In this injury, the fracture line is diagonal to the column of the bone (see Figure 8.12).
- **Spiral fractures:** Spiral fractures are complete fractures of the bone where the fracture line curves around the bone column, cutting the column at different locations and producing a spiral staircaselike lesion (see Figure 8.13).
- **Joint dislocations (luxation):** In articular joints, a dislocation pushes the bone off the articular surface of the other bone, preventing normal movement of the joint and producing swelling and pain (see Figure 8.14).

Exposure to the Outside
In open fractures, the bone has punctured through the skin and is exposed to the outside. It has an increased chance of infection. Open fractures may require increased care and long-term medications.

A closed fracture has no communication with the environment.

Number of Bone Fragments Involved
Simple fractures usually contain two bone fragments (see Figure 8.15). Comminuted fractures contain multiple bone fragments, usually suggestive of severe traumatic injury (i.e., gunshot wound, hit by a car). These types of fractures generally require major orthopedic fixation (see Figure 8.16).

Obtaining a History in Orthopedic Cases

It is very important to take a thorough history of when and how the orthopedic concern occurred and if any other body systems are affected. Some factors to consider are discussed next.

The Signalment
Although fractures and general orthopedic disease can be seen in both young and older dogs and cats, there are some specific conditions to consider, depending on the age of the animal, the species, and in some cases the breed.

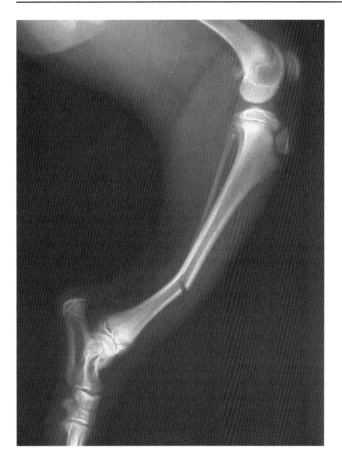

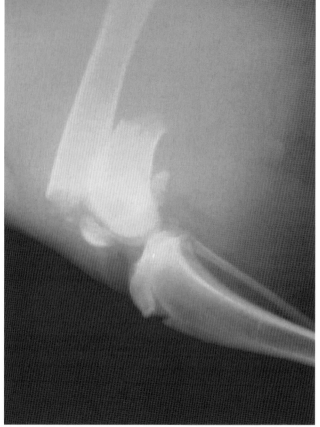

Figure 8.10. A greenstick fracture is a fracture of one the side of the bone column. This fracture is a greenstick midshaft diaphyseal fracture.

Figure 8.11. Transverse fracture of the distal femur. This is a distal diaphyseal or epiphyseal fracture of the distal femur.

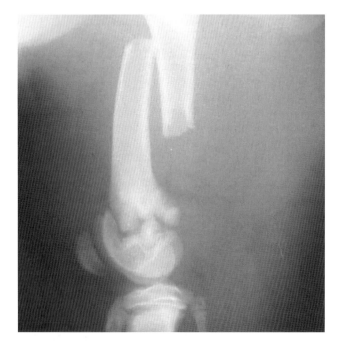

Figure 8.12. This radiograph reveals an oblique mid-diaphyseal fracture of the femur.

In general, cats do not have specific orthopedic diseases. Their injuries are generally secondary to trauma or injury.

In general small breed dogs tend to have more problems with their stifle, having both possibilities of cruciate ligament injury and luxating patella.

Young dogs may have congenital patellar disease, and middle age to older dogs may have cranial cruciate injuries in which the ligament within the stifle ruptures (see below).

Large Breed Dogs

Larger breed dogs tend to have hip and elbow injuries and disease as well as long bone disease.

Young Animals

There are some problems specific to young animals.

- **Hip/elbow dysplasia:** Congenital misalignment of the hip and elbow joints potentially produce an arthritic joint (see below).
- **Panosteitis:** An inflammation of the medullary canal in the long bones in rapidly growing large to giant dog breeds (see below).

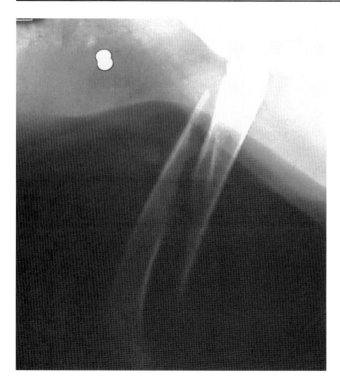

Figure 8.13. Spiral fractures produce sharp, pointed fractures of the bone. This is a spiral mid-diaphyseal fracture of the humerus.

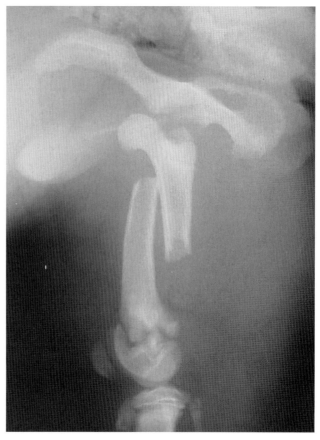

Figure 8.15. Image shows a simple, closed, transverse mid-diaphyseal fracture of the femur and a femoral head dislocation.

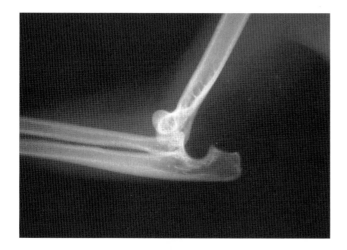

Figure 8.14. This radiograph shows a dislocation of the elbow.

- **Osteochondritis dissecans**: A disease of improper cartilage formation within specific joints (see below).
- **Epiphysitis:** An inflammation of the growth plate in young, rapidly growing large to giant breed canines.

Middle-Aged to Geriatric Animals
There are some problems specific to older animals.

- Arthritis
- Anterior cruciate injury/rupture
- Neoplasia

History Questions

Although a full history should always be discussed (see Chapter 5), the following questions should be documented:

- **What was the onset of disease?** Acute lameness can suggest sudden injury or trauma. Some examples are
  — fracture,
  — anterior cruciate rupture,
  — torn toe nail,
  — soft tissue injury,
  — sting/bite, and
  — pad injury.
- Is this a chronic progressive lameness?: Chronic lameness can suggest a slow progressive infectious or inflammatory disease.
  — Infectious disease: coccidiomycosis (a chronic fungal infection), Lyme disease
  — Arthritis
  — Tumor
- **Is the pet three-legged lame?** Non-weight-bearing limbs can suggest serious injury, such as fractures or tendon/ligament injury.

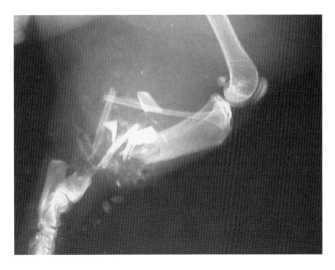

Figure 8.16. Image of a severely comminuted fracture of the tibia/fibula.

- **Does animal warm out of lameness or get worse with exercise?**
  — If an animal can warm out of lameness, it suggests a chronic or mechanical injury that begins sore and gets better as the pet warms up.
  — If animals become lame with exercise, it suggests a serious, painful injury that may also be reinjuring itself with activity.
- **What is the pet's level of activity?**
  — Very active and exercising pet can suggest athletic injury
  — More sedentary animals with an injury can suggest injury due to chronic infectious, inflammatory, or **neoplastic** (cancerous) disease.
- **Are other limbs affected?** When other limbs are affected with a constant or waxing and waning lameness, this can suggest systemic inflammatory, infectious, or immune-mediated disease. An immune-mediated disease is one in which the body's white blood cells attack a specific region or tissue of the patient as if it is foreign bacteria. In this case, the patient's immune system attacks the joints, producing pain, swelling, and lameness (i.e., **rheumatoid arthritis**). Some other disease examples are
  — panosteitis
  — infectious diseases: coccidiomycosis, Lyme disease, etc.
- **Is there a previous history of the disease to that limb?** Previous fracture or injury can sometimes set up chronic arthritis or injury in later life.
- **Has the animal been given anti-inflammatory medication and has it been effective?**
  — Many pets may have already been on anti-inflammatory medication and the lameness may still be present.
  — If an animal responds to anti-inflammatory medication, it can suggest a soft tissue injury or chronic inflammatory disease.

- **Is there any history of travel?** Some animals who travel to specific geographic regions could contract systemic disease, which can produce signs of lameness and bone pain weeks to months after travel. Some examples of such disease are
  — New England/Midwest: Lyme disease, and
  — Southwest: Coccidiomycosis
- **Are there any signs of systemic disease?** There are systemic diseases that can produce secondary bone pain and lameness. Specific signs of systemic disease are coughing, sneezing, vomiting, diarrhea.

Initial Assessment

The assessment of the musculoskeletal system is based on observation and palpation of the pet. The goal of the physical examination is to locate and appreciate the severity and location of the lameness. However, some injured animals may not show signs of lameness while in the office. Nervous animals can withhold any evidence of pain in the office if the cause of the lameness is not too severe. This is a beneficial test in itself. If the lameness is not apparent in the room, it may be a subtle or mild lameness. Furthermore, it is important to be mindful of the pet's pain sensitivity. It is important to make sure the pet is as pain free as possible while in the exam room.

- Make sure the pet can stand on a good traction surface while waiting in the exam room.
- If the pet is unable to stand, help the pet to lie down comfortably on soft bedding with good traction.

When initially assessing the animal and obtaining the medical history, simply **observe the pet as it moves or is brought into the exam room,** and document the following:

- Is the pet toe touching, unable to move the limb or limbs, or is the pet non-weight bearing? (See Figure 8.17.)
- Is the pet rotating the limb unusually inward or outward, or does the limb have an abnormal configuration? (See Figure 8.18.)
- Does any part of the limb appear swollen? And if so, at which joint? (See Figure 8.19.)

Diagnostics
After observing the pet, a light palpation may be performed starting at the bottom of the limb, beginning by palpating the toes with a light pressure. Care should be taken not to produce pain or discomfort for the pet. The limb should be palpated from the toe proximally, checking for heat, swelling, or changes in the muscle mass of the leg. While doing the light palpation, the team member should compare the injured limb to the other leg (see Figure 8.20.)

Clinical diagnostics for the orthopedic system largely focus on imaging of the bone, blood work to check for systemic disease, joint taps, and bone marrow aspirates to detect infections and changes in the bone marrow.

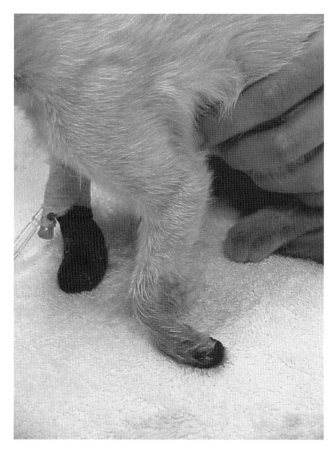

Figure 8.17. This pet is unable to use its left front leg.

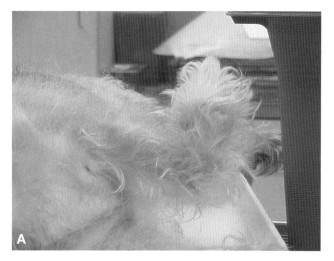

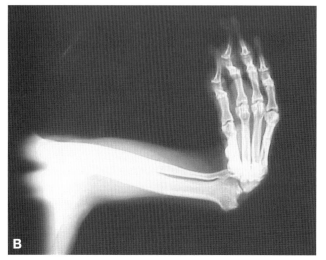

Figure 8.18. Abnormal rotation or configuration of the limb can suggest fracture or possibly a ruptured ligament or tendon (a). Note the fracture of the carpus in this radiograph (b).

Radiology is the most common diagnostic tool used for bone disease. Proper radiographic studies of the bone can help detect

- changes in bone density,
- fractures,
- masses,
- joint architecture,
- growth plates, and
- bone deformities.

It is always important to take two views when assessing bones. Furthermore, with some lesions in the limbs, it may be necessary to radiograph the nonaffected limb so the veterinarian can compare the affected limb to the normal limb and check for pathology (see Figure 8.21). Radiographic diagnostics are discussed in Chapter 25.

Clinical blood work is often collected to assess if there are any changes in the complete blood count that could suggest an infection or inflammation. Increases in blood calcium levels can sometimes suggest serious cancerous or hormonal diseases. Finally, blood titers of regional diseases can help detection of illnesses that can produce bone or muscle lameness.

How to Explain the Necessity of Blood Work in Orthopedic Cases to Clients
- The doctor is recommending blood work to see if there are changes in the complete blood count that may suggest chronic infection or inflammation that may be occurring due to the orthopedic disease.
- The doctor would like to assess the organs and body calcium levels, which could suggest a hormonal or cancerous disease process.
- Finally, in specific geographic regions, there are diseases for which the animal should be tested that can produce limping and bone and muscle pain.

A **surgical joint tap** is used to detect infection, inflammation, or neoplasia in the joint. A joint tap is indicated with chronically swollen joints that typically do not respond

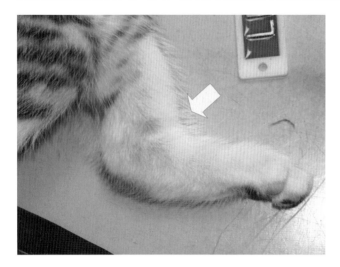

Figure 8.19. Swelling at a specific joint (joint effusion) can suggest a traumatic injury, an infectious process, an inflammatory process, a neoplastic process, or a fracture. In this picture swelling of the hock (ankle) occurred secondary to a distal diaphyseal fracture of the tibia.

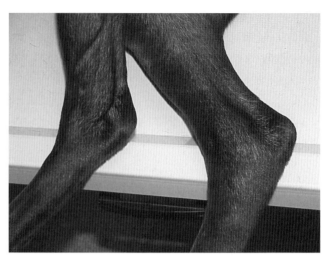

Figure 8.20. When trying to determine if mild or moderate swelling occurs, it is important to compare that limb to the other leg.

to medication and rest and when x-rays and other diagnostics are not helpful in indicating the pathology of the disease. The procedure is usually completed with the pet in mild to moderate sedation or placed under anesthesia. Once sedated, the needle is placed into the joint capsule and joint fluid is harvested. The fluid is then prepared for evaluation. Changes in joint fluid can suggest inflammatory joint disease (i.e., arthritis, rheumatoid arthritis), infection (septic joint), or cancer.

How to Explain the Necessity of a Joint Tap in Orthopedic Cases to Clients

- A joint tap is being recommended to obtain a sample of fluid and cells from the joint to aid the veterinarian in detecting disease that could be causing the chronic lameness and joint swelling.
- A joint tap is done with the pet under light sedation with general anesthesia; this depends on the pet and the pain associated with the procedure.
- The region over the joint capsule is shaved and surgically prepared for the procedure.
- A sterile needle is then placed into the joint, and samples are taken to test for infection and for cytology.

A radiographic abnormality in the bone density can suggest infection or cancer. With these concerns, a biopsy of that section can be taken with the animal under anesthesia. The biopsy is then submitted to a histopathologist (see Figure 8.22).

How to Explain the Need for Bone Marrow Aspirate in Orthopedic Cases to Clients

- A bone marrow aspirate is being recommended to obtain a sample of bone to detect infection, inflammation, or cancer within the bone because there are concerns regarding changes in bone density in the radiograph.
- A bone marrow aspirate is done with the pet under general anesthesia.
- The region over the bone is shaved and surgically prepared for the procedure.

Diseases of the Skeletal System

Fractures

A fracture is a break in a bone or multiple bones due to trauma, infectious disease (rarely), or neoplasia. Fractures can occur in both dogs and cats at any age.

Common Points in History
- Sudden onset of lameness
- Pet is not bearing weight on leg
- Can be associated with trauma
- Common in outside animals

Common Observations on Initial Assessment
- Swollen limb (see Figure 8.23).
- Pet is not bearing weight.
- Limb is abnormally deviated.
- Pet is in pain.

Complications

If the fracture goes untreated, it can lead to chronic pain, lack of use, and muscle atrophy. Due to the location of the

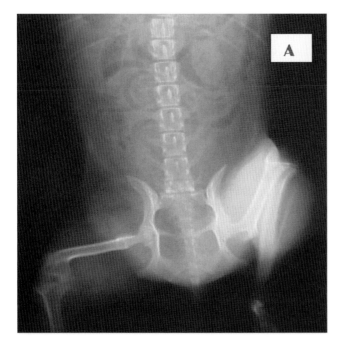

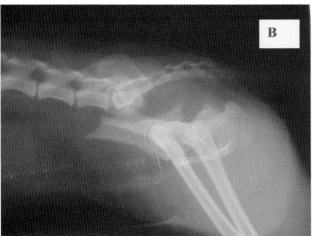

Figure 8.21. These x-rays are of a dog that was hit by car. The first x-ray (a) shows a ventro-dorsal view of this pet's back and hips. This view appears normal. It is only until a lateral view (b) is taken that there is a pelvic fracture.

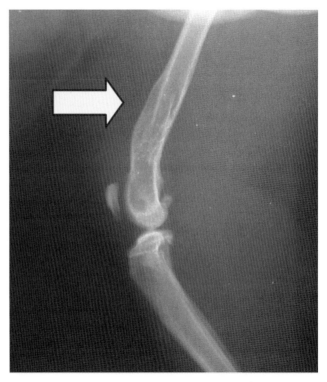

Figure 8.22. Image of questionable region within the femur of a cat.

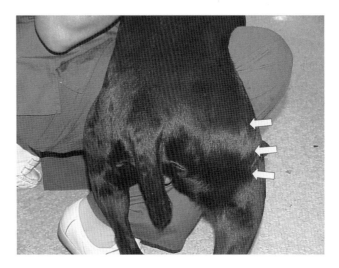

Figure 8.23. The right upper limb shows moderate swelling with the hip and gluteal muscles (white arrows). This may suggest a fracture of the femur or hip.

fracture, there may be nerve damage, inhibiting the ability of the limb to move or bear weight properly.

Diagnosis
Diagnosis is made on physical exam, palpation, and radiographs of the limbs. Radiographs are necessary to help characterize the type of fracture and the fixation needed to repair the fracture.

Treatment
There are many types of external and internal repairs available to the veterinarian. The type of repair is based on the

nature and location of the fracture, the preference of the veterinarian, and the financial constraints of the client.

External fixation uses an external device such as a Robert Jones Bandage, bandage and splint, hemi cast, or cast. This type of fixation isolates and confines the limb for a period of 4–8 weeks to allow the bones to heal properly (see Figure 8.24). Some guidelines for this type of fixation follow.

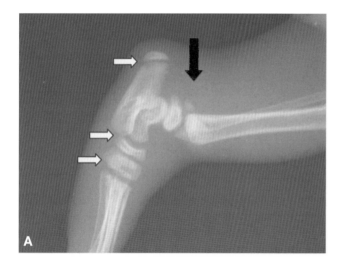

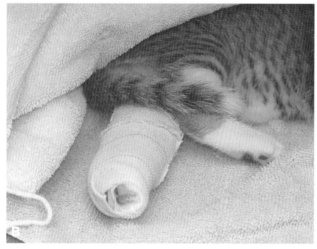

Figure 8.24. Radiograph of a young kitten with a fracture of the distal epiphyseal region of the tibia. The fracture (dark arrow) shows a cranial movement away from the bone. The other lines (white arrows) are normal growth plates in a young cat (a). A Robert Jones bandage and splint are placed to help stabilize the fracture (b).

- The device is used to isolate movement in a fracture by limiting the movement of the joint above and below the fracture site. Thus these devices can only be used to isolate fractures below the knee or elbow.
- Casts and splints cannot properly isolate fractures of the femur or humerus, since they are unable to isolate the shoulder or hip.
- Casts and splints work best with simple fractures; the highly comminuted fractures (multiple pieces) cannot be stabilized by this method.
- Generally, the animal needs to be rechecked throughout the 4–8 week period with x-rays and bandage changes.
- The animal needs to be limited to cage rest to properly heal the fracture and keep the bandage or splint from slipping or excessive wear.

Internal fixation devices are placed surgically to help isolate and stabilize a fracture. Types of internal fixators are cerclage wire, intramedullary (IM) pins, bone plates, and screws (see Figure 8.25). Some guidelines for this type of fixation follow.

- More advanced fractures, which have multiple pieces or are at an uncastable region, can be isolated and stabilized.

How to Discuss Fracture with the Client
Disease
A fracture is caused by a sudden, acute trauma of the bone, producing a break or multiple breaks of the bone column. The trauma can sometimes be a significant injury (i.e., hit by a car or a fall from a height); however, depending on the animal, the injury can occur from a fall out of owner's hands to the floor 3 feet below.

Clinical Diagnostics
Fractures are diagnosed primarily with radiographs. The radiograph allows the veterinarians to

- assess the location and type of injury,
- assess the best options for medical or surgical fixation,
- assess if the fracture involves a joint surface, or
- observe if the location of the fracture could injure other structures (i.e., nerves).

Treatment
The goal of treatment is to isolate and stabilize the injury until the bone heals properly. Fracture repair options are cage rest, external fixation, and surgical treatment.

With some minor fractures where there is reasonable alignment of the break, the veterinarian may suggest to simply cage rest the animal for a period of 4–8 weeks. The animal will need strict confinement for the fracture to stabilize.

External fixation largely uses casts, splints, and support wraps to help stabilize the fracture. To do this the fixation method must isolate the joint above and below the fracture site. Casts and splints

- work well on simple fractures below the elbow and knee;
- require cage rest confinement;
- often require rechecks, follow-up radiographs, and changes of the bandage under anesthesia or surgery; and
- can cause significant muscle loss after the cast or splint comes off, producing increased recuperation time. *(continued)*

How to Discuss Fracture with the Client (*continued*)

Surgical fixation uses orthopedic hardware such as plates, screws, and wires to stabilize the fracture. These procedures are generally used with more complex fractures or with fractures that cannot be isolated with a splint or cast. Orthopedic surgery

- allows for quicker recovery without significant muscle loss from the pet;
- allows a quicker return to function as the limb can maintain moderate weight bearing and movement after surgery;
- repair is generally more expensive than other procedures; and
- may require additional surgery to remove the plate or pin after the limb has healed.

Client Compliance

The most important part of successful fracture repair lies in proper client compliance.

- It is very important that all rechecks and rebandaging appointments are maintained to properly assess the fixator and the progress of bone healing.
- Many animals will want to resume normal levels of activity once the limb is pain free. The owner must restrict activity of the pet; even the best plate and cast can fail.
- The cast or splint must be carefully monitored for signs of swelling, slippage, or bandage tightening to make sure the external fixator is doing the proper job.
- The surgery site should be monitored for regions of swelling, pain, or discharge, which suggests a break or movement of the internal screw, wire, or pin.

- Generally, after surgery, the pet can begin bearing light to moderate weight on the limb, preventing muscle loss and decreasing recovery time.
- The pet must not return too quickly to normal activity while the internal fixation device is used, since movement or breakage of the device can occur leading to failure of fracture stabilization.
- When dealing with IM pins or surgical plates, these devices may have to be removed surgically after the bone is properly healed.
- Generally, surgical repair is more costly than the use of external fixation.

Prognosis

Prognosis for the fracture depends upon

- the age of the animal,
- the location and extent of the injury,

- if there is any nerve damage, and,
- most importantly, the client's compliance with the discharge information.

Prevention

Limiting animals' access to areas that could produce a trauma can prevent fracture occurrence (i.e., outside animals that roam freely).

Arthritis

Arthritis is an inflammation of the fluid-filled (synovial) joints caused by a wearing down of the normal articular cartilage of the joint until bone begins to rub on bone.

Articular cartilage damage is produced from

- congenital malformation/poor articulation of bones (i.e., hip dysplasia),
- chronic injury/fracture to the joint (i.e., ruptured cranial cruciate ligament injury),
- congenital disease of the cartilage (i.e., osteochondritis dissecans), and
- chronic infection/inflammation of the joint (i.e, septic joint infection, rheumatoid arthritis).

Once the injury begins, articular damage occurs until the bone surface becomes raw and swollen. The body responds by sending inflammatory cells (i.e., WBC, neutrophils) to the joint. The white blood cells migrate through the bone in response to inflammation and pain. Over time, from chronic inflammation, the bone remodels irregularly, producing sharp, irritating bone spicules on articular surfaces. The sharp bony ends produce pain and lameness.

Arthritis from malformation and injury is an underlying condition in which the bones in the joint are poorly aligned, producing an overall weakened conformation. This weakened architecture makes the joint less stable, making it easier to injure the cartilage with normal activity and wear and tear. For example, with hip dysplasia, the following can occur (see Figure 8.26).

- In young, rapidly growing dogs, the femoral head should fit into the hip like a ball in a socket joint.
- When the head of the femur is not very well seated into the socket of the pelvis, the leg moves easily in and out of the joint.
- The chronic movement produces damage to the articular cartilage and starts inflammatory change.

Common Signalment

Although arthritis can occur at any age, there are some specific generalizations. Arthritis can be prevalent in both dogs and cats. Predisposing factors can be

- genetic predisposition in certain breeds,
- athletic or working dogs,
- obese animals, and

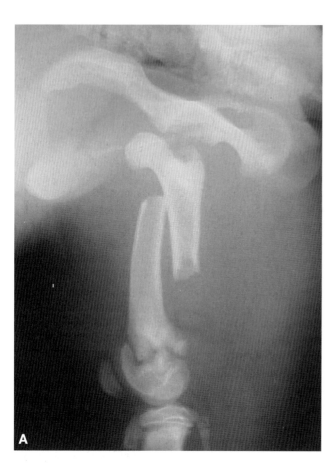
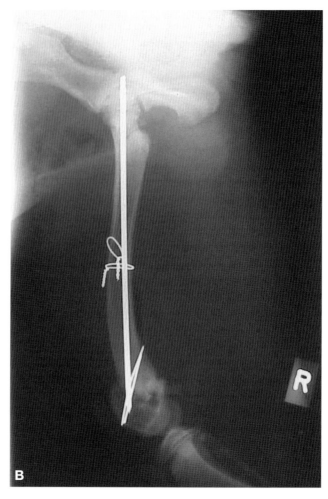

Figure 8.25. Radiograph of a mid-diaphyseal transverse femoral fracture, a distal femoral epiphyseal fracture, and a hip luxation (a). This type of fracture cannot usually be stabilized by a cast or splint. In this procedure, a combination of IM pin and cerclage wire were used to stabilize the fracture (b).

- animals with hormonal diseases (such as Cushing's disease, diabetes mellitus).

Common Breeds Affected by Arthritis

For felines there is no breed specificity.

In canines, hip dysplasia and elbow dysplasia can occur. Although more common in large breed, rapidly growing dogs, any size or breed of dog can have poor hips. Some breeds predisposed to hip dysplasia are

- St. Bernards,
- Labrador retrievers,
- Rotteweilers,
- German shepherds, and
- Golden retrievers.

Elbow dysplasia is a highly inheritable disease of large breed dogs in which there is improper formation of the bones of the elbow. Due to joint instability, acute inflammatory changes are set up within the joint producing an arthritic condition. Common breeds for which this is most common are

- St. Bernards,
- Labrador retrievers,
- Rotteweilers,
- German shepherds,
- Golden retrievers,
- Bernese mountain dogs,
- Chow chows,
- Bearded collies, and
- Newfoundlands.

Age of Onset/Incubation

Usually, arthritis is seen in middle-aged to older animals due to chronic damage to joints. However, this can occur in young animals as young as 4–5 months of age.

Common Points in History

- Animals worsen with exercise or activity.
- Animals cannot get up as well, or move as well, especially in the hind end.
- Patients lose their ability to jump on furniture.
- The lameness responds to aspirin or aspirin-like drugs.

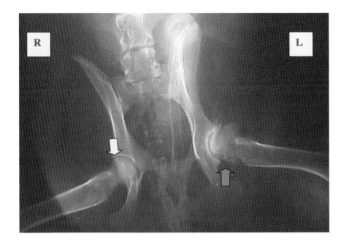

Figure 8.26. A comparison of hip joints. In this picture, the right head of the femur (white arrow) is well seated within the socket of the pelvis, and there is little movement and therefore very little arthritis. In the left leg (red arrow), the femoral head sits much shallower in the pelvic socket. As the animal moves, the leg rubs and irritates the bone and begins the inflammatory process. Notice the changes in the femoral head and neck from arthritis. This limb is painful to the pet because the sharp jaded edge digs into the joint capsule as the pet moves.

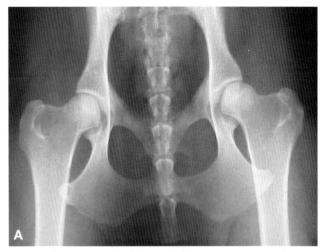

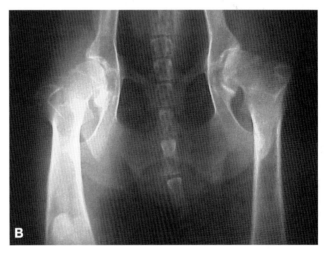

Figure 8.27. X-ray of mild hip dysplasia with slight squaring of the femoral heads. The heads are well seated into the hip (a). X-ray of severe hip dysplasia with severe arthritic change in the femoral heads and neck (squaring of the neck). Notice the poorer seating of the femoral heads into the hip socket (b).

- Animals walk abnormally, noticeable particularly in the hind end.
    — Chronic lameness that progressively gets worse with time
    — Bunny hopping (young dog)
    — Shifting their weight from side to side in the hind end
    — Unable to walk well on slick surfaces
    — Weakness in the hind end
    — Non-weight bearing in limbs
    — Lameness, which is made worse with exercise, long periods of lying down, rapid changes in weather (barometric pressure)

History of Previous Joint Injury
- Ruptured cranial cruciate ligament
- Osteochondritis dissecans (OCD)
- Poorly healed fracture of the joint

Common Observations on Initial Assessment
- The animal may be weak or slow in the hind end.
- They may keep the hind limbs underneath them and be reluctant to walk a full stride.
- There may be specific muscle wasting of the upper hip muscles or gluteal muscle range.
- With severe hip arthritis, animals may fall down or collapse on a slippery or angled surface.
- They may have a stiff walk or run, sometimes getting better as the dogs warms up.
- Bunny hopping may occur in young dogs, with animals that move their hind end like a rabbit running

Complications
- **Chronic pain/unable to use limb:** With severe chronic arthritis, animals can become increasingly immobile, pain filled, and less active.
- **Muscle loss:** As the pet continues to use the affected limb less and less, the muscle associated with movement of that limb becomes decreased (**disuse muscle atrophy**).

Diagnosis
The initial diagnostics for a lame animal generally use radiographs of the affected limb and possibly the unaffected limb. Generalized blood work may be indicated if there are concerns of infectious or neoplastic process in the bone. With chronic disease, joint taps or bone biopsies may be performed due to physical exam signs, diagnostics, and response to treatment (see Figure 8.27).

Treatment

There are both medical and surgical options in the treatment of arthritis. Determination of which type of surgical and medical treatment is chosen is based upon physical signs, clinical diagnostics, and response to treatment.

Medical treatment is generally done initially with mild to moderate lameness or done chronically in the nonsurgical cases.

- **Diet:** Making sure obese animals lose weight and keeping other animals lean makes the wear and weight on the joints much less.
- **Nonsteroidal anti-inflammatory medication:** These medications are a class of nonsteroidal drugs that reduce inflammation in the body. In this category are aspirin, Ascriptin, carprofen, meloxicam, and other drugs. They can be extremely effective but can cause gastrointestinal upset, and some may affect the kidneys and liver in sensitive animals. This type of drug should be used with extreme caution in the cat (see Chapter 26).
- **Chrondroprotective agents:** These drugs help increase joint fluid while protecting the cartilage. In general, they have mild to no side effects and can be reasonably effective in controlling inflammation. Drugs in these categories are chondroiten sulfate and glucosamine hydrochloride.
- **Other types of anti-inflammatory medication:** DMSO is a potent anti-inflammatory that is generally given in pill or powder form. It has minimal side effects to the body, but may need to be given for some time before it takes effect.

Surgical repairs are typically done with hip dysplasia or hip arthritis. The procedure can be done as a prophylactic surgical procedure for animals with hip dysplasia or as a treatment for the animals with chronic hip arthritis. The surgical procedures are discussed next.

Triple Pelvic Osteotomy

This procedure is done prophylactically in young animals with evidence of early hip dysplasia and poor hip conformation, where the femoral head is not well seated within the hip. The goal of surgery is that when young animals are detected with femoral heads that sit superficially within the acetabulum and are easily movable within the joint, the acetabular region of the hip can be repositioned so that it more fully covers the femoral head. The veterinarian surgically fractures the pelvis in three different locations, and the bone is repositioned such that it more fully covers the femoral head. Once positioned, the pelvic bone is plated. The procedure can be done bilaterally or unilaterally. A total hip surgery can be done later if the joint destruction continues. This procedure is generally done by a board-certified veterinary surgeon.

Femoral Head and Neck Excision (FHO)

This surgery removes the femoral head from the hip joint out of the acetabulum and then severs the femoral head from the femur. The procedure allows the removal of the inflamed, irritated bone from the hip joint, instantly relieving the pain. Over time, the hip muscles tighten up, forming a false joint around the upper femur (**pseudoarthrosis**). The animal is then able to bear weight and walk. The procedure is typically done on the worst leg and can later be done on the remaining leg, after the animal begins to be mobile again.

The procedure is extremely effective in cats and small dogs that bear little weight on each leg. The procedure is harder on larger animals that must support a larger amount of weight per limb.

Complete Hip Replacement

When the joint is severely inflamed and shows extreme bony change and pain, a new hip joint can be implanted.

In this procedure, the affected head and neck is removed and replaced with a plastic prosthesis. The hip socket (**acetabulum**) is also replaced. The new femoral head is then placed within the new hip joint. It produces a painless well-moving joint.

This surgery can be done on both hips, generally starting on the worst hip. The surgery is fairly expensive but is one of the most effective treatments for severe hip arthritis. This procedure is generally done by a board-certified veterinary surgeon.

The prognosis is good to poor, depending on the physical signs, clinical diagnostics, and response to treatment.

Prevention

Because in some large breed dogs this disease has a congenital basis, prevention can focus on the following.

Reproduction

If a pet is going to be used as a sire or dam, hip radiographs (OFA or PennHIP) should be taken and reviewed for dogs more than 2 years old for evidence of hip dysplasia. Animals who have marginal hips should not be bred.

Diet

Young animals on high-energy/high-protein diets can grow to be young adults that are slightly obese. These animals with hip dysplasia can have early onset of hip arthritis (8 months of age or older).

- Keeping large and giant breed canines lean as young adults by switching them to an adult diet when they reach 6–8 months or 75 pounds (giant breeds) is recommended.
- This will not stop the pet from reaching its normal size and weight, but it will slow the growth curve slightly, preventing the pet from becoming a slightly obese (paunchy) pup in the 6- to 12-month interval.

How to Discuss Arthritis with the Client

Arthritis is a degenerative, painful change in the bone and cartilage of the normal joint due to congenital abnormalities or chronic injury. The abnormal architecture of the joint causes increased destruction of the normal protective cartilage. As an exposed section of bone begins to rub on the bone in the joint, sharp bony spicules occur, producing pain, lameness, and a decreased use of the limb. In some breeds of animals, because of congenital abnormalities in the pet's joint, early onset of arthritis can occur.

Clinical Diagnostics

Arthritis is diagnosed primarily with radiographs. Other diagnostics, such as joint taps or general blood work, may also be used. (See above for client discussion points on this topic.)

Treatment

Treatment is based on the severity of the pet's arthritis, the clinical diagnostics, and the response to treatment. However, there are two overall medical protocols.

- **Medical Treatment:** Medical treatment of arthritis is focused on the use of aspirin-like drugs to reduce inflammation and pain, nutritional supplementation (i.e., chondroiten sodium and glucosamine hydrochloride) to increase joint fluid and protect cartilage, and an exercise and weight-loss regime. Medications may only be used when the pet is in pain and may be needed for the lifetime of the animal.
- **Surgical Treatment:** With significant arthritic disease or arthritis that has not responded significantly to medication, surgical treatment is indicated. It will be up to the veterinarian to recommend which procedure would best help the pet based on size of the animal and changes in the joint.

Prevention

Prevention of the disease should be focused on pre-breeding radiographic screening of large breed dogs that have a genetic predisposition for hip dysplasia and careful control of the diet of the young, rapidly growing giant and large breed dogs.

Panosteitis

Panosteitis is a benign, painful condition of the long bone affecting young, rapidly growing dogs. At this time, the cause of this disease is unknown. Pain and limping is thought to be caused by disruption of the normal architecture of the bone.

Common Signalment

The disease typically affects dogs from 5 to 18 months of age; however, it has been reported in dogs from 2 months to 5 years of age. German shepherds and German shepherd mixes are most commonly affected. Males tend to be more affected than females.

Common Points in History

- No history of trauma.
- The pets show a mild to moderate lameness.
- The limping can affect more than one limb, and signs can wax and wane from one leg to the other.
- On occasion there can be other mild systemic signs, such as
  — Decreased appetite,
  — Depression,
  — Weight loss, and
  — Fever.

Common Observations on Initial Assessment

On initial assessment, a team member may note that the

- animal can be mildly to severely lame,
- animal can be non-weight-bearing to toe-touching lame, and
- animal can have mildly swollen lower limbs.

Complications

There are usually no long-term complications for animals being treated with panosteitis.

Diagnosis

As with arthritis, the diagnosis of panosteitis is largely made based on radiographic changes in the diaphysis of the long bones. The medullary canal of the affected bone shows and increased grainy appearance in comparison with the other limbs (see Figure 8.28).

Treatment

Panosteitis is a benign self-limiting disease. The goal of treatment is to reduce pain and soreness until the dog grows out of the condition. There are two overall goals in medical treatment: medication and activity.

Nonsteroidal anti-inflammatory medication such as Carprofen is used to control pain and inflammation during severe episodes.

Decreased activity may decrease pain associated with panosteitis; however, decreased exercise has not been shown to help with remission of the disease.

Prevention

There is no way to prevent panosteitis.

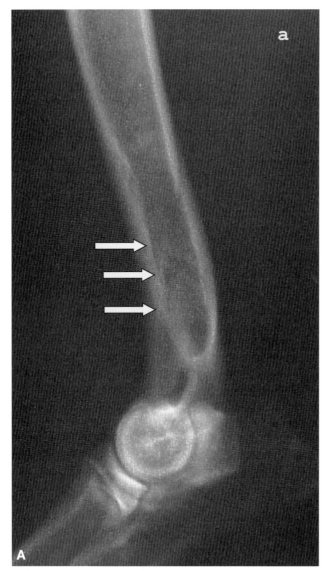
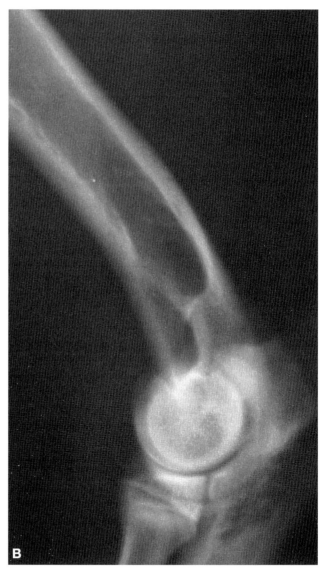

Figure 8.28. An x-ray comparison. A radiograph image of a humerus affected with panosteitis. Note the grainy appearance of the bone above the joint (a). Note the unaffected bone (b).

How To Discuss Panosteitis with the Client
Panosteitis is a self-limiting disease of the long bone. It produces mild pain and inflammation of the inside column of the long bones of the limbs. This inflammatory change produces lameness in possibly one to all four limbs. The disease produces no long-term change in the bone or growth of your pet. The disease usually is outgrown by 12–18 months of age.

Clinical Diagnostics
Panosteitis is diagnosed primarily with radiographs and presentations of physical signs. (See above for client discussion points on this topic.)

Prevention
There is no prevention available for this disease process.

Cranial Cruciate Ligament Rupture Release
The cranial cruciate is a ligament that attaches from the femur (long bone of the upper rear leg) to the tibia (long bone of the lower hind leg, below the knee). It prevents the grating of the femur on the tibia when an animal bears weight on the leg. It also prevents internal rotation of the joint. The rupture of the ligament causes instability in the knee and decreases the ability of the animal to bear weight on its hind leg. Partial rupture of the ligament is also possible, causing a chronic degenerative lameness.

There are many possible causes of rupture of the cranial cruciate ligament; however, the most common is caused by trauma due to hyperextension or flexion of the joint. An immune-mediated degenerative arthritis can also predispose the ligament to rupture. Animals with conformational problems in the knee are also likely to have a cruciate rupture (e.g., animals with severe luxating patella). Predisposing factors for a cruciate rupture are obesity, animals with

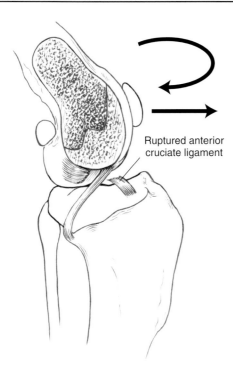

Ruptured anterior
cruciate ligament

Figure 8.29. In this diagram the cranial cruciate is ruptured. This allows increased forward and medial rotational movements (arrows) as the pet bears weight on the leg. To prevent this movement, pets often come in with their limbs pulled upward and rotated medially.

poor conformation, or animals with luxating patella (see Figure 8.29).

Signalment

Rupture of the cranial cruciate ligament is common in all dogs; however, it is more common in rotteweiler and Labradors, where ligament rupture can occur in dogs less than 4 years old. In other breeds, cranial cruciate ligament rupture occurs in dogs older than 5 years. It is more common in female dogs and rare in cats.

Common Points in History

- The pet usually presents with a sudden acute non-weight-bearing lameness.
- There can be a history of trauma, a fall, or increased activity.
- The pet may have a history of patellar luxation.

Common Observations on Initial Assessment

- Inability to stand on the leg
- Leg rotated inward
- Toe-touching lameness without bearing weight
- Swelling of the knee joint
- Heat and pain on the knee

Complications

If the joint instability created by the ruptured cruciate is not corrected adequately with rest and medication, there is a good chance that severe arthritis can occur within a few months.

Diagnosis

Diagnoses is based on orthopedic examination and radiographs. Diagnosis is generally made by a thorough orthopedic veterinary exam with a sedated or anesthetized patient. The key to diagnosis is to observe an increased forward movement in the tibia when the bone is pulled cranially as the femur is held in place. This movement is called a **cranial draw sign** and suggests the cruciate is damaged. Nonsedated/anesthetized patients can lock the muscle around the knee to prevent this forward motion, which is why sedation is recommended.

Radiographs are sometimes suggested to help assess the bony components of the stifle joint for fractures, signs of infection, or the beginnings of arthritis. **Radiographs will show only the bony structures of the joint and cannot show a ruptured cranial cruciate ligament.**

Treatment

In small breed dogs, especially with a partial tear of the cranial cruciate ligament, conservative treatment of rest, heat, and anti-inflammatory medications may allow for joint contracture and a return to partial to full function. However, with a complete rupture, especially in a larger dog, surgical repair of the ligament may be necessary. There are a few surgical repair options available.

Cranial Cruciate Ligament Repair Using Allograft or Suture Prosthesis

This surgical repair uses a thick-gauge suture or thick tissue above the knee to act as a false ligament (**prosthesis**). During surgery, the veterinarian will also open the joint to make sure there has not been any other injury to the internal architecture of the knee, especially the menisci. The menisci (see Figure 8.8) are thick, cartilaginous structures within the joint that help hold the joint in place. With a destabilized joint, the cartilage can tear or fold up as the bone moves abnormally against it. A folded meniscal cartilage can produce a severe inflammatory response that can lead to severe arthritis. Damaged cartilage is removed to prevent further arthritic change in the joint.

Complications to the procedure are possible. If the animal is obese, extremely active, or young at the time of injury, it is possible for the prosthesis to break. It may need to be replaced over time. It is also possible for the other knee to have a cranial cruciate rupture.

Tibial Plateau Leveling Osteotomy Procedure (TPLO)

Tibial plateau leveling osteotomy is a newer procedure that allows the transposition of a section of the tibia bone (tibia plateau) into a new position on the bone. It allows the joint to be stabilized without the need to open up the joint and inspect the internal structures. This procedure is thought to be an improved stabilizing procedure in the larger-breed dogs.

How to Discuss Ruptured Cranial Cruciate Ligament with the Client

There are two thick, fibrous ligaments in the knee of your pet that help stabilize the movement of the knee joint. The first ligament helps prevent forward motion of the upper bone (the femur) that may cause it to grate and rub on the lower bone (the tibia) as your pet bears weight. When the ligament snaps, the bones begin to grate on each other, producing pain, swelling, and lameness. Once this ligament is completely ruptured, the body cannot repair it. If the joint is not stabilized over time (months), the joint can become severely arthritic and painful to the animal.

Clinical Diagnostics

- A ruptured anterior cruciate ligament is diagnosed primarily with an orthopedic examination and radiographs.
- The orthopedic exam is usually done on a sedated or anesthetized animal so the doctor can fully appreciate the movement in the pet's joint without the pet feeling too much pain.
- Radiographs will not show the ruptured cruciate ligament, but they will allow the doctor to assess if there are any fractures or disease of the bony components of the joint.

Prevention

Prevention of the disease should be focused on the following.

- **Preventing obesity in the pet:** Obese pets have a great deal more weight on their limbs, increasing the chance of joint injury.
- **Decreasing activities that could injure the knee:** Animals that climb and jump down or play in activities with a great deal of up and down movement (i.e., Frisbee play) have an increased chance of cruciate injury.
- **Proper fixation of previous joint injury:** Cruciate injuries can occur from a previous congenital condition (i.e., patellar luxation) or a bony injury of the stifle joint that is not properly repaired.

Prevention

Preventing cranial cruciate ligament damage should focus on

- weight control in the pet,
- decreasing activities with a large vertical component (i.e., Frisbee), and
- properly stabilizing the knee joint from congenital or traumatic injury (i.e., congenital patellar luxation; see below).

Patellar Luxation

The **patella** (kneecap) is a small bone (**sesamoid**) within the pet's knee that sits within a small groove (**the patellar groove**) on the large long bone called the femur. The muscular attachments to the patella and the patellar attachments to the bones of the leg (the femur and the tibia) allow the patella to act as a hinge so that the animal can bear full weight on its hind legs. With patellar luxation, the small bone can move in and out of the patellar groove causing mild to profound lameness.

Medial patellar luxation is a congenital abnormality in the formation of the patellar groove, the position of the tibia and femur in respect to the patella, or the attachments of the muscle bodies on the patella. Medial luxation is typically seen in young toy and small breed dogs. Medial patellar luxation is graded I–IV, depending on the severity of the disease (see Figure 8.30).

- **Grade I (mildest form)**: Here the patella moves out of the groove when pressure is placed on the kneecap, but the patella quickly moves back into position.
- **Grade II**: The patella can be manually removed from its groove and the kneecap will remain out until it is placed back in or the animal flexes its legs.
- **Grade III**: The patella spontaneously moves out of its groove but will replace itself when replaced manually or the animal extends or flexes its knees.
- **Grade IV (most severe)**: The patella freely moves out of its groove and does not reposition itself normally.

Lateral patellar luxation is also possible in small and toy breeds in middle to older patients and is also observed in young large to giant breed dogs.

Signalment

Medial patellar luxation occurs often in dogs but is rare in cats. It has been associated more commonly with miniature and toy breeds of dogs, especially

- Yorkshire terriers,
- Pomeranians,
- Pekingese,
- Chihuahuas, and
- Boston terriers.

Medial patellar luxation tends to be more prevalent in females. Clinical signs are typically seen shortly after birth.

Common Points in History

- Pet has waxing and waning lameness.
- Pet has a history of three-legged lameness and then spontaneously soundness.
- Pet will run with limb extended, locked in position.
- Usually pet has no other physical signs.

Common Observations in Initial Assessment

- The animal will present as non-weight bearing but may produce a normal gait.
- As animal walks, the limb may be unable to bear weight for a few strides and then pop back into a normal stride.

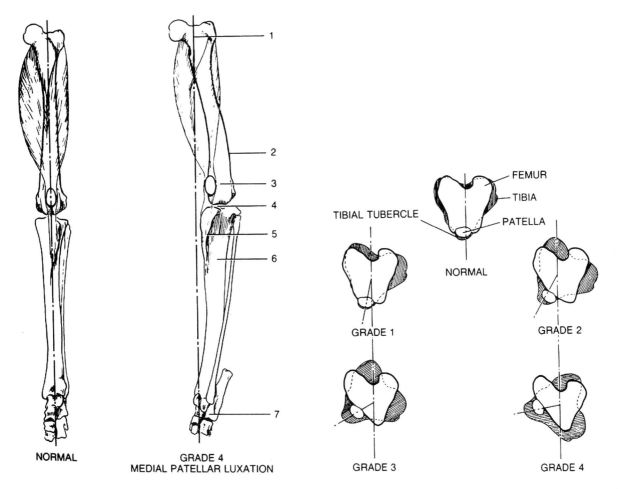

Figure 8.30. Illustration of a normal patella compared with a limb with abnormal architecture producing advanced degrees of patella luxation. (Courtesy of *Handbook of Small Animal Orthopedics,* 2nd edition. Brinker, W., Piermattei, D., and Flo, G. W.B. Saunders, Philadelphia, PA, 1990.

- On **light** palpation of the knee, the patella moves in and out of the groove.
- The patella may be palpated on the medial or lateral side of the joint

Complications

If severe patellar luxations are not properly repaired, chronic arthritis and further joint injury (i.e., cranial cruciate ligament damage) can occur, causing the pet severe pain and requiring more serious surgery that may leave the affected limb with decreased function.

Diagnosis

Diagnosis of patellar luxation is based largely on history, physical examination, and radiographs. The radiographs will allow the veterinarian to see how severely the joint is affected and what medical or surgical treatment may be needed to correct the underlying problem.

Treatment

Treatment is based on the presentation of the animal and the severity (grade) of the disease noted. Some medical protocols may require the following.

- **Medications:** Anti-inflammatory medication may be prescribed, focused on reducing inflammation and pain produced from the chronic movement of the patella in and out of the patellar groove.
- **Diet:** Obesity can make patellar luxation occur more often and increase the damage caused by the movement of the bone. Weight loss may be suggested to help decrease the amount of weight the pet needs to carry on the leg and decrease the joint instability.
- **Cage rest:** With mild luxations, if the lameness is acute and the joint inflamed, the pet may need to be cage rested to decrease movement and injury in the joint.
- **Surgery:** Depending on the severity of the luxations and the persistence of lameness, a surgical repair may be indicated. The repairs depend on how severe are the luxation and the congenital changes in the bones and muscles. Surgery can involve
  — deepening of the patellar groove,
  — repositioning the attachment of the patella onto the tibia, and
  — tightening of the tissue around the kneecap.

Other procedures may also be suggested.

How to Discuss Patellar Luxation with the Client

- The patella (kneecap) is a small bone (sesamoid) within the pet's knee that sits within a small groove (the patellar groove) on the large, long bone called the femur.
- When properly held in place, it allows the pet to bear full weight on the leg.
- Patellar luxation is a congenital disease in which the patella can freely move in and out of its groove, producing a waxing and waning lameness.
- The pet usually will become three-legged lame acutely, and then just as suddenly become sound on the leg as the patella moves in and out of the joint.

Clinical Diagnostics

The diagnosis of patellar luxation is based on its presence on physical exam and changes noted on rear-limb radiographs. The radiographic changes help the medical team recommend medical and surgical treatment protocols for the pet.

Prevention:

Prevention of the disease should be focused on

- early detection of patellar luxation in the pet and repair if necessary, and
- prevention of obesity in mildly affected animals.

Complications

In severe cases, if the patellar luxation continues, the joint will be destabilized, setting the joint up for cruciate ligament rupture and arthritis.

Prevention

Preventing patellar luxation injury should focus on early detection of congenital problems and repair that can prevent continued damage to the joint. Weight control in the pet is also important.

Osteochondritis Dissecans

In all moveable joints of the body, there is a soft spongy cartilage, called **hyaline cartilage,** that produces a thick, viscous lubricant called **hyaluronic acid.** The purpose of this tissue is to act as a lubricant to decrease the chance of irritation, inflammation, and bony change in the joint.

In osteochondritis dissecans (OCD), there is change in the normal laying down of cartilage lining the joint, producing areas of thickened irregular cartilage prone to injury and breaking loose. When this occurs, a nonhealing ulcer results, which produces chronic pain upon movement of the joint.

Also, the small irregular piece of cartilage (called a **joint mouse**) that has broken off can lodge itself between the moving bones, causing severe pain and inflammation (see Figure 8.31).

The cause of OCD in not yet fully understood. It is

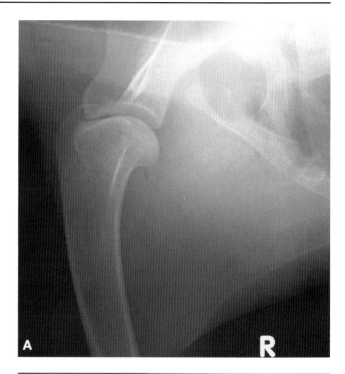

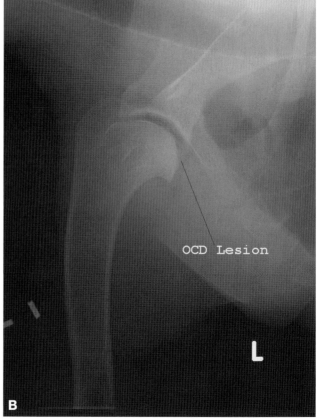

Figure 8.31. Illustration of a normal shoulder joint (a) and one that had an OCD lesion in the proximal humerus (b). This exposed bone has a ulcerative sore evident that causes pain and lameness as the scapula moves. Furthermore, the free-floating cartilage (joint mouse) can lodge in the moving joint, causing pain, swelling, and further lameness.

thought that there may be changes in the normal nutrition of the cells that produce the forming cartilage, thus causing the improper formation of the tissue. There is also a genetic component to this disease.

OCD commonly affects

- the shoulder,
- the knee,
- the ankle,
- the elbow, and
- possibly the back.

Signalment
The disease has been reported with a high incidence in large breed dogs.

- Labrador retriever,
- Newfoundland,
- Rotteweiler,
- Great Dane,
- Bernese mountain dog,
- English setter, and
- Old English sheep dog

OCD of the shoulder is seen more in male animals (2:1 over females).

Common Points in History
- The pet is usually a young adult large breed dog.
- The pet presents for ongoing progressive lameness affecting one or multiple limbs.
- The lameness generally becomes worse with exercise.
- The lameness can begin acutely and may come and go over weeks to months.

Common Observations in Initial Assessment
On physical examination,

- the animal will show a mild to severe (usually unilateral) lameness;
- the affected leg has decreased range of motion when walking, or the animal may not be weight bearing;
- if the lameness is severe enough, muscles around the joint may be atrophied **(muscle atrophy)**; and
- the joint itself may be swollen and hot to touch (acute episode).

Complications
If OCD lesions are not properly repaired, chronic arthritis and further joint injury can occur, causing the pet severe pain and requiring more serious surgery that may leave the affected limb with decreased function.

Diagnosis
Diagnosis is largely made based upon physical signs and radiographic changes in the joint. OCD lesions have specific

locations where the defect in the bone can be seen. Specific locations of OCD within the joint are as follows.

- **Shoulder:** Typical lesion is a lucent or darker area of the humerus overlying the caudal dorsal aspect of the greater tubercle.
- **Hock (talus):** Typical lucent lesions can be noted on the medial aspect of the trochlea of the talus.
- **Stifle:** The typical lesion is seen on the medial aspect of the lateral femoral condyle.
- **Elbow:** A lesion can be seen on the distal humerus on the cranial/medial aspect. The lesion can represent itself as a small triangular wedge that has broken off from the main bone.

How to Discuss Osteochondritis Dissecans with the Client
- All bones that make up joints are covered with a soft spongy cartilage called hyaline cartilage.
- In some young dogs, there is a problem with the normal maturation of the joint cartilage.
- In specific areas of the joint, a piece of cartilage can break away from the bone, producing an ulcerative lesion and making the bone painful and sore.
- Furthermore, the free-floating piece of cartilage, also called a joint mouse, floats free within the joint. If this cartilage moves into the bone as the joint moves, the pet can also have pain and become lame.
- Osteochondritis dissecans usually presents as a progressive lameness that can alternate from mild to severe in the rapidly growing large breed dog.
- Although there is suggestion of a congenital component of the disease, the cause of the disease is unknown at this time.

Clinical Diagnostics
The diagnosis of OCD is based on its presence on physical exam and changes noted on joint radiographs. The radiographic changes help the medical team recommend medical and surgical treatment protocols for the pet.

Complications
If the OCD lesion is not repaired, the joint can become arthritic and the pet can have chronic pain and be unable to bear weight on the leg.

Treatment
Treatment is based upon the presentation of the animal and the severity of the disease noted on physical examination and radiograph. Although the use of anti-inflammatory medications and cage rest may help decrease physical signs of lameness, often surgical exploration of the joint and clean-

ing out the joint mice and affected flaps of cartilage to allow for proper healing is one of the best options to prevent arthritic change in the joint.

Bone Neoplasia—Osteosarcoma

Bone neoplasia is a cancerous condition of the bone, which is the primary tumor of the bone in the dog. These types of tumors can carry a poor prognosis due to their high rate of spread into other tissues of the body (**metastasis).** This is less common in the cat and carries a slightly better prognosis due a decreased rate of metastasis.

There is no known cause for osteosarcoma.

Signalment

Tumors tend to be more common in large and giant breed dogs with a median age of 7 years. It has been reported in patients as young as 6 months of age. It has also been reported in older domestic short hair cats.

Common Points in History

The patient presents with a history of lameness with moderate to severe pain. Owners may also report mild to moderate swelling of the affected leg.

Common Observations in Initial Assessment

On physical examination, the animal will show

- swollen limb or
- swelling that can often be firm to hard on palpation and very painful, and
- non-weight-bearing lameness.

Complications

With aggressive osteosarcoma, decalcification of the bone can be so severe that the leg can break without any trauma (**pathologic fracture**). Without aggressive treatment, metastasis of the tumor to other organ systems (i.e., lungs) may occur. In many cases, metastases have already occurred even prior to the tumor mass being identified.

Diagnosis

Diagnosis is largely made based upon physical signs and radiographic changes in the bone. Bone density can be increased, decreased, or a mixed pattern (see Figure 8.22). In more advanced cases bony loss can be so severe that a fracture may occur. The diagnosis is confirmed through bone biopsy of the suspected site. Further chest radiographs may be suggested by the veterinarian to detect any obvious metastatic masses within the lung fields.

Treatment

Treatment is based upon the location of the mass (limb versus body), the physical status of the patient, and if there is obvious metastatic masses detected elsewhere. With tumors of the limbs, treatment options are as follows.

- **Limb amputation:** With aggressive tumors, removal of the affected limb is recommended to reduce the chance of metastasis of the tumor and reduce pain and immobility of the patient. The owner must understand that there is still a high potential that metastasis has already occurred prior to surgery.
- **Chemotherapy:** The use of aggressive chemotherapeutic medication can help extend quality of life. Owners will need to be educated on the strict schedule of the chemotherapy drugs, the follow-up clinical diagnostics needed, potential side effects, and cost before beginning therapy.

Prognosis

In canines prognosis is poor. Most pets that do not have amputation and chemotherapy succumb in the first 4 months after diagnosis. With amputation alone, mean survival time is 4 months. With amputation and chemotherapy survival time can be as high as 1 year. It is important to understand that these survival times are averages of animals diagnosed with osteosarcoma, and patients can live longer or succumb much quicker than expected.

In cats with treated with amputation only, the mean survival time is greater than 4 years.

How to Discuss Osteosarcoma with the Client
Disease

Osteosarcoma is a cancer of the bone, causing swelling, pain, and lameness. Osteosarcoma can occur on any bone in the body. These tumors can spread aggressively into other organ systems of the body, especially the lungs. It is more common in large to giant breed dogs. It is rare in cats.

Clinical Diagnostics

Diagnosis is made by physical examination, radiographic changes in the bone, and bone biopsy. If osteosarcoma is suspected, chest radiographs may also be recommended to evaluate for any potential spread of tumors to the lung fields.

Complications

If not diagnosed, osteosarcoma can spread aggressively to other tissues of the body and lead to death of the patient.

CD-ROM 1 reviews material presented in this chapter. Please try the cases for Section 2 (Anatomy and Physiology—The Science behind the Diseases) to help reinforce the information presented here.

Chapter 9

Teeth and the Oral Cavity

In a busy general practice, a great deal of energy and time are spent with the client and patient in implementing a strong dental wellness program. In recent years, dental health and preventative medicine has become a large part of general practice. With the advent of more advanced and affordable dental x-ray machinery, equipment, advanced procedures (i.e., root canals and crowns), and more choices of antibiotics and pain medications, the medical team can offer a more progressive dental program. Furthermore, with clients able to sympathize with dental disease and tooth pain, client education about dental treatments can be straightforward and easily accepted by the pet owner.

Dental and Oral Anatomy

Mouth
The **mouth** (oral cavity) is the beginning of the digestive process. The overall function of the mouth and early digestive tract is to break down food into smaller molecules that can be digested. Proteins are broken down into smaller amino acid chains, fats are broken down into triglycerides, and complex sugars are broken down into simple small-unit sugars. To complete this function, the animal relies on its teeth to break down the large foodstuffs into smaller units so that the intestinal system can facilitate digestion.

Furthermore, to help facilitate digestion the salivary glands secrete saliva to help emulsify food into a liquid solution. There are four sets of **salivary glands.** Each gland is named for the anatomical region of the face where the glands lie. The four glands are the **parotid gland, submandibular gland, sublingual gland,** and the **zygomatic gland**. These glands function to produce saliva, which homogenizes the food into a liquid chyme. It is then transported into the stomach and small intestine. Saliva also contains chemicals (**enzymes**) that begin breaking down the food stuffs to start the digestive process, (e.g., **trypsin**).

Teeth
Each tooth has its own function.

- **Incisors** are smaller teeth in the front of the jaw. They are meant to rip and tear skin and meat.
- **Canines** are next to the incisors and are meant for tearing, piercing, and catching prey.
- **Premolars and molars** are used to grind and shear the food.

The teeth number and type vary from species to species. However, basic anatomy of the small animal tooth is similar (see Figure 9.1). They contain the following.

- **Cusp**: Top surface of the tooth also known as the **occlusal surface**
- **Crown**: Part of the tooth that protrudes above the gum line
- **Neck**: A constriction of the tooth where the crown meets the root as it dips below the gum line
- **Root**: Part of the tooth embedded in the tooth socket (alveolus) of the jaw
- **Pulp cavity**: Central cavity in the tooth extending from the root a variable distance toward the crown. The pulp cavity narrows as the animal ages.

The architecture of the teeth depends on the animal's diet and evolution. Felines are strict **carnivores** (eat meat only), so their teeth are meant for ripping and tearing, their jaw movement is sharp and scissorlike, and the table surfaces of the teeth are sharp angles.

On the other hand, canines are **omnivores** eat meat and vegetables). Their jaws function for both carnivore and herbivore diets; their incisors and canines are sharp and can tear, and their molars have a flat surface for grinding. Their jaws have both scissor motion and grinding circular motion.

Animals have specific dental formulas that help to quantitate and describe their teeth type and number. The canine formula enumerates half the skull's upper and lower teeth and is as follows (see Figure 9.2).

Canine Teeth
Deciduous teeth number 28 total (baby teeth):

$$\frac{3 \text{ incisors (I); 1 canine (C); 3 premolars (P)}}{3 \text{ incisors (I); 1 canine (C); 3 premolars (P)}} \; (\times 2 \text{ for entire skull})$$

Permanent teeth number 42 total:

$$\frac{3 \text{ incisors (I); 1 canine (C); 4 premolars (P); 2 molars (M)}}{3 \text{ incisors (I); 1 canine (C); 4 premolars (P); 3 molars (M)}} \; \times 2$$

(See Table 9.1.)

Feline Teeth
Felines have a slightly different dental architecture compared with dogs (see Table 9.2). Their first premolar and second molar

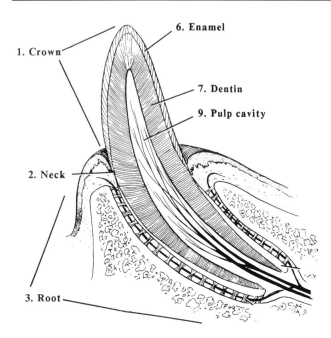

Figure 9.1. Anatomy of the tooth. (Courtesy of *Anatomy of Domestic Animals*, 7th Edition. Pasquini, Chris, and Pasquini, Susan. Sudz Publishing, Pilot Point, Tx 1989. Used with permission from Sudz Publishing.)

Table 9.1. The canine's tooth eruption schedule.

Teeth	Eruption of Temporary Teeth	Eruption of Permanent Teeth
Incisor 1	3–4 weeks	3–5 months
Incisor 2	3–4 weeks	3–5 months
Incisor 3	3–4 weeks	3–5 months
Canine	3–5 weeks	4–6 months
Premolar 1		4–6 months
Premolar 2	4–12 weeks	4–6 months
Premolar 3	4–12 weeks	4–6 months
Premolar 4	4–12 weeks	4–6 months
Molar 1		5–7 months
Molar 2		5–7 months
Molar 3		5–7 months

Note: Eruption times may vary depending on the breed and size of the individual animal.

are missing from the upper jaw. Also, their first and second premolars and second and third molars are missing from the lower jaw (see Figure 9.3). Their dental patterns are as follows:

$$\frac{3I1C3P}{3I1C2P} \times 2 \text{ (26 total)} \qquad \frac{3I1C3P1M}{3I1C2P1M} \times 2 \text{ (30 total)}$$

Oral and Dental Diseases

Dental disease in dogs and cats can take many forms. The obvious forms include broken, infected, or decayed teeth.

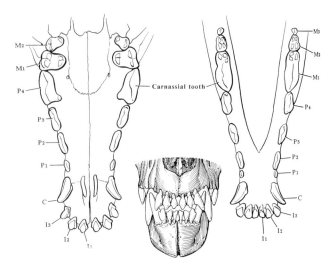

Figure 9.2. Illustration of canine skull with teeth. (Courtesy of *Anatomy of Domestic Animals,* 7th Edition. Pasquini, Chris, and Pasquini, Susan. Sudz Publishing, Pilot Point, Tx 1989. Used with permission from Sudz Publishing.)

Table 9.2. The feline's tooth eruption schedule.

Teeth	Eruption of Temporary Teeth	Eruption of Permanent Teeth
IIncisor 1	2–4 weeks	3–4 months
Incisor 2	2–4 weeks	3–4months
Incisor 3	2–4 weeks	3–4 months
Canine	3–4 weeks	4–5 months
Premolar 2	3–6 weeks	4–6 months
Premolar 3	3–6 weeks	4–6 months
Premolar 4	3–6 weeks	4–6 months
Molar 1		4–5 months

Note: Eruption times may vary depending on the breed and size of the individual animal.

However, many other disease processes are frequently seen affecting the teeth and oral cavity, the most common of which is periodontal disease. This disease affects the gums (**gingiva**) and other tissues in the mouth that surround and support the teeth. Periodontal disease affects over two-thirds of all adult dogs and cats, making it one of the top diseases seen in pet dogs and cats.

Dental Disease Terminology

- **Plaque** is the soft "slime" layer of material found on tooth surfaces and comprises salivary proteins, decayed food materials, and bacteria. It is hard to see with the naked eye and is easy to remove with brushing, but it returns quickly.
- **Calculus** is mineralized plaque deposits that are often yellow to brown in color. It adheres to teeth and is diffi-

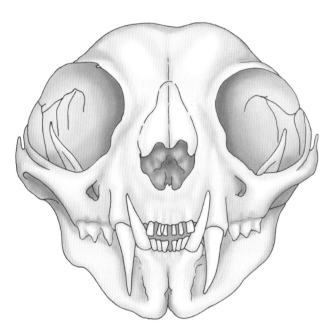

Figure 9.3.   Image of feline skull from below with upper arcade.

cult to remove, requiring professional cleaning under anesthesia. It is often called **tartar** by laypersons.

- **Gingiva** is the term used to describe the soft tissue that lines the oral cavity and surrounds the teeth. It is generally pink in color but may be dark pigmented in some breeds. It is often called the **gums** by laypersons.
- **Gingivitis** is considered to be inflammation of gums (gingiva). It is the first stage of periodontal disease. Gingivitis causes the gum tissue to be swollen, red, and bleed easily when touched.
- **Prophylaxis** is a term used to describe the process of cleaning a patient's teeth under anesthesia in the veterinary hospital. It can also be called professional dental cleaning or professional dental prophylaxis.

Systemic Manifestations of Dental Disease

The physical manifestations of dental disease are not just limited to the health of the mouth and teeth. The dental calculus that is seen so often with chronic dental disease contains pathogenic bacteria. The chronic infection of the teeth and gums can produce heavy bacterial loads that can seed to other parts of body, potentially producing life-threatening and life-limiting disease. Common sites of secondary infection can be in the following areas.

- **Sinuses**: The tooth roots in the upper jaw communicate with the nasal sinuses. Heavy bacteria-laden dental calculus can lead to chronic sinusitis that can respond to antibiotics initially, but then will reoccur. These animals will show
  — chronic sneezing,
  — nasal discharge (blood and pus),
  — weight loss,
  — decreased appetite, and
  — trouble breathing (occasional).

- **Heart:** Some medical studies suggest that a heavy bacteria load can enter the bloodstream and cause infections in the heart. A common site for bacterial buildup is on the mitral valve or left atrial/ventricular valve between the left atrium and left ventricle. If enough bacterial debris builds up on this valve, the mitral valve will not close properly and **mitral regurgitation** can occur (see Chapter 12).
- **Kidneys:** Increased bacterial load can infect the filtering devices of the outer kidney (the **glomeruli**) and produce a chronic underlying infection that can lead to chronic kidney disease or kidney failure (see Chapter 13).
- **Liver:** Just as with the kidneys, increased bacterial buildup can set up a bacterial infection of the liver (**hepatitis**), which can seriously affect the ability of the liver to metabolize toxins and produce necessary body proteins (see Chapter 14).

It is important to realize that these disease processes do not typically occur quickly with light dental calculus and mild oral disease, but rather occur over years with significant buildup of periodontal disease. Regular professional dental cleanings will help prevent these disease processes.

Obtaining a History for Dental Disease

Dental disease can produce a vast array of physical signs and complaints.

- **Anorexia**: With dental disease animals may stop eating due to dental pain, although some animals with severe dental disease still continue to eat normally.
- **Halitosis**: Animals may have mild to severe bad breath.
- **Changes in appetite**: The pet may also stop eating dry food and eat only soft food because this type of food will produce less dental pain.
- **Weight loss**: This is secondary to anorexia and dental disease.
- **Vomiting:** Animals who have severe dental disease typically do not chew their food well enough to have the stomach continue the digestion process; the large remaining food pieces may be vomited back up.
- **Excessive drooling:** Drooling associated with eating can be in response to dental disease and pain.
- **Sneezing/sinusitis, nose bleeds, and nasal discharge:** Many of the large premolars and molars have deep roots that communicate with the nasal sinuses. Chronic infection of these tooth roots can seed, causing a progressive sinusitis.
- **Facial swelling/chronic abscess formation in the jaw:** Many animals with chronic dental abscesses may have reoccurring facial swelling as well as abscess formation in the lower and upper jaws.

- **Eating abnormally:** Animals with dental pain and sensitivity may roll their food or push the food to one side of the mouth while eating.

The goal of the history and physical examination is to discover if the cause of the medical complaint is from the teeth and oral cavity or if the problem is located lower in the gastrointestinal tract. To help the medical team accomplish this task, the following questions should be asked.

- **What is the duration of illness?** Dental disease is usually a chronic on-going progressive problem where the clinical signs start mildly and then become more significant.
- **Does the pet eat hard or unusual substances?** Certain substances (i.e., rocks) can cause the increased wear or fractures of the teeth. The incisors may show wear from chronic chewing, and the premolars are commonly fractured from hard chew bones or rocks.
- **Does the pet show pain when eating?** Oral pain or abnormal eating patterns can suggest dental disease. Certain eating patterns to ask the client about are as follows:
  — Does the pet roll the food in its mouth?
  — Is there excessive drooling when eating?
  — Is there facial swelling?
  — Is there trouble swallowing?
  — Does the pet chew on only one side of the mouth?
- **Is the pet a chronic vomiter?** Vomiting can sometimes suggest dental disease, since the pet is not adequately breaking down food for digestion. If the pet is vomiting, other questions to ask the client to help identify the cause of the problem can be as follows.
  — How many times does the pet vomit per day?
  — Is it associated with eating or drinking?
  — Is there any blood or foreign debris present in the vomitus?
- **Is the pet chronically sneezing or having nasal discharge?** With chronic severe dental disease, the nasal sinuses can be infected. Pets may have waxing and waning purulent and/or bloody nasal discharge and chronic sneezing.
- **Does the pet have bad breath?** Bad breath (**halitosis**) can be a symptom of dental infection and periodontal disease.

Observation on Initial Assessment

The main focus of the initial assessment should be to determine if there is significant dental disease evident to account for the patient's symptoms. Care should always be exercised to make sure the pet will allow its mouth to be evaluated.

Generally, with severe oral disease, there are significant changes within the oral cavity. The factors that should be observed and documented in an oral examination to help determine if significant dental disease is present are as follows.

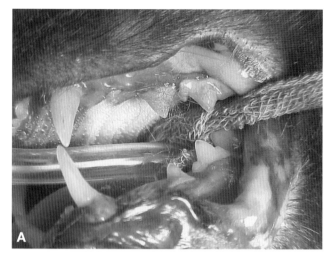

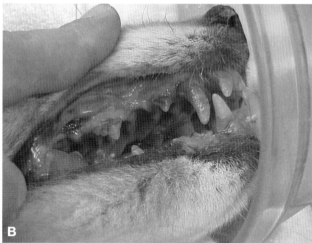

Figure 9.4. Images of mild dental tartar (a) and severe dental disease (b). Based on simple observation, it is understandable that the pet in (b) has significant dental disease, dental pain, and may have secondary disease (i.e., heart, kidney, or liver disease) from chronically infected teeth.

- **Dental calculus**: By carefully examining the teeth, the amount of dental calculus present, the severity of halitosis, and the health of the gums, a dental problem can be identified (see Figure 9.4).
- **Evidence of dental pain:** Dental pain can be appreciated by carefully examining the gum regions through the lips for sensitivity on the lower and upper dental arcades.
- **Evidence of oral and dental lesions**: Abnormalities in the teeth or jaw can predispose the pet to increased dental calculus and dental disease. Furthermore, oral masses and changes in the gums can also suggest serious pathology. The mouth should be examined for the following: normal bite (see Figure 9.5), underbite (see Figure 9.6), overbite (see Figure 9.7), retained baby (deciduous) teeth (see Figure 9.8), broken teeth (see Figure 9.9), gingival inflammation (see Figure 9.10), and oral masses/growths (see Figure 9.11).

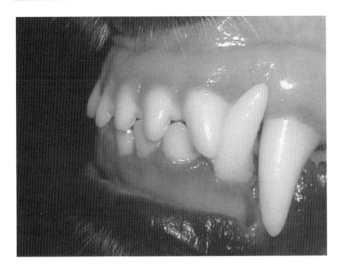

Figure 9.5. This dog has a normal bite and occlusion of the incisor and canine teeth. This is often called a scissors bite or class 0 occlusion.

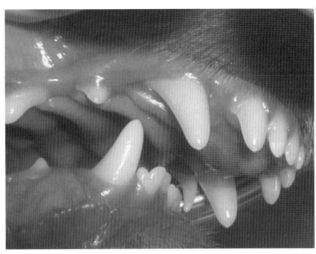

Figure 9.7. In this dog the upper jaw is much longer than the lower, causing misalignment of the teeth. This is commonly called an overbite or a class 2 malocclusion. (Reprinted by permission of Curt Coffman, DVM ACVD, Aid Animal Clinic, 7908 E. Chapparral, Suite 108, Scottsdale, Az 85250.)

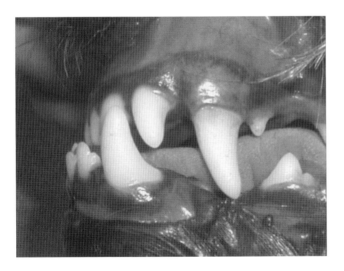

Figure 9.6. In this dog the lower jaw is much longer than the upper, causing misalignment of the teeth. This is commonly called an underbite, or a class 3 malocclusion. (Reprinted by permission of Curt Coffman, DVM ACVD, Aid Animal Clinic, 7908 E. Chapparral, Suite 108, Scottsdale, Az 85250.)

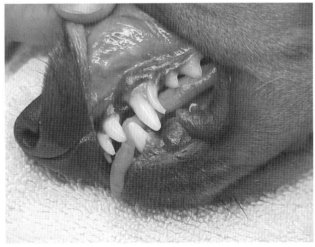

Figure 9.8. Note how much calculus is evident due to the presence of the retained baby tooth, which causes an abnormal region where plaque can build easily.

- **Temperature**: A fever **(hyperthermia)** can suggest infection or inflammation caused by chronic dental infection or dental abcessation.
- **Focal facial swelling or discharge:** Focal facial swelling and purulent (pus) discharge can suggest dental root abcessation. Usually, the swelling occurs over the larger premolars and molars causing a focal swelling ventral to the eye or on the lower mandible (see Figure 9.12).

- **Enlargement of the submandibular lymph nodes:** The submandibular lymph nodes located ventral to the mandible drain infection from the head and neck. With chronic infection of the oral cavity or teeth these nodes may be enlarged and observed by palpation.
- **Evidence of a heart murmur:** Severe periodontal disease can produce a secondary bacterial infection of the heart valve leaflets, especially affecting the mitral valve, producing mitral valve regurgitation (see Chapter 12).

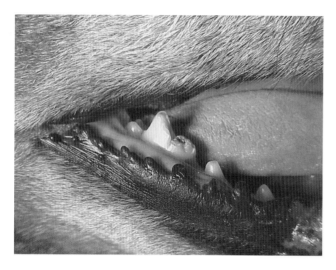

Figure 9.9.   Note the broken right lower first molar. The break is exposing the pulp cavity, opening the tooth for pain and a tooth root abscess.

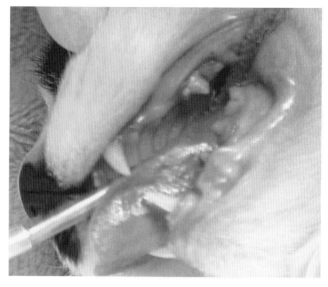

Figure 9.10.   Evidence of both dental calculus and red swollen gums indicate gingivitis and periodontal disease, suggesting that the teeth, roots, and the surrounding tissues are affected. (Reprinted by permission of Curt Coffman, DVM ACVD, Aid Animal Clinic, 7908 E. Chapparral, Suite 108, Scottsdale, Az 85250.)

Key Points in Discussing Dental Disease with a Client

There are several points to discuss with a client when dealing with dental disease.

- Dental disease is usually a chronic problem that develops into an acute problem.
- If not properly treated, severe dental disease can produce kidney, liver, and heart diseases.
- Even if the animal does not show physical pain or other symptoms, they can have significant disease that could be life limiting over the pet's normal lifetime.
- With severe dental infection and periodontal disease, professional dental cleanings and periodontal treatment requires more time and care as well as potential removal of teeth.

Clinical Diagnostics for Pets with Dental Disease

Diagnostic test recommendations depend upon the history, the presenting medical complaint, and the physical examination findings. Some diagnostics that may be suggested are discussed next.

Baseline Diagnostic Blood Work and Urinalysis

Most patients with chronic dental disease are middle-aged and older animals. Because chronic dental disease can be associated with heart, kidney, and liver disease, baseline blood work and urinalysis should be recommended.

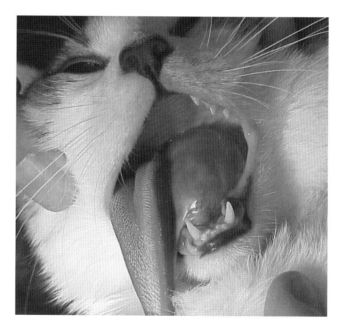

Figure 9.11.   Evidence of an abnormal mass associated with the gums or tongue can suggest serious oral disease or cancer. (Reprinted by permission of Curt Coffman, DVM ACVD, Aid Animal Clinic, 7908 E. Chapparral, Suite 108, Scottsdale, Az 85250.)

- **Complete blood count**: Severe chronic infectious disease can produce significant changes in the complete blood count in the following parameters.
  — **Low red blood cell count (anemia)**: Both chronic infection and bleeding from infected teeth can produce

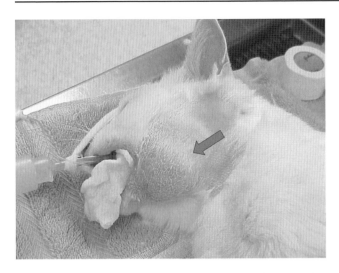

Figure 9.12.   Image of a focal facial abscess secondary to an infected lower molar.

mild to moderate red blood cell decrease that should be observed and monitored.

— **Increased white blood cell count:** Chronic infection can produce elevations in the white blood cell populations that suggest mild to moderate infection.

- **Clinical chemistry:** As discussed previously, chronic dental disease can be associated with kidney, liver, and cardiac changes. The medical team should evaluate the blood work for changes in the kidney or liver enzymes that may suggest early organ disease. Since many of these pets are in the middle- to geriatric-age interval, evaluations and early detection for other organs and hormonal disease (i.e., diabetes mellitus, hyperthyroidism, etc.) is important to document.

- **Urinalysis:** Early changes in urinary components (i.e., protein, blood glucose, etc.) and the kidney's abilities to concentrate urine and filter the bloodstream properly may be an early indicator of renal or hormonal diseases (see Chapter 13).

Key Points in Discussing the Need for a Complete Diagnostic Baseline with a Client

- With moderate to severe dental disease, the accumulation of calculus represents a large accumulation of bacteria that the body must deal with on a daily basis.

- Over years, these bacteria can seed into the bloodstream, producing disease in other organs of the body, primarily the heart, kidneys, and liver.

- To properly evaluate the effect of the dental disease and establish if the patient is a good candidate for anesthesia, general blood work is recommended to detect early changes in the kidneys and liver as well as the other organ systems in the body.

- **Dental radiography:** With dental radiography technology and equipment becoming less expensive and more available, many medical teams are finding dental radiography units a necessary diagnostic tool. Dental x-rays can be used to evaluate broken and chipped teeth, periodontal disease, oral masses (tumors), and jaw fractures (see Figure 9.13).

  — The ability to assess the tooth and roots radiographically can help detect the presence of early infection and abcessation.

  — The pet can then be spared chronic dental infection and tooth loss when these changes are noted early and proper cleaning and medical treatment is completed.

Key Points in Discussing the Need for Dental X-Rays with a Client

- Just as with the human dentist, dental radiographs allow the veterinarian to evaluate the teeth for early dental changes, as well as examine regions below the gum line that may have infection and abcessation.

- Because pets cannot tell us about teeth sensitivity and pain, routine dental radiography allows the medical team to evaluate and detect problems early to prevent chronic dental pain, tooth loss, and infection.

- The pet must be under general anesthesia to take dental x-rays. The pet will not remain still and hold the film in the mouth while awake.

The Professional Dental Prophylaxis

Performing a professional **dental prophylaxis (cleaning)** is an important part of preventative care and prolonging the life span of the pet. Chronic dental disease can cause weight loss, chronic pain, and decrease in their quality of life, leading to secondary disease in the heart, kidney, or liver. Even with such long-term health concerns, severe dental health problems often go completely unnoticed by the owner. The following parameters should be used when discussing dental disease with the owner and recommending a dental procedure.

When to Recommend a Dental Procedure

Although dental disease can affect any breed at various stages in life, the following factors may help distinguish which patients are most likely to need dental care.

Predisposing Factors

- **Age of animal**: Dogs and cats as young as 3 years of age can form cavities, get tooth root infections, and develop infections of the gums (**periodontal disease**).

- **Signalment:** Short-faced (**brachiocephalic**) breeds (i.e., pug, bulldog, etc.) can have increased dental calculus and disease due to improper alignment and crowding of teeth in the shortened muzzle.

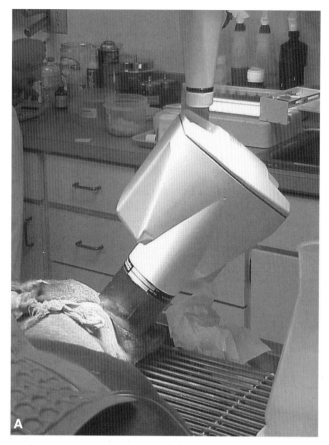

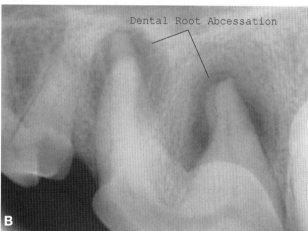

Figure 9.13. With more dental radiography units available, it becomes easier to detect dental disease and infection (a). The radiograph of the fourth premolar shows a dark halo around the roots, indicative of root abcessation (b). (Reprinted by permission of Curt Coffman, DVM ACVD, Aid Animal Clinic, 7908 E. Chapparral, Suite 108, Scottsdale, Az 85250.)

- **Health status of the animal**: Animals with immunosuppressive diseases (feline leukemia virus, feline immunodeficiency virus, etc.) will have accelerated dental disease since the normal protective mechanisms of the body are slowed or impeded by their infection.

- **Diet**: Animals that eat only canned food may have increased dental disease because there is very little abrasive contact of the diet with the teeth.
- **Abnormal dietary elements**: Animals that are chronic rock eaters and tennis ball players can have increased dental wear and fractured teeth, leading to pain and infection.

Evidence of Dental Disease
As outlined earlier in the chapter, animals with mild to moderate changes in dental calculus, gingivitis, or evidence of significant dental lesions should have professional dental prophylaxis.

The Components of a Thorough Dental Examination
Anesthesia
Anesthesia allows complete cleaning and examination of all the surfaces of the teeth above and below the gum line. This is not possible in an awake animal. Professional dental prophylaxis involves the use of ultrasonic scalers that use small particles of water to clean the teeth. The patient is placed under full anesthesia with an endotracheal tube in place to prevent the water particles and bacteria from passing into the trachea and lungs.

Protective Gear
As the veterinary technician/assistant is cleaning the heavy dental calculus and bacteria from the teeth, the ultrasonic cleaner produces a fine mist of bacteria-laden water. It is important to wear protective equipment covering the eyes, nose, and mouth. Further protective gloves should be used to prevent exposure of cuts and scrapes that could allow the bacteria to seep into the body (see Figure 9.14).

Dental Cleaning
The components of a thorough professional dental prophylaxis should include a thorough oral examination in which the oral cavity is checked for dental lesions and pathology. Each tooth is probed and checked for pockets that could suggest the beginning of periodontal disease, early tooth abcessation, or weakening of the teeth (see Figure 9.15).

- **Rinsing:** The mouth should be rinsed with an antibacterial solution such as chlorhexidine prior to the prophylaxis. This will reduce the bacterial levels that the technician and patient are exposed to during the prophylaxis.
- **Ultrasonic cleaning and hand scaling:** Plaque and calculus are cleaned from the tooth surfaces using ultrasonic and hand-scaling instruments.
- **Polishing:** Dental polishing removes the microscopic scratches produced from the dental cleaning to help prevent new calculus formation (see Figure 9.16).
- **Dental radiographs:** After the pet's teeth are cleaned, dental x-rays are taken of any abnormal teeth, regions of periodontal disease, or any other diseased oral tissue.
- **Perioceutic treatments:** If there are periodontal pockets

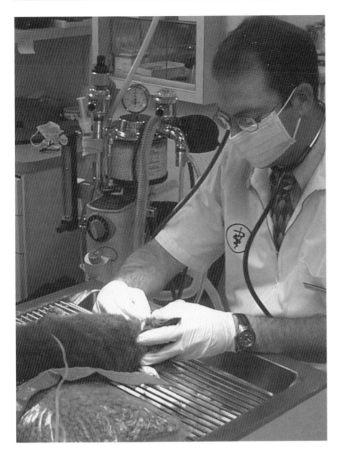

Figure 9.14. The proper protective eyewear, gloves, and mask should worn to protect the team member performing dental procedures. (Reprinted by permission of Curt Coffman, DVM ACVD, Aid Animal Clinic, 7908 E. Chapparral, Suite 108, Scottsdale, Az 85250.)

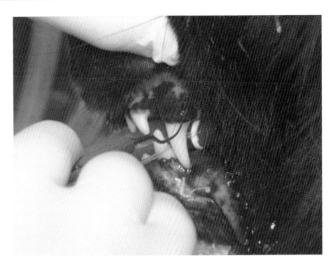

Figure 9.15. Careful probing of the gums around the tooth can suggest early disease.

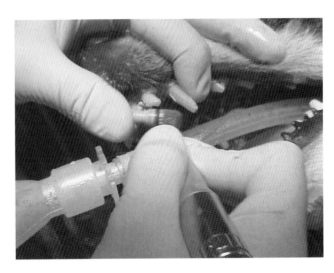

Figure 9.16. Polishing the teeth after an ultrasonic cleaning is very important for preventing a premature formation of calculus on the microscopic scratches produced by the ultrasonic cleaner. (Reprinted by permission of Curt Coffman, DVM ACVD, Aid Animal Clinic, 7908 E. Chapparral, Suite 108, Scottsdale, Az 85250.)

within the gums around the pet's teeth, these regions may be treated with a long-acting antibiotic polymer that helps control infection and decrease the pocket size.

- **Tooth extraction:** Some teeth can be severely infected and mobile and may be so weakened that they must be extracted to reduce pain and infection.
- **Dental charting:** Problems identified during the dental prophylaxis are recorded on a dental chart. Treatments performed, such as extractions or perioceutic treatments, are also recorded. The dental chart becomes part of the patient's medical record.
- **Dental aftercare:** Dental aftercare can take many different forms, including pain management, antibiotics, and tooth brushing to help prevent reoccurring dental problems.
  — **Antibiotic medications:** With moderate to severe dental disease, large amounts of bacteria can be released into the bloodstream when the teeth are cleaned. Antibiotics can be prescribed to help heal the mouth and reduce the amount of bacteria that can enter the system circulation.
  — **Pain medications:** Pain management is especially important when dealing with dental extractions. Pain con-

trol should be prescribed using pain medications (i.e., buprenorphine or other opioids) or anti-inflammatory medications (i.e., carprofen, meloxicam)

- **Preventative care:** There are many types of dental preventative care that aid in decreasing recurrence of dental disease and maintaining good oral health. Some available dental products are:
  — dental toothbrush and toothpaste,
  — antiseptic oral rinses,
  — enzymatic dental chews, and
  — diets and biscuits.

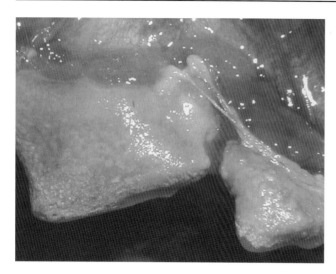

Figure 9.17. Clinical signs of swollen inflamed gums, pus and debris around the teeth, receding gums, and potential pockets under the gum line all suggest periodontal disease is present in these upper premolars in a dog. (Reprinted by permission of Curt Coffman, DVM ACVD, Aid Animal Clinic, 7908 E. Chapparral, Suite 108, Scottsdale, Az 85250.)

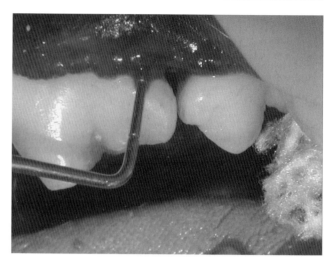

Figure 9.18. Image of red swollen gums bleeding when the gum line is probed. This indicates gingivitis and a periodontal pocket. (Reprinted by permission of Curt Coffman, DVM ACVD, Aid Animal Clinic, 7908 E. Chapparral, Suite 108, Scottsdale, Az 85250.)

Periodontal Disease

Periodontal disease is a process that causes destruction of the supporting structures around the teeth. These supporting structures include the gums (**gingiva**), the bone that forms the tooth socket (**alveolar bone**), and the connective tissue that attaches the tooth into the tooth socket (**periodontal ligament**). In people, periodontal disease is often called gum disease.

Etiology
The primary cause of periodontal disease is bacteria. As plaque and calculus build on the teeth, it forms an ideal environment in which disease-causing bacteria multiply. These bacteria gradually invade the gums and other supporting tissue around the teeth. When the bacteria invade below the gum line, they cause infection and inflammation leading to the destruction of the periodontal tissues (see Figure 9.17).

Common Signalment
All breeds of dogs and cats can develop periodontal disease. Many of the smaller breeds of dogs may be predisposed due to crowding and malocclusion of the teeth. Some purebred cats also seem to be more commonly affected.

Common Points in History
In the early stages of the disease the pet may show no signs other than mild redness of the gums. As the disease progresses the buildup of calculus on the teeth becomes easily visible. Pet owners may describe symptoms of:
  — oral pain,
  — bleeding from the gums (see Figure 9.18),

  — swollen gums,
  — bad breath (halitosis),
  — anorexia or decreased appetite, and
  — salivation.

Common Points on Initial Assessment
- Visible calculus on the teeth
- Bad breath (halitosis)
- Swollen gums
- Bleeding from the gums
- Teeth that appear loose
- Pus and debris around the teeth

Complications
In advanced cases periodontal disease can weaken the gum tissue and bones surrounding the teeth, leading to recession of the gums, bone loss, and eventually tooth loss.

Diagnosis
Diagnosis of periodontal disease is based on the presence of the clinical signs listed above and the diagnostics discussed next.

Radiographs
Dental x-rays are essential in determining the extent of periodontal disease once it progresses below the gum line. Dental x-rays will show destruction of the supporting bone around the teeth in areas of moderate to severe periodontal disease (see Figure 9.19).

Periodontal Probing
A special instrument called a periodontal probe is used to evaluate for periodontal disease and to measure periodon-

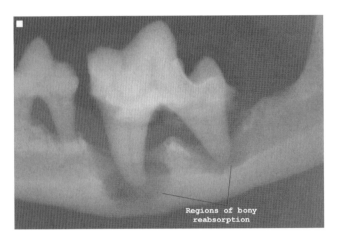

Figure 9.19. A dental x-ray shows advanced periodontal disease around the lower first molar in a dog. (Reprinted by permission of Curt Coffman, DVM ACVD, Aid Animal Clinic, 7908 E. Chapparral, Suite 108, Scottsdale, Az 85250.)

tal pockets and areas of gum loss around the teeth (see Figure 9.20).

Treatment of Periodontal Disease

- **Dental cleaning**: Early stages of periodontal disease need thorough, professional teeth cleaning above and below the gum line.

> ### How to Discuss Periodontal Disease with the Client
> - Periodontal disease is a disease of the gums and other tissues surrounding the teeth. Studies have shown that over two-thirds of dogs and cats over 2 years of age have some level of periodontal disease.
> - If untreated, periodontal disease will lead to painful, bleeding gums, chronic infection, and tooth loss.
> - Common breeds affected are small and miniature breed dogs and purebred cats.
> - Periodontal disease can be prevented by keeping the pet's teeth clean. Although home tooth brushing, dental chews, and dry food are very important, professional teeth cleaning while the pet is under anesthesia is the only way to ensure all surfaces of the tooth are cleaned.

Clinical Diagnostics
Periodontal probing and dental x-rays are necessary to determine of the extent of periodontal disease.

Prevention
Good dental hygiene to prevent plaque and calculus buildup is the goal for prevention of periodontal disease. Daily tooth brushing at home, as well as regular professional teeth cleaning at the veterinary hospital are necessary.

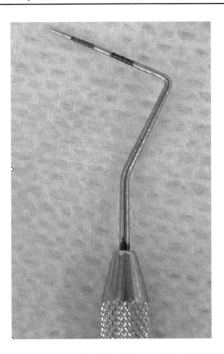

Figure 9.20. Periodontal probe with a graduated tip for measuring periodontal pockets. (Reprinted by permission of Curt Coffman, DVM ACVD, Aid Animal Clinic, 7908 E. Chapparral, Suite 108, Scottsdale, Az 85250.)

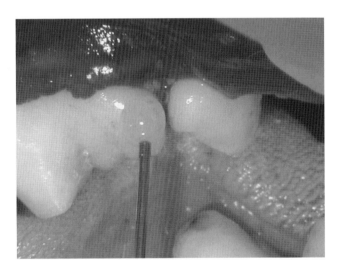

Figure 9.21. Perioceutic treatment of a periodontal pocket in a dog. (Reprinted by permission of Curt Coffman, DVM ACVD, Aid Animal Clinic, 7908 E. Chapparral, Suite 108, Scottsdale, Az 85250.)

- **Medications: Perioceutic antibiotics** are used for treatment of periodontal pockets (see Figure 9.21). **Oral antibiotics** are often prescribed after professional cleaning with moderate to severe dental periodontal disease.
- **Home care:** The pet owner must perform tasks such as daily tooth brushing and oral rinsing to prevent recurrence of the disease.

- **Prevention:** Good dental hygiene and home tooth brushing will help prevent periodontal disease. Even pets with no established periodontal disease need their plaque and calculus removed by professional prophylaxis to prevent the onset of periodontal disease.

Retained Deciduous Teeth in the Young Animal

Dogs and cats can begin to lose baby (deciduous) teeth at 3–4 months of age and should lose all remaining baby teeth by 6–8 months of age. In some pets, baby teeth can take longer than 8 months to fall out. Retained teeth can cause malocclusions, periodontal disease of the gums, and trauma and injury to the mouth. These retained teeth can also cause accelerated plaque formation on surrounding teeth as well as be painful or irritating to the gums. If deciduous baby teeth are present in the pet's mouth once the adult teeth begin to erupt, they should be removed surgically (extracted).

Retained baby teeth are a developmental problem caused by improper alignment of jaws or teeth that produces crowding and malocclusions, leading to periodontal disease and pain.

Common Signalment

Retained teeth are more common in smaller breeds of dogs (i.e., pugs, Lhasa apsos, poodles, etc.). They are less common in large breed dogs and cats.

Common Points in History

These pets may have no physical complaints or symptoms of the retained teeth. Occasionally, pets may show dental pain or sensitivity if the deciduous teeth are cutting into the gums.

Common Points on Physical Exam

- Presence of a deciduous tooth once the adult tooth has already erupted
- Increased plaque and calculus on adult teeth
- Halitosis (due to calculus buildup)
- Irritated red gums
- Indents or holes in gums and jaw secondary to misplaced teeth
- Malocclusions

Complications

If the retained teeth are not removed at a young age, they can increase dental calculus formation on the adult teeth. They also will cause malocclusion of the adult teeth, leading to increased dental wear and continued oral pain.

Diagnosis

The presence of baby teeth in a pet's mouth at the same time as the counterpart adult tooth indicates the abnormality.

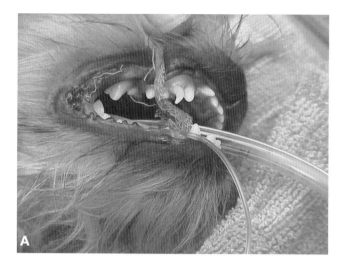

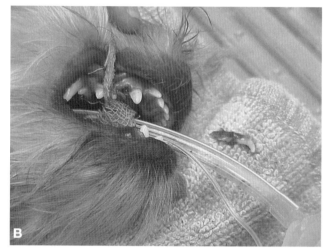

Figure 9.22.   Image of retained canine tooth on the side of mouth (a). Image of retained tooth removed (b). (Reprinted by permission of Curt Coffman, DVM ACVD, Aid Animal Clinic, 7908 E. Chapparral, Suite 108, Scottsdale, Az 85250.)

Treatment

With the pet under general anesthesia, the deciduous teeth are extracted (see Figure 9.22).

Prevention

There is no way to prevent retained baby teeth. Treatment is indicated as soon as the problem develops.

Carnassial Tooth Root Abscess

The upper fourth premolars and lower first molars are the largest teeth in an animal's mouth and are called **carnassial teeth**. Each tooth has two to three roots and can become severely infected if injured, broken, or affected with advanced periodontal disease. The upper carnassial teeth have tooth roots close to a large sinus, called the **maxillary sinus.**

Discussing Retained Deciduous Teeth with the Client
- Retained deciduous teeth occur in pets with overbites, underbites, and poor teeth alignment in which the baby teeth are not in a normal position to be pushed out when the adult teeth erupt.
- Retained deciduous teeth frequently occur in small and miniature breeds where jaw malalignments are more common (i.e. pugs, Lhasa apsos, teacup poodles).
- Without proper care and treatment, these baby teeth can cause dental pain, irritation of the gums, and accelerate the formation of dental calculus and periodontal disease.
- The presence of a baby tooth in the mouth at the same time as the adult counterpart tooth is abnormal and treatment is recommended.
- Treatment is focused on removal (extraction) of the baby teeth under anesthesia.

Etiology

The large carnassial teeth can be injured as the pet chews on bones, rocks, or other hard materials. If the tooth is cracked or fractured, bacteria from the mouth may invade inside the tooth, causing infection leading to a root abscess. A root abscess can also be caused by advanced periodontal disease around the tooth. The infection can progress from the root to the maxillary sinus, causing a swelling or open sore below the eye.

Common Signalment

Carnassial tooth root abcessation can occur in any feline or canine with moderate to severe periodontal disease or broken, fractured teeth.

Common Points on Medical History

As with general dental disease, the pet will show a common history of dental pain and infections, including these symptoms.

- Halitosis
- Chronic nasal discharge
- Change in appetite (not eating dry food as well as/or only wet food)
- Complete anorexia
- Chronic weight loss
- Chronic vomiting
- Eating abnormally, such as
  — rolling food to other side of mouth,
  — excessive salivation while eating, and
  — wincing while eating.

Common Points in Initial Assessment

When the pet develops a severe infection of these roots, the sinus also becomes infected and fills with pus and debris, causing the following signs.

- Focal facial swelling around eye and cheek area
- A swelling with an area of purulent (pus) drainage
- Salivating
- Bad odor present
- Pain on palpation of tooth or side of the face
- Obvious fracture of the fourth premolar or first molar

Complications

Without proper treatment and care, root abscess can produce chronic nasal and sinus infection, dental pain, and chronic periodontal disease. These complications can cause anorexia, weight loss, and other organ diseases.

Diagnosis

Diagnosis of a carnassial tooth root infection is based on physical signs, diagnostic blood work, and dental radiographs.

Treatment

- **Professional dental prophylaxis:** A thorough dental cleaning and oral examination are performed to remove the calculus, polish the teeth, and explore the oral cavity for evidence of infection or disease.

How to Discuss Carnassial Tooth Root Abscess with the Client
- Carnassial tooth root infection is an infection of the root of the large premolar or molar teeth of the cat or dog.
- The large teeth roots are closely associated with the nasal passage and sinuses.
- Chronic infection from dental disease produces a focal swelling and draining tract above the upper premolar or below the lower tooth and produces chronic swelling and purulent discharge.
- Diagnosis of a carnassial tooth abscess depends on the history and physical signs, as well as blood work and dental x-rays (see above discussion on diagnostics).
- Proper dental prevention, such as brushing the teeth, oral rinses, and special diets or treats can help reduce dental plaque and calculus. This can aid in the reduction of periodontal disease. Avoiding hard bones, chews, or toys that can cause tooth injury will prevent fractures of the teeth.

- **Dental extraction**: In some cases, due to severe root abscesses and damage to the tooth, the veterinarian may recommend extraction of the affected tooth.
- **Root canal and crown:** Another option is to remove the nerves and infected pulp from the affected tooth by performing root canal treatment and crown restoration.
- **Antibiotics and pain medications**: Long-term antibiotics are indicated to help resolve the infection. Pain medication is needed to reduce pain or sensitivity after the oral surgical care.

Gingival Hyperplasia

Gingival hyperplasia refers to excessive growth or enlargements of the pet's gums (gingiva). The size of the growth may be small to large and may appear vegetative to firm and/or solid. There can be single or multiple masses.

Etiology
The exact cause of the disease is unknown. The surrounding teeth usually have plaque and calculus buildup. Although the gums do not have to be inflamed, inflammation is typically associated with chronic dental disease.

Common Signalment
There is a predisposition shown in the boxer and possibly the great Dane, collie, Doberman pinscher, and Dalmatian. It has been shown in association with administration of primidone and cyclosporine.

Common Points on Medical History
Often the pet will show no signs, but lesions are seen either on the preanesthetic exam or during the oral exam while the pet is under anesthesia. However, symptoms can occur if the pet bites down on the swollen tissue, producing

- oral pain,
- bleeding from the mouth,
- halitosis,
- anorexia, and
- salivation.

Common Points in Physical Exam
- Bad breath
- Presence of an enlarging gum or masses around the teeth
- Bleeding from the gums
- Teeth that appear loose around the mass area

Complications
Gingival hyperplasia can lead to periodontal disease weakening tissue surrounding the teeth. This can cause recession of the gums, bone loss, and ultimately tooth loss.

Diagnosis
Diagnosis is based on the presence of excessive gum tissue, gingival mass, or swelling of the gums and the following further diagnostics.

- **Radiographs:** Both dental and skull x-rays aid in determining if teeth are affected and if any of the surrounding bone is also showing changes.
- **Biopsy:** Depending on the size and location of the gingival mass or gingival swelling, your veterinarian may suggest attaining a biopsy to diagnose the disease.

Treatment
Initially, if the pet is on any drugs that may make them predisposed to this type of disease, the medication should be discontinued. Surgery is then generally elected to remove the excessive gingiva or mass for biopsy and diagnosis (see Figure 9.23). Repeat procedures may need to be performed because gingival hyperplasia often reoccurs.

Prevention
Good dental hygiene to reduce dental infection may help prevent gingival hyperplasia.

> **How to Discuss Gingival Hyperplasia with the Client**
> - Gingival hyperplasia is a redundancy or overgrowth of the gums typically associated with chronic dental disease.
> - Although typical masses of gingival hyperplasia are benign, these regions can enlarge, leading to periodontal disease, and can become focally destructive to the surrounding teeth and underlying bone.
> - Common breeds affected are the boxer, great Dane, collie, Doberman pinscher, and Dalmatian.
> - Also, pets that have been on primidone or cyclosporine (Atopica) may be prone to the disease.
> - Diagnosis of gingival hyperplasia is based on physical presence of excessive gingiva or gingival mass, dental radiographs, and biopsy of the growth.
> - Good dental hygiene to prevent chronic dental infection can help slow the recurrence of gingival hyperplasia.

Root Canal Treatment and Crown Restoration

In cases where a large tooth, such as a canine, large molar, or premolar tooth, is infected or damaged, the medical team may suggest a root canal and a crown restoration.

This endodontic procedure performed by veterinarians with advanced training in dentistry can be less traumatic and invasive than extraction and maintains a functional nonpainful tooth. The procedure involves removing the sensitive part of the tooth (pulp) from the center of the tooth (root canal).

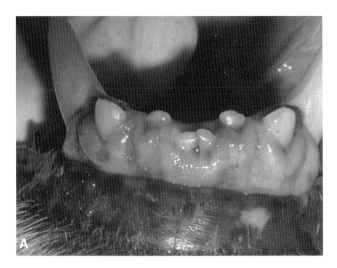

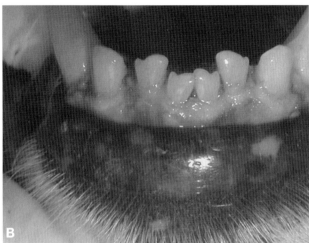

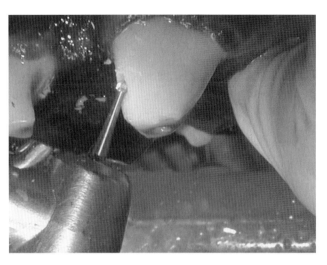

Figure 9.24. A broken canine is opened using a dental drill to remove the diseased pulp. (Reprinted by permission of Curt Coffman, DVM ACVD, Aid Animal Clinic, 7908 E. Chapparral, Suite 108, Scottsdale, Az 85250.)

Figure 9.23. Gingival hyperplasia in a dog (a). Image of the same gums after treatment (b). (Reprinted by permission of Curt Coffman, DVM ACVD, Aid Animal Clinic, 7908 E. Chapparral, Suite 108, Scottsdale, Az 85250.)

The root canal procedure involves several steps.

- The root canal is opened and the nerve (pulp) is removed. (see Figure 9.24).
- The tooth is disinfected, dried, and a filling material is applied to seal the inside of the root canal (see Figure 9.25).
- The tooth surface is then restored with a hard dental filling material (see Figure 9.26).
- In some cases a metal crown is placed to further protect the tooth (see Figure 9.27).

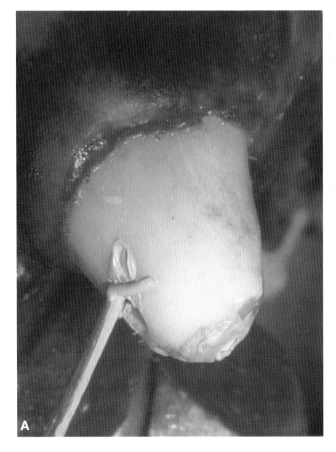

Figure 9.25. A filling material called gutta percha is added to seal the disinfected canal (a).

Discussing Root Canal Treatment with the Client

- When dealing with larger infected or broken teeth, such as a canine or larger molar or premolar, there are dental treatment options other than removal of the tooth.
- Just as in humans, the root canal can be treated and the nerve (pulp) removed to block pain and sensitivity.
- Once completed, a crown can be placed over the tooth to maintain dental strength and prevent further breakage.
- After a crown is in place, the tooth must be monitored and cleaned regularly to ensure the long-term success of the root canal and crown restoration.

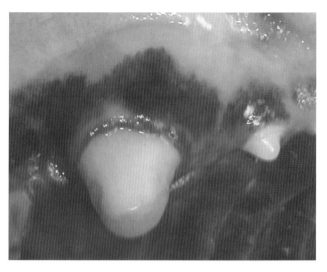

Figure 9.26. This tooth has been restored with a tooth-colored dental composite filling. (Reprinted by permission of Curt Coffman, DVM ACVD, Aid Animal Clinic, 7908 E. Chapparral, Suite 108, Scottsdale, Az 85250.)

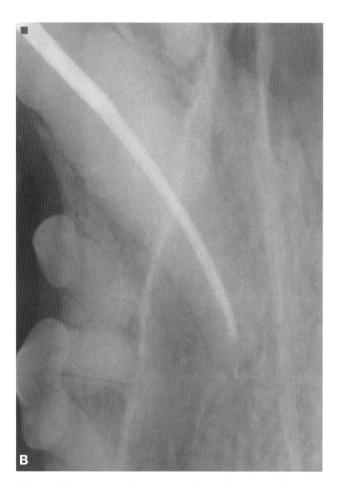

Figure 9.25. (*continued*) A radiograph is taken to visualize the pulp cavity and prepped root canal (b). (Reprinted by permission of Curt Coffman, DVM ACVD, Aid Animal Clinic, 7908 E. Chapparral, Suite 108, Scottsdale, Az 85250.)

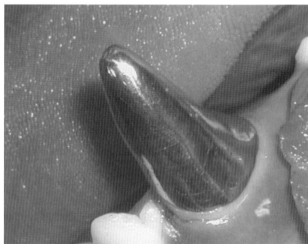

Figure 9.27. Image of the metal crown over the canal-treated tooth. (Reprinted by permission of Curt Coffman, DVM ACVD, Aid Animal Clinic, 7908 E. Chapparral, Suite 108, Scottsdale, Az 85250.)

CD-ROM 1 reviews material presented in this chapter. Please try the cases for Section 2 (Anatomy and Physiology—The Science behind the Diseases) to help reinforce the information presented here.

Chapter 10

Gastrointestinal System

Introduction

As discussed in the last chapter, the gastrointestinal system is a specialized tube running from the animal's mouth to its rectum. The main functions of this system are to break down and absorb foodstuffs, reabsorb water to form well-formed feces, and excrete toxins from the kidneys and liver. Closely associated with the intestinal system are specific glands to aid in absorption of nutrients and toxin removal.

- The **pancreas** (Chapter 15) produces pancreatic enzymes that facilitate the breakdown of foodstuffs. Enzymes such as **lipase,** which breaks down fats, and **amylase,** which aids in the breakdown of sugars, gain access to the small intestine through a common tubular system, the **pancreatic duct** and the **accessory pancreatic duct**, which drains the pancreas and the liver**.**
- The **liver** (Chapter 14) secretes toxins that are stored in the gallbladder and are then excreted into the intestines through the **common bile duct**.

The intestinal tract is innervated by a complex nervous system. This organization of intestinal muscles and nerves is as complicated as the central nervous system and is responsible for complex movements of food through the intestinal tract. A special muscular lining of smooth muscle within the muscle wall helps propel and churn the food by a process called **peristalsis.**

Anatomy of the Gastrointestinal System

The gastrointestinal system is broken down into common regions: mouth, esophagus, stomach, small intestine, and large intestine. Each region has its own specific anatomy, function, and disease processes. It is important to gain understanding of the unique anatomy and physiology of each region to better understand the diseases that can affect each area.

As discussed in Chapter 9, the **mouth (buccal cavity), teeth,** and the **salivary glands** are the beginning of the digestive process. The overall function of the mouth and early digestive tract is to break down food into smaller molecules that can then be digested. Thus proteins are broken down into smaller amino acid chains, fats are broken down into triglycerides, and complex sugars are broken down into simple, small-unit sugars. To do this, the animal relies on its teeth to break down the large foodstuffs into smaller units where the intestinal system can facilitate digestion. Also, the mouth secretes saliva to help emulsify food into a liquid solution and contains chemicals (enzymes) to begin the breakdown process.

Once the food leaves the mouth (**oral cavity**), it enters the **esophagus (see Figure 10.1)**. The esophagus is a muscular tube that stretches from the back of the mouth (**pharynx**) to the stomach. It is divided into three segments covering the neck (**cervical region**), the chest (**thoracic region**), and the stomach (**abdominal region**). The esophagus is a thick, well-muscled section of striated muscle where the lumen is closed by deep, lengthwise longitudinal folds that constrict and propel food into the stomach. The esophagus enters the stomach by a thick muscular sphincter called the **cardiac sphincter,** which prevents stomach acid and contents from flowing back into the esophagus.

The **stomach** is a large dilation of the gastrointestinal tract between the esophagus and small intestine. It lies between the diaphragm and liver on the left side of the abdomen (see Figure 10.2). The stomach produces hydrochloric acid (HCl), which helps to break up food's chemical bonds. The food then passes into the small intestine for further digestion. The stomach also produces other enzymes, which further break down foodstuffs into smaller molecules. Overall, the stomach has limited absorptive abilities, but rather moves food into the small intestine for absorption. Food leaves the stomach through a thick muscular sphincter called the **pyloric sphincter.**

The **small intestine** is a tube that connects the stomach to the cecum and large intestine. It consists of three parts: the **duodenum,** the **jejunum,** and the **ileum**. The **duodenum** is a short S-shaped tube leaving the stomach from the pylorus. It contains the opening of the common bile duct, and pancreatic ducts empty into this region, bringing digestive enzymes from the pancreas and waste from the liver (see Figure 10.2)**.** The **jejunum** makes up about 90% of the total length of the small intestine and serves as a major site of absorption. Its internal lining (**mucosa**) has many repeating surface folds that increase surface area to help increase the amount of nutrients the jejunum can absorb. Finally, the **ileum** is a shortened section of intestines that runs from the jejunum to the large intestine (colon and cecum). The ileum has limited absorptive ability but can serve as a site of bac-

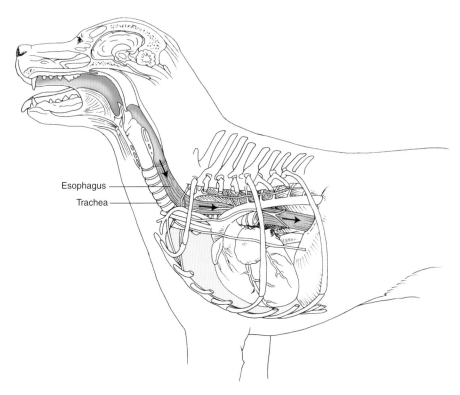

Figure 10.1. Image of the esophagus as it moves from the back of the mouth, through the neck, and into the chest, where it meets the stomach in the cranial abdomen.

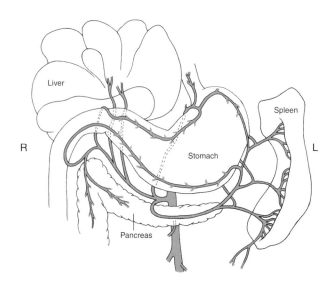

Figure 10.2. Normal anatomy of the liver, stomach, spleen, and pancreas. The gallbladder empties its toxins and the pancreas empties its digestive enzymes through a common small duct, the common bile duct, which empties into the duodenum.

terial fermentation. The entire intestinal system is suspended from the top of the abdomen by a sheet of connective tissue called the **mesentery** (see Figure 10.3).

The ileum empties into a small vestigial region of the intestines called the **cecum,** which is closely related to the human appendix. It is a blind sack situated between the ileum and large colon and is virtually inactive in the small animal (with exception is the rabbit).

The cecum then enters into the **colon** or **large intestine.** The large intestine is broken into the ascending loop, the transverse loop, and the descending loop. Overall, it functions to absorb water from the remaining ingesta to produce well-formed fecal material. This function helps prevent dehydration. The large intestine also can serve as a site of limited microbial fermentation, producing the B vitamins and vitamin C.

Obtaining a History for Gastrointestinal Disease

The goal of obtaining a history and performing a physical examination is to determine the location of the intestinal disease and choose proper diagnostic tools to aid in diagnosis. There are many diseases that secondarily affect the intestines causing vomiting and diarrhea (e.g., kidney disease, liver disease, diabetes, etc.) However, this chapter is concerned with determining the diseases that primarily affect the gastrointestinal system. Due to the complexity of the types of gastrointestinal disease, it becomes extremely important to get a detailed history from the client. Guidelines for obtaining an accurate history are discussed next.

What is the Duration of the Illness?
Acute onset of severe disease suggests animals are suddenly affected by an infectious, obstructive, or metabolic disease

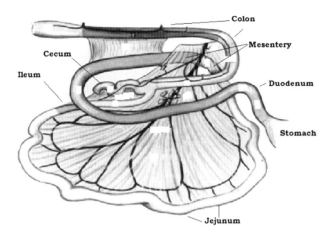

Figure 10.3. Normal intestinal anatomy. (Courtesy of *Anatomy of Domestic Animals,* 7th Edition. Pasquini, Chris, and Pasquini, Susan. Sudz Publishing, Pilot Point, Tx 1989. Used with permission from Sudz Publishing.)

that produces a wide progression of vomiting, diarrhea, or anorexia. Although the pet can be severally dehydrated and sick, most of these pets do not show chronic signs of weight and muscle loss, emaciation, or wasting.

In a **chronic disease** state animals can have a long-time history of vomiting, diarrhea, and decreased appetite to periods of anorexia. Chronic disease can also be produced from long-term inflammatory, metabolic, or neoplastic disease of the intestinal system. Due to the length of illness, these pets usually have history of weight loss and emaciation.

What Is the Pet's Diet or Has There Been a Sudden Change in Diet?

Many gastrointestinal upsets can start with sudden changes in diet or improper diets; therefore, it is important to get a full understanding of exactly what the pet is eating. Some guideline questions follow.

What Brand, Type, and Form of Diet Is Fed?

Each veterinary team may have their favorite type of diet they recommend. Whether it is IVD, Iams/Eukanuba, Hills, etc., is not the overall concern. However, clients who switch from one brand to another of the same type of diet (i.e., adult, puppy) may randomly produce gastrointestinal signs due to the difference in the dietary components.

Diet types can be puppy, adult, senior, or hypoallergenic diets. Some diseases can occur or be made worse when the pet is being fed the wrong type of diet for its life stage or medical condition.

For example, some clients may bring a pet in for chronic weight loss. When questioning the client, they inform the team member that the pet is on a weight-reducing diet because another pet in the household has chronic obesity issues. This pet is on the wrong type of diet.

Some prescription diets for health conditions are only meant for short-term administration. Over months to years,

these diets can produce serious health issues. Understanding the goal of the diet and the health concerns of the pet are key to making sure the pet is on the correct prescription.

Forms of diet can be dry, canned, or semimoist.

- Canned and semimoist diets are highly palatable and easily digestible. These types of diets are high in carbohydrates and can accelerate dental disease and obesity issues.
- A dry diet is better for oral and dental health, overall. On occasion, in smaller pets, larger chunks of dry food can become obstructive to the oral cavity or esophagus.

Sudden changes in diet, even from one similar type of food to another, can produce serious gastrointestinal disease: vomiting, diarrhea, anorexia, and flatulence.

Does Your Pet Get Human Food or Table Scraps and If So, What?

It is very important to ask, specifically, how much and how often human food is available to the pet. Clients vary dramatically on what they feel is reasonable for their pet (i.e., a teaspoon of ice milk once in a while versus splitting a half-gallon of banana ice cream with their pet).

Did the Animal Get into the Trash?

Many animals have access to trash and debris. Exposure to trash, bones, and other debris can lead to serious gastrointestinal and pancreatic disease. Furthermore, if the pet does get into the trash, is it a kitchen trash, bathroom trash, or trash from another room? Kitchen trash can contain food remains, wrappers, and other consumables; bathroom trash may contain medication, razors, and other dangerous goods.

Has the Pet Been Given a Bone or Had Exposure to Bones?

Pets with exposure to bones can have severe irritation to the intestines, possible obstruction, or even perforation from the sharp edges.

Does the Pet Eat Unusual Things?

Animals that eat abnormal things can easily become obstructed. Some common materials causing obstructions are

- toys,
- shoes,
- strings/tinsel/yarn (especially cats),
- balls,
- underwear/stockings,
- baby nipples,
- corn cobs, and
- foam packing material.

Are There Any Poisons or Plants That the Pet Could Get Into?

Many clients do not understand that many plants and medications that are commonly available in a household may be severely toxic to animals. Being as specific as possible with the client helps the client understand what type of toxic agents may be of concern.

Poisons

There are numerous poisons that produce gastrointestinal signs; some are

- antifreeze,
- cleaners,
- fertilizer,
- rat poison,
- gopher bait, and
- snail bait.

Medications

There are many over-the-counter and prescription medications that owners give their pet that may produce severe gastrointestinal signs, especially in the cat. Some of these drugs are

- aspirin,
- acetaminophen (i.e., Tylenol),
- ibuprofen,
- naproxen, and
- prednisone.

Plants

Almost all plants can produce gastrointestinal signs; however, some plants with some more serious side effects include

- mushrooms,
- oleander,
- poinsettia, and
- dieffenbachia.

Is There Pain When Eating?

As discussed in Chapter 9, pain or sensitivity while eating can suggest dental or oral disease. Some questions to help determine oral pain or sensitivity are as follows:

- Does the pet roll the food in its mouth?
- Is there excessive drooling when eating?
- Is there facial swelling?
- Is there trouble swallowing?
- Did the patient stop eating dry food and is now eating only canned food?

Is the Pet Regurgitating or Vomiting?

This is one of the most important questions when beginning a medical case.

Regurgitation

- Regurgitation is the mechanical process of food being brought back up that has remained in the esophagus.

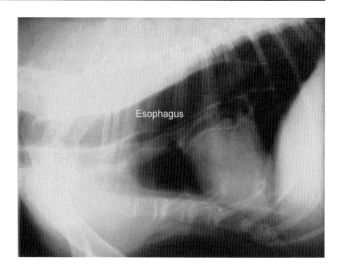

Figure 10.4. Radiographic image of a dilated megaesophagus above the trachea and heart; this animal would present regurgitating, not vomiting.

- It is a passive process, where the animal simply opens the mouth and the food comes out with abdominal contraction.
- **Regurgitation suggests esophageal disease,** not stomach or intestinal disease.
- Typically, regurgitation is a sign of a pathologically dilated esophagus (**megaesophagus**) that is unable to contract to push food down into the stomach (see Figure 10.4).
- Megaesophagus can be secondary to chronic gastrointestinal disease or other systemic diseases.
- With chronic megaesophagus, food lies in the esophagus for hours until the pet opens its mouth and the food comes out.
- Many affected pets can have severe secondary **aspiration pneumonia,** because food particles can enter the trachea and lung fields as the pet regurgitates.

Vomiting

Unlike regurgitation, vomiting is an active contracture of the abdomen and stomach producing a violent forceful return of food. When determining if there is vomiting, the following guidelines are also important to document.

- **How many times per day is the pet vomiting?** As a general rule, animals that vomit multiple times per day (more than five times) can suggest severe disease. Repeated multiple vomiting can quickly overwhelm a patient and produce dehydration.
- **Is the vomiting associated with eating or drinking?** When animals vomit spontaneously without an association of food and water, it can suggest a severe gastrointestinal (i.e., intestinal foreign body/obstruction) or metabolic disease. These pets have a severely inflamed intestinal tract that continues the vomiting reflex without oral stimulation.

Table 10.1. Comparing small vs. large bowel disease.

Signs	Small Intestine	Large Intestine
Consistency	Cow patty to liquid	Liquid or squishy
Force	Nonstraining	Straining
Amount	Increased	Normal to decreased
Blood	Black/tarry	Fresh
Mucus	No	Yes

Table 10.2. Triage concerns in the gastrointestinal patient.

Systems	Signs Indicating an Emergency
Mentation	Depressed or lethargic animals that are mildly to nonresponsive
Fever	Temp >104.5° or <99.5° Fahrenheit
Hydration	Dehydration >5–7%
Gum color	Pale pink
	White
	Yellow
	Red
	Blue or gray
Capillary refill time (CRT)	CRT >2–3 seconds
Abdominal pain	Any animal that vocalizes, winces or becomes aggressive when the abdomen is lightly palpated

- **Is any blood present in the vomit?** The evidence of blood suggests moderate inflammation and ulceration of the stomach and intestinal mucosa. Blood in the vomit can suggest a more serious intestinal disease.
- **Is any foreign debris present in the vomit?** Evidence of foreign material in the vomit can suggest the cause of the irritation and symptoms.

Is Diarrhea Evident and If So, What Type?

When assessing gastrointestinal disease with diarrhea, it becomes imperative to differentiate large bowel and small bowel disease, since diagnostic tests and treatment can be dramatically different. The nature and consistency of the diarrhea can tell us the location and, potentially, the types of disease occurring. Although a pet may have disease of both the small or large bowel, it is important to document what the main type of diarrhea seen is (see Table 10.1).

Small Bowel Diarrhea

As stated previously, the small intestine's main function is to digest and absorb nutrients. When the small intestine is unable to complete this task, the following symptoms are noted:

- Soft cow patty diarrhea to liquid
- Increased odor
- Black or tarlike feces suggesting digested blood
- Ravenous appetite
- Weight loss
- Normal to increased amounts of feces

Small bowel diarrhea can be associated with chronic disease of the pancreas or small intestine. These pets usually present as bright, alert, and responsive, but eat ravenously and can be very thin to emaciated because of their inability to digest food normally.

Large Bowel Diarrhea

The large bowel's primary function is to reabsorb water from the ingesta to produce well-formed stool. When the colon is not functioning properly, the following symptoms are noted:

- Liquid
- Fresh/frank blood
- Mucus
- Straining

Although large bowel diarrhea can be seen chronically, an inflammation of the large bowel (**colitis**) is typically associated with an acute inflammatory change brought on by gastrointestinal or systemic disease.

Is Coughing, Sneezing, Increased Thirst, or Increased Urination Evident?

Coughing, sneezing, increased thirst, and increased urination can suggest infectious disease or other system disease that produces secondary gastrointestinal signs.

What Is the Vaccination Status of the Pet?

Young pets with no to limited vaccination history are more prone to parvovirus infections.

Observations on Initial Assessment

The main goal of the initial assessment is to ascertain if the pet is in an emergency status and how seriously the pet is affected (see Table 10.2). The basic tenets of the initial assessment for the gastrointestinal system are discussed next.

Mentation

The less responsive the dog, the more potentially serious and life threatening is the case. Animals with depression, stupor, or coma should be evaluated immediately by the medical team.

Temperature

Changes in body temperature can suggest both cause and severity of the underlying disease.

- A **fever (hyperthermia)** can suggest infection or inflammation resulting from massive whole-body infections (**sepsis**) caused by parvovirus infection, ruptured intestines, and ingestion of toxins and poisons, and other causes.

- **Low body temperature (hypothermia)** can be an even greater concern, because the animal is unable to fully maintain its metabolic process to keep body temperature normal. In this case, hypothermia can be caused by
  — shock or massive infection,
  — massive dehydration, and
  — metabolic disease, such kidney disease, liver disease, diabetes.

Dehydration

With gastrointestinal disease, dehydration can be an important indicator of serious pathology. Animals that have significant gastrointestinal acute losses can become life-threateningly dehydrated in a few hours.

- All animals with moderate diarrhea/vomiting are assumed to be **at least 3–5% dehydrated.**
- Most dehydrated animals do not adequately eat and drink secondary to depression. With persistent vomiting and diarrhea, these animals can become life-threateningly dehydrated.

Gum Color/Capillary Refill Time

With severe dehydration from gastrointestinal losses, capillary refill time (CRT) could be prolonged and may suggest serious underlying disease. **CRTs of more than 2–3 seconds should be reported to the medical team immediately.**

Abdominal Pain/Palpation

Increased abdominal tenderness can suggest severe abdominal disease. If the abdomen is extremely painful, the medical team should be notified, and the patient should be evaluated quickly by the veterinarian.

Clinical Diagnostics of the Gastrointestinal System

Diagnostic tests depend on the history, physical signs the pet presents with, and the physical examination findings. Not all clinical tests are indicated with each case.

Getting a Fecal Sample and Doing a Fecal Examination

Any time there is a diarrheal condition, taking a fecal sample is strongly recommended. There are many ways of doing a fecal examination. The most common are discussed here.

Fecal Floatation

One of the most common fecal screenings done allows the feces to be examined for parasite eggs (see Chapter 23).

- The feces are placed in a tube with a very dense liquid (i.e., with zinc sulfate) solution and mixed thoroughly and allowed to sit for 15 minutes.
- Any intestinal parasite eggs will float to the top of the solution and be trapped on a coverslip.

Fecal Smear

A small amount of feces is mixed with saline on a microscope slide and a coverslip is applied (see Chapter 23.). The fecal material is examined for specific protozoa (i.e., giardia) and other microscopic single-cell parasites that can be seen only in the wet saline preparation.

Fecal Cytology

The feces are spread on a slide and heat fixed (see Chapter 23). The slide is then stained with Wright-Giemsa or Gram stain preparation. The feces are then examined for abnormal bacteria and white blood cells that could suggest infection or disease.

Fecal Culture

Occasionally, the medical team will obtain multiple fecal samples to culture for fecal bacterial pathogens (e.g., salmonella, campylobacter, etc.) that can cause bacterial enteritis.

Enzyme-Linked Immunoassay Tests

Enzyme-linked immunoassay (ELISA) tests allow the feces to be checked for the presence of surface molecules (**antigens**) on specific pathogens that are being shed within the feces. The meaning of the results follow.

- A positive result suggests that the pet has been exposed to and is currently infected with the infectious agent.
- A negative test does not rule out the infection, because the pet may not have enough antigen of the infectious agent to produce a positive test.
- Multiple ELISA tests may be necessary to confirm an infection.

Key Points in Discussing the Need for a Fecal Exam with the Client

- If a pet is coming in for a diarrhea or gastrointestinal problem, recommend they bring in a fresh fecal sample (less than 2 hours old).
- Fecal exams are generally recommended to detect parasites and other abnormalities in the feces.
- There are several different types of fecal diagnostic tests that aid the veterinarian in detecting intestinal parasites or infection.
- Some animals may need repeated fecal exams to allow proper detection of the parasite or problem since some infections can be chronic and evident only in low numbers in the intestinal tract.
- When checking a fecal ELISA test, a negative result does not always rule out the possibility of the disease. ELISA tests help to confirm the disease, but at times the pet may not be shedding sufficient antibody levels against the infectious agent to turn the test positive.

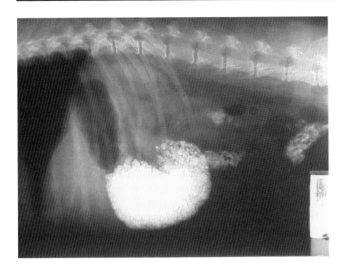

Figure 10.5.   X-ray of the stomach and small intestines filled with a radio-dense foreign material (rocks).

ELISA tests are now available to check for the presence of

- giardia,
- *Clostridium perfringens,*
- cryptosporidium, and
- parvovirus.

Radiographs
Radiographs are a key diagnostic tool of gastrointestinal disease (see Chapter 25). There are two basic radiographic studies that aid in assessment of the abdomen.

Study I: Plain Film Radiograph
The plain abdominal radiograph will help detect the following (see Figure 10.5):

- Radio-dense foreign body (rock, metal)
- Dilation in the intestines suggestive of obstruction by non-radio-dense material (i.e., clothing, plastic, wood)
- Abdominal masses
- Organ enlargement
- Other abnormalities

Study II: The Upper Gastrointestinal Radiographic Series
The upper gastrointestinal radiographic series is a further diagnostic test that allows the intestines to be evaluated for an obstruction, mass, or ulceration that would not show up on a normal radiograph.

- Initially, after the two plain abdominal films are taken, the animal is administered barium, a radio-dense liquid that will show up on radiographs (see Figure 10.6).
- Radiographs are taken over the next 0–8 hours at regular intervals, and the flow of barium is monitored through the intestinal tract.
- If the barium gets to a specific location and stops, an obstruction or mass may be suggested.

- It is important to understand the lack of advancement of the barium is not always suggestive of an obstruction.
  - With some severe intestinal disease, the normal peristaltic movement of the intestine is interrupted (**ileus**). In some cases, severe ileus prevents normal flow of the barium through the intestines, making it appear as if there is a foreign body present.

Key Points in Discussing the Need for a Radiographic Evaluation with the Client
A radiograph study is being recommended

- to address concerns regarding abdominal tenderness;
- to appreciate the region of the abdomen behind the rib cage that cannot be effectively palpated by the veterinarian for any changes suggestive of obstruction or abdominal disease; and
- to appreciate changes to organs and the abdomen (i.e., stones, areas of enlargement, masses, fluid, etc.) that cannot be evaluated without a radiographic image.

Radio-dense material such as stones, bones, and metal will be visualized in the intestines. There are certain materials and items that will not show up on a plain film x-ray. Items such as cloth, plastic, wood, and other non-dense items may not be seen. However, the veterinarian is also examining for changes in the intestinal pattern, that could suggest a soft tissue obstruction.

If your pet still is vomiting and a plain film radiograph does not conclusively show an obstruction, a barium series (an upper gastrointestinal test) may be needed.

- Barium is administered to the pet orally or by stomach tube.
- Barium is an opaque radio-dense liquid that will accentuate the stomach and intestines and allow the veterinarian to evaluate the barium's flow through the intestines over time.
- If the barium fails to move through the intestines in a set amount of time, or if there are areas that continue to have uptake from the barium, it could be suggestive of a mass or obstruction.

Ultrasound Examination
An abdominal ultrasound can aid in the detection of abnormalities within the intestines or the accumulation of abdominal fluid that could be suggestive of a intestinal perforation (see Chapter 25; see also Figure 10.7).

Endoscopy
Under anesthesia, a fiber-optic camera can be passed into the stomach/early duodenum or large colon (see Chapter

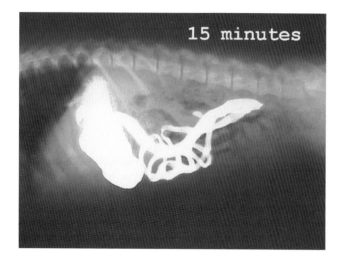

15 minutes

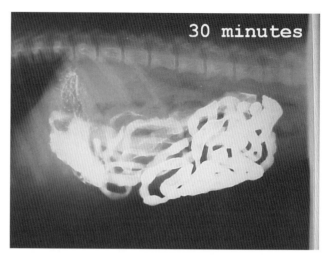

30 minutes

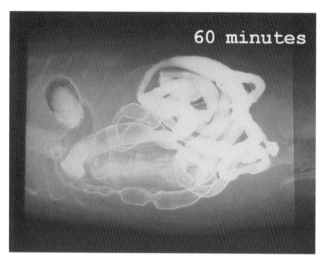

60 minutes

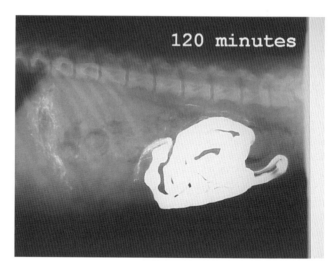

120 minutes

Figure 10.6. Radiograph of an upper gastrointestinal study. Note how the barium accentuates the stomach and small intestines.

25). Images of these regions can then be produced and small sections of masses or intestinal wall can be taken for biopsy.

Abdominal Tap

The abdominal tap is performed when there is suspicion of fluid in the abdomen. If there is an intestinal perforation, abdominal fluid can be greenish brown with a fetid odor. On microscopic examination, there can be the presence of degenerate white blood cells, bacteria, and food particles.

Diseases of the Intestinal System

Although not all diseases are mentioned below, the common diseases are discussed, with the main goal being to understand and be able to explain to the client what the diseases are, how they can present themselves, and what can be the overall short- and long-term concerns of each disease. Any discussion of overall diagnostic and treatment protocols should be discussed based on the recommendations of the doctor and the medical team. Please use the following infor-

mation as a basis to discuss and educate the client, **but never to diagnose a patient.**

Intestinal Parasites

Intestinal parasites are responsible for significant disease and death in animals. Parasites that live within the intestines are called **endoparasites.** Some common endoparasites are

- protozoa: giardia, cryptosporidium;
- cestodes: tapeworms;
- trematodes: flukes; and
- nematodes.
  - — roundworms
  - — hookworms
  - — strongyles
  - — whipworms

Life Cycle

Certain parasites can survive and reproduce in only one species (**host specific**), whereas others are capable of infect-

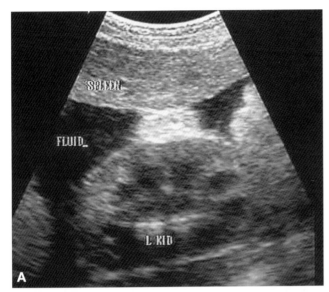

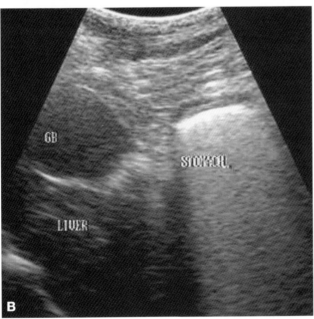

Figure 10.7. Ultrasound images allow the evaluation of the internal architecture of organs, thickness of intestines, and checking for other abnormalities within the abdomen.

ing many species. The basic parasitic **life cycle** has multiple life stages.

- Stages are egg → larval form (L_1 → L_6) → adult phases → eggs.
- The third larval form (L_3) is usually the infectious life stage.
- Most life cycles have a phase where they live in the environment (**environmental phase).**

Vectors

A vector is a third-party organism that carries the larval stage to allow proper maturation to its infectious state. The parasite is then introduced to the host by ingestion of the vector or bite/sting of the vector to the primary host. For example, tapeworms must mature in small fleas or rodents before becoming infectious to the dog or cat. The infected flea or rodent is ingested by the pet, and the pet begins to shed tapeworms in their stool.

Expression of Disease

The damage to the host from the infection is dependent upon parasite load on the intestine, location of the parasite in the host, production of toxins from the parasite, and interference with normal physiological processes within the intestine.

There are many animals with asymptomatic infections of parasites. These pets are still shedding the parasite and infecting the environment. Furthermore, these pets can be more severely affected by other gastrointestinal disease if a parasite is also involved.

Parasitic Infections

Hookworms (Ancylostoma caninum, Uncinaria steno-cephala)

Hookworms are a collection of nematode parasites that cause moderate to severe gastrointestinal infection and potentially severe anemia.

Life Cycle

1. The hookworm is transmitted by ingestion of the parasite or by skin penetration from a contaminated environment.
2. The eggs hatch in the environment and produce a small larval parasite, which burrows into the skin or is swallowed.
3. The parasite then migrates through the body into the bloodstream and into the lung fields.
4. It then matures into adult and migrates up the bronchi and trachea, where it is coughed up and then swallowed.
5. Once in the intestinal tract, the parasite latches on to the lining of the small intestine, absorbs the partially digested nutrients, and upsets the stable beneficial bacteria in the gut.
6. As it feeds, it begins to shed eggs into the environment to begin the entire cycle again.
7. The parasite causes the pet to not absorb food properly (**malabsorption syndrome**), and the hookworm's sharp, pointed mouth piece attached to the intestine produces moderate to severe hemorrhagic disease.

Etiology

The cause of the disease is a collection of small microscopic parasites (6–20 mm) from the genera *Ancylostoma* and *Uncinaria.*

- The parasite is commonly found in dogs and cats and is more likely in young pups than adult dogs.
- Kenneling situations increase the prevalence of the disease.
- Pregnant animals can pass the infections to their young through the placenta.

Signalment

Canines and felines can have hookworm infection without any age, sex, or breed predilection. Younger animals are more prone to acute severe disease, whereas older patients may have chronic, more subtle disease.

Common Points in History

These animals can be severely depressed and weak with general complaints of:

- vomiting,
- diarrhea (usually with blood),
- anorexia, and
- dry cough.

Common Points in Initial Assessment

The parasite generally causes acute disease in young animals so severe it can mimic parvoviral infection (see below). In the older pet, hookworms can produce more chronic or intermittent signs. Common signs of hookworm infection are

- dark, tarry stools;
- pale gum color;
- constipation;
- debilitation (secondary to diarrhea), especially in the young or newborns;
- decreased appetite;
- dry cough;
- severe bloody diarrhea with or without vomiting;
- severe anemia; and
- **sudden death.**

Complications: Zoonotic Disease

In contaminated areas, this parasite can infect humans. The larval form burrows through the skin, causing erosive paths usually seen in the feet or legs (**cutaneous larval migrans**).

Diagnosis

- Diagnosis of hookworm infections is based largely on the observation of the hookworm eggs in the feces (see Figure 10.8).
- Young animals with severe infections usually have large numbers of eggs present on the fecal floatation.
- Because hookworms can produce a severe hemorrhagic diarrhea, the veterinarian may also suggest other diagnostics (i.e., parvoviral ELISA test) to make sure the pet isn't dealing with multiple infections.

Treatment

The goal of treatment is to **deworm** the patient with medications that will eradicate the adult worms and to provide supportive care, as follows:

- **Fluid support**: Due to severe fluid losses producing dehydration, some patients may require some form of fluid therapy (i.e., intravenous fluids, subcutaneous fluids).

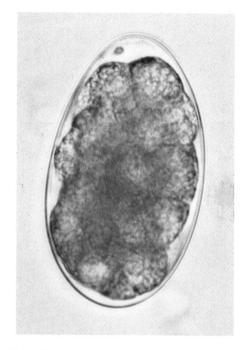

Figure 10.8.   Image of the hookworm egg under high magnification.

- **Blood products:** In very young small pets, the blood loss may be so severe that the pet may require a transfusion of blood products to help replace the losses that have been sustained.

Prevention

Prevention is focused on routine fecal screening in adult and young pets to detect hookworms in asymptomatic animals to prevent disease and contamination of the environment. Further monthly heartworm preventatives (Heartguard Plus, Interceptor) can also help to eliminate low-lying infection and prevent reinfection.

Roundworms (Ascariasis)

Roundworms are serious infections that cause moderate to severe gastrointestinal infection, especially in newborn puppies and kittens.

Life Cycle

1. The parasite is transmitted by ingestion of eggs from a contaminated environment.
2. The eggs hatch in the small intestine and produce a small larval parasite.
3. It then matures into a large adult, which decreases intestinal movement and utilization of food, causing diarrhea and poor body condition.
4. **A pregnant animal can pass the infection to its offspring through the placenta, causing newborn animals to be born with a preexisting infection.**

5. The eggs can also be passed by the ingestion of infected rodents.

Etiology

The cause of the disease is a collection of a small microscopic parasite from the ***Toxocara*** genus.

- The parasite is commonly found in dogs and cats and is more likely in young pups than adult dogs.
- Kenneling situations increase the prevalence of the disease.
- **The larva can cross the placenta and infect embryonic pups and can be passed in milk as well.**

Common Points of History

Toxocara infection can produce mild to moderate intestinal disease. However, older animals can have mild to moderate numbers of roundworms without evidence of an infection. Common complaints are,

- anorexia,
- bloating, and
- small amount of fecal production.

Common Points in Initial Assessment

The parasite generally causes acute disease in young animals and more chronic or intermittent signs in adults. Common signs are

- abdominal distention,
- poor body condition—emaciation,
- gas pain,
- passing adult worms in the feces (looks like spaghetti),
- vomiting adult worms, and
- **sudden death in neonates.**

Complications: Zoonotic Disease

- There is a serious zoonotic potential for the parasite to infect humans in contaminated areas through the ingestion of the eggs.
- People that ingest contaminated feces (especially raccoon or other wild carriers) may develop the disease.
- The larva migrates through tissue and organs potentially causing a serious liver or kidney disease (**visceral larval migrans**).

Diagnosis

Diagnosis of roundworm infections is based largely on the observation of the roundworm eggs or adult worms in the feces (see Figure 10.9).

Treatment

The goal of treatment is to **deworm** the patient with medications that will eradicate the adult worms and to provide supportive care. Due to severe fluid losses producing dehydra-

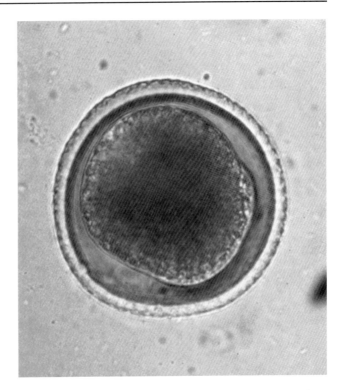

Figure 10.9. Image of the roundworm egg under high magnification.

tion, some patients may require some form of fluid therapy (i.e., intravenous fluids, subcutaneous fluids).

Prevention

Prevention is focused on routine fecal screening in adult and young pets to detect roundworms in asymptomatic animals to prevent disease and contamination of the environment and reduce the zoonotic potential to humans. Further, monthly heartworm preventatives (Heartguard Plus, Interceptor) can also help eliminate low-lying infection and prevent reinfection.

Whipworms

Whipworms are a serious infection that causes moderate to severe gastrointestinal infection.

Life Cycle

1. The parasite is transmitted by ingestion of eggs from a contaminated environment.
2. The eggs then hatch in the small intestine and produce a small larval parasite.
3. The worm matures into a large adult, which decreases intestinal movement and utilization of food, causing bloody diarrhea and poor body condition.
4. The adult worms begin producing eggs that are then passed into the feces and into the environment.

5. **The eggs have a thick outer coating, which can make them survive in the environment for months to years.**

Etiology
The cause of disease is a collection of small microscopic parasites from the *Trichuris* genus.

- The parasite is commonly found in the cecum of dogs, foxes, coyotes, and other canines and is more likely in young pups than adult dogs.
- Kenneling situations increase the prevalence of the disease. The eggs are passed into the environment and have a very thick shell, making them survive in the environment for years.

Common Points in History
- The parasite generally causes acute disease in young animals, producing a history of diarrhea, anorexia, and poor condition.
- Chronic or asymptomatic disease can be evident in the older pet without significant symptoms.

Common Points in Initial Assessment
Common signs of whipworm infections are

- abdominal distention,
- gas pain,
- bloody diarrhea, and
- poor body condition.

Complications
Without proper deworming and environmental control, whipworm infestation can be a long-standing problem.

Diagnosis
Diagnosis of whipworm infections is based largely on the observation of the eggs in the feces (see Figure 10.10).

Treatment
The goal of treatment is to **deworm** the patient with medications that will eradicate the whipworms and provide supportive care. Some form of fluid support may be needed in young pups that become dehydrated and malnourished secondary to infection.

Prevention
Prevention is focused on routine fecal screening in adult and young pets to detect roundworms in asymptomatic animals to prevent disease and contamination of the environment. Further, monthly heartworm preventatives (Heartguard Plus, Interceptor) can also help eliminate low-lying infection and prevent reinfection.

Giardia (Giardiasis)
Giardia is a microscopic protozoal parasite that causes mild to moderate gastrointestinal infection.

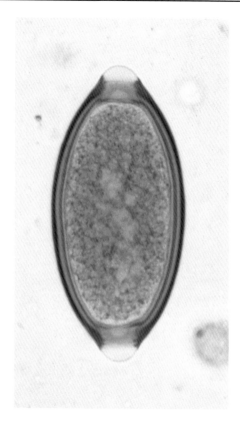

Figure 10.10. Image of the whipworm egg under high magnification.

Life Cycle
1. Giardia exists in the environment in small eggs called **cysts** that live in contaminated water and soil.
2. Once ingested, the cysts then produce a motile protozoon, which infects the small intestine (see Figure 10.11).
3. The parasites absorb the partially digested nutrients and upset the stable, beneficial bacteria in the gut.
4. These cause the pet to not absorb food properly (**malabsorption syndrome**).

Etiology
The cause of the disease is a small microscopic one-celled bacterium-like parasite called **giardia**.

- The parasite is more commonly found in dogs than cats and more likely in young pups than in adult dogs.
- The parasite can also be seen in contaminated water and soil sources.
- Kenneling situations increase the prevalence of the disease.

Common Points in History
The parasite can cause acute, chronic, or intermittent signs of disease. In general, when the pet is affected by giardia, common medical complaints can be

- diarrhea, soft or liquid;
- vomiting (occasionally);
- anorexia; and
- increased flatulence or gas.

Common Points in Initial Assessment
Common signs of animals with clinical giardiasis are

- increased flatulence or gas,
- diarrhea, and
- dehydration (occasionally).

Complications
Giardiasis can affect humans; however, human infections largely come from contaminated water supplies.

Diagnosis
Diagnosis of giardia infections is based largely on the observation of the protozoa in fecal smear or on a giardia ELISA test (see Figure 10.11).

Treatment
The goal of treatment is to **deworm** the patient with medications that will eradicate the giardia and to provide supportive care. Occasionally dehydrated pets will need fluid support.

Prevention
Prevention is focused on routine fecal screening in adult and young pets to detect protozoa.

Cleaning up standing water and puddles can decrease the transmission of giardia into the environment.

Tapeworms
Tapeworms are a minor intestinal infection that causes small tapeworm segments to be passed in the stool and some hind end pruritis.

Life Cycle
- The parasite is transmitted by ingestion of fleas or rodents (**vectors**) infected with the larval form of the tapeworm.
- Once ingested, the larva infects the dog and cat and grows to adult in the large intestine.
- The worms are passed into the environment and picked up by the vector to become infective to a new host.
- The eggs are stored in the worm segments and are very rarely seen in a fecal exam.

Etiology
The cause of the disease is collection of a small microscopic parasite from the genera **Taenia** and **Diplydium**. The parasite is commonly found in dogs and cats.

Common Points in History
Since tapeworm infection causes low-lying or asymptotic disease, generally the only complaints are

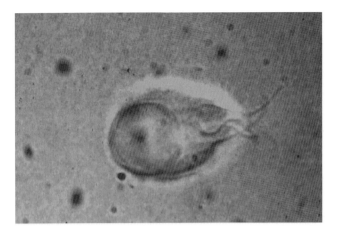

Figure 10.11. Image of giardia adult protozoa under high magnification.

- seeing the adult "rice-shaped" worm, and
- pets scooting on their hind ends.

Common Points on Initial Assessment
Generally the pet shows no evidence of physical change except the observation of the tapeworms themselves.

Complications
Animals can become reinfected if re-exposed to the vector (flea or rodent).

Diagnosis
Diagnosis of tapeworms is based on the presence of the adult worm in the feces or tapeworm egg seen on fecal float (rare) (see Figure 10.12).

Treatment
The goal of treatment is to deworm the patient with medications that will eradicate the tapeworms. It is possible for clients to see dead tapeworms passed days after deworming.

Prevention
The goal of prevention is to

- control and eliminate flea populations, and
- prevent animals from hunting rodents.

Coccidia
Coccidia are a collection of parasites that cause mild to moderate gastrointestinal infection.

Life Cycle
1. Eggs are passed into the environment.
2. The eggs are ingested and the larvae hatch within the intestinal system.
3. The larvae grow into adults and begin to pass eggs into the feces.

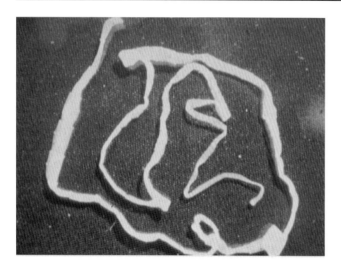

Figure 10.12. Image of an adult tapeworm. The tapeworm eggs are carried in the body segments of the adult.

Etiology

Coccidial infections are from the genus **Isospora**. Canines carry *Isospora canis* and felines carry *Isospora felis*. These parasites are host specific and are not infectious to other species. **Cryptosporidium** is a very small parasite that is also being found to produce severe diarrhea in young animals.

Common Points in History

Coccidial infections cause general mild signs of diarrhea, anorexia, and bloated abdomen.

Common Points on Initial Assessment

Except in very young patients, animals appear to be within normal limits. Young neonates may appear weak.

Complications

Animals can become reinfected by ingesting ova in contaminated environments.

Diagnosis

Diagnosis of *Isospora* is made by demonstration of the small ova on fecal cytology and smear. Due to the minute size of *cryptosporidium*, diagnosis is done by ELISA antigen testing of the feces (see Figure 10.13).

Treatment

The goal of treatment is to **deworm** the patient with medications that will eradicate the tapeworms.

Prevention

Coccidia infections can be reduced through reducing environmental contamination of fecal debris.

Key Points in Discussing Intestinal Parasites with Clients

- Most intestinal parasites cause a mild to moderate gastroenteritis, producing diarrhea, anorexia, and sometimes vomiting.
- In younger animals, hookworms and roundworms can produce a more life-threatening disease with dramatic vomiting and diarrhea that can sometimes mimic parvoviral infection.

Recommending a Fecal Sample

- Even when no worms are seen, most parasites are microscopic and infections can be severe.
- Even though newborns are not exposed to the environment, they can get an infection from their mother in utero or from her milk.
- With diarrhea and, sometimes, vomiting, a fecal sample should always be examined.
- Even if the animal is wormed with a general wormer, there are parasites (giardia, coccidia, and tapeworms) that will respond only to prescription medication.
- Even if other fecal examinations have been done, it sometimes takes multiple fecal exams to identify a disease-producing parasite. Some chronic infections can be produced by low numbers of parasites.

Zoonotic Disease

Hookworm (cutaneous larval migrans) or roundworm infections (visceral larval migrans) are produced by either oral ingestion (roundworms) or physical contact with contaminated feces. These syndromes can produce skin damage or internal injury. The best way to control these diseases is by limiting contamination of the environment through a regular parasite control program for the patient.

Intestinal Obstructive Disease

Esophageal Foreign Bodies

An esophageal foreign body is a foreign nondigestible item that gets lodged within the esophagus.

Etiology

The cause of disease is swallowing a nondigestible foreign material that becomes lodged within the esophagus. Objects can vary vastly: bones, toys, balls, and other items (see Figure 10.14).

Signalment

Although any pet can get an esophageal obstruction, it is most commonly seen with young dogs.

Common Points in History

Patients with an esophageal foreign body can show mild to severe signs. The pet's symptoms can be subtle with a possible

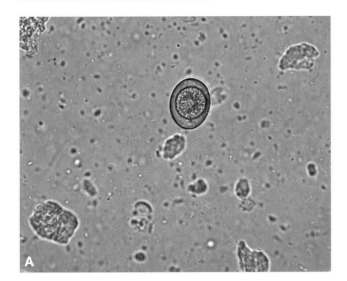

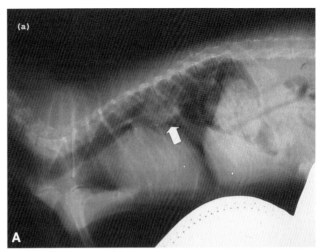

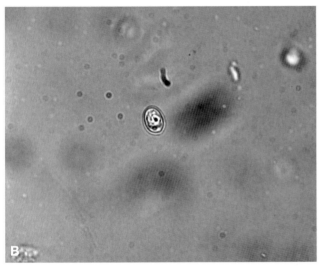

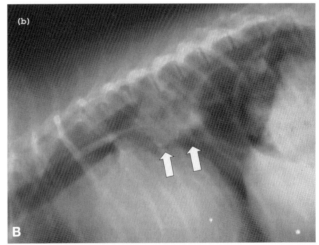

Figure 10.14. Radiograph of esophageal foreign body above the heart base (a). Enlargement of the same image of object stuck within the esophagus (b).

Figure 10.13. Image of the coccidia oocyte under high power (a). Image of cryptosporidium under high magnification (b).

change in temperament, attitude, or a history of swallowing foreign material. Common complaints with this disease are

- regurgitating (not vomiting);
- drooling;
- extending the neck;
- trying to swallow hard, having pain while swallowing; and
- anorexia.

Common Points on Initial Assessment
Common symptoms are

- trying to swallow repeatedly,
- drooling,
- respiratory distress,
- pain while swallowing, and
- extending the neck.

Complications
If the esophageal foreign body is not removed, the mass can produce esophageal perforation or can produce severe scarring and narrowing of the esophagus (**esophageal stricture**).

Diagnosis
Diagnosis of esophageal foreign bodies is based on the history, physical examination, and radiographs.

- **Plain film radiographs:** These radiographs can often detect dilation of the esophagus and the foreign body.
- **Barium swallow**: If the foreign material does not show, the barium, flow will stop or outline the potential obstruction. Barium should only be used if regurgitation is not of concern.

Treatment

The goal of treatment is removal of the foreign body from the esophagus. The approaches to removal are by endoscopy and/or surgery.

Ideally, removal of the foreign material with the use of an endoscope is highly recommended.

- This is a noninvasive anesthetic procedure where the endoscope shows the foreign material and either removes it through the mouth or pushes the material into the stomach.
- The endoscope can also inspect the esophagus for perforation, ulceration, or strictures.
- The owner will need to be informed that if the mass cannot be removed with the endoscope, surgery may be indicated.

Depending on the location of the foreign body (neck, chest, or abdomen), surgery may be required and entry may be through the chest and ribs. This procedure, called a **thoracotomy**, is a very complicated procedure. Furthermore, the esophagus does not heal well after surgery, and esophageal strictures can be common side effects.

Prevention

The goal of prevention is to limit access of foreign material for animals that have a history of eating unusual objects.

Gastrointestinal Foreign Body (Gastric/Intestinal)

A gastrointestinal foreign body is an acute syndrome brought on by the consumption of foreign material that is obstructing the stomach or small intestine.

Etiology

The cause is a soft or rigid obstruction that partially or completely obstructs the stomach or small intestine (see Figure 10.15).

Signalment

Although any pet can get an intestinal obstruction, it is most commonly seen with young dogs.

Common Points in History

Classically, animals with an obstruction of their stomach or small intestine have the following complaints:

- Vomiting
- Anorexia
- Depression

Common Points on Initial Assessment

Animals with potential foreign bodies have the following physical changes:

- Depression
- Vomiting (usually excessive)

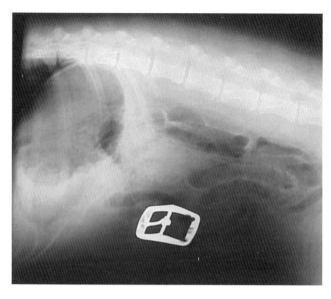

Figure 10.15. Radio-dense foreign bodies are easy to detect on plain film radiographs.

- Tender painful abdomen
- Constipated and straining to defecate
- Unable to hold down food or water
- Dehydrated and weak

Complications

If not properly treated, the obstruction can wear through the intestine causing intestinal rupture and massive infection of the abdomen (called **peritonitis**). Peritonitis can be life threatening.

Diagnosis

Diagnosis is made based upon history, physical exam, plain film radiographs, and/or a barium series.

Treatment

The goal of treatment is removal of the foreign body from the stomach or small intestine. Approaches to removal are as follows:

- **Inducing vomiting:** If caught early, with some soft tissue foreign bodies (i.e., clothing, paper products) the veterinarian may induce vomiting to bring up the foreign material before an obstruction can occur.
  — Care must be taken by the veterinarian to select the proper candidates for induction of vomiting.
  — Inducing vomiting on jagged or irregular material may risk esophageal obstruction.
  — Furthermore, inducing vomiting in patients that have swallowed petroleum products (i.e., gas) may produce a stomach or intestinal rupture.
- **Endoscopy:** In some cases, with specific foreign material, a fiber-optic endoscope can be passed into stomach

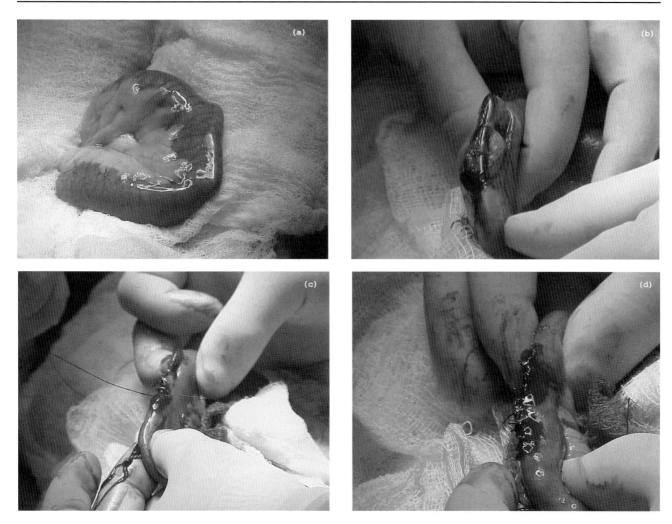

Figure 10.16.   When removing a foreign body from the intestines, the section of intestine is packed off with "lap" sponges from the rest of the abdomen (a), the intestine is then opened, and the foreign body removed (b). The intestine is then surgically closed with absorbable sutures (c), and the intestines are evaluated for damage or leakage from the incision site (d).

to remove a foreign body. As with the esophageal procedure, the owner will need to be informed that the mass may not be able to be removed with the endoscope and surgery may be indicated.

- **Surgery:** Exploratory surgery is recommended for obvious (radio-dense) masses of the stomach and small intestines that are not removable by endoscopy. Further surgery is indicated if the pet has undergone a barium study and the barium is suggestive of an obstruction. Key points to exploratory surgery are discussed next.

With a radio-dense foreign body (stones, rocks, bones, etc.) the following procedure is followed (see Figure 10.16).

- The abdomen is entered surgically and the veterinarian exteriorizes and visualizes the intestine and stomach and locates the foreign body obstruction.
- The affected intestine is isolated and opened and the foreign body is removed.

- The intestine is then surgically closed and the abdomen copiously rinsed (**lavaged**) with sterile fluids to decrease the risk of infection.
- The veterinarian will assess the intestinal tract for evidence of severe damage or perforation. Any severely injured intestine may require surgical removal of the affected section.

With possible non-radio-dense foreign bodies (i.e., fabric, plastic, plant material, etc.),

- the goal of surgery is to evaluate the stomach and intestinal tract for possible obstruction;
- if an obstruction is found, then the material will be removed as discussed in the section above; and
- if there is no obvious obstruction, the veterinarian may elect to take intestinal tissue for biopsies to determine the cause of the disease.

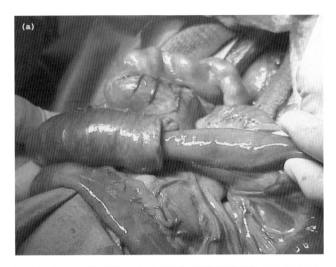

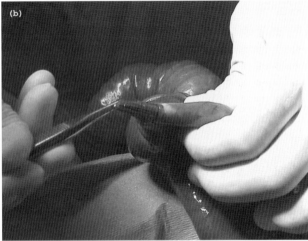

Figure 10.17. Image of an intestinal intussusception (a) caused by a sock foreign body (b).

Prevention
The goal of prevention is to limit access of foreign material for animals that have a history of eating unusual objects.

Intussusception
An intussusception is an invagination of a section of small intestine into another adjoining section, causing an obstruction. These areas of intussusception can occur in the small or large intestine (see Figure 10.17).

Etiology
In most cases, there is no known cause of the disease (**idiopathic**). However, it has been associated with

- inflammation of the intestines (**enteritis),**
- intestinal foreign bodies,
- abdominal surgery,
- heavy intestinal parasites,
- intestinal masses,

- parvoviral infection, and
- other causes.

Signalment
Intussusceptions are most common in animals less than 1 year of age. Specific types of intussusception (gastroesophageal intussusception) can be seen in German shepherds and Siamese cats.

Common Points in History
With an intussusception, animals are usually acutely ill and depressed. Common medical complaints are

- depression (usually acute),
- anorexia, and
- vomiting (usually excessive).

Common Points on Initial Assessment
Clinical signs of this disease depend on the location of the intussusception.

With high intussusception (in the small intestines close to the stomach), animals display

- depression,
- anorexia,
- tender, painful abdomen,
- vomiting blood,
- shortness of breath, and
- collapse.

With lower intussusception (in the large intestine, close to rectum), animals display

- constipation and straining to defecate,
- bloody and mucosal diarrhea,
- intermittent vomiting, and
- weight loss.

Complications
If not properly treated, an acute intussusception can perforate, causing intestinal rupture and massive infection of the abdomen (called peritonitis). Peritonitis can be life threatening.

Diagnosis
Diagnosis is made based on history, physical exam, plain film radiographs, a barium series, and/or an ultrasound examination.

Treatment
The general goal of treatment is the removal of the affected section of intestines. Simple reduction of the intestines back to normal presentation does not prevent a reoccurrence of the intussusception.

Prevention
There is no known prevention for this disease.

Key Points in Discussing Foreign Body Obstruction with Clients

- A foreign body is a solid mass or collection of debris that obstructs the normal flow of ingesta through the intestines.
- Foreign material can vary from a collection of hair and plant material that has been accumulating over months to a solid metal object (i.e., belt buckle).
- If an animal has swallowed something acutely, inducing vomiting should never be recommended until the veterinarian is consulted. Potentially, some foreign bodies can become lodged within the esophagus or lacerate the intestines or esophagus if vomiting is induced.
- All foreign bodies are a potential emergency and the client should be advised that a physical examination by the doctor is necessary.
- Some foreign bodies may pass; however, some foreign bodies can become lodged and produce a perforation that could start a life-threatening infection.
- Not all foreign material shows up on x-rays (i.e., cloth, plastic, wood, hairballs, and other nonmetal/nondense debris).
  —Radiographs are generally recommended.
  —If an obstruction is suspected and does not show up as an obvious foreign body, a barium series may be recommended (see diagnostic section).
- All foreign bodies are potential surgical emergencies.

Infectious Intestinal Disease

Parvoviral Infection

Parvoviral infection is a potentially lethal infection of the stomach and small intestines in dogs.

Etiology

- Parvo is a viral infection that attacks the cells that absorb food in the small intestine, slowing the body's ability to absorb food or water.
- Furthermore, the virus attacks white blood cell populations, causing the pet to be unable to fight off secondary infection (**immunosuppression**).
- Food and water are unable to be properly absorbed and this produces vomiting and diarrhea.
- Often there is blood in the vomit and diarrhea, secondary to bleeding from infected sites along the intestines.
- The dog becomes dehydrated secondary to fluid loss and is more prone to secondary infection. These animals can debilitate rapidly and die suddenly, looking almost like a poisoning.
- Parvoviral infection can be lethal.
- **Long-term environmental contamination** occurs because the virus is very hearty and will live in the environment through the heat of summer and cold of winter.

Signalment

- All dogs from 6 weeks to 18 months can be affected.
- Dobermans and rotteweilers are more sensitive to the disease.
- Vaccinated animals have increased resistance to the disease; however, they can still be affected.
- Older animals (2 years and older) that are unvaccinated can be also infected.
- The length of time it takes from exposure to clinical signs (**incubation period**) is generally 10 or more days, but can range from 24 hours to days.

Common Points in History

The disease usually produces an acute severe intestinal disease. In general, these pets have limited to no vaccine status. Common medical complaints are

- anorexia,
- depression,
- vomiting, and
- diarrhea (usually with blood).

Common Points on Initial Assessment

Clinical signs of this disease can be

- depression (sometimes to comatose),
- vomiting (possibly with blood),
- diarrhea (usually liquid with blood),
- abdominal pain,
- seizing (secondary to septic shock),
- coma, and
- death.

Patients that come in with symptoms suggestive of this disease should be isolated immediately due to its infectious potential to other patients.

Complications

Septic shock (see Chapter 30) and intussusception (rare) can be complications of parvoviral infection.

- Because of the viral-induced immunosuppression, bacteria can build up in the bloodstream and actively reproduce.
- The infection begins to consume large amounts of the patient's blood sugar level.
- The brain requires adequate sugar levels to maintain normal function. With decreasing sugar levels, the pet may show
  — increasing depression to the level of coma,
  — seizures, and
  — death.

Diagnosis

Diagnosis is made based on medical history, physical examination, and diagnostics. Some possible diagnostics are a fecal ELISA parvo test and a complete blood count.

- Many pets will show a decreased total white blood cell count.
- Pets with a total white blood cell count of less than 1000 cells per microliter are at high risk for massive infection and sepsis.

Treatment

Treatment is focused on supportive care while the animal overcomes the virus.

- It is recommended that the dog have some form of fluid therapy to maintain hydration, antibiotics for secondary infection, and monitoring of electrolytes and blood sugar levels.
- Overall, it is strongly recommended that the dog be hospitalized for intravenous fluids and antibiotics and careful monitoring for dehydration, electrolyte imbalances, and low blood sugars.

Prevention

- **Vaccination:** Multiple vaccinations of pups beginning at 6–8 weeks of age are recommended. Further isolation of the pet from large populations of dogs until the pet is fully vaccinated will limit exposure to the virus.
- **Environment**: Because parvo virus can live in the environment for years, cleaning the areas where the pet has

---

Key Points in Discussing Parvoviral Infection with Clients

- Parvovirus is potentially lethal.
- Parvovirus can infect young dogs from 6 weeks to 18 months.
- Even vaccinated dogs can be infected with the disease.
- Vaccines usually help produce a less severe form of the disease, but no vaccination prevents 100% of all diseases.
- Parvoviral infection destroys the cells that absorb food and water and also secondarily lowers the animal's immune response so it cannot fight off infection.
  —Pets become dehydrated from massive vomiting and diarrhea.
  —Animals can potentially succumb to massive infection from secondary bacterial pathogens (sepsis).
- Some animals can get over the infection in a few days, and some require days to a week plus of treatment. Response is variable.
- Once an animal recovers from a parvoviral infection, it can live a normal healthy life span without any long-term problems from the infection.

---

vomited and had diarrhea with a 10% bleach solution, Parvosol, or other hospital disinfectant is recommended.

Feline Panleukopenia (Feline Distemper)

Feline Panleukopenia is a severe viral infection of the gastrointestinal system of cats.

Etiology

Feline panleukopoenia, which is closely related to canine parvovirus infection, attacks the intestinal cells that absorb food and water.

- These cells temporarily are unable to function, and the unabsorbed food and water are removed from the body by vomiting and diarrhea.
- The virus also temporarily causes a decreased response by the immune system, making the animal much more prone to secondary infection.
- Infections of pregnant cats can cause infections of the central nervous system of the kittens, resulting in permanent changes within brain.

Signalment

The disease is evident in cats and minks. It is usually apparent in young, unvaccinated cats, typically between the ages of 2 to 6 months.

Incubation Period

Incubation period of this disease is 10+ days.

Common Points in History

Feline panleukopenia is an acute disease producing severe gastrointestinal signs and depression in young cats with variable levels of vaccination. Common medical complaints for this disease are

- vomiting,
- diarrhea,
- anorexia,
- nasal and ocular discharge, and
- an inability to stand properly (in newborns).

Common Points on Physical Exam

- Dehydration (severe)
- Nasal and ocular discharge
- In newborns, the inability to stand properly and falling over easily
- Loss of balance
- Blindness (retinal detachment)

Complications

The infection of kittens in utero can cause permanent damage to the cerebellum and eyes. Animals will be born blind and unable to properly balance themselves and walk normally.

Diagnosis

Diagnosis is made on medical history, physical exam, and fecal ELISA parvoviral (canine) test.

- Even though the test is used largely for canine parvoviral infection, cats with high virus levels will show positive with the same diagnostic exam.
- As with canine parvovirus, there are times when the virus is shed in the feces. A positive test is strongly suggestive of parvoviral infection; however, a negative test does not rule out the disease.

Treatment

As with most viral infections, treatment is focused on supportive care while the animal overcomes the virus.

- It is recommended that the cat have some form of fluid therapy to maintain hydration, antibiotics for secondary infection, monitoring of electrolytes and blood sugar levels.
- Overall, it is strongly recommended that the cat be hospitalized for intravenous fluids and antibiotics and careful monitoring for dehydration, electrolyte imbalances, and low blood sugars.
- **There is a very high percentage of fatality associated with this disease**.

Prevention

Proper vaccination of kittens with the FVRCP vaccine can help prevent or minimize the disease.

Key Points in Discussing Panleukopenia Viral Infection with Clients

- Although feline panleukopenia is called feline distemper, the virus is related to canine parvovirus.
- The feline virus typically attacks unvaccinated kittens from 2 to 6 months of age.
- Feline panleukopenia viral infection destroys the cells that absorb food and water and also secondarily lowers the animals' immune response so they cannot fight off infection.
  —Pets become dehydrated from massive vomiting and diarrhea.
  —Furthermore, the animals can potentially succumb to massive infection from secondary bacterial pathogens (sepsis).
- Some animals can get over the infection in a few days, and some require days to a week of treatment. Response is variable, but mortality from the infection can be high.
- Once an animal recovers from panleukopenia, they can live a normal, healthy life span without any long-term problems from the infection.
- Pregnant queens that are infected with the virus during early pregnancy can produce kittens with central nervous system dysfunction. These kittens can be blind and unable to walk and balance properly.

Chronic Disease of the Intestine

Constipation/Obstipation

Constipation is an obstruction of the large colon with an incomplete ability to pass dry, hard, firm feces. Obstipation is a severe obstruction with an inability to defecate at all.

Etiology

Constipation can occur with any disease that impairs fecal transit through the colon, produces profound dehydration such that large amounts of water are removed from fecal material slowing transit, or with diseases that slow or stop intestinal movement (**ileus**). Some suggested causes of disease are discussed next.

Dietary Changes

Animals that ingest large quantities of bones, hair, and foreign bodies can produce a large colon obstruction.

Environment

When there are changes in environment (such as new pet added to a household, changes in litter box location, changes in litter), animals may defecate less, leading to possible obstruction.

Drugs

Certain types of medications can be constipating:

- Antihistamines
- Pain medications
- Antacids
- Diuretics
- Other medications

Animals with **rectal disease** that causes pain while defecating will decrease the amount of time it defecates, leading to constipation. Some diseases are

- anal gland abcessation,
- rectal strictures, and
- rectal trauma.

Animals with mechanical obstruction of the outflow tract can also obstipate. Some types of diseases are

- tumors pushing down on colon,
- tumors of the large intestines, and
- polyps of the large colon.

Neurologic Disease

Older animals can lose nervous control of their large colon (**megacolon**). The colon cannot propel food forward out of the rectum; instead, the feces builds up until severe constipation occurs.

Hormonal Disease

Animals suffering from specific hormonal disease that can chronically dehydrate the pet and lead to dry hard feces can produce obstipation/constipation. Some of these diseases are

- hyperthyroidism,
- hypothyroidism,
- kidney disease, and
- liver disease.

Signalment
Obstipation/constipation can occur both in dogs and cats, but it is more common in cats.

Common Points in History
Common medical complaints from chronic constipation are

- straining to defecate,
- defecating small amounts of dry hard firm stool,
- straining with small amounts of liquid stool,
- occasional vomiting, and
- not wanting to eat.

Clinical Points on Initial Assessment
Common physical exam findings can be

- depression,
- lethargy,
- dehydration, and
- abdominal tenderness.

Complications
Chronic constipation can lead to loss of innervation of the large bowel. Furthermore, constipation can produce dehydration, chronic vomiting, and, in severe cases, intestinal perforation.

Diagnosis
Because there are many potential causes of constipation, the clinical diagnostic workup can vary depending on the medical history and physical examination. Some diagnostics that may be recommended are:

- **Radiographs**: Abdominal x-rays can aid in detection of the potential underlying cause and severity of the constipation in the large colon.
- **Complete blood count/chemistry**: Blood work may be suggested to determine if there are any underlying metabolic, infectious, or neoplastic diseases that may be the cause of the constipation.
- **Colonoscopy/biopsy**: Sometimes with chronic constipation, an endoscope is used to explore the large bowel and take intestinal wall tissue to biopsy for possible masses and polyps. Furthermore, sections of the intestinal wall can be taken to determine if there is an underlying disease process.

Treatment
The goal of treatment is to relieve the cause of the constipation/obstipation while treating the primary underlying disease. Some treatment options may be as follows:

- **Enemas**: The repeated use of soap and water and other chemical enema solutions is used to help break up the hardened fecal material.
- **Fluid therapy/hospitalization**: Severely dehydrated pets may require some form of fluid therapy to aid in rehydration and help intestinal motility.
- **Medication**: There are specific medications available that aid in stool softening and help intestinal motility. Some types of medications can be
  — **Dietary supplementation**: Addition of some fiber form to the diet can help increase water inflow into the large bowel producing soft, well-formed stool.
  — **Lubricants/emollients**: The veterinarian may suggest oral medications that aid in the lubrication and movement of ingesta through the intestinal system.
  — **Motility modifiers**: When dealing with constipation not associated with obstructions, these drugs aid in increasing motility of the intestines.

Prevention
Prevention of chronic constipation/obstipation is dependent on the cause of the symptoms. Prevention can be focused on

- preventing dehydration,
- early detection of systemic disease that produce constipation,
- limiting exposure to foreign bodies that can be obstructive,
- changing environmental conditions that could prevent normal bowel movements in animals, and
- other treatment options.

Inflammatory Bowel Disease
Inflammatory bowel disease refers to an inflammatory process that can affect the stomach, small intestine, or the large bowel. The affected areas of the gastrointestinal system become infiltrated with white blood cells at a microscopic level causing these areas to malfunction.

Etiology
- Inflammatory bowel disease is caused by a local sensitivity within the affected section of intestine to some component of the diet, which produces a localized infiltration of white blood cells at a microscopic level.
- The dietary component usually is something common to most commercial diets (i.e., wheat, chicken, meat, pork, corn, etc.) and generally produces sensitivity over the long term (i.e., a sudden change in one commercial diet for another diet does not typically produce an inflammatory response.)

Signalment

This syndrome can affect both dogs and cats of any age but generally begins once the animal is over 2 years old. Commonly affected breeds are

- Irish setters,
- boxers,
- French bulldogs,
- basenjis, and
- Lundehunds.

Common Signs in History

Inflammatory bowel disease can be very subtle and chronic and can mimic other intestinal and systemic ailments. Physical symptoms depend on the section of the gastrointestinal tract affected.

With areas of the stomach and early small intestines affected, the chief complaints are

- weight loss;
- diarrhea, with soft stool (cow patty-like), and increased amounts, with possible dark blood;
- flatulence;
- vomiting; and
- ravenous appetite.

With areas of the lower small intestine and large intestine affected, the chief complaints are

- chronic watery diarrhea,
- straining while defecating,
- frank blood or mucus present, and
- producing feces more often with small amounts each time.

Common Points on Initial Assessment

Animals can be unaffected to severely ill. Some common signs are

- dehydration,
- depression,
- anorexia,
- vomiting (sometimes severe), and
- abdominal sensitivity to abdominal pain.

Complications

Complications to chronic inflammatory bowel disease can produce moderate to severe weight loss, severe vomiting, and profuse waxing and waning diarrhea.

Diagnosis

Diagnosis of inflammatory bowel disease is made by a **diagnosis of exclusion**, because other gastrointestinal disease must be first ruled out. Some possible clinical diagnostics examination can be as follows:

- **Fecal examination/fecal ELISA**: These diagnostics are used to rule out possible parasitic infections that could cause chronic diarrhea and weight loss.
- **Radiographs**: Abdominal x-rays can aid in detection of the potential underlying cause, masses, or changes in organ size.
- **Complete blood count/chemistry**: Blood work may be suggested to determine if there are any underlying metabolic, infectious, or neoplastic disease that may be the cause of the constipation.
- **Infectious titer screens**: Depending on the geographic region and the species, the veterinarian may suggest blood work to check for infectious disease (feline leukemia, feline immunodeficiency virus, fungal infections, etc.).
- **Endoscopy/biopsy**: Sometimes with chronic gastrointestinal disease, an endoscopic procedure to explore the early small intestine or large bowel and to take tissue to biopsy the intestinal wall for possible masses and polyps can determine if there is an underlying disease process occurring.

Treatment

With concerns of inflammatory bowel disease, the patient is treated with a combination of medicine and diet change to help reduce the microscopic inflammation within the intestinal tract. Some treatment options are as follows:

- **Medications:** Medications for inflammatory bowel disease focus on using anti-inflammatory doses of steroids or immunosuppressants to reduce the white blood cell response and return normal function to the affected sections of intestines.
- **Diet:** Hypoallergenic diets (such as fish and potato, lamb and rice, venison and potato, and rabbit and potato) can aid in reducing the inflammatory process by eliminating the component of the food that is stimulating the white blood cell response.

Prevention

There is no known way to prevent inflammatory bowel disease.

Key Points in Discussing Chronic Intestinal Disease with Clients

- Diseases such as obstipation/constipation and inflammatory bowel disease are usually chronic long-term problems that can affect a pet for a majority of its life span.
- Animals with chronic constipation, vomiting, and diarrhea may need extensive workups to help diagnose the overall cause of disease.
- Specific hospitals have in-depth questionnaires to help get a detailed history and help isolate the causes of chronic disease.
- Doctors may need more appointment time with clients to discuss, perform physicals, and do advanced diagnostics that are required for a thorough workup.

Emergencies of the Gastrointestinal System
Gastric Dilation-Volvulus
Gastric dilatation-volvulus (GDV) is a serious life-threatening disease of the large and giant breed dog, although it can occur in smaller breed dogs as well.

Etiology
The underlying cause of the disease is unknown; however, there are predisposing factors, such as

- eating food too quickly,
- exercising too close to a meal,
- having one large meal per day instead of more frequent small feedings, and
- sudden changes in diet.

The mechanisms of the disease are as follows:

- The disease is caused by an increase of gas content in the stomach with or without rotation of the stomach on its longitudinal axis.
- As the gas increases it causes the stomach to shift on its own axis and rotate out of normal position.
- The rotation of the stomach decreases normal blood flow to the stomach and spleen and makes the animal unable to vomit.
- The enlarged rotated stomach decreases normal blood flow back to the liver and heart and produces a severe shock and metabolic upset to the system.
- The ensuing disease can be life threatening.

Signalment
GDV tends to occur in large to giant breed dogs; however, the disease has occurred in small dogs (dachshunds, schnauzers).

Common Points in History
This disease is an acute onset of a life-threatening process producing depression, shock, and death in a matter of a few hours (30 minutes–120 minutes). Common medical complaints can be that the pet

- has a bloated abdomen ,
- is retching–**or is *trying to vomit but cannot*,**
- is salivating and drooling heavily,
- is uncomfortable, and
- is unable to get up.

Common Points on Initial Assessment
Physical signs can be severe, rapid in onset, and life threatening. These signs can include

- retching, trying to vomit;
- salivating;
- weak and unable to get up;
- abdomen distended, sometimes severely;
- poor, rapid pulses;

- poor gum color;
- lying on side; and
- coma.

Complications
If not treated immediately and aggressively the patient will die. After the GDV has been corrected, due to the severity of the metabolic upset produced from this disease, there are many possible postoperative concerns.

- **Irregular heart rhythm**: The ventricles can misfire causing a **premature ventricular contraction (PVC).**
- **Infection of the abdomen (peritonitis).**
- **Severe temporary stasis of the gut** (ileus).
- **Disseminated intravascular coagulopathy (DIC)**: DIC is a severe metabolic upset that stimulates clot formation in all vessels, exhausting the chemicals (**clotting factors**) that produce the clot. With the clotting factors gone, the patient begins to bleed spontaneously.

Diagnosis
Diagnosis is based upon the medical history, the physical symptoms, and abdominal radiographs. When the stomach bloats and rotates, there is a specific pattern seen in the cranial abdomen on radiographs. The stomach, which has rotated on its own axis, shows two distinct distended regions: one region representing the normal stomach, the second region representing the outflow tract of the stomach, the **pylorus,** that has rotated above the normal position of the stomach (see Figure 10.18).

Treatment
- Initially, in the first few minutes, treatment is geared toward stabilizing the patient with intravenous fluids and medications (see Chapter 30).
- Once stabilized, the dog is placed under anesthesia, and a stomach tube is passed to help decompress the stomach and expel the gas and ingesta.
- Once the stomach tube is passed, the stomach is lavaged with water to help bring out any thickened stomach contents.
- If a stomach tube cannot be passed, then a surgical repair is indicated.
- After the stomach is decompressed, permanent surgical attachment of the stomach to the abdominal wall (**gastropexy**) is recommended. This procedure will help prevent the stomach from rotating in the future. **However, the stomach can still bloat.**
- If surgical repair is not done, there is increased chance of the stomach bloating and rotating again.
- While in surgery, the stomach, spleen, and esophagus will be explored for any damage or injury they may have sustained due to the rotation process.
- If there is severe extension and rotation of the stomach, there can be permanent damage to the spleen, stomach, and\or the esophageal wall.

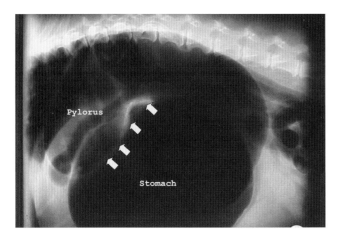

Figure 10.18. X-ray image of a rotated stomach. The arrows indicate where the free end of the stomach (pylorus) moves as the stomach rotates, blocking off the arteries and veins. This rotation is often called "the double bubble," indicating the two obvious sections of the stomach.

- Sometimes removal of the spleen and/or affected areas within the wall of the stomach must be done for the overall health of the animal.
- Rarely, damage is too extensive to repair.

Prevention

To help prevent pets from bloat and stomach rotation, the following recommendations can be made to the owner:

- Offer smaller feedings multiple times during the day rather than one large feeding.
- Try to avoid abrupt changes in diet.
- Do not let your pet exercise heavily an hour before or an hour after eating.

Key Points in Discussing GDV/Bloat with Clients

- GDV is one of the true veterinary emergencies where every second counts.
- Key symptoms are large breed dogs that are acting lethargic, depressed, trying to vomit but can't, or any other signs of bloat. If present, the dog should be evaluated immediately.
- Dogs that actually have bloat gastropexy surgery can still bloat. They generally do not rerotate, but the stomach can fill with air and distend.
- Bloated animals are open to numerous postoperative complications that may require the pet to be hospitalized for days.
- Dogs with a gastric distention volvulus will die if not treated.

CD-ROM 1 reviews material presented in this chapter. Please try the cases for Section 2 (Anatomy and Physiology— The Science behind the Diseases) to help reinforce the information presented here.

Chapter 11

Respiratory System

Anatomy of the Respiratory System

At all times mammalian cells require oxygen to produce energy for normal function and growth. In order to produce energy, these cells take 1 unit of sugar molecules and, through a process called **cellular respiration,** convert sugar into energy (**ATP**), water, and carbon dioxide (CO_2). The chemical formula for this reaction is:

$$6\ O_2 + C_6H_{12}O_6 \text{ (sugar)} \rightarrow 6\ CO_2 + 6\ H_2O + \text{Energy (ATP)}$$

Once the chemical reaction has occurred, the produced CO_2 must be excreted. CO_2 becomes toxic and can inhibit breathing centers of the central nervous system if the concentration becomes too high. In order to exchange gases, mammals have developed an extensive tubular system to bring air in to absorb oxygen and expel CO_2. The anatomy of the respiratory system (see Figure 11.1) includes the

- nasal cavity/sinus,
- pharynx,
- trachea,
- primary bronchus,
- secondary bronchus,
- terminal bronchus,
- alveolar ducts,
- alveolar sacs, and
- alveolus.

The upper respiratory system comprises the nasal cavity, nasal sinuses, and the common region of the nose and mouth called the **pharynx**. These air passageways are lined with hair and nasal mucosa to filter debris and bacteria to keep them from entering the body. Once the air moves through the nasal passageways, it enters the trachea and the lung fields of the thoracic cavity.

The lungs occupy the greater part of the chest cavity and communicate with the outside air via the trachea and bronchial system. The lungs are divided into lobes. Each lobe contains a series of ducts that get smaller and smaller until they reach the alveoli. The pathway of the air through the ducts is as follows:

- Primary bronchus
- Secondary bronchus
- Terminal bronchus
- Alveolar sacs
- Alveolar ducts
- Alveolus

At the end of the duct system, the alveoli are structures of specialized cells that are closely associated with small capillary and venous beds. These are the sites where oxygen enters the bloodstream and binds to hemoglobin within the red blood cell. **Hemoglobin** is a special iron-based chemical that has the ability to carry oxygen and CO_2 through the body. At the same time oxygen is absorbed by the red blood cells, CO_2 is released from the hemoglobin into the lungs and expired (see Figure 11.2).

The act of respiration is controlled by the autonomic nervous system, which is part of the central nervous system. Initiation of breathing is stimulated by the respiratory center in the brain that monitors CO_2. Increasing blood CO_2 stimulates the autonomic nervous system to increase respiration. Abnormally high levels of CO_2 suppress respiration.

The muscles that produce an inspiration are the smooth muscles around the alveoli, the muscles between the ribs (**intercostal muscles**), and the diaphragm. The **diaphragm** is a musculoskeletal partition that completely separates the thoracic cavity from the abdomen.

The lungs are able to expand and contract because they exist within a vacuum. As the diaphragm and chest expand and increase the volume within the chest cavity, the volume of lungs also increases proportionally. This action forces the air to rush into the lungs. As the diaphragm and chest relax, the volume decreases and air is expelled from the chest.

The rate at which the animal breathes normally while at rest is called the normal **respiration rate**. It can vary dramatically, depending on the size, species, and sex of the animal. In general, female animals breathe faster than males, younger animals breathe faster than older animals, and smaller animals breathe more rapidly than larger animals. Some examples are

- horses: 8–16 breaths per minute,
- dogs: 20–40 breaths per minute, and
- cats: 24–42 breaths per minute.

Although these are the accepted respiratory rates of these species, stress, pain, and nervousness can greatly increase respiratory rates.

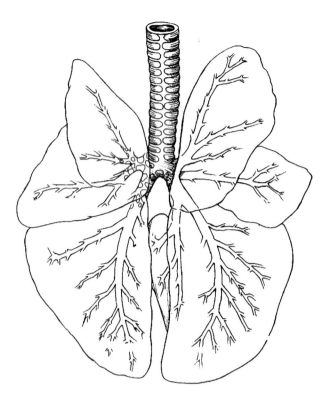

Figure 11.1. Image of the respiratory system from the trachea into the bronchi and the alveolar duct system.

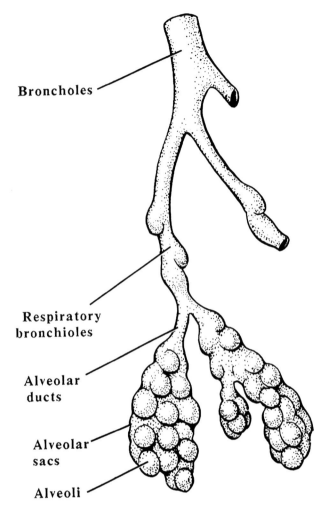

Figure 11.2. Image of alveolar sacs, where oxygen is absorbed into the blood stream and carbon dioxide is expelled. (Courtesy of *Anatomy of Domestic Animals*, 7th Edition. Pasquini, Chris, and Pasquini, Susan. Sudz Publishing, Pilot Point, Tx 1989. Used with permission from Sudz Publishing.)

Pathology of the Respiratory System

Like the gastrointestinal system where physical symptoms occur due to the abnormal function of the stomach and intestines to digest food stuffs and absorb nutrients and water, the respiratory symptoms occur due to the impedance of gas exchange at the alveolar level of the lungs. Primary respiratory signs occur from the causes discussed next.

Physical Obstruction of the Airways and Alveolus

If fluid, cells (i.e., pus), or masses physically fill and obstruct normal bronchioles and alveolar tissue, oxygen exchange cannot occur. As the airways are obstructed, the animal begins to cough reflexively, trying to clear and bring up debris and fluid.

As further obstruction continues, the animal's respiratory rate increases in response to increasing CO_2 levels in the body.

Finally, as oxygenation ability is severely impaired, the pet's peripheral mucus membrane (i.e., gums) becomes **cyanotic** (blue), the animal becomes weak, has trouble breathing, breaths abdominally, and can faint or pass out. Causes for obstruction of airways are discussed next.

Pulmonary Edema/Congestion

Although discussed more thoroughly in Chapter 12, pulmonary edema refers to a filling of the airways with fluid. The excess fluid accumulates in the lung fields secondary to drowning, heart disease, electrical injury, and other causes.

Pneumonia

Pneumonia refers to the accumulation of white blood cells, infectious agents, and inflammatory debris that fills the airways secondary to a bacterial, fungal, rickettsial, or viral infection.

Mass/Tumor

In this case a solid tumor or mass begins to invade the lung fields and physically destroys normal tissue as it grows larger.

Narrowing of the Trachea/Bronchioles

There are specific chronic diseases that can, over time, produce profound narrowing of the trachea and bronchioles. As the disease progresses, the airways become thickened with fibrous tissue that continues to limit normal airflow. Some diseases that can produce these changes are

- feline asthma,
- collapsing trachea,
- chronic obstructive pulmonary disease, and
- allergic/anaphylactic reactions.

Thoracic Disease

Diseases that affect the chest cavity can inhibit normal respiration and exchange of gases within the lungs. These disease syndromes produce signs identical to the first category and must be differentiated by clinical diagnostics. The following syndromes can produce primary thoracic disease.

Pleural Effusion

A pleural effusion, as discussed later in the chapter, is an accumulation of fluid within the chest, surrounding the lungs and heart. If enough fluid accumulates, the normal expansion of the lungs can be affected. Pleural effusions can be associated with heart disease, infection/foreign body, tumors, trauma, and systemic disease.

Pleuritis

Pleuritis is a viral, bacterial, fungal, or rickettsial infection of the lining of the chest (**pleura**). It can be associated with a severe pneumonia that can rupture out from affected lung tissue, producing an infection within the chest cavity.

Mass/Tumor

Cranial and caudal to the heart, between the lungs, is a region called the **mediastinum**. If a tumor or mass occurs in this region and grows to significant size, lung expansion may be affected.

Pneumothorax

Although discussed later in the disease section of this chapter, a pneumothorax is an injury to the chest or lung fields that allows the introduction of air into the thorax. The chest exists in a vacuum, and the lungs are able to expand and contract only as long as this vacuum exists. If air is introduced into the chest from an injury, the lungs will begin to collapse and respiration will become seriously affected.

Obtaining a History for Respiratory Disease

The key to a thorough evaluation of a potential respiratory or cardiovascular patient is to try to isolate the cause of the physical symptoms based upon history, auscultation examination, and a thorough physical examination. There are key points in the history that can help the medical team determine if the disease is an upper or lower respiratory problem or a cardiovascular disease. Some important questions to ask when taking a history follow.

What Is the Duration of Illness?

Acute onset of respiratory disease suggests the pet has been rapidly affected by a bacterial or viral infectious agent, for-

eign body, or an allergenic condition (i.e., acute asthma, severe allergic reaction, etc.) producing respiratory symptoms of a short-term duration (usually fewer than 3–5 days).

Chronic respiratory disease can be a more complicated progressive disease that produces waxing and waning or persistently worsening signs. Chronic diseases of the respiratory system can be chronic long-term infection (i.e., fungal infection) and obstructive (collapsing trachea), parasitic (heartworm disease), or cancerous (neoplastic) disease.

Is a Cough Present?

Identifying the type and nature of the cough is very important to help distinguish its cause. Some basic questions are as follows.

- **How often does the cough occur?** Is this a mild infrequent cough or is the pet coughing regularly?
- **Is the cough becoming worse or more frequent?** Worsening coughs can suggest a more progressive problem.
- **Is the cough worse with excitement?** Coughs that become worse with exercise or excitement can suggest heart or respiratory problems severe enough to affect the pet's ability to exercise normally.
- **Is the cough productive?** Purulent debris (pus) that comes up when the pet is coughing can suggest an infectious disease.
- **Is the cough worse at night?** When air cools at night, water droplets can condense and pool in the lung fields. Healthy lungs can handle the increased fluid condensation. Animals with chronic conditions, such as heart disease patients that have decreased ability to remove fluid from the lung fields, can have a more productive cough at night.

Does the Pet Tire More Often and Require Rest More Frequently?

If pets cannot maintain normal levels of activity (exercise intolerance), it suggests that their tissues cannot be oxygenated adequately and can suggest severe disease. If this is noted, further questions may need to be documented.

Have There Been Any Episodes of Collapsing or Fainting?

Animals that have a history of collapse or weakness can have severe cardiac disease.

- These pets should be handled with extreme caution since their heart is so severely affected that the pet collapses or loses consciousness with any exertion.
- Furthermore, these patients may need to be placed on oxygen and the medical team notified immediately.

Does the Pet Have Periods of Increased Respiratory Effort?

Patients that seem to have episodes of increased rigor while breathing, breathing abdominally (see below), breathing with their head and neck extended, or making abnormal sounds while breathing may have serious respiratory or cardiac disease.

Is Sneezing Evident?

Just as with coughing, the nature and occurrence of the sneezing can help distinguish the types of disease. Sneezing can be seen with infection of the respiratory tract, a foreign body, or an allergic reaction.

Is There Nasal Discharge?

The type and location of nasal discharge can significantly help distinguish between different types of respiratory disease. Some key points are as follows:

- Is the discharge bilateral or unilateral? **Unilateral discharge** suggests a localized problem within the upper airway. **Bilateral discharge** suggests that the discharge is from a problem with the trachea or lower respiratory system or a systemic disease.
- What is the type of discharge present?
  — **Mucopurulent (pus) discharge** generally suggests a bacterial or fungal infection or a foreign body.
  — **Clear (serous) discharge** generally suggests a viral infection or allergy. However, it is important to note that with canine distemper virus, a mucopurulent discharge can be noted.
  — **Bloody discharge** may suggest a foreign body, infectious disease, bleeding problem, trauma, or tumor.

Is the Pet on Heartworm Prevention?

In specific geographic regions of the country, heartworm disease (see Chapter 12) is endemic for both felines and canines. In these regions, animals that are not on a program of prevention may be at increased risk.

What Is the Vaccination Status of the Pet?

Young pets with no to limited vaccination history are more prone to canine distemper viral infections.

Obtaining an Initial Assessment on a Patient with Respiratory Disease

When assisting in a clinical evaluation of a pet affected with a possible respiratory disease, it becomes important to be able to fully auscultate the animal for abnormalities. A technician must be able to practice listening to normal and abnormal chests with the stethoscope to aid in proper evaluation of the sick and hospitalized pet.

The most important concept is that these are potential life-threatening diseases that may need quick assessment and treatment. *If a team member is unsure if a pet may have a life-threatening respiratory difficulty, oxygen is never contraindicated* (see Chapter 30). If the pet seems stable enough, initial assessment may include the important concepts discussed next.

What is the Respiratory Rate and Nature of the Breathing Cycle?

Normal respiratory rates in a hospital situation can be slightly more elevated:

- Canines: 30–60 breaths per minute
- Felines: 40–70 breaths per minute

Is the Pet Tachypneic?

Animals can breath more rapidly (tachypnea) when nervous; however, rates above the following parameters can suggest abnormality:

- Canines with more than 80–100 breaths per minute
- Felines with more than 100–120 breaths per minute

Is the Pet Dypsneic?

The normal respiratory pattern is a slow expansion and relaxation of the chest. Animals that are having trouble breathing (dyspneic) and with altered breathing styles can suggest compromised respiratory systems. Some concerns to observe are the following.

Is the Pet Breathing Abdominally?

Although panting can appear to have an abdominal component, if animals must use their abdomen to drive air in and out of their lung field, it can suggest serious respiratory disease. These pets also tend to open-mouth breath to help maximize the amount of air entering the respiratory system.

Is There Respiratory Noise?

Is the dog making respiratory noise that can be heard without a stethoscope? Animals with a respiratory noise (also called a **stridor**) can suggest a potential obstruction of the upper airway or bronchial constriction of the lower airway. It is important to note if the stridor is occurring during inhalation, exhalation, or both.

Are the Neck and Head Extended While Breathing?

If pets extend their neck and head upward in conjunction with increased respiratory effort, it suggests life-threatening respiratory or cardiac disease. These pets are so severely affected that they must keep their trachea in an absolutely straight line to maximize airflow into the lungs. Many patients will have their elbows held away from their body as well (see Figure 11.3).

Does the Pet Have Decreased Shallow Breathing?

Severely depressed animals with a slow, shallow respiratory cycle are animals that may be severely life threatened and may need the full attention of the medical team.

What Is the Color of Gums and the Capillary Refill Time (CRT)?

Patients with respiratory difficulty, who are having problems oxygenating their tissue, have cyanotic mucus membranes.

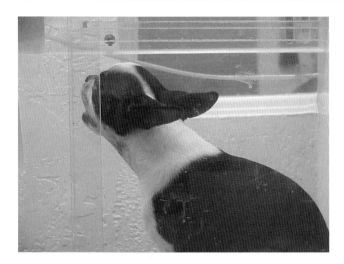

Figure 11.3. Image of a dog in an oxygen cage with severe respiratory disease. Note the pet is extending his neck and head upward while open mouth breathing.

Their gums, whites of their eyes, rectum, and other tissue can be light purple to blue to gray.

The CRT is often hard to assess because the gum color is cyanotic.

Auscultation

Whether initially assessing a respiratory patient or reevaluating a hospitalized patient, auscultation is the most important part of the respiratory examination.

Auscultating the Chest

Auscultation should be done in a quiet region of the hospital where slight changes in chest sounds can be ascertained. To fully appreciate the lung sounds, a team member should start auscultating in the cranioventral aspect of the right or left lung field, starting where the elbow meets the chest wall (see Figure 11.4). Slowly sweep caudally, moving dorsally to ventrally until the entire field is auscultated.

The goal of auscultation is to differentiate a region where the sounds become abnormal and different.

Normal sounds of the lungs are represented by air flowing through unobstructed airways. When the flow of air encounters narrowing or fluid, the sounds change.

Abnormal Sounds

- **Crackles:** The sound is best represented as the sound of crumpling cellophane paper. It is produced as air goes through fluid or cells, such as with pneumonia. The normal airways and alveoli are filled with cells and fluid. The crackle sounds are produced as air passes through the cramped region.
- **Rasps:** This sound is best represented as air flows through narrowed/constricted airways, producing a musical whistle. Diseases that produce fibrosis or narrowing of the bronchi (e.g., feline asthma, allergic reaction, and others) produce this whistle (see Figure 11.5).

Table 11.1. Triage concerns in the respiratory patient.

Systems	Signs Indicating an Emergency
Mentation	Stressed, eyes dilated
Fever	Temp >104.5° (due to increased respiratory effort or infection
	Temp <99° (due to shock, DIC, coma)
Hydration	Dehydration >5–7%
Gum color	Blue, purple, or gray
Capillary refill time (CRT)	CRT >2–3 seconds
Respiratory nature, auscultation, and	Nature: Pet's open mouth breathing, abdominally breathing with head and neck elevated
	Auscultation: Severely increased respiratory noise, evidence of rasps, rubs, or crackles
	Rate: Respiratory rates >80–100 breaths per minute
Heart rate and pulse	Rate: Heart rate <80 bpm or >180–200 bpm
	Pulse: Weak or decreased pulse quality, pulse deficits, or paradoxical pulses (see Chapter 12)

- **Rubs:** This sound is best represented as a friction rub produced when there are adhesions between the lungs and the chest wall causing a sound like sandpaper rubbing on wood.
- **Referred sound from the upper airway:** These are sounds produced from the trachea and the upper airway.
  — These sounds are produced from the obstructions of debris, masses, or fluid in the upper airway and are heard slightly decreased deeper in the chest.
  — In short-nosed breeds (i.e., pug, English bulldog, etc.), there can be significant upper-airway sounds that are normal due to the shortened compressed airways of the nostrils.

See Table 11.1 for a summary of signs indicating an emergency.

Clinical Diagnostics of the Respiratory System

In general, diagnostics of the chest are focused on blood and urine screens to check for bacterial, fungal, or viral infection, diagnostic imaging of the chest and heart, and chest tapping to remove fluid for treatment and diagnosis.

Blood Work Diagnostics

General blood work helps determine if there are changes in the complete blood count suggestive of bacterial or fungal infections. Furthermore, specific blood testing for infectious agents or bloodborne parasites are also done based on the geographic endemic diseases. Blood chemistry and urinalysis may also be recommended if there are concerns about organ or hormonal disease affecting the respiratory or cardiovascular systems

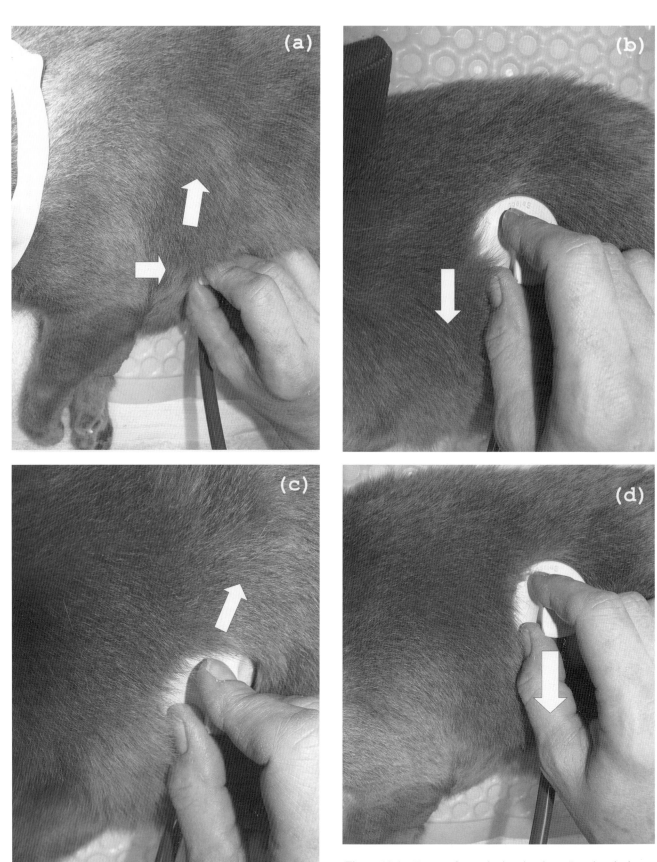

Figure 11.4. Image of auscultating the chest. Start by placing the stethoscope behind the elbow (a), sweep the lung fields from dorsal (b) to ventral (c), moving caudally until the entire region is auscultated (d). Then repeat it for the other side of the chest.

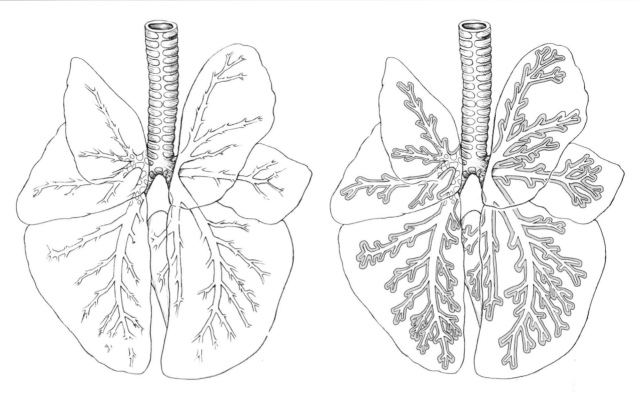

Figure 11.5. Illustration of normal lungs (left) and lungs affected by thickened bronchi (right) producing mechanical rasps that are perceivable by auscultation.

(i.e., renal disease producing a secondary hypertension; see Chapter 13). Some possible clinical diagnostics are

- a complete blood count and chemistry,
- urinalysis,
- infectious disease titer screens, and
- fungal screens:
  — coccidiomycosis
  — aspergillosis
  — blastomycosis
  — histoplasmosis
  — cryptococcus
- parasite screens:
  — ehrlichia
  — toxoplasmosis
  — heartworm

Key Points in Discussing the Need for a Blood and Urine Evaluation with the Client
- General changes in blood work can help the medical team evaluate the possibility of infectious, metabolic, inflammatory, or parasitic respiratory diseases.
- Depending on the geographic region, there are specific clinical diagnostics that will help evaluate the pet for a disease (i.e., heartworm test).
- These clinical diagnostics, in combination with other imaging studies, will help evaluate the overall health of the pet.

Radiography

A large part of clinical testing of respiratory disease is diagnostic imaging of the chest and heart. Plain film radiographs are often the first screening procedure in thoracic disease. Chest films allow the veterinarian to detect obvious pathology or changes within the heart, trachea, and mediastinum. The chest should be assessed when the lungs are fully inflated (see Figure 11.6).

A **metastatic chest protocol** is used when there are concerns of possible masses or tumors of the lung field. With this protocol, three chest views (**right lateral, left lateral, and a back to front view [V/D]**) are taken because small tumors are not always seen with the patient down on only one lateral side. When imaging the animal in lateral recumbency, the down side of the chest is always slightly compressed. This accentuates the up side's lung field and may show a small mass in comparison with the lower field. If the animal was placed in an opposite view, a small mass may be lost due to the slight compression of the lower lung field (see Figure 11.7).

When concerned about tracheal disease or collapse, imaging the neck and chest on both inspiration and expiration helps distinguish whether there is abnormal narrowing in the trachea at the height of inspiration. Once the inspiratory/expiratory study is completed, a comparison of the tracheal diameter on both films helps determine if there is pathology evident. However, since tracheal collapse is an ongoing, dynamic process, plain film radiographs do not always capture the extent of narrowing (see Figure 11.8).

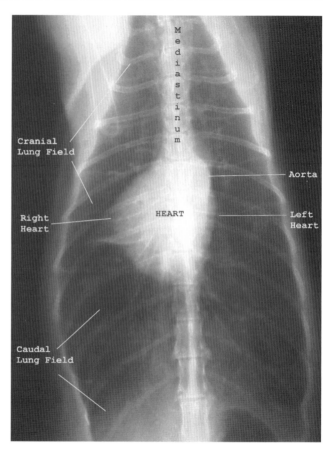

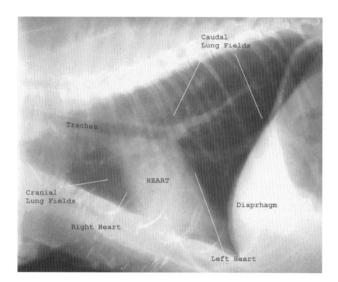

Figure 11.6. Radiographic images of normal thoracic cavity anatomy in both views of the chest.

Key Points in Discussing the Need for a Radiographic Evaluation with the Client

A radiograph study is being recommended for the following reasons.

• Symptoms of coughing, respiratory distress, or changes in the physical examination suggest disease of the chest and lungs.
• The study will help the medical team assess changes in the trachea and lung fields that could suggest infection, obstructive disease, fluid accumulations within or around the lung fields, or masses in the chest cavity.
• Finally, the study will help assess changes in the heart and large vessels of the chest.

With specific concerns, advanced radiographic studies may need to be performed to help evaluate the pet for functional tracheal disease or concerns of masses or tumors within the lung fields.

Advanced Diagnostics

A **thoracic ultrasound** has limited applications in the diagnosis of respiratory disease because ultrasound waves do not carry in air. Therefore, an ultrasound exam of the chest can help diagnose fluid within the chest cavity or masses in between the lungs (mediastinum) but cannot aid in diagnosis of lung lesions or masses, unless the lesions are in direct contact with the chest wall (see Chapter 25).

A chest tap (**thoracentesis**) is a diagnostic and therapeutic procedure focused on removing air or fluid from the chest. When radiographic studies suggest a fluid accumulation around the lung fields (**pleural effusion**), a needle is inserted into the chest cavity to help remove the excess fluid and obtain a diagnostic sample (see Figure 11.9).

Diagnostically, a chest tap is used to gain a sample of fluid that has accumulated within the chest around the lungs (pleural effusion) in order to determine the cause of the fluid accumulation. The type of fluid can help suggest the type of disease process.

• **Clear:** A clear or straw-colored fluid can suggest an accumulation of fluid due to
  — heart disease (especially in the cat; see Chapter 12),
  — feline infectious peritonitis (FIP), and
  — a thoracic mass/tumor.

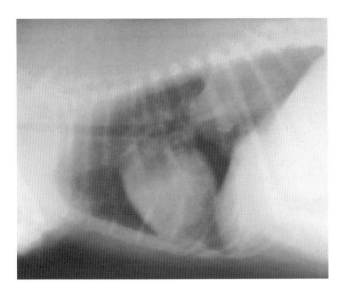

Figure 11.7. Image of a small to medium chest mass in the caudal dorsal lung fields

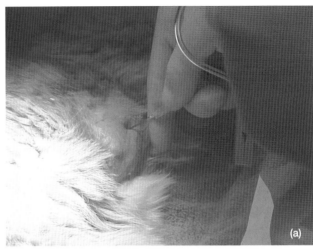

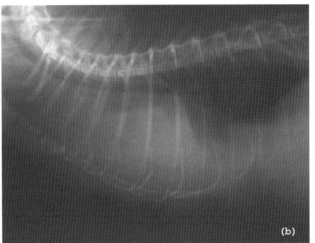

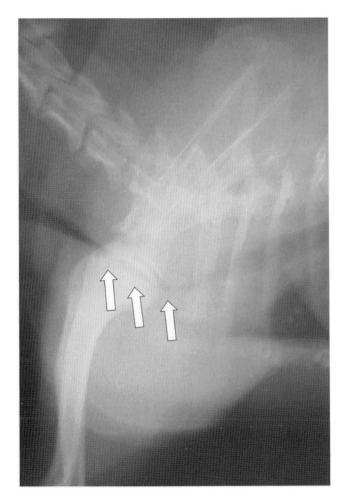

Figure 11.8. Image of an inspiratory thoracic radiograph with evidence of tracheal narrowing (white arrows)

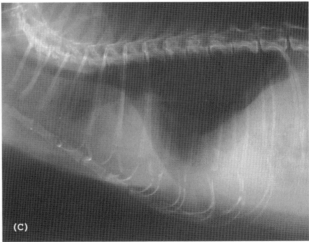

Figure 11.9. Image of a chest tap: A needle is inserted into the chest to help relieve fluid accumulations around the lung fields and heart (pleural effusion) that accumulate secondary to serious disease (a). In the first radiograph (b), the heart and lower lung fields are obstructed by a gray fluid line. The second radiograph (c) was taken after the fluid was removed from the chest, note that the ventral heart and lungs are more easily visualized.

> **Key Points in Discussing the Need for a Chest Tap with the Client**
> - The chest tap is used when there is concern that there is a fluid accumulation within the chest surrounding the heart and lungs.
> - A chest tap cannot remove fluid within the lung fields (pulmonary edema).
> - Some pets may require light sedation or anesthesia.
> - A small, square region of the chest is surgically shaved and prepared on both sides of the chest wall.
> - A needle is introduced under the skin and then enters the chest cavity.
> - As much of the fluid as possible is removed. Samples are kept for diagnostic evaluation.
> - The consistency and color of the fluid helps the medical team assess the nature of the disease affecting your pet.

- **Purulent (pus):** Purulent debris can suggest an infection of the thoracic cavity (pleuritis) or a foreign body that may have penetrated into the chest.
- **Milky and pink/white:** These effusions suggest a possible tumor of the thoracic cavity or a rupture or injury of the **thoracic duct**. The thoracic duct is a vessel that brings digested fat and triglycerides through the chest cavity and into the caudal vena cava. Once the fat enters the bloodstream it moves to the liver for utilization and storage.
- **Blood:** Blood can suggest a trauma or a tumor within the chest, or a pet with a generalized bleeding disorder.

A **transtracheal wash** uses a sterile catheter or red rubber feeding tube placed between the tracheal rings of a sedated animal. The catheter is run down the trachea as far as possible, and a small amount of sterile fluid is flushed into the trachea and lower airways. This stimulates the animal to cough and bring up debris. The sterile fluid and debris are then aspirated for culture and cytology. This procedure allows the veterinarian to get a better assessment of the disease process occurring within the lower bronchi and lungs.

Tracheoscopy/bronchoscopy is performed by passing a fiber-optic camera down the trachea into the lung fields; the doctor can better see changes in the bronchi that can suggest infection or neoplasia. Tissue and brushings of the bronchi can be obtained for biopsy evaluation and culture and sensitivity.

Finally, a **computeraxial tomography (CAT) scan** and **magnetic resonance imaging (MRI) scan** may be performed because not all masses can be imaged with x-ray or ultrasound; an advanced imaging technology may help distinguish smaller masses within the lung fields that may be hidden by the heart or trachea.

> **Key Points to Discuss about Other Advanced Procedures with the Client**
> - **Transtracheal wash:** A transtracheal wash is being recommended to obtain pathogenic bacteria and cells from the trachea and bronchi that can suggest the disease process affecting your pet. The pet will be placed under light sedation, and a small 1- to 2-inch square prepared over the trachea. A small incision is made through the skin and into the trachea, and a small sterile rubber catheter is inserted. A small amount of sterile fluid is flushed into the trachea and bronchi, which stimulates the pet to cough. Upon coughing, the fluid is aspirated, and the samples are used for cytology and culture to help determine the disease affecting your pet.
> - **Tracheoscopy/bronchoscopy:** A tracheoscopy/bronchoscopy is a surgical procedure in which a fiber-optic camera is passed into the trachea and down the large bronchi to help examine the lower lung fields. Although the smallest bronchioles and alveoli are too small for the endoscope to enter, cell samples and cultures of the lower airway can be obtained to help the medical team determine the disease process.
> - **A MRI/CAT scan:** A scan has been recommended by the medical team due to concerns that there may be a small mass or tumor evident in the lung fields that cannot be seen through a radiograph or identified through other procedures. The scan can distinguish normal lung tissue from that of a mass or tumor.

Diseases of the Respiratory System

Although not all diseases are mentioned below, the common diseases are discussed with the main goal being to understand and be able to explain to the client how these diseases can present themselves and what may be the overall short- and long-term concerns of each disease. Any discussion of overall diagnostic and treatment protocols should be based on the recommendations of the veterinarian. Please use the following information as a basis to discuss and educate the client, *but never to diagnose a patient.*

Obstructive Disease of the Lungs
Collapsing Trachea
The syndrome of collapsing trachea refers to a chronic condition of imperfect cartilage formation within the trachea causing the trachea to collapse as the pet inhales, which results in a temporary repeating obstruction.

Etiology
The condition in dogs is thought to be linked to a decrease of necessary elements within the cartilage. Causes of carti-

lage loss may be secondary to chronic lower airway disease, a nutritional deficiency, or even a genetic abnormality.

Signalment
This disease affects mainly dogs, and rarely cats, and has been associated with

- miniature poodles,
- Yorkshire terriers,
- Chihuahuas,
- Pomeranians, and
- other small and toy breeds

Collapsing trachea has been seen in animals from 4 to 14 years of age. Obesity may predispose an animal to this condition.

Common Points in History
Pets with collapsing trachea may show mild to severe signs. The syndrome produces a deep honking (gooselike) nonproductive cough. The cough can be made worse with excitement or exercise and can occasionally be severe enough to cause the patient to collapse. Patients may have a history of obesity as well. Common complaints with this disease are

- coughing (honking),
- respiratory difficulty (dyspnea),
- retching, and
- inability to exercise.

Common Points on Initial Assessment
Common signs are

- coughing (honking),
- respiratory difficulty (dypsnea),
- retching,
- increased respiratory rate,
- pale gums,
- weakness/collapse (**syncope**) in severe cases,
- an inspiratory chest sound in severe cases, and
- cyanotic mucus membranes (blue to purple to gray).

Complications
If not properly treated and controlled, this syndrome can produce a life-threatening obstructive disease.

Diagnosis
Diagnosis of collapsing trachea is based on radiographic or endoscopic examination of the trachea collapsing on inspiration. An inspiratory/expiratory radiographic study is usually recommended to help see changes in the tracheal diameter (see Figure 11.8).

Treatment
Treatment is focused on decreasing tracheal irritation and predisposing factors that produce tracheal collapse. The veterinarian may suggest the following:

- **Cough suppressants:** Oral cough medication may help decrease the coughing response. Most of these medications also have a mild sedative effect (i.e., butorphanol, Hycodan, etc.).
- **Bronchodilators:** Drugs such as theophylline and terbutaline help increase lower bronchial dilation to aid in increasing the lower airways to allow the maximum flow of air in and out of the body. Although these drugs do not work on the trachea itself, they increase air inflow so animals do not have to work as hard to breath.
- **Steroids:** The veterinarian may suggest regular dosing of medications such as prednisone to decrease inflammation in the airway and help prevent the chronic collapse.
- **Weight loss:** Obesity is a major contributor to this condition, and over weight animals should be placed on a calorie-restricted diet to help decrease body size.
- **Activity and environment:** Over excitement, especially in a humid environment, can cause crisis. Owners should monitor activity closely, especially during the hotter months of the year. Lastly animals should have harnesses on rather then collars since this can decrease chronic irritation over the trachea caused by a neck collar.
- **Surgical correction:** In severe cases, surgical repair replacing diseased cartilage rings with artificial replacements can be completed. This type of procedure is generally done at a surgical referral center.

Prevention
The best prevention in small breed dogs with concerns of collapsing trachea is to maintain the normal weight of the pet.

Key Points in Discussing Collapsing Trachea with Clients
- Collapsing trachea is a syndrome of increasing amounts of tracheal cartilage loss affecting generally middle-aged, small breed dogs.
- The loss of cartilage allows the trachea to collapse on itself on inspiration, producing a significant honking cough.
- As the disease progresses, the pet may not be able to exercise normally, may collapse (rarely), or even faint.
- The disease has been linked to congenital abnormalities with the formation of cartilage, chronic respiratory disease, and nutritional deficiency.
- If not controlled, collapsing trachea may produce a life-threatening respiratory syndrome.

Feline Asthma
Feline asthma is an allergic condition in the cat that is very similar to human asthma. In this condition, allergens cause a spontaneous constriction of the bronchi in the airways, causing mild to severe clinical signs.

Etiology

The cause of the disease is a reaction of the tissue (**epithelium**) lining the bronchi to a noxious chemical or chronic allergen, causing swelling of the tissue (**bronchoconstriction**), production of mucus and other excretions, and infiltration of white blood cells (inflammatory cells) into the lumen of the bronchi, causing an obstruction.

Signalment

The disease generally affects cats of any age and is more common in the Siamese and Himalayan breeds.

Common Points in History

Cats with asthma can have mild to severe attacks of respiratory difficulty (**dypsnea**), open-mouth breathing, collapse, fainting, and occasionally, death. Common medical complaints are

- respiratory wheeze or noise,
- collapse, and
- exercise intolerance during episodes.

Common Points on Initial Assessment

The initial assessment reveals a cat with mild to severe trouble breathing.

- The patient may be open-mouth breathing with a wheeze audible without a stethoscope.
- The patient may have an increased respiratory rate or effort.
- Auscultation reveals mild to severe wheezing over localized or generalized sections of the chest.
- Further, the pet may be syncopal or have severe tachypnea.
- Mucous membrane color can be light pink to severely pale gum color
- Finally, the pet may have a chronic mild to severe cough.

Complications

With severely affected animals, an asthma attack may produce a respiratory emergency.

Diagnosis

There is no one absolute diagnostic test for feline asthma; it is a diagnosis of exclusion. Clinical diagnostics are recommended to rule out other forms of infectious, obstructive, cardiac, cancerous, and other disease forms. Some diagnostics follow:

- **Complete blood count/chemistry/urinalysis:** Allows the medical team to evaluate any changes in the blood work that could suggest infectious, metabolic, or hormonal diseases.
- **Infectious screens:** Allows the evaluation of the pet for specific viral (i.e., Felv, FIV, FIP) or fungal diseases that can produce respiratory symptoms.

- **Radiographs:** Can help determine if there are significant changes and thickening in the bronchioles and lung fields that can suggest asthma.

Treatment

Treatment options are focused on reducing bronchial swelling and controlling reactions to inhalant irritants. Some possible treatment options are discussed next.

- **Steroids:** The veterinarian may suggest short-term oral steroid medications to longer-term steroid injections. This allows good control of the inflammatory process that stimulates the bronchoconstriction as well as reducing bronchial swelling. Steroids are handled well by most cats, with very few side effects. *However, over long-term use, steroids can cause liver disease and promote diabetes mellitus.*
- **Bronchodilators:** Bronchodilators, such as theophylline or terbutaline, may be suggested to help in bronchodilation to increase the amount of air coming into the lung fields.
- **Antihistamines:** Antihistamines such as cyproheptadine may be suggested to decrease the possible allergic reactions that stimulate the asthma condition. Response to antihistamines is more variable than response to steroids.
- **Inhaler therapy:** In severe cases, the use of a specialized inhaler with steroidal or bronchodilator medication to deliver microscopic levels of drugs into the bronchial ducts may also be suggested.

Prevention

There is no known protocol to prevent feline asthma; however, keeping the cat indoors in a clean environment may help decrease severity of the attacks.

Key Points in Discussing Feline Asthma with a Client

- Much like human asthma, feline asthma is an allergic condition of the cat that produces chronic bronchial airway thickening.
- The disease is episodic, producing mild to severe coughing, open-mouth breathing, and an evident respiratory wheeze.
- Animals with severe disease can have acute life-threatening episodes that may require critical care hospitalization, oxygen, and medications to help reduce the severity of bronchial constriction.
- There is no cure for feline asthma; the goal of treatment is controlling and minimizing the severity of the episodes.

Infectious Diseases of the Respiratory System

Pneumonia

Pneumonia is a bacterial, fungal, or viral infection involving the lung fields, the bronchi, and the trachea. The infection produces an infiltration of white blood cells and fluid into these areas.

Cause of Disease
The cause of the disease is a bacterial, fungal, or viral infection arising from the upper airway (trachea, mouth, or nasal passages), or, less often, from the blood.

Signalment
Pneumonia is more common in dogs than in cats and has been reported in higher incidence in sporting breeds, hounds, working dogs, and larger breed dogs. It has been reported in animals from 2 months to 15 years of age.

Common Points on Medical History
Depending on the causative agent producing the pneumonia, the disease can progress slowly to a very acute stage, and symptoms can be mild to severe. Common complaints with animals suffering from pneumonia can be

- weight loss,
- depression and lethargy,
- not wanting to eat or drink,
- inability to exercise,
- productive deep cough,
- sneezing, and
- nasal discharge.

Common Points in Initial Assessment
Pneumonia produces the following clinical signs:

- Fever
- Increased breathing rate (tachypnea)
- Extending the head and neck when breathing
- Inability to exercise
- Discharge of the eyes and nose
- Wheezing or crackling noise present on auscultation

Complications
If left untreated, pneumonia can cause a life-threatening whole-body infection (sepsis), producing severe illness, shock, and death.

Diagnosis
Diagnosis of generalized pneumonia is based on changes in the complete blood count, suggesting infection, thoracic radiographs, and aspirates of the trachea and bronchi collected through advanced procedures (i.e., transtracheal wash/bronchoscopy).

Treatment
Treatment is based on the presentation of the animal and the severity of the disease noted.

- **Hospitalization/supportive care:** In some cases if the pet is dehydrated, unable to eat or drink, or has a high fever, the veterinarian may suggest that the pet be hospitalized for intravenous fluids, intravenous antibiotics, and possibly oxygen support.
- **Medications:** Medications are focused on controlling or eliminating the infection, opening up the airways, and decreasing severe coughing or irritation. The following medications may be discussed.
  — **Antibiotics** are indicated if there is a concern regarding bacterial pneumonia.
  — **Antifungals** are indicated if there is a concern regarding fungal infection (see below).
  — **Bronchodilators** (i.e., theophylline, terbutaline, etc.) are used to help open up bronchi and increase the amount of air brought into the lungs.

> **Key Points in Discussing Bacterial Pneumonia with a Client**
> - Bacterial, fungal, or viral pneumonia is generally an acute infection of the bronchial and lung tissue of the pet.
> - The infection fills normal airways and lung tissue with purulent debris (pus) and infection, decreasing the ability of the lungs to oxygenate the tissue.
> - Animals will typically present with a moist, productive cough, fever, depression, anorexia, and increased breathing difficulty.
> - If enough lung tissue is affected, pneumonia can be a life-threatening condition.

Prevention
To help prevent bacterial pneumonia, try to maintain animals in a thermoneutral environment (70° Fahrenheit or more) during colder winter months.

Coccidiomycosis (Valley Fever)
Coccidiomycosis is a fungal infection that can affect the respiratory, skeletal, abdominal organs; integumentary system (skin); central nervous system; and other systems of the body. The disease is very slow growing and can take weeks to months to start showing symptoms.

Etiology
The cause of the disease is a fungal arthrospore from the species *Coccidiodes immitis,* which exists in warm dry environments (the Southwest of the United States) and typically affects only canines.

Signalment
Boxers and Doberman pinschers can be most sensitive to the infection. The disease is very rarely seen in cats.

Common Points in Medical History
Valley fever is a slowly progressing disease in which symptoms worsen over weeks to months, and initial signs may be very mild. Common medical complaints are

- weight loss,
- depression and lethargy,
- coughing,
- limping, and
- seizures.

Common Points on Initial Assessment
Since valley fever can affect multiple body systems, physical exams can show multiple system symptoms. Some changes in the physical exam can be

- chronic fever that is not responsive to antibiotics,
- depression and lethargy,
- coughing,
- increased lung sounds, crackles to rasps,
- limping,
- draining purulent (pus) tracts in the skin,
- infections within the eye (**uveitis**), and
- disease of the central nervous system, including seizures and depression.

Complications
Complications can vary depending on the systems affected, the animal, and the severity of infection. In some cases, untreated valley fever can produce life-threatening disease.

Diagnosis
Diagnosis of valley fever can be based on changes in the complete blood count suggesting infection, thoracic radiographs suggesting a pneumonia, and clinical serology testing for antibodies evident against valley fever (i.e., **coccidiomycosis titers**).

Treatment
- Treatment is focused on use of long-term antifungal drugs, supportive care, and anti-inflammatory medication for pain while the animal overcomes the fungus.
- The treatment of this disease can be extremely long term, and may take months to a year to treat.
- Overall, it is strongly recommended that the pet have restricted activity for the first 1–2 months of treatment.
- Valley fever is spread in the air throughout the Southwest, is not usually directly contagious from animal to animal, and is not considered zoonotic.

Blastomycosis
Blastomycosis is a fungal infection caused by the fungus *Blastomycosis dermatitidis* and can affect the respiratory, skeletal, integumentary (skin), central nervous, and other systems of the body. The disease is very slow growing and can take weeks to months to start showing symptoms.

Etiology
The cause of the disease is a fungal arthrospore, which exists in warm/high-humidity environments. Growth is associ-

ated also with moist, rotting organic debris, such as bird droppings. Areas of decreased sunlight also help the spore to proliferate (i.e., old barns).

Signalment
Male canines between 1–5 years of age, especially Doberman and Labrador retriever breeds, are the most susceptible. Felines (no sex predisposition) between 2–7 years are most commonly at risk.

Common Points in Medical History
Blastomycosis is a slowly progressing disease in which symptoms worsen over weeks to months, and initial signs may be very mild. Common medical complaints are

- inability to exercise (exercise intolerance),
- anorexia/weight loss (chronic),
- lameness,
- cough, and
- seizures.

Common Points on Initial Assessment
Since blastomycosis can affect multiple body systems, physical exams can show multiple system symptoms. Some changes in the physical exam can be

- fever,
- chronic cough/shortness of breath,
- lymph node enlargement,
- skin lesions—abscesses or fluid-filled granulomas,
- lameness,
- hind limb paralysis (cats), and
- eye problems—infections inside the eye (uveitis).

Complications
Complications can vary depending on the system affected, the animal, and the severity of infection. In some cases, untreated blastomycosis can produce life-threatening disease.

Key Points in Discussing Fungal Pneumonia with a Client
- Fungal pneumonia is a chronic, slowly progressing disease affecting the lung fields and possibly other body systems (i.e., eyes, central nervous system, organs, intestine).
- The disease may start with mild, subtle signs of cough, weight loss, anorexia, and depression and then may develop into severe systemic disease.
- Because fungal infections grow very slowly, treatment may take months to cure.
- If untreated, fungal infections can produce whole-body life-threatening systemic infections.

Diagnosis
Diagnosis of blastomycosis can be based on changes in the complete blood count suggesting infection, thoracic radiographs suggesting pneumonia, and clinical serology testing for antibodies evident against blastomycosis (i.e., **blastomycosis titers**).

Treatment
Treatment is focused on use of long-term antifungal drugs, supportive care, and anti-inflammatory medication for pain while the animal overcomes the fungus. **The treatment of this disease can be extremely long term and may take months to a year to treat.** Overall, it is strongly recommended that the pet have restricted activity for the first 1–2 months of treatment.

Canine Distemper Virus (CDV)
This disease is passed by airborne exposure or from direct contact of nasal or ocular discharge. The disease does not exist in the environment for long. The disease can have two phases: acute, which is the upper respiratory form, and chronic, which is the neurologic form.

If neurologic signs occur, there is a poor prognosis for recovery.

Etiology
The cause of the disease is a virus affecting dogs and other carnivores. Often the acute form will occur within 10 days of exposure initially, with neurologic signs showing up possibly 30 or more days later.

Signalment
All dogs can be affected with the disease. However, with regular vaccinations adult dogs have a better chance of resistance.

Incubation Period
Once exposed, the dog may begin to show signs within 10–28 days.

Common Points on Medical History
Since canine distemper virus can produce two distinct syndromes, either simultaneously or separated by a few weeks, the chief medical complaints can vary.

In the acute, or respiratory, form complaints may be

- depression,
- anorexia,
- sneezing,
- coughing, and
- purulent nasal or ocular discharge.

In the chronic, or neurologic, form the disease may occur in conjunction with the acute form or be seen up to 30 or more days later. Common signs are

- a history of chronic upper respiratory disease, sometimes within the last 30 days;
- seizures, focal to grand mal; and
- changes in behaviors.

Common Points on Initial Assessment
Clinical signs can vary depending on what systems are being infected by the virus.

In the acute/upper respiratory form, signs may be

- fever (usually high, more than 104°);
- purulent (pus) nasal and ocular discharge;
- dehydration; and
- vomiting and diarrhea (rare).

In the chronic/neurologic form, signs may occur in conjunction with the acute form or be seen up to 30 or more days later. Common signs are

- seizures, focal to grand mal;
- changes in behavior;
- increased sensitivity to pain (**hyperesthesia**);
- coma; and
- death (up to 90% mortality).

Patients that come in with symptoms suggestive of this disease should be isolated immediately due to its infectious potential to other patients.

Complications
There are some common complications to CDV.

- **Seizures:** If the patient recovers from the neurologic phase of the disease, the patient may have seizures for its lifetime.
- **Dental lesions:** In juvenile patients, the high fever can produce enamel lesions to the adult teeth, causing breaks in the surface of the enamel on the teeth.
- **Hard pad:** Some juvenile pets will have hardening of their pads secondary to the virus.

Diagnosis
In general, the tentative diagnosis of CDV is based on the presence of physical signs and changes in the blood work. Some clinical diagnostics are as follows.

- **CDV blood titers:** This is a clinical diagnostic test for the presence of antibodies in the blood against the distemper virus. **However, any vaccinated animal will have some positive titer level to CDV.**
- **CDV titer—cerebral spinal fluid:** This test of the cerebral spinal fluid for antibodies against CDV can suggest a distemper viral infection of the central nervous system.
- **Conjunctival smear:** As with many viral infections, CDV does leave intracellular remnants called **inclusion**

bodies in specific cells of the body. With CDV, inclusion bodies can be found in the cells of the inner eyelid (the **conjunctiva**) during the acute upper respiratory phase of the infection. Observation of these inclusion bodies suggests CDV infection.

Treatment

The treatment is focused on supportive care while the animal overcomes the virus. It is recommended that the dog have some form of fluid therapy to maintain hydration and antibiotics for secondary infection. Overall, it is strongly recommended that the dog be hospitalized for intravenous fluids and antibiotics and careful monitoring for dehydration, electrolyte imbalances, and low blood sugar.

Prevention

Most patients that have gone through their entire puppy series of vaccinations and are up to date on adult vaccinations have high immunity against CDV.

Environmental

Clean the exposed area with a 20% bleach solution, Parvosol, or other hospital disinfectant. The virus lives in the environment for only a short period of time (days).

Key Points in Discussing Canine Distemper Virus with a Client
- CDV is an acute upper respiratory viral infection that generally infects unvaccinated young dogs.
- Physical signs of the upper respiratory disease are severe nasal and ocular discharge, fever, anorexia, depression, and coughing.
- Fifty percent of animals infected with CDV will also have infection of the central nervous system as well.
- Physical signs of the neurologic system are seizures, increased sensitivity to pain, behavior changes, and death.
- There is a high mortality rate (approximately 90%) associated with animals that have central nervous system infections.
- Neurologic signs can occur up to 30 days after the upper respiratory phase of the disease.
- Most dogs that have gone through their full set of puppy vaccinations and that are up to date on their adult vaccinations are highly resistant to CDV infection.
- Distemper virus exists for only a short time in the environment (days).

Canine and Feline Kennel Cough—Tracheobronchitis

Tracheobronchitis is a highly infectious upper respiratory and bronchial infection that is a combination of a viral and bacterial or fungal infection affecting most dogs and cats, especially in a shelter environment.

Etiology

Kennel cough is caused by an initial viral infection that develops into a secondary bacterial component.

Signalment

All dogs and cats can be potentially affected. Dogs and cats from 6 to 30 weeks are at highest risk for the most severe form of the disease. The incubation time is 4–10 days.

Common Points in Medical History

Kennel cough is a mild to moderate upper respiratory infection producing the complaints

- coughing,
- sneezing,
- depression, and
- anorexia (occasionally).

Common Points on Initial Assessment

Kennel cough generally produces mild upper respiratory signs producing

- coughing,
- sneezing,
- nasal discharge,
- ocular discharge,
- increased respiratory effort with increased lung sounds, and
- fever.

Patients that come in with symptoms suggestive of this disease should be isolated immediately due to its infectious potential to other patients.

Complications

If gone untreated, a mild to severe bacterial or fungal pneumonia may occur.

Diagnosis

There is no obvious diagnostic test for kennel cough. Diagnosis is made on physical signs, history, blood work diagnostics to rule out other disease, and response to treatment.

Treatment

Unless the disease is severe, the animal should be placed on a broad spectrum of antibiotics and kept in a thermoneutral vaporized environment. If the pet develops dehydration and anorexia, hospitalization, fluids, and other medication may be indicated.

Prevention

There are intranasal and subcutaneous vaccines that offer protection for 3–6 months.

Keeping infectious dogs isolated from the general population and maintaining ample disinfection to exposed cages, pans, and other environmental regions are important to decrease the infectious potential of disease.

Key Points in Discussing Kennel Cough with a Client
- Kennel cough is generally a mixed viral and bacterial infection producing a mild to moderate upper respiratory infection/sore throat complex in cats and dogs.
- Common symptoms of kennel cough infection are a deep productive cough, sneezing, nasal discharge, and occasionally depression and anorexia.
- Animals with exposure to other pets in shelters, dog parks, grooming salons, and other locations are at higher risk to infection.
- There are vaccines that help decrease the risk of disease and physical signs of disease.
- Kennel cough disease is rarely a life-threatening disease.

Trauma to the Respiratory System
Pneumothorax

A pneumothorax occurs when there is an injury or trauma to the chest that allows air into the thoracic cavity. When the vacuum of the chest is interrupted, air rushes into the chest, collapsing the lungs and preventing normal respiration. How quickly the air enters the chest and the amount of air present determines how severe and acute the signs are. The condition can become life threatening 12–24 hours after the initial injury as air slowly accumulates within the chest cavity.

Etiology

A pneumothorax occurs when an acute trauma either punctures a hole in the thoracic cavity or produces severe bruis-ing and trauma to the lungs such that air spontaneously leaks from the lungs themselves. Some possible types of trauma are

- being hit by car,
- falling,
- animal attack,
  - — direct bite wounds into the chest,
  - — a smaller animal shaken by a larger one (i.e., a big dog–little dog attack),
- gunshot/BB wound.

Signalment

There is no age, sex, or breed predilection to a pneumothorax.

Common Points in Medical History

Animals may present with just a history of trauma and initially may show very limited symptoms. With more advanced pneumothorax, some complaints may be

- increased respiratory difficulty,
- restlessness,
- weakness, and
- collapse.

Common Points on Physical Examination

Signs depend on the severity of the pneumothorax. With a slow accumulation of air, the pet may appear to be normal on the initial triage examination. As the pneumothorax worsens, common physical concerns are

- open-mouth breathing,
- increased respiratory rate and difficulty,
- abdominal breathing,
- purple to blue to gray mucus membrane color,
- bounding pulses,
- generalized increased lung sounds,
- evidence of air under the skin (subcutaneous emphysema),
- collapse,
- shock, and
- death.

Complications

If gone untreated, pneumothorax can produce a life-threatening emergency.

Diagnosis

Diagnosis of pneumothorax is based on history, physical examination, and thoracic radiography (see Figure 11.10).

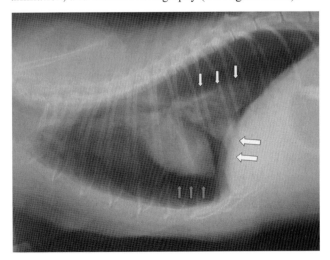

Figure 11.10. Thoracic radiography of a pneumothorax demonstrates three overall concerns: (1) The heart is floating off the sternum on a cushion of air (red arrow); (2) lungs look consolidated and lung margins can be appreciated. (yellow arrow); (3) There is flattening of the diaphragm (white arrow).

Key Points in Discussing a Pneumothorax with a Client

- The chest cavity exists in a vacuum, which allows the lungs to expand and contract when the pet breathes.
- If air is introduced into the chest cavity from a puncture of the chest wall or from an injury to a lung, the lungs may collapse.
- This process can occur suddenly, producing symptoms of severe shortness of breath, blue to purple gum color, collapse, weakness, and even death.
- This process can also be a slow condition over 12–24 hours, and symptoms may not occur for several hours after the trauma.
- **If not treated quickly, these conditions can be fatal**.
- Types of traumas that can produce a pneumothorax are
  —being hit by car,
  —chest trauma/bite,
  —falls, and
  —small animals shaken by larger animals (animal fight).
- Pneumothorax is diagnosed by thoracic radiographs, and radiographs are often recommended after a pet has had a serious injury or attack, **even if the pet is asymptomatic at the time of exam**.
- It is strongly recommended that animals with pneumothorax be hospitalized for monitoring and treatment.

Treatment

Treatment depends on physical signs.

If a mild pneumothorax is detected on thoracic radiography after a trauma, but there are no physical symptoms, the veterinarian may simply recommend monitoring.

With mild to moderate physical symptoms, the pet may need a chest tap to remove the air accumulated, and the pet hospitalized and monitored.

With severe pneumothorax that does not improve with a single tap, a chest tube may need to be placed and maintained under critical care hospitalization.

Prevention

Preventing possible trauma can help decrease the chance of pneumothorax.

———

CD-ROM 1 reviews material presented in this chapter. Please try the cases for Section 2 (Anatomy and Physiology—The Science behind the Diseases) to help reinforce the information presented here.

Chapter 12

Cardiovascular System

Anatomy of the Cardiovascular System

In mammals, the heart is a four-chambered structure, with each chamber separated by valves. The heart lies on the floor of the thoracic cavity surrounded by the lungs. It is divided into two halves (see Figure 12.1).

The Overall Anatomy of the Heart

Right Heart

The right heart receives deoxygenated blood from the body and carries it to the lungs for oxygenation. The right side of the heart is further separated by two valves:

- The **right AV (tricuspid or right A/V valve)** separates the right atrium and the right ventricle.
- The **pulmonic valve** separates the right ventricle from the pulmonary artery, which takes blood to the lungs for oxygenation.

Left Heart

The left heart receives oxygenated blood from the lungs and distributes the blood to the rest of the body. The left side of the heart is further separated by two valves:

- The **left atrioventricular valve (mitral valve** or **left AV valve)** separates the left atrium from the left ventricle and opens to push oxygenated blood from the lungs into the lower ventricle.
- The **aortic valve** separates the left ventricle from the aorta and opens to push oxygenated blood into the entire body.

Pericardium

The heart is surrounded by a sheet of clear tissue called the **pericardium**. It separates the heart from the rest of the chest, preventing an infection of the heart. It produces a small amount of clear sterile fluid, which normally keeps the heart slightly moist and prevents bacteria from setting up an infection.

The heart is composed of specialized striated muscle that works collectively to stimulate its own contractions and contracts as one unit strongly enough to pump blood through the body. Blood flows through the heart and into the body in a dynamic cycle to meet the demands of oxygenation. A normal cardiac cycle begins as follows.

1. Deoxygenated blood from the **cranial** and **caudal vena cava** enters the right atrium.
2. As the right atrium contracts, blood is then passed through the right AV valve (**tricuspid valve**) into the right ventricle.
3. Next, the right ventricle contracts, pushing blood into the lungs to be oxygenated via the pulmonic artery.
4. Once the blood is oxygenated at the alveolar level, blood then moves back into the left atrium from the lungs via the pulmonic vein.
5. As the left atrium contracts, the blood is pushed through the left AV valve (**mitral valve**) into the left ventricle.
6. Finally, as the left ventricle contracts, the blood is pushed into the body via the largest artery, the **aorta.**

Heart contraction is divided into two phases; the first phase, the **diastole,** describes the phase of contraction of the atriums. The goal of this phase is to move blood from atria into the ventricles.

1. Both atriums contract at the same time to pass the blood from the atriums into the ventricles.
2. Here the AV valves open and then snap shut at the end of diastole.
   - The right atrium pushes deoxygenated blood into the right ventricle.
   - The left atrium pushes oxygenated blood into the left ventricle.
3. At the end of the diastolic cycle, the AV valves snap shut. This action produces the **first heart sound ("lub")** or S_1 (see Figure 12.2).

The next phase of the heart beat is **systole** and describes the phase of contraction of the ventricles (see Figure 12.3).

1. Contraction of the left and right ventricles pushes blood into the body at the same time.
   - The right ventricle pushes deoxygenated blood through the pulmonic valve toward the lungs.
   - The left ventricle pushes oxygenated blood through the aortic valve to bring oxygenated blood into the general circulation.
2. The action of the closing of the aortic and pulmonic valves at the end of the systolic phases produces the **second heart sound ("dub")** or S_2.

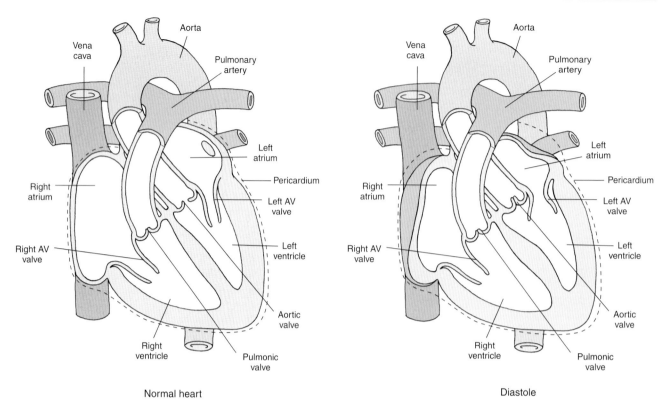

Normal heart

Figure 12.1.   An illustration of the normal heart.

Diastole

Figure 12.2.   An illustration of the normal heart during diastole.

For each successive normal diastolic and systolic cycle, blood is pushed out of the aorta into the body. This pressure causes a wave of blood flow through the elastic arteries, which produces

- a perceivable strong pulse,
- pink mucous membranes, and
- a capillary refill time (CRT) of less than 2 seconds.

Heart disease occurs when blood is unable to flow through the heart at a normal rate to meet the demands of the body. This chapter will discuss many potential causes of heart failure. Cardiac pathology can occur in either the left, right, or both sides of the heart. However, when the normal flow of blood is slowed or inhibited, the following pathologic changes can occur.

In a chronic condition, the contractions of the ventricles with a leaking AV valve produce a retrograde flow of blood back into the atrium. Over time, this increased volume causes atrial enlargement.

As the atrium enlarges and the blood continues to have decreased flow, an accumulation of blood in the tissue immediately caudal to the right and left atriums occurs. On the right side, the blood will back up into the liver; on the left side the blood backs into the lung fields.

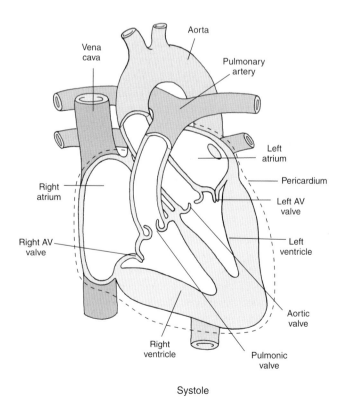

Systole

Figure 12.3.   An illustration of the normal heart during systole.

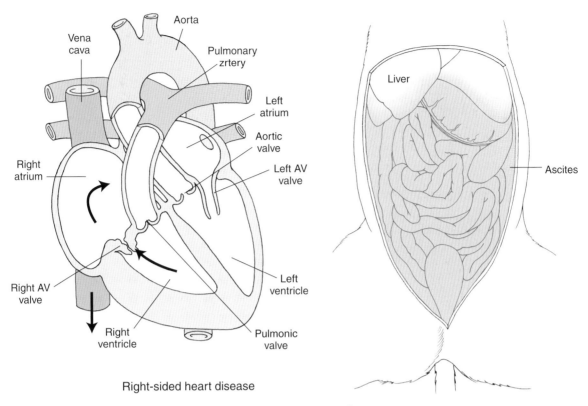

Figure 12.4. An illustration of right-sided heart disease with hepatic congestion.

As there is decreased flow through these organs, the fluid component of blood may begin to move out of the vessels and collect within the organs and/or the body cavity. This is called **congestion**. Depending upon which side of the heart is affected, pathologies may occur.

In **right-sided heart congestion**, the blood begins to pool within the liver (**hepatic congestion)** and collect in the abdominal cavity. This fluid is called **ascites** (see Figure 12.4).

In **left-sided heart failure,** in the dog, the fluid begins to accumulate in normal airways. This is called **pulmonary edema** (see Figure 12.5). In the cat, fluid builds up around the lungs and heart; this is called **pleural effusion** (see Figure 12.6).

Although discussed in detail in Chapter 13, a common secondary component to chronic heart disease is kidney disease and failure. The kidneys require a constant rate of blood flowing through them at all times. With decreased blood flow, the kidneys have decreased ability to filter blood at an acceptable rate. Over time, kidney tissue becomes damaged and chronic renal disease can occur. **Since many of the medications (i.e., furosemide, enalapril, etc.) for heart disease increase the kidney's output, it is very important to have the medical team inform the pet's owner of potential secondary renal disease and monitor the animal regularly for changes in blood work results.**

Obtaining a History of Cardiac Disease

The most important key to getting a thorough history regarding cardiac disease is to understand the basic difference between canine and feline heart disease.

In canines, heart disease is generally a **slowly progressive chronic disease** that presents with worsening symptoms over time until the animal enters a cardiac failure state. Typically, chief complaints are weakness, lethargy, inability to exercise properly (**exercise intolerance**), coughing, and shortness of breath.

In felines, heart disease generally presents as a sudden and acute process with little to no previous history or symptoms. The cat can act completely normally just hours before it presents with acute signs of cardiac failure. The disease itself has been going on for months to years, but felines rarely show chronic evidence of heart problems until they are in an acute failure episode.

As with respiratory disease (see Chapter 11), the focus of obtaining a history is trying to differentiate if the symptoms are stemming from pathology of the respiratory or cardiac systems. At times it is impossible to differentiate the signs. However, some key questions to help indicate if there is cardiac disease are presented here.

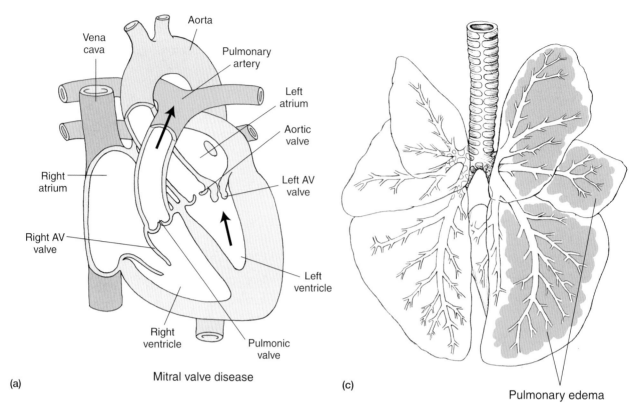

(a)   Mitral valve disease

(c)   Pulmonary edema

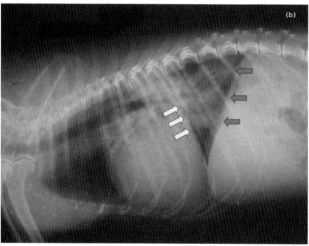

Figure 12.5. An illustration of left-sided heart disease with hepatic congestion (a). The radiograph (b) shows enlargement of the left atrium as noted by extension of the caudal heart silhouette dorsally and caudally (white arrows) and fluid accumulation in the caudal dorsal lung lobes (dark arrows) and (c).

Is a Cough Evident?

In general, coughing produced by heart disease is due to pulmonary congestion or enlargement of the heart, which pushes upward on the trachea, producing a significant cough. This type of cough is generally associated with the following.

- **Excitement:** Coughs that are made worse with exercise or excitement can suggest heart problems severe enough to affect the pet's ability to exercise normally.
- **Exercise:** Animals that cough when exercised or with increased activity may have cardiac disease. These animals' hearts cannot keep up with the demands that are associated with increased activity.

Is the Cough Worse at Night?

At night when the air cools, water droplets condense and pool in the lung fields. Healthy lungs can handle the increased fluid condensation. Animals with chronic conditions, such as heart disease patients that have decreased ability to remove fluid from the lung fields, can have a more productive cough at night.

Does the Pet Show Exercise Intolerance?

When pets cannot maintain normal levels of activity, it suggests that they cannot oxygenate their tissue adequately and they may have cardiac disease. If this is noted, further questions may need to be asked.

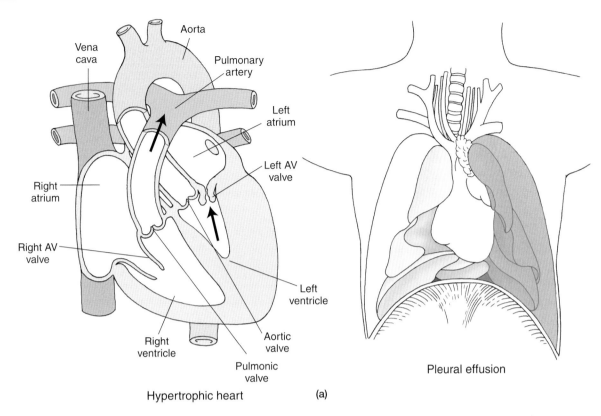

Hypertrophic heart   (a)

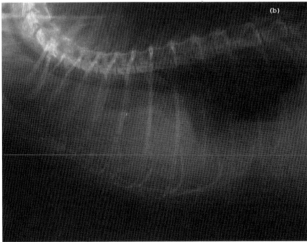

Figure 12.6. Illustration and radiograph of pleural effusion in the cat (a). Compare this radiograph to the one in Figure 12.5. Note the loss of detail (line) of the ventral lung fields and cardiac silhouette (b). This is caused by the buildup of fluid in the ventral chest.

Has There Been an Episode of Collapse or Fainting?
- These pets should be handled with extreme caution because their heart is so severely affected that the pet collapses or loses consciousness with any exertion.
- These pets should be placed in oxygen and the medical team notified immediately.

Does the Pet Have Periods of Increased Respiratory Effort?
When patients seem to have episodes of increased rigor while breathing, breathe abdominally, breathe with their head and neck extended, or make abnormal sounds while breathing, it suggests serious disease (see Figure 12.7).

Is the Pet on Heartworm Prevention?
In heartworm-endemic regions, heartworm testing and medication status is important to document. Furthermore, it is important to determine if the pet has traveled to any heartworm-endemic regions in the last 6 months, especially in the spring and summer months (see below in disease section).

Obtaining an Initial Assessment with Cardiac Disease

Just as discussed in the last chapter, when assisting in the initial assessment of a pet affected with a possible cardiac disease or failure, it becomes important to be able to fully

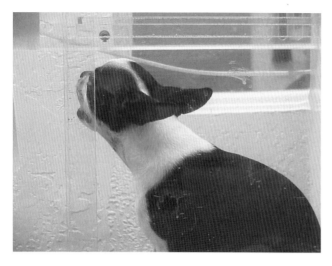

Figure 12.7. Image of a dog in an oxygen cage with severe respiratory disease. Note the pet is extending his neck and head upward while open-mouth breathing.

Table 12.1. Triage concerns in the cardiology patient.

Systems	Signs Indicating an Emergency
Mentation	Stressed, eyes dilated
	Nonresponsive/comatose
Fever	Temp >104.5°
	Temp <99° (due to shock, DIC, coma, sometimes due to aortic thrombo-embolism)
Hydration	Dehydration >5–7%
Gum color	Blue, purple, or gray
Capillary refill time	CRT >2–3 seconds
Respiratory nature, auscultation, and rate	Nature: Pet's open-mouth breathing, abdominally breathing with head and neck elevated.
	Auscultation: Severely increased respiratory noise, evidence of rasps or crackles.
	Rate: Respiratory rates >80–100 breaths per minute
Heart rate/pulse	Rate: Heart rates <80 bpm or >180–200 bpm
	Pulse: Change in pulse quality
	• Weak pulse
	• No pulse
	• Paradoxical
	• Pulse deficits
Limbs (feline)	Animal is unable to bear weight on limbs that are cool, painful, swollen, and without a pulse, or has decreased pulses (thromboembolism).

auscultate the animal for abnormalities. A technician must be able to practice listening with the stethoscope to normal and abnormal cardiac sounds in order to properly evaluate the sick and hospitalized pet.

The most important concept is that these are potentially life-threatening diseases that may need quick assessment and treatment.

> Practice Point: If a team member is unsure if a pet may have life-threatening cardiac failure, oxygen is never contraindicated (see Table 12.1).

Pulse

The pulse is one of the most important indicators of heart disease. It represents cardiac output and efficiency. There are animals that may present in an emergency or anesthetic situation with reasonable heart rates, but have abnormal or missing pulse rates. Changes in the pulse do not always indicate heart disease; however, the pulse must always be evaluated when there are concerns of cardiac problems. The pulse should be evaluated as follows.

Pulse Rate

Changes in pulse rate can be suggestive of a cardiac or systemic disease.
- Normal pulse rates are generally as follows.
  Canines: 80–120 beats per minute
  Felines: 100–140 beats per minute
- **Tachycardia** is defined as an abnormally rapid or accelerated heart rate. Tachycardic rates are defined as follows.
  Canines: >200 beats per minute
  Felines: >220 beats per minute

- **Bradycardia** is defined as an abnormally slow rate. Bradycardia rates are defined as follows.
  Canines: <60 beats per minute
  Felines: <80 beats per minute

Pulse Quality

Evaluation of pulse quality is extremely important in the differentiation of cardiac disease. Evaluating overall quality requires the team member to practice determining what a normal pulse feels like on numerous healthy animals. All members of the hospital team should be able to determine what a normal versus an abnormal pulse feels like.

Weak Pulse

Pulses that are diminished or not perceivable suggest that the heart cannot adequately perfuse tissue. This always suggests a life-threatening emergency and can be caused by many disease entities:

- Heart disease/failure (see below)
- Shock (see Chapter 30)
- Severe dehydration
- Partial arterial thrombus (see below)

Pulse Deficit

For each heartbeat there should be a definable pulse. Each team member should place his or her hand on the femoral ar-

Abdominal aorta

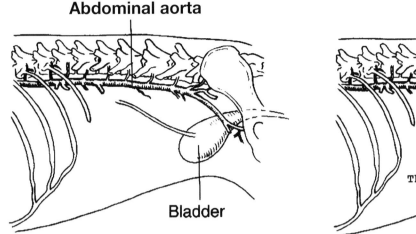
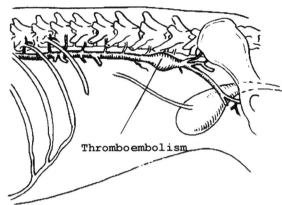

Figure 12.8.   An illustration of a saddle thrombus (thromboembolism) in the terminal aorta.

tery (or brachial, digital, or other arteriole) while auscultating the heart. For every heartbeat there should be a pulse. If not, this is a pulse deficit.

- This is an extremely important observation to make since detection of a pulse deficit can be the first indication of a life-threatening cardiac arrhythmia or shock situation.
- *Animals with severe pulse deficits can be in life-threatening cardiac failure.*
- Any pulse deficits should be reported to the medical team immediately.

Paradoxical Pulse
Another important distinction of pulse quality is the **para-doxical pulse**. This is a syndrome in which the pulse weakens and strengthens as the patient inhales and exhales. This change suggests a fluid accumulation around the heart, a **pericardial effusion**.

- As the heart is surrounded by large amounts of fluid, it tries to push blood out while fighting increasing pressure within the pericardial sack.
- As the pet breathes in, the interthoracic pressure increases, and the heart is unable to maintain normal cardiac output.
- This causes the pulses to weaken as the pet inspires and strengthen as the pet expires, due to the changes of interthoracic pressure.
- Although there are other diagnostic tests that help the medical team determine if there is a pericardial effusion, detection of a paradoxical pulse is an important observation of serious disease.

No Pulse
Lack of a pulse is a life-threatening condition suggestive of cardiovascular shock, cardiovascular collapse, and thromboembolism in the feline.

Cardiovascular Shock—No Cardiac Output
In cardiovascular shock there is still an evident heartbeat, but the heart is unable to maintain any cardiac output. *If not treated immediately, the pet will go into complete cardiovascular collapse.*

Cardiovascular Collapse—Code
In cardiovascular collapse, there is no pulse or respiration evident. *Cardiopulmonary resuscitation must be initiated immediately* (see Chapter 31).

Thromboembolism—Feline
With severe feline heart diseases the ventricles and atria can be enlarged, causing abnormal blood flow within the heart. As this occurs, a clot can form, attaching itself to the heart muscle.

The clot can break loose (called a **thromboembolism**) and begin moving through the arteries until it lodges within a smaller artery. A common site for an embolism to lodge is where the aorta splits to become the femoral artery, which feeds the hind legs (see Figure 12.8). If the limbs have no pulse and are cool, it can suggest an arterial thromboembolism.

Breathing
As discussed in Chapter 11, respiratory rate and quality can be significantly altered in animals with left-sided heart disease. The following parameters should be noted.

Is the Pet Tachypnic?
Animals can breathe more rapidly (be **tachypnic**) when nervous; however, rates above the following parameters can suggest abnormality:

- Canines with respiratory rates greater than 80–100 breaths per minute

- Felines with respiratory rates greater than 100–120 breaths per minute

Does the Pet Have Decreased Shallow Breathing?
Severely depressed animals with a slow, shallow respiratory cycle are animals that may be severely life threatened and may need the full attention of the medical team.

Does the Pet Have Abnormal or Noisy Respiration?
The normal respiratory pattern is a slow expansion and relaxation of the chest.

- **Abdominal breathing:** Although panting can appear to have an abdominal component, if animals must use their abdomen to drive air in and out of their lung field it can suggest serious respiratory disease. Increased abdominal breathing can suggest trouble breathing (**dyspnea.**)
- **Respiratory noise:** Is the pet making respiratory noise that can be appreciated without a stethoscope? If so, respiratory noise (also called a **stridor**) can suggest a potential obstruction of the upper airway. It is important to note if the stridor is occurring during inhalation, exhalation, or both?

Is There Extension of the Neck and Head While Breathing?
Pets that extend their head and neck upward in conjunction with increased respiratory effort may have life-threatening respiratory or cardiac disease. These pets are so severely affected that they must keep their trachea in an absolutely straight line to maximize air flow into the lungs (see Figure 12.7).

Color of Gums/Capillary Refill Time
Pets with respiratory disease that are having problems oxygenating their tissues have cyanotic mucous membranes. Their gums, whites of their eyes, rectum and other tissues are light purple to blue to gray.

CRT is often hard to assess because the gum color is cyanotic.

Auscultation of the Heart
Proper auscultation techniques of the cardiac system are described in Chapter 6. Murmurs occur when there is an abnormal flow of blood through a valve or a septal defect. The irregular flow of blood produces abnormal sounds as the blood flows in an altered path, masking the normal heart sounds. The most important concept is to identify if the pet has an altered heart sound. With practice, the team member should be able to identify the types of murmurs discussed next.

Valvular Murmurs
Valvular murmurs usually occur at one phase of heart contraction (systole versus diastole) as blood flows retrogradely through a narrow or damaged valve. The altered flow produces a high-pitched trill that masks the sounds of valve closure. When auscultated, the murmur is loudest over the valve. These types of murmurs are produced two ways.

Over time AV valves can become leaky, allowing blood to reflux when the valve is normally closed (see Figure 12.9).

In **pulmonic/aortic valves,** there is typically a narrowing of the area in front, at the valve level or above the valve. This is called a **stenosis**. The sound is produced as the blood increases speed going through the narrowed region.

Other murmurs are produced when there is an abnormal opening in the septal wall or between blood vessels. This pathology usually produces a constant flow of blood from the right to the left side of the heart (see Figure 12.10).

- When auscultated, the murmur has a constant machine-like sound without the normal sounds of valve closure.
- *The murmurs are usually during both the diastole and systolic phases of contraction.*

Auscultation of the Lung Fields
As discussed in Chapter 11, changes in the lung fields can also suggest cardiac disease.

Respiratory Crackles
Of all the respiratory sounds discussed, the one of most concern in connection with cardiac disease is **respiratory crackles.** The sound is best represented as the crumpling of cellophane paper.

In this situation, the sound is produced because air must go through pulmonary edema (fluid) caused by left-sided heart disease. The normal airways and alveoli are filled with cells and fluid. The crackle sounds are produced as air passes through the cramped region.

Lack of Sound
The inability to hear the heart can be as important as auscultating an abnormal heart sound. Inability to hear a normal heart sound can suggest

- the presence of a pleural effusion or a pericardial effusion, which can produce decreased heart sounds, or
- a mass in a lung field or near the heart that can obscure normal sounds.

Also, in some deep-chested dogs the heart can sit to one side or the other side of the chest and decrease heart sounds on one side.

Diagnostics for the Cardiovascular System

Because heart disease can occur in conjunction with many other systemic inflammatory, infectious, metabolic, and hormonal diseases, a cardiac evaluation may involve in-depth clinical diagnostic procedures. An overview of these procedures are presented next.

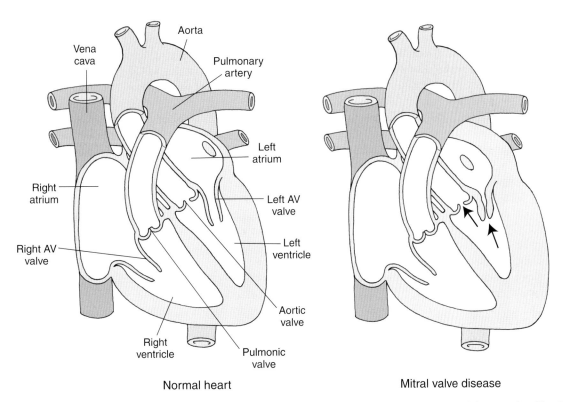

Vena cava

Aorta

Pulmonary artery

Left atrium

Right atrium

Left AV valve

Right AV valve

Left ventricle

Aortic valve

Right ventricle

Pulmonic valve

Normal heart

Mitral valve disease

Figure 12.9. Image of blood flow through a normal heart and a heart with mitral valve disease. The normal heart pushes blood through the left AV valve during diastole and then pushes blood through the aortic valve during systole, producing a normal "lub-dub" as the valves close. With mitral valve disease, the blood flows into the ventricle during diastole, but then flows through both the aorta and the partially closed mitral valve. This would produce a "lub-swish" sound, which would be heard loudest over the mitral valve during auscultation.

Blood flow through a septal defect

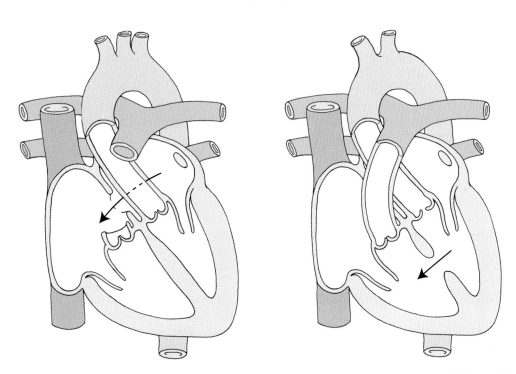

Figure 12.10. Image of flow of blood through an atrial or ventricular septal defect. The blood flows constantly through the opening, producing a constant machinelike murmur in both diastole and systole.

Diagnostic Blood Work

Blood diagnostic tests help determine if there is underlying organ, infectious, or hormonal disease that could predispose the pet to worsening an existing heart disease. Furthermore, it allows the veterinarian to evaluate if there is existing organ disease that may limit medical treatment options.

Complete Blood Count

A complete blood count allows the veterinarian to determine if there is any underlying anemia (low red blood cell count), increased white blood cell count, or low platelet count that may be adding additional stress to the pet.

Chemistry

A blood chemistry test is recommended to ensure there is no other organ, such as kidney, liver, or pancreas, affected. There are several general health concerns that can be evaluated with a blood chemistry workup.

- Kidney disease is a common secondary concern with any heart disease due to decreases in blood flow to the kidney.
- Severe alterations in normal electrolyte concentrations (calcium, potassium, sodium, magnesium, etc.) can have a profound effect on normal electrical rhythms of the heart.
- Increased thyroid hormone levels in the body can cause an increase in metabolism that can make the heart more prone to arrhythmias. This could apply to hyperthyroid cats (see Chapter 16) and dogs on thyroid supplementation.

Key Points in Discussing the Need for a Blood and Urine Evaluation with the Client
- There are serious underlying organ and hormonal diseases that can make heart disease worse. General blood work and urinalysis can allow the veterinarian to assess the overall health status of the pet.
- Furthermore, heart disease can cause secondary kidney disease. Since many of the medications increase the workload of the kidneys, it is important to ascertain normal organ function through routine blood work.
- Depending on the geographic region, there are specific clinical diagnostic tests that will help evaluate the pet for disease that can affect the heart and lungs (i.e., heartworm test).
- These clinical diagnostics in combination with other imaging studies will help evaluate the overall health of the pet.

In addition to a blood chemistry workup, a **urinalysis** is important as well. It allows the veterinarian to evaluate the patient for early changes that could suggest kidney disease. Changes in urine protein, concentrating ability, and urine sediment may indicate early renal pathology.

An additional diagnostic test, the heartworm test, is discussed below.

Diagnostic Imaging of the Chest and Heart

New advances in veterinary medicine allow us to view the chest, heart, and lungs. These newer technologies allow the veterinarian to image the internal architecture of the heart and measure changes in wall thickness and overall contractility of the heart. Some imaging diagnostics are discussed next.

Thoracic Radiography

Chest films allow the veterinarian to detect changes within the chest, heart size, tracheal position, mediastinum (region between the lungs), fluid in the chest, air in the chest, or possible masses or tumors (see Figure 12.11).

- When evaluating the heart, the thoracic cavity should be assessed on inspiration, when the lungs are fully inflated, with the pet on its right side; another radiograph should be taken with the animal on its back.
- Care must be taken with animals with cardiac disease. Some animals cannot comfortably be positioned for radiographs without producing severe respiratory distress.
- *Radiographic procedures should never be attempted in pets that are having severe respiratory difficulty.*

Key Points in Discussing the Need for a Radiographic Evaluation with the Client
- A radiograph study is being recommended because of concerns about coughing, respiratory distress, or changes in the physical examination that suggest disease of the heart and lungs.
- The study will help the medical team assess changes in the heart, chest, and lung fields that could suggest the difference between heart and pulmonary disease and will allow the veterinarian to make other diagnostic and treatment choices.

Ultrasound

Ultrasound of the heart allows the veterinarian to assess if there is fluid within the heart sack (**pericardium**) around the heart and if there are changes in the size of the ventricles, thickening of the heart wall, changes in the valves of the heart, and masses within the heart (see Figure 12.12). Furthermore, the veterinarian can take ultrasound measurements of the

- left atrium,
- left ventricle, and
- contractility of the heart.

These measurements allow the veterinarian to assess the degree of heart damage and, in future ultrasounds, the response to heart medications and treatments.

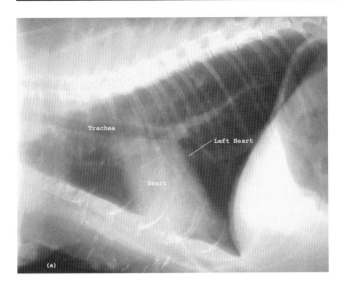
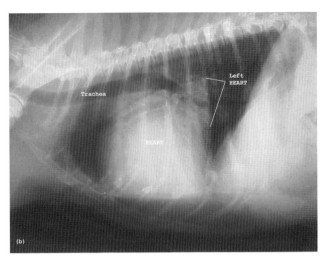

Figure 12.11.   Radiograph of a normal heart (a) and a heart affected with mitral valve disease (b). Notice that as the disease worsens, the left atrium enlarges, elevating the trachea and in time produces pulmonary edema (left heart disease). The changes in the heart and thorax allow the veterinarian to decide on further diagnostic and treatment options.

Key Points in Discussing the Need for an Ultrasound Evaluation with the Client

- Because there is concern regarding underlying heart disease from evidence found on physical exam or other diagnostic tests, a cardiac ultrasound is being recommended.
- The cardiac ultrasound allows the medical team to create an image of the internal architecture of the heart, its chambers, and its movement.
- This allows the veterinarian to evaluate changes in the heart wall and valves that could suggest disease or cancer.
- Furthermore, diagnostic measurements can be taken to evaluate the severity of the heart disease and the heart's ability to pump blood. These measurements can also be used as a baseline for further studies to see the effectiveness of treatment and the progression of disease.

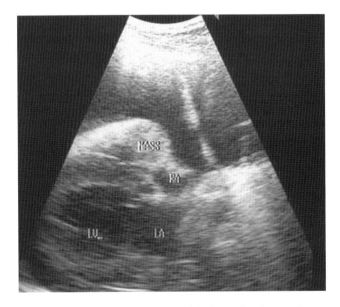

Figure 12.12.   Ultrasound image of the heart showing an abnormally large heart with a possible mass associated with the right atrium. The darkened region above the heart represents evidence of a pericardial effusion.

Electrocardiogram

An electrocardiogram (EKG) allows the medical team to assess the electrical rhythm of the heart. The heart acts as an electrical pump producing a specific electrical rhythm that initiates normal contraction of the atria and ventricles. Abnormal electrical rhythms are possible in many cardiac diseases and secondary to other systemic concerns. An abnormal EKG rhythm suggests an abnormal contraction of the heart. If these abnormal rhythms occur often, the animal's life can be threatened. (EKGs are fully discussed in Chapter 24.)

Pulse Oximetry

Pulse oximetry determines the oxygen-carrying capacity of the blood. A decrease in blood oxygen levels can suggest poor oxygenation of tissue or decreased ability of the lungs to properly bring in oxygen. A pulse oximetry with a rectal or tendon probe can be an excellent tool to monitor changes in the oxygen-carrying capacity of the body. Normal pulse oximetry should be 90% or greater oxygen saturation for canine and feline blood.

Blood Pressure

Because heart disease can occur from systemic hypertension (high blood pressure) and cause systemic hypertension, blood pressure monitoring is of key importance in diagnosing and treating cardiac patients. Increasing blood pressure can increase the strain on the heart's ability to perfuse the body and can make the disease condition worse. (See Chapter 13 for more information on blood pressure.)

Key Points in Discussing the Need for Further Diagnostics in a Cardiac Patient

EKG

- An EKG measures the heart's electrical impulses that stimulate normal contraction.
- If the electrical impulse is abnormal, it suggests the heart is not contracting normally.
- Abnormal cardiac rhythms can greatly affect the heart's output and can endanger the pet.
- The medical team needs to evaluate the heart's electrical impulses to ensure there are no underlying abnormal cardiac contractions.

Pulse Oximetry

When there are concerns that the heart cannot meet the demands of the body for oxygenating tissue, a pulse oximetry allows the medical team to quantitatively evaluate the oxygen saturation in the blood. A normally functioning heart can maintain 90–100% oxygenation of the blood at all times. Decreases in the result of a pulse oximetry can suggest the severity of heart disease.

Blood Pressure

Blood pressure measures the overall resistance to blood flow in the arteries that the heart pumps against to produce a normal pulse. Abnormally high blood pressure (hypertension) from underlying disease can make the heart work much harder than necessary. If the pet suffers from borderline to severe high blood pressure, the veterinarian can suggest courses of medications to reduce hypertension and reduce the workload on the heart.

Diseases of the Cardiac System

Although not all diseases are mentioned in this discussion, the common diseases are presented with the goal being to understand and be able to explain to the client what the diseases are, how they can present themselves, and what the overall short- and long-term concerns of each disease can be. Any discussion of overall diagnostic and treatment pro-

tocols should be discussed based on the recommendations of the doctor and the medical team. Please use the following information as a basis to discuss and educate the client, *but never to diagnose a patient.*

Before discussing specific cardiac disease, understanding congestive heart failure is critical. Although cardiac disease can affect the heart valves, cardiac muscle, and rhythm, all these diseases can end in the syndrome of congestive heart failure and cardiovascular shock.

Cardiovascular shock (congestive heart failure) is the loss of the normal ability to perfuse the body and maintain normal blood pressure and cardiac output due to an obstructive, functional, or metabolic disease process. Symptoms and pathology of the disease depend on which side of the heart is most affected. In general,

- **left-sided** heart failure produces an acute respiratory cardiac collapse even in the presence of chronic disease, and
- **right-sided** disease produces a chronic progressive hepatic and abdominal disease.

Left-Sided Heart Failure

Pathology

With left-sided heart disease, the heart is unable to advance blood at a rate adequate to meet the body's metabolic needs. This syndrome may be caused by

- pressure overload of the left heart,
- impediment of the left heart filling, and
- rhythm disturbances.

Heart failure may be caused by a combination of disease of the muscle, cardiac arrhythmias, and valvular disease. Congestive heart failure may be produced by one or all of these components. Not all heart failures will have a cardiac murmur, an arrhythmia, or a disease of the cardiac muscle.

Etiology

There are many potential causes of congestive heart failure caused by underlying disease of the heart, metabolic disease, hypertension, and other diseases. Some underlying diseases that can potentiate left-heart failure are

- cardiomyopathy (see below),
- hyperthyroidism (see Chapter 26),
- systemic hypertension (see Chapter 13),
- mitral valve disease (see below),
- cancer of the heart,
- narrowing of the outflow tract of blood leaving the heart (aortic stenosis), and
- any other disease entities that increase the heart output (e.g., hyperthyroidism, anemia, etc.) that can make heart disease more severe until there is a potential failure.

Signalment

There is no breed or sex predilection with cardiovascular shock.

Common Points in Medical History

In canine disease, congestive heart failure is a slowly progressing chronic disease that presents with worsening symptoms over time until the animal enters a cardiac failure state. Common medical complaints are

- weakness,
- lethargy,
- inability to exercise properly,
- coughing, and
- shortness of breath.

In feline disease congestive heart failure generally presents itself as a sudden and acute process, with little to no previous history or symptoms. The cat can act completely normally hours before the syndrome occurs.

Common Points on Initial Assessment

These animals present in a life-threatening syndrome of respiratory and cardiac failure, which may progress to cardiopulmonary arrest.

If the pet seems severely challenged, you may not be able to complete a thorough triage exam and emergency treatment may be indicated immediately.

There are several common physical signs of cardiovascular shock.

Dyspnea

Respiratory rates greater than 80–100 breaths per minute (canine) and greater than 100–120 breaths per minute (feline) indicate cardiovascular shock. Open-mouth breathing, with head extended and ears back, and abdominal breathing are other signs.

Color of Gums

Blue, purple, or blue coloration of gums suggest poor oxygenation of tissue (cyanosis).

Pulse

The pulse should be monitored for both rate and quality to help determine the cause and magnitude of the cardiac disease evident. Some common factors to observe are the pulse rate and quality.

In tachycardia, in early heart failure, the pulse rates are as follows.

- Feline: >220 beats per minute
- Canine: >200 beats per minute

In bradycardia, in later failure, the pulse rates are as follows.

- Feline: <80 beats per minute
- Canine: <60 beats per minute

The quality of the pulse observed includes the categories

- weak pulse,
- paradoxical,
- pulse deficit, and
- no pulses.

Auscultation

As with the pulse rate, auscultation can give the medical team an indication of the cause of disease. Common characteristics to observe while auscultating are

- valvular murmurs,
- lack of sound, and
- respiratory noise—crackles and wheezes.

Complications

Congestive heart failure can be a life-threatening disease even with complete medical support.

Diagnosis

Because cardiovascular shock can occur secondary to disease of the cardiac valve, heart muscle, cardiac arrhythmia, or other systemic disease, a thorough workup as discussed in the diagnostic section may be indicated. *Clinical diagnostics must be completed as the pet stabilizes and can handle the stress.*

Treatment

The goal of treatment of heart failure is to reduce the burden and stress on the animal while treating the underlying heart disease.

Oxygen is frequently used in treatment. In fact, *there is never a contraindication to oxygen therapy.* The animal may greatly improve simply by the increased oxygenation of the bloodstream and decreased demands on the heart. Administration of oxygen should be done with as little stress as possible. There are many ways to administer oxygen to a patient:

- Oxygen cage
- Anesthetic induction chamber
- Open face mask
- Oxygen e-collar
- Nasal oxygen (best way)

Catheter

Once the animal is stable enough to handled, an intravenous catheter should be set to allow venous access for medications and possible fluids.

Fluids

Large fluid boluses to stabilize for this kind of shock are not indicated! Excess fluid is already accumulating in the lung fields. The key to treatment is to try to move the excess fluid out of the lungs and body.

Medications

- **Diuretics:** The goal of diuretics such as furosemide (Lasix) is to produce a diuresis within the kidneys to increase the outflow of fluid through the urine. A high dose of furosemide may be key to help decrease pulmonary congestion. Although this will challenge the kidneys and could make an early to moderate kidney disease worse, this may be of secondary concern to the pet in this critical syndrome.

- **Venodialators:** Drugs such as nitroglycerine help dilate venules in the lungs, causing decreased left atrial filling pressure and reducing the factor that produces pulmonary congestion. The drug is generally applied topically and absorbed transdermally. *Latex gloves should be used when applying this medication or systemic uptake can occur in the medical staff.*
- **Antiarrhythmics:** Drugs such as digoxin or lidocaine are used in the presence of specific types of cardiac arrhythmias.
- **ACE inhibitors:** Drugs such as enalapril can aid in decreasing blood pressure, thus decreasing the amount of work the heart must do to move blood.
- **Sedating drugs:** In some cases, animals require light sedation to decrease their concern about the severe dypsnea and oxygenation of tissues. The patient's hyperventilation can actually can increase pulmonary edema.

Monitoring
Because left-sided congestive heart failure is an emergency situation, monitoring the critical care patient is important. *It is always important to remember that no monitoring or clinical diagnostics should be attempted if the pet is unstable and cannot handle the stress of the procedures.*

Animals should be monitored regularly (potentially every 15–60 minutes), at least visually, for

- respiratory effort,
- mentation (i.e., attitude, responsiveness), and
- urine output.

If possible, perform the following tasks with the least amount of stress possible every 1–3 hours, depending on the patient's stability.

- Auscultate the heart.
- Monitor pulses: check for pulse deficits.
- Auscultate the lungs: Check for moist lung sounds and crackles.
- Check mucous membrane color.
- Check the capillary refill time.
- Check hydration.

The following concerns should be observed, documented, and discussed with the medical team:

- Cool limbs—no pulse
- Increased respiratory effort or rate
- Change in pulse quality and rate
- Poor mucus membrane color
- Pulse deficit
- Nonresponsive or decreased responsivity

Fluid Monitoring
Fluids must be carefully monitored in animals with severe heart conditions. Because the heart's ability to move blood adequately is compromised, pulmonary and hepatic congestion can occur. These animals must be carefully monitored for fluid overload.

Diagnostic Monitoring
With continued care and hospitalization, regular diagnostic checks of the following may be necessary.

- **EKG:** A regular check for abnormal rhythms, slow, or rapid heart rate is indicated.
- **Pulse oximetry:** In some cases with poor oxygenation of tissue or decreased ability of the lungs to properly bring in oxygen, a pulse oximetry with a rectal or tendon probe can be an excellent tool to monitor changes in perfusion.
- **Electrolytes:** Animals on long-term fluids or on diuretics (i.e., Lasix [furosemide]) may become depleted in specific electrolytes, especially potassium. With low potassium, heart arrhythmias can be more common.
- **Kidney function:** As discussed previously, a common sequelae to heart disease can be renal disease due to decreased perfusion of the kidneys over time. Especially during an acute episode, with patients already on medications that can stress kidney function (i.e., enalapril, furosemide), function should be assessed.

Prevention
Through careful screening of susceptable breeds and geriatric animals, cardiac disease may be identified before congestive heart failure occurs. Many forms of heart disease are not curable but can be controlled with medications and diet. There may be periods of time when any pet with cardiac disease may still go through episodes of congestive heart failure.

Right-Sided Heart Failure
With right-sided heart disease, the heart is unable to advance blood at a rate adequate to meet the body's metabolic needs. This can be caused by pressure overload of the right heart, impediment of the right heart filling, or a rhythm disturbance. Right-sided heart failure produces a chronic disease, producing moderate to severe abdominal ascites, distention, and respiratory difficulty. It is less likely to produce an acute life-threatening crisis.

Etiology
There are many potential causes of congestive heart failure, including underlying disease of the heart, metabolic disease, hypertension, and other diseases. Some underlying diseases that can potentiate right heart failure are

- cardiomyopathy (see below)
- heartworm disease (see below)
- pulmonary hypertension
- tricuspid valve disease
- cancer of the heart
- narrowing of the outflow tract of blood leaving the right heart (pulmonary stenosis)
- any other disease entities that increase the heart output (e.g., hyperthyroidism, anemia) and that can make heart disease more severe until there is a potential failure.

Signalment
There is no breed or sex predilection with cardiovascular shock.

Common Points on Medical History
Right-sided heart disease is a more chronic condition that can have both symptoms of right- and left-sided disease. The decreased blood flow through the right heart produces hepatic congestion and ascites. Common medical complaints can be

- weakness,
- lethargy,
- abdominal distention,
- decreased ability to exercise, and
- weight loss.

Common Points on Initial Assessment
These animals can present with large distended abdomens and minimal to severe respiratory symptoms. Some pets can have increased respiratory disease secondary to severe abdominal distention inhibiting normal movement of the diaphragm. Common physical signs of cardiovascular shock are

- abdominal distention,
- dyspnea,
- cyanotic gums,
- changes in pulse quality and rate, and
- auscultation shows
  — valvular murmurs
  — lack of sound

Complications
Right-sided congestive heart failure can be a chronic life-threatening disease, producing severe ascites and respiratory difficulty from the abdominal fluid load.

Diagnosis
Because cardiovascular shock can occur secondary to disease of the cardiac valve, heart muscle, cardiac arrhythmia, or other systemic disease, a thorough workup as discussed in the diagnostic section may be indicated. *Clinical diagnostics must be completed as the pet stabilizes and can handle the stress.*

Key Points in Discussing Cardiovascular Shock/Congestive Heart Failure with Clients
- Congestive heart failure/cardiovascular shock is a syndrome produced from an underlying heart disease.
- The pet's heart cannot keep up with the demands placed upon it, and the patient cannot properly oxygenate their tissues.
- This produces a life-threatening respiratory and cardiac syndrome.

Canine
- Cardiac disease is a slowly progressing condition that produces a chronic cough that worsens with excitement or activity, weight loss, decreased ability to exercise, and possibly collapse.
- As the pet enters congestive heart failure, fluid begins to accumulate within the lung fields due to decreased blood flow through the lungs.
- This fluid, called pulmonary edema, further decreases the animal's ability to oxygenate its tissues and increase demands upon the heart and lungs.

Treatment focuses on the following

- Treatment is focused on supporting the pet through the crisis with medications that decrease the fluid accumulations within the lung fields and decrease the amount of work the heart must do.
- Furthermore, the pet is generally placed in a rich oxygen environment to help increase oxygen concentration within the body.
- With this disease, the fluid accumulations cannot be physically removed from the lungs, but require medication to decrease the fluid level.

Feline
- Cardiovascular disease is a chronic condition and the feline may show no obvious symptoms until *the pet is in an acute cardiac crisis*.
- Unlike the canine, the decreased movement of blood through the lungs and heart produces an accumulation of fluid within the chest cavity itself.
- This fluid, called pleural effusion, begins to further decrease the ability of the heart and lungs to expand and contract, worsening the overall disease process.

If not treated, the pet can progress into cardiovascular arrest. Treatment of the feline focuses on the following.

- As with the canine, the goal of treatment is to support the pet in an oxygen-rich environment with medications that help decrease the overall workload of the heart.
- Unlike the canine, the pleural effusion can be removed from the chest cavity through a medical procedure called a chest tap.

Dilative Cardiomyopathy

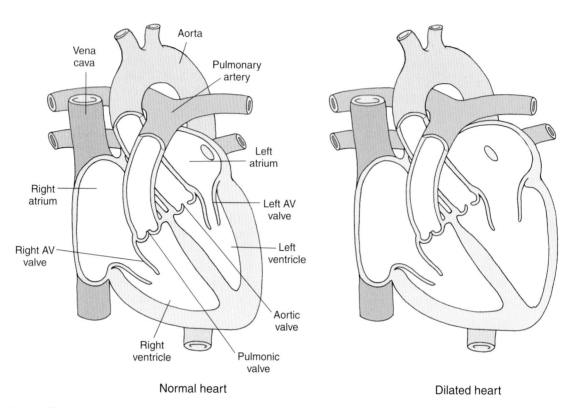

Figure 12.13.   Illustration of a normal heart (left) in comparison to one affected by dilatative cardiomyopathy.

Treatment

Treatment is focused on treating the underlying cardiac or systemic disease producing the hepatic congestion. Furthermore, with severe hepatic congestion, removal of large amounts of abdominal fluid (**ascites**) may need to occur at regular intervals.

Prevention

Through careful screening of susceptible breeds, routine diagnostic testing for heartworm disease, and monitoring of geriatric animals, cardiac disease may be identified before congestive heart failure occurs.

Diseases of the Cardiac Muscle

Canine Dilatative Cardiomyopathy

Dilatative cardiomyopathy is a degenerative disease of the heart in which the muscles of the ventricles become thin and weakened. The weakened muscle is unable to contract with the same force, decreasing the amount of blood that can be expelled from the ventricles (see Figure 12.13).

This produces decreased contractility of the left and right ventricle, increasing the amount of blood that is retained in both ventricles after each ventricular contraction. Over time, the ventricles enlarge. As this process continues, the blood

begins to build back into the left and right atrium and into the lungs and liver. The heart then tries to pump more blood at an increased rate to make up for the decreased amount of blood ejected. The enlarging ventricles can also pull the AV valves apart, causing them to leak (**mitral valve** or **tricuspid insufficiency**).

If the process of canine dilatative cardiomyopathy goes untreated, it can progress to heart failure and secondary kidney disease.

Etiology

The cause of the disease is unknown; however, viral, protozoal, genetic, and nutritional causes have been suggested.

Signalment

Dilatative cardiomyopathy can be prominent in all breeds of dogs, especially the Doberman pinschers, boxers, cocker spaniels, Irish wolfhounds, great Danes, and other giant breed dogs. The average age of onset is from 4 to 10 years. This disease is more common in males than females.

Common Points in Medical History

Unlike most forms of canine heart disease, *the Doberman and boxer forms of this disease can come on acutely without any previous history or symptoms of cardiac disease.* These pets may be admitted to the hospital in cardiovascular shock. However, some pets may show a chronic progressive disease. Some medical complaints can be

- weakness, lethargy, and collapse;
- decreased ability to exercise;
- coughing; and
- weight loss.

Common Points on Initial Assessment

Physical signs depend on the severity of the disease; if right, left, or both ventricles are affected; and how rapidly the changes in the heart occurred. Care should be taken with these pets because with severe disease, *pets can collapse and enter cardiopulmonary arrest with minimal stress.* Possible physical signs of disease are as follows.

- A cough is present that worsens at night. Pets may find it hard to lie down and get comfortable.
- Pets may have increased respiratory difficulty with
  — head extended,
  — elbows abducted,
  — abdominal breathing, and
  — increased respiratory rate.
- Pets may have changes in pulse rate and quality (pulse deficits).
- There may be changes in capillary refill time and mucous membrane color (cyanosis).
- Auscultation reveals
  — murmur,
  — lack of heart sounds, and
  — respiratory crackles.
- Pets may have a bloated abdomen with ascites present.

Complications

If not diagnosed and treated, dilatative cardiomyopathy can progress into congestive heart failure and cardiopulmonary arrest.

Diagnosis

Dilatative cardiomyopathy can also affect the cardiac valves, produce cardiac arrhythmias, and lead to secondary organ disease. A thorough workup as discussed in the diagnostic section may be indicated.

Treatment

Treatment is focused on reducing the amount of work the heart must do, correcting irregular heart beats, reducing the amount of fluid on the lungs caused by the buildup of fluid, and restricting activity. Some therapies are discussed next.

Medications commonly prescribed fall into the following categories.

- **Diuretics:** These drugs help decrease the amount of fluid within the lung fields. They accomplish this by stimulating the kidneys to push out more fluid from the body (e.g., furosemide, chlorothiazide).
- **Bronchodilators:** These drugs help dilate the bronchi to maximize the flow of oxygen into the lungs (e.g., theophylline, aminophylline, terbutaline).
- **ACE inhibitors:** This category of drugs helps lower the blood pressure in the body, decreasing the amount of work the heart must do to pump blood through the body. (e.g., enalapril, benazepril).
- **Antiarrhythmics:** These drugs help prevent irregular heart rhythms (e.g., lidocaine, procainimide).

Diet is an important part of treatment.

- **A low-salt/low-protein diet** is recommended. Low-salt diets decrease the amount of fluid retained in the body, decreasing the amount of dietary salt can slow the buildup of fluid within the lung tissue. Low-protein diets decrease the amount of work the kidneys have to do in clearing toxins produced from protein metabolism.
- **Amino acid supplementation:** Some heart conditions can be linked to low dietary levels of specific amino acids, taurine or carnitine. These amino acids can be supplemented to help slow continuing heart damage.
- **Vitamin supplementation:** The vitamin supplement coenzyme Q10 has been used as a dietary supplement and aids the heart in conduction of energy within its muscle fibers.

Prevention

Through careful screening of susceptiable breeds, routine diagnostic testing for signs of early heart disease, and monitoring geriatric animals, cardiac disease may be identified before congestive heart failure occurs.

Discussing Canine Dilatative Cardiomyopathy with the Client

- Dilatative cardiomyopathy is a disease of the heart muscle in which the muscle itself becomes thin and irregular.
- The heart's large ventricles that pump blood to the lungs and the body become dilated and unable to pump with enough force to move blood adequately through the body.
- The disease can affect the muscle, valves, and rhythm of the heart.
- As the disease progresses, the pet becomes less and less able to keep up with the demands of the body and can show signs of weakness, coughing, inability to exercise, and potential collapse.
- In some cases, symptoms may not become evident, even with severe disease, until the pet is in a life-threatening syndrome.
- The cause of canine dilatative cardiomyopathy is unknown.
- Common breeds that are more susceptible to this disease are the boxer, Doberman, and cocker spaniel.

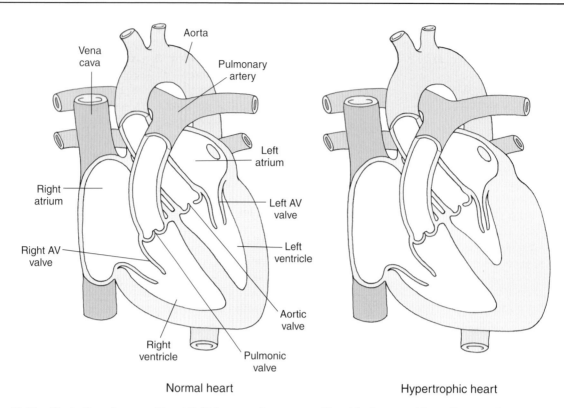

Vena cava
Aorta
Pulmonary artery
Right atrium
Left atrium
Left AV valve
Right AV valve
Left ventricle
Aortic valve
Right ventricle
Pulmonic valve

Normal heart   Hypertrophic heart

Figure 12.14.   Illustration of a normal heart (left) in comparison to one affected by hypertrophic cardiomyopathy.

Feline Dilatative Cardiomyopathy
Feline dilatative cardiomyopathy is a rare disease of the heart muscle secondary to an **amino acid (taurine) deficiency**. When adequate levels of taurine are supplemented in the diet, this form of heart disease is rarely observed. Almost all feline diets have sufficient levels of taurine. Cats on non-feline diets (i.e., human tuna fish diets) are at risk for developing dilatative cardiomyopathy. Although taurine deficiency is thought to be a component of canine dilatative disease, it is not the only factor in producing canine disease.

Canine Hypertrophic Cardiomyopathy
Canine cardiac hypertrophic cardiomyopathy is a disease of the muscle wall, where the ventricular muscle wall becomes thickened, narrowing the ventricles severely, decreasing the amount of blood that can fill the ventricular area (see Figure 12.14). This produces increased blood volume retained in the atria after each diastole. Over time, the atria enlarge because they have to handle a larger amount of blood. As this occurs, pulmonary and hepatic congestion can occur. The heart then tries to pump more blood at an increased rate to make up for the decreased amount of blood ejected through the narrowed ventricle. The enlarging ventricle can also pull the AV valves apart, causing it to leak (mitral valve or tricuspid insufficiency).

If this process goes untreated, it can progress to heart failure and possibly secondary kidney disease.

Etiology
The cause of the disease is unknown.

Signalment
Usually predominant in large breed dogs (i.e., German shepherd), it is seen on average from 10 weeks to 13 years of age. This disease is more common in males than females.

Common Points in Medical History
The disease can come on rapidly or chronically. Common medical complaints can be as follows:

* A cough that worsens at night. Pets may find it hard to lie down and get comfortable.
* Trouble breathing.
* Collapse.
* Weakness/inability to exercise.
* Bloated abdomen/ascites.
* Weight loss.

Common Points on Initial Assessment
Physical signs depend on the severity of the disease; if right, left, or both ventricles are affected; and how rapidly the changes in the heart occurred. Care should be taken with these pets because, with severe disease, *pets can collapse and enter cardiopulmonary arrest with minimal stress*. Possible physical signs of disease are

- changes in pulse rate and quality (pulse deficits);
- moist, deep cough;
- changes in capillary refill time and mucus membrane color (cyanosis);
- increased respiratory difficulty with
  — head extended,
  — elbows abducted,
  — abdominal breathing, and
  — increased respiratory rate
- dypsnea/abdominal breathing;
- respiratory crackles;
- murmur;
- lack of heart sounds;
- bloated abdomen/ascites; and
- collapse.

Complications

If not diagnosed and treated, hypertrophic cardiomyopathy can progress into congestive heart failure and cardiopulmonary shock.

Diagnosis

Because hypertrophic cardiomyopathy can also affect the cardiac valves, produce cardiac arrhythmias, and lead to secondary organ disease, a thorough workup as discussed in the diagnostic section may be indicated.

Treatment

Treatment is focused on reducing the amount of work the heart must do, correcting irregular heart beats, reducing the amount of fluid on the lungs, and restricting activity. Some therapies include the following:

- **Diuretics:** These are drugs that help decrease the amount of fluid within the lung fields. They accomplish this by stimulating the kidneys to push out more fluid from the body (e.g., furosemide, spirolactone, chlorothiazide).
- **Calcium channel blockers:** Drugs such as Cardizem and verapamil help slow the flow of calcium into the heart muscle, slowing the rate of contraction of the heart, increasing the amount of fluid filling the ventricle, improving oxygenation to the heart muscle, and controlling irregular heart rhythms.
- **Beta-blockers:** This group of drugs (i.e., propranolol, atenolol) help slow down rapid, bounding heart rates, making the heartbeat slower but more effective.
- **A low-salt/low-protein diet:** Dietary changes are recommended. Low-salt diets decrease the amount of fluid retained in the body. Decreasing the amount of dietary salt can slow the buildup of fluid within the lung tissue. Low-protein diets decrease the amount of work the kidneys have to do in clearing toxins produced from protein metabolism.
- **Activity:** Decreasing and limiting activity may also be necessary to decrease the amount of work the heart must do.

Prevention

Through careful screening of susceptiable breeds, routine diagnostics, and monitoring of geriatric animals, cardiac disease may be identified before congestive heart failure occurs.

Discussing Canine Hypertrophic Cardiomyopathy with the Client

- Hypertrophic cardiomyopathy is a disease of the heart muscle in which the muscle itself becomes thickened and irregular.
- The heart's large ventricles that pump blood to the lungs and to the body become narrowed and smaller by the abnormally thickened cardiac muscle.
- The disease can affect the muscle, valves, and rhythm of the heart.
- As the disease progresses, the pet becomes less and less able to keep up with the demands of the body and can show signs of weakness, coughing, inability to exercise, and potential collapse.
- In some cases, symptoms may not become evident, even with severe disease, until the pet is in a life-threatening syndrome.
- The cause of canine hypertrophic cardiomyopathy is unknown.
- The breed that is more susceptible to this disease is the German shepherd.

Feline Hypertrophic Cardiomyopathy

Feline cardiac hypertrophic cardiomyopathy is one of the more common forms of feline heart disease. As with canine disease, the ventricular heart muscle becomes abnormally thickened, which can produce AV valve murmurs and arrhythmias. However, there are specific differences seen only in the feline.

- Ventricular thickening can occur symmetrically as with the dog, or asymmetrically within just the intraventricular septum, or irregularly through the ventricle wall.
- Furthermore, due to abnormal blood flow, small clots can form in the ventricle, which can be pushed into the aorta as the ventricle contracts. These clots are then called **embolisms** or **thromboembolisms**.
  — The **embolism** can lodge in the lower aorta where it divides, obstructing blood to the legs (see Figure 12.8).
  — The emboli can also lodge within another arteriole in another limb, the lungs, the central nervous system, or other organs (see Figure 12.15).
- Finally, feline hypertrophic cardiomyopathy can be associated with feline hyperthyroid disease (see Chapter 16).

Etiology

The cause of the disease is unknown, but it can be associated with feline hyperthyroidism.

Signalment

Feline hypertrophic cardiomyopathy can be prominent in all breeds, especially the Maine coon cat. It has been reported in animals from 5 to 7 years of age, but has been seen in patients from 6 months to 16 years. This disease is more common in males than females.

Common Points in Medical History

Medical complaints can be similar to canine disease; however, feline disease is generally seen only when the patient is in an acute crisis of chronic disease. The owner may report that the pet was completely normal 12–24 hours prior to the crisis.

Common Points on Initial Assessment

Commonly these patients are seen in acute emergency due to accumulation of pleural effusion or an arterial thromboembolism.

Signs of heart disease without thromboembolism are as follows:

- Severe respiratory difficulty
- Open-mouth/abdominal breathing
- Cough (occasionally)
- Cyanotic mucous membrane color
- Changes in pulse rate and quality
- Increased lung sounds
- Possible murmur
- Lateral recumbency
- Respiratory/cardiac arrest
- Death

Often the pet will show no signs of cardiac disease as described above. Instead, the pet will show an inability to use the hind limbs, although other limbs, organs (i.e., lungs), or the central nervous system can be affected. *It is important to note that in the canine embolisms are rare and do not occur secondary to heart disease.*

Physical signs are

- acute inability to use the limbs (typically hind limbs; see Figure 12.15);
- cold, painful, and possibly swollen legs;
- trouble breathing—panting;
- vocalization;
- anxiety;
- poor color of the gums; and
- weak to no pulses in the limbs.

Complications

With untreated feline hypertrophic cardiomyopathy, the feline can decompensate into cardiovascular failure and/or throw an aterial thromboemolism. Untreated feline hypertrophic cardiomyopathy with thromboembolic disease carries an extremely poor prognosis.

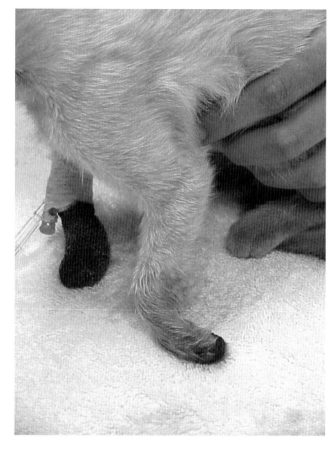

Figure 12.15. Image of a front limb affected by a thromboembolism.

- *The pet can produce another emboli at any time in other places in the body.* These animals can push clots into the lungs, central nervous system, and other organs, causing death.
- Furthermore, even with successful treatment of this condition and the heart disease, emboli can reoccur causing another potential obstruction.

Diagnosis

The clinical diagnostic protocols for uncomplicated feline disease is similar to the canine workup. Diagnosis of thromboembolism is made largely based on the physical signs and history of the patient.

Treatment

With uncomplicated feline disease, treatment options are similar to canine disease. With hypertrophic disease with thromboembolism, the goal of treatment is to support the animal until the body is able to degrade and destroy the obstructive clot. At the same time, the goal is also to prevent more clots from forming. *Prognosis for response to treatment and recovery is generally very poor.* Overall treatment options may include the following.

Supportive Care

These animals are in need of intensive care. The veterinarian may suggest oxygen therapy, catheter and fluids, and blood work to help monitor the pet's condition. The pet must be very closely monitored until the clot has been reabsorbed and there is a response to treatment. This may take several days.

Medications are focused on slowing the clotting process to help prevent further emboli formation. These medications include the following.

- **Heparin:** Heparin is a drug that helps slow the blood-clotting process. While on this drug, the pet must be closely monitored due to increased chance of bleeding.

Discussing Feline Hypertrophic Cardiomyopathy with the Client
- Hypertrophic cardiomyopathy is one of the most common cardiac diseases of the cat.
- In this disease, the muscle itself becomes thickened and irregular.
- The heart's large ventricles that pump blood to the lungs and to the body become narrowed and smaller by the abnormally thickened cardiac muscle.
- The disease can affect the muscle, valves, and rhythm of the heart.
- As the disease progresses, the pet becomes less and less able to keep up with the demands of the body.
- In some cases, symptoms may not become evident until the pet is in a life-threatening syndrome.
- The cause of feline hypertrophic cardiomyopathy is unknown.
- The common breed that is more susceptible to this disease is the Maine coon cat.
- A possible life-threatening complication to feline heart disease is the formation of a thromboembolism.

Thromboembolism
- Due to turbulent flow of blood through a diseased heart, the blood itself can begin to clot.
- The small clot can remain attached to the heart wall or break free and move through the blood vessels (thromboembolism).
- The emboli will lodge in a blood vessel, occluding that vessel and inhibiting normal blood flow.
- The most common location for this to occur is at the end of the aorta where the blood supply feeds the hind legs.
- This produces an inability to use the hind end.
- The limbs are generally cold, painful, and stiff.
- Emboli can also lodge within the central nervous system and lungs, causing acute death.
- The presence of thromboembolism is a very poor prognosis for the longevity of the pet.

- **Aspirin:** Aspirin therapy must be given very carefully to cats because they can handle only a small amount of the medication every 2–3 days. The aspirin helps slow platelet function that initiates clotting.
- **Sedatives:** These drugs are an antianxiety medication given to lightly sedate the pet and decrease pain and anxiety.
- **Cardiac medication:** The veterinarian may suggest cardiac medications to make the heart work more effectively. These medications may need to be started after a complete cardiac consultation and diagnostic workup are completed.

Prevention

Through careful screening of susceptible breeds, routine diagnostic testing, and monitoring geriatric animals, cardiac disease may be identified before congestive heart failure occurs.

Valvular Disease of the Heart: Mitral Insufficiency

Cardiac mitral insufficiency is a disease of the mitral valve (left AV valve), which separates the left atrium and left ventricle of the heart. The mitral valve becomes thickened and does not close properly, allowing the valve to leak. This allows blood to be ejected back into the atrium and lungs each time the ventricle contracts. Over time, the atrium enlarges, because it must handle a larger amount of blood. The ventricle also enlarges as the heart tries to pump more blood into the body to make up for the blood ejected backward due to the leaky valve. As the disease progresses, the left heart becomes enlarged and the blood begins to build up in the left atrium and lung fields.

The disease can occur secondarily to dilatative or hypertrophic cardiomyopathy.

Etiology

The disease can either be a primary congenital malformation of the mitral valve or an acquired disease secondary to thickening of the valve leaflets. The thickening of the valve can occur secondary to chronic bacterial infection (i.e., severe dental disease; see Figure 12.16).

Signalment

Cardiac mitral insufficiency is usually predominant in small breed dogs. This disease is more common in males than females.

Common Points in Medical History

The disease can come on rapidly or it can be chronic. Common medical complaints can be as follows.

- A cough is present that worsens at night. Pets may find it hard to lie down and get comfortable.
- The pet has difficulty breathing and has labored breathing.
- The pet has decreasing ability to exercise (exercise intolerance).

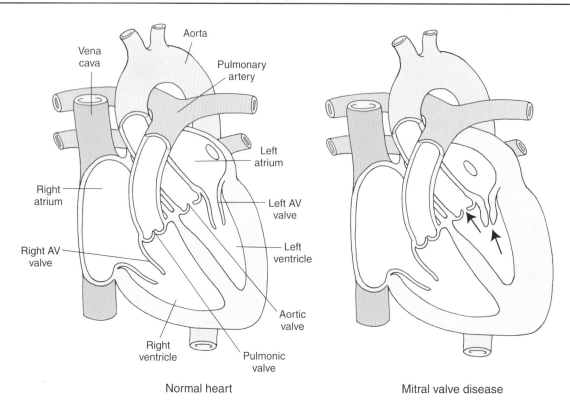

Figure 12.16.   Image of a normal heart in comparison with a heart with mitral valve disease.

- Secondary kidney disease develops (as the disease progresses), with
  — weight loss,
  — vomiting,
  — decreased appetite, and
  — increased urination/thirst.

Common Points on Initial Assessment
Physical signs depend on the severity of the disease and how rapidly the changes in the heart occurred. Care should be taken in handling these animals and collecting samples from them because, with severe disease, *pets can collapse and enter cardiopulmonary arrest with minimal stress.* Possible physical signs of disease are

- coughing (deep moist productive cough),
- changes in mucous membrane color (cyanosis),
- increased respiratory difficulty, with
  — head extended,
  — elbows abducted,
  — abdominal breathing,
  — increased respiratory rate, and
  — changes in capillary refill time and mucous membrane color (cyanosis).

Upon auscultation, murmur and respiratory crackles are evident.

Complications
If not diagnosed and treated, mitral valve disease may progress into congestive heart failure and cardiopulmonary shock. *However, there are many patients with mitral valve murmurs that do not progress into physical symptoms.*

Diagnosis
Because mitral valve disease can be secondary to other heart diseases and produce secondary organ disease, a thorough workup as discussed in the diagnostic section may be indicated.

Treatment
Treatment is focused on reducing the amount of work the heart must do and decreasing the amount of fluid on the lungs caused by decreased blood flow and congestion. Some therapies used are as follows.

- **Diuretics:** These are drugs (e.g., furosemide, spirolactone, chlorothiazide) that help decrease the amount of fluid within the lung fields. They accomplish this by stimulating the kidneys to push out more fluid from the body.
- **ACE inhibitors:** This class of drugs (i.e., enalapril, benazepril) decreases blood pressure and decreases the amount of work the heart must do to move blood through the body.

- **Diet:** A low-salt/low-protein diet is recommended to decrease fluid buildup on the lungs while also decreasing the amount of work the kidneys need to do.
- **Activity:** Decreasing and limiting activity may also be necessary to decrease the amount of work the heart must do.

Prevention
Through careful screening of susceptible breeds and geriatric animals, mitral valve disease can be diagnosed in its early phases. Furthermore, routine dental care and cleanings can decrease the amount of bacteria in the body and slow or stop the progression of bacterial thickening and infection of the mitral valve.

Discussing Mitral Valve Insufficiency with the Client
- Mitral valve insufficiency is a disease of the valve separating the left atrium from the left ventricle of the heart.
- Over time this valve can become leaky, and every time the left ventricle constricts, blood also is pumped into the left atrium.
- Furthermore, the blood backs up into the fields behind the left atrium, and fluid begins to collect in the lung tissue secondary to decreased blood flow (pulmonary edema).
- As the disease progresses, the pet becomes less and less able to keep up with the demands for oxygenated blood and can show signs of weakness, coughing, inability to exercise, and potential collapse.
- The disease can be secondary to diseases of the cardiac muscle.
- The disease is typically caused by chronic bacterial infection causing thickening of the mitral valve.
- Small breed dogs more commonly have mitral valve disease.

Infectious Diseases of the Heart

Heartworm Disease
Heartworm disease is a parasitic infection of a bloodborne parasite, *Dirofilaria immitis*. The disease is spread by mosquitoes, which feed on an infected dog. The mosquitoes pick up larval heartworms (microfilaria), which they in turn inject into an uninfected animal the next time they feed.

- The parasite is injected into the tissue, and over the next 3–6 months it migrates through the tissue to the blood supply and to the right heart (see Figure 12.17).
- There the worms mature and reproduce, causing obstructive heart disease in the right heart and lung fields.
- The disease can be asymptotic initially (especially in felines), but as the infection worsens, the right side of the heart begins to obstruct and potentially fail.

Etiology
The cause of the disease is the bloodborne parasite, *Dirofilaria immitis*. The bloodborne parasite must mature within a mosquito for 15–17 days at a temperature greater than 58° Fahrenheit.

Signalment
The infection affects dogs and cats (rarely) in mosquito-endemic regions, along the Atlantic and Gulf coasts, and other parts of the United States. Outside, unprotected animals are at the highest risk.

Common Points in Medical History
In canines the disease produces a chronic progressive disease. In felines, the disease can be asymptotic until the pet enters acute cardiac failure. Common medical complaints can be

- sudden death (cats);
- weakness, lethargy, collapse;
- decreased ability to exercise;
- coughing (rare in cats);
- shortness of breath;
- weight loss; and
- fluid buildup in the abdomen (ascites) in a severely affected animal due to obstructive right heart disease.

Common Points on Initial Assessment
Physical signs depend on heartworm burden, length of disease, age of the pet, and other underlying disease conditions. Signs are species dependent.

In **canines**, patients may present with a mild to worsening cough. In severe cases animals may be unable to exercise properly. There may be evidence of a right tricuspid murmur with increased lung sounds. The pet may be coughing up blood.

In **felines**, pets may not show any physical signs until the pet is in cardiovascular failure or death.

Complications
Without proper treatment, heartworm disease can cause right-sided obstructed heart disease, kidney disease, disease of the lung, and possibly death.

Diagnosis
Diagnosis is largely based on screening patient blood for specific proteins (**antigens**) on the surface of the adult heartworm. In canines, there are many excellent in-hospital tests to determine potential exposure. In feline patients, there are tests available through many outside animal health laboratories. Once diagnosed with heartworm disease, the medical team may follow up with general blood work and radiographs to help determine the extent of the damage to the heart and lungs.

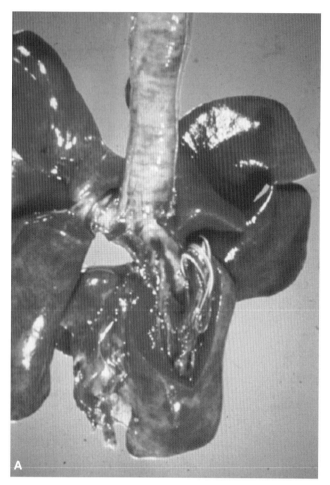

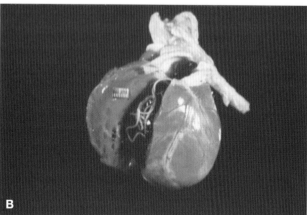

Figure 12.17.   Image of heart and lungs. Heart is infested with heartworms (a). Image of heart with right ventricle filled with heartworms (b).

Discussing Heartworm Disease with the Client

- Heartworm disease is a bloodborne parasite infection that is spread by mosquito bites.
- The disease is endemic in warm climates where there are active mosquito populations.
- However, specific geographic regions are more endemic for the disease (i.e., north and southeast coastal states, Texas, and parts of the Midwest).
- The disease is transmitted by the mosquito that feeds on a currently infected animal and then bites an unaffected pet.
- The mosquito injects a small larval form of the parasite into the tissue, which over 4–6 months migrates into the right heart and lung fields.
- There the parasite begins to reproduce and become obstructive to the heart and lungs.

Physical Signs
- In the canine, pets generally develop a persistent, worsening cough that can develop into weakness, inability to exercise, and collapse in severe cases.
- In feline heartworm disease, the worm loads can be much less, with infections having only a few worms evident. Physical symptoms are mild to nonexistent until the feline enters a cardiovascular shock crisis.

Clinical Diagnostics
Although there are many diagnostic tests used to diagnose and confirm the extent of heartworm disease, the initial clinical test is a simple blood test that evaluates the pet's blood for the presence of specific proteins (antigens) from the adult heartworm. Many of these tests can be run in a few minutes within the hospital setting.

Treatment and Control
Although once diagnosed with heartworm there are treatment options available. The simplest way to control heartworm disease is through prevention. Through annual to biannual heartworm testing and placing the pet on heartworm prevention, the pet is highly unlikely to develop the disease. The preventatives are monthly tablets that kill any of the larval parasites that the pet comes in contact with.

Treatment
Treatment is focused on reducing the adult worms within the heart and lung field gradually so that the decreased worm load does not overwhelm the pet. A general protocol for heartworm follows.

- The animal is placed on 2 days of a medication that destroys the adult heartworm infection present in the body. The drug used is called Immiticide. Animals may be hospitalized while being treated with Immiticide.
- The pet is sent home under strict rest and confinement as the body begins to break down the dead heartworms.

- In 3–4 weeks, the pet is brought into the hospital and given a medication, called ivermectin, to destroy any remaining baby heartworms (microfilaria) still evident in the system.
- In another 3–4 weeks, a test to check for microfilaria in the body is conducted. If positive, another course of ivermectin is completed.
- Once the pet tests negative for the microfilaria, the pet can be started on a heartworm preventative.
- Ninety days after beginning the heartworm preventative, another adult heartworm test should be run.

Prevention

Annual to biannual heartworm testing and routine heartworm prevention (every month) can greatly reduce the chance of heartworm infection in endemic regions.

CD-ROM 1 reviews material presented in this chapter. Please try the cases for Section 2 (Anatomy and Physiology—The Science behind the Diseases) to help reinforce the information presented here.

Chapter 13

Urogenital System

Introduction

The urogenital system compromises the kidneys, ureters, bladder, urethra, and reproductive organs of the animal. This chapter will deal with the kidneys and urinary system; other chapters will discuss the reproductive anatomy and physiology. The urinary system's main function is to control the elimination of waste and toxins from the body. In order to accomplish this, the kidneys function to

- filter out toxins and waste through specialized structures called **glomeruli (renal cortex)**, and
- concentrate the urine by reabsorbing water in the **loops of Henle (renal medulla)** to prevent fluid loss producing dehydration.

Furthermore, the kidneys also play a key role in other body functions.

- Control of blood pressure through the **renin–angiotensin system**
- Acid/base control of the blood
- Balance of electrolytes (sodium and potassium) within the body

The body cannot survive without normal kidney function, and kidney disease is one of the most common diseases in the geriatric animal**.**

Each animal is born with two kidneys, the right and the left. The kidneys sit close to the spine in the middle of the abdomen. The left kidney is slightly more caudal than the right kidney, which is positioned behind the last rib. The right kidney lies within the rib cage. The right and left adrenal glands are positioned at each kidney's cranial poll (see Figure 13.1).

The internal anatomy of the kidneys is split into several sections, each section having its own anatomy and function (see Figure 13.2). The anatomical sections are

- renal cortex,
- renal medulla,
- renal pelvis, and
- ureter (leading to the bladder).

The **renal cortex** is the outer most tissue region of the kidney, which houses hundreds of thousands of specialized structures called **glomeruli** (**Bowman's capsules**). The glomeruli are a set of tubules closely interdigitated with small arterioles that serve as filters for the body. The beginning of the glomeruli has very fine openings (called **fenestrations**) that allow small molecules to filter into the tubules from the bloodstream. Initially, as blood filters through the small arterioles and glomerular region, all of the small molecules within the blood flow passively into the glomeruli. The smaller molecules are sugar, amino acids, waste products, and electrolytes (sodium, potassium, chloride, etc.). Larger molecules such as proteins (e.g., albumen, globulin, etc.) cannot pass through the healthy glomerular membranes (see Figure 13.3).

Once the molecules and fluid have been passed into the beginning of the glomerular capsule, the liquids move on into the **proximal convoluted tubules**. The function of these tubules is to actively reabsorb all of the necessary nutrients the body needs back into the bloodstream. This process is an active process accomplished by cellular pumps within the walls of the proximal and distal tubules. Once the necessary nutrients are reabsorbed, the fluid within the convoluted tubule moves into the loops of Henle within the renal medulla (see Figure 13.4).

The renal medulla houses a section of the nephron called the **nephrotic loops (loops of Henle)**, which function to reabsorb most of the fluid component of the urine. *This system of fluid reabsorption is key to maintaining adequate hydration in the animal.* To reabsorb the water, the cells of the nephrotic loops actively absorb sodium ions (Na^+) and move them into the medullary tissue around the nephrotic loops. Water passively diffuses into this space to try to balance the salt gradient. As the urine moves through the medulla**,** up to two-thirds of the fluid within the nephrotic loops is passively reabsorbed (see Figure 13.5). Pets that cannot reabsorb most of the fluid within the urine can dehydrate and become acutely ill.

The glomeruli, the convoluted tubules, and the nephrotic loops are called a **nephron** and represent the smallest functional unit within the kidney. Once the urine leaves the loops of Henle, it enters the collecting ducts and enters the **renal pelvis**. The renal pelvis sits in the middle of the kidney and collects all the urine produced before moving into the **ureters.** The ureters run dorsally within the abdomen until they enter the bladder at the bladder's neck in the area called the **trigone.** Once urine collects in the bladder, it then moves

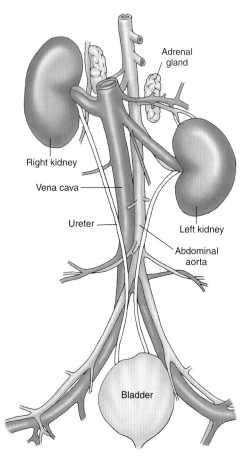

Figure 13.1. Illustration of the dorsal abdominal anatomy. Note the location of the kidneys and adrenals on the ventral spine.

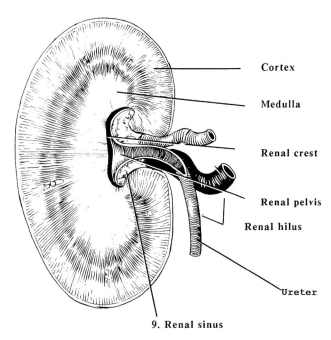

Figure 13.2. Illustration of cross section of the kidney. (Courtesy of *Anatomy of Domestic Animals*, 7th Edition. Pasquini, Chris, and Pasquini, Susan. Sudz Publishing, Pilot Point, TX 1989. Used with permission from Sudz Publishing.)

through the urethra into the penis or vagina and exits from the urethral opening (see Figure 13.6).

The kidneys also play an extremely important part in the control of blood pressure in the body. At any one minute, over 20% of the blood of the body is pumped through the kidneys. When this percentage decreases, the kidneys are not able to maintain the normal rate of filtering (**glomerular filtration**) of the blood, and over time the kidneys can begin to deteriorate. To help prevent a decrease in blood volume, the kidneys have their own mechanism called the **renin–angiotensin system** that increases blood pressure. This mechanism operates as follows.

- Specialized cells, called **juxtoglomerular cells,** are present within the arterioles of the glomeruli. These cells stretch, depending on the blood pressure.
- As blood pressure decreases, which produces a decrease in glomerular filtration, the juxtoglomerular cells shrink. This process stimulates the release of a chemical called **renin.** Renin circulates within the bloodstream and activates angiotensin I, which then activates angiotensin II.
- Angiotensin I is then changed into angiotensin II within the lungs.

- Angiotensin II is a potent constrictor of blood vessels, thus causing a whole-body arteriole constriction.
- With increased constriction of the blood vessels, blood pressure rises, increasing blood through the kidneys and increasing glomerular filtration.

One of the primary causes of hypertension (high blood pressure) is chronic renal disease. As glomeruli begin to fail and their ability to filter blood decreases, the active glomeruli continue secreting renin in response to decreased glomerular filtration. This continued process can produce constant hypertension (see Figure 13.7).

The kidneys also play a key role in the production of red blood cells from the bone marrow. A normal healthy kidney secretes a hormone called **erythropoietin,** which stimulates red blood cell production from the bone marrow. In chronic renal disease, erythropoietin levels drop, decreasing the normal production of red blood cells and producing chronic anemia.

Expression of Renal Disease

Generalized renal disease can take the following forms:

- Glomerular disease, producing a buildup of toxins within the bloodstream
- Tubular disease, producing the inability of the kidneys to concentrate urine normally
- A combination of glomerular and tubular disease

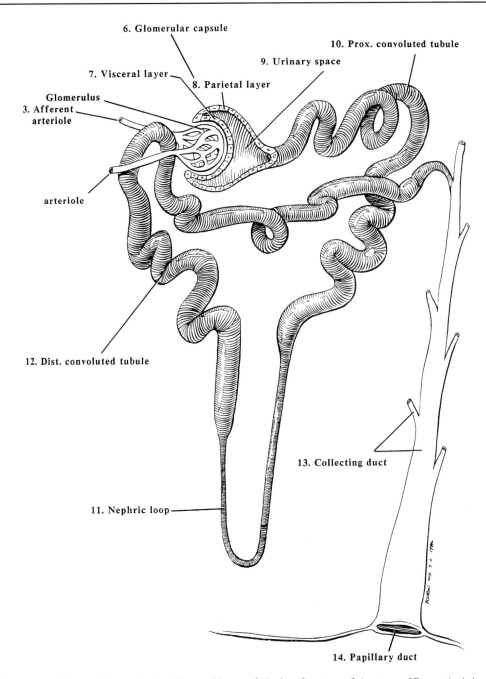

6. Glomerular capsule

10. Prox. convoluted tubule

9. Urinary space

7. Visceral layer

8. Parietal layer

Glomerulus

3. Afferent
   arteriole

arteriole

12. Dist. convoluted tubule

13. Collecting duct

11. Nephric loop

14. Papillary duct

Figure 13.3. Illustration of glomeruli, proximal tubules, and loops of Henle. (Courtesy of *Anatomy of Domestic Animals*, 7th Edition. Pasquini, Chris, and Pasquini, Susan. Sudz Publishing, Pilot Point, TX 1989. Used with permission from Sudz Publishing.)

Renal Glomerular Disease

Glomerular disease produces an inability of the kidneys to filter out toxins from the bloodstream into the urine. The severity of the disease is directly proportional to the amount of toxins within the bloodstream. In general, it takes 65–70% of the glomeruli of both kidneys to be affected before there is a rise in renal toxins (**azotemia**). Causes of glomerular disease can be

- infections of the kidneys: **pyelonephritis;**
- inflammation within the kidneys: **chronic interstitial nephritis;**
- neoplasia: **renal lymphoma, adenocarcinoma**; and
- kidneys that have lost their ability to function with age (end-stage kidneys).

Glomerular disease is monitored by changes in the toxin level within the bloodstream. Although glomerular disease

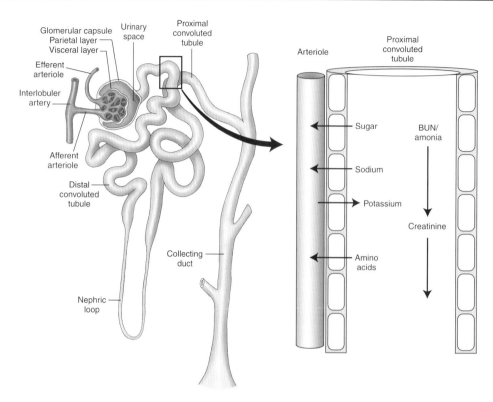

Figure 13.4.   A magnified section of a proximal tubule of a nephron illustrating reabsorption of nutrients into the blood supply.

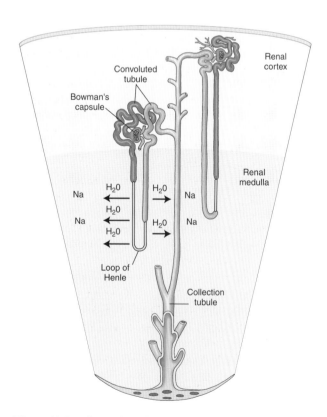

Figure 13.5.   Illustration of water reabsorption from the nephrotic loops.

can occur secondary to other systemic diseases (see below), the changes in blood work discussed next can suggest a renal component.

Blood Urea Nitrogen

Blood urea nitrogen (BUN) is a form of conjugated ammonia produced within the liver that is to be excreted by the kidney. Although BUN does elevate secondary to a kidney problem, elevations in BUN can also be seen in animals that are having episodes of intestinal bleeding (e.g., gastrointestinal ulcerations, parvo, disseminated intravascular coagulopathy) and dehydration.

Creatinine

Creatinine is a small amino acid excreted primarily by the kidneys. In general, the more glomerular filtration is affected, the higher the blood creatinine level.

Phosphorus

Phosphorus is an electrolyte excreted by the kidneys. With severe renal disease, elimination can be very difficult, and phosphorus levels can increase dramatically.

Proteinuria

Proteinuria is defined as the presence of abnormally high amounts of protein in the urine. The presence of protein in the urine can reflect damage to the glomerular filters.

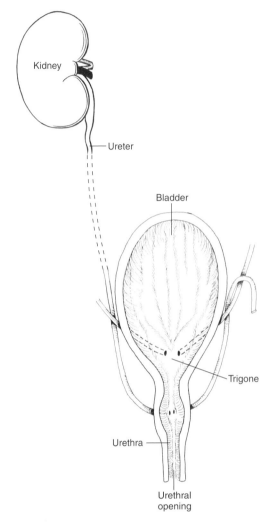

Figure 13.6.   Image of the lower urinary tract.

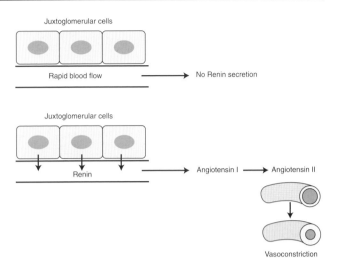

Figure 13.7.   An illustration of the renin–angiotensin system. As blood pressure drops through the nephron and the juxtomglomerular cells are not stretched, renin is released. the renin activates angiotensin I, which then in turn activates angiotensin II, a potent constrictor of blood vessels. The generalized constriction of the vessels increases overall blood pressure.

severe potassium-depleting disease such as chronic renal failure (see Figure 13.8).

Renal Medullary Disease

Renal medullary disease affects the animal's ability to concentrate urine. These animals have lost the ability to actively reabsorb sodium, thus are unable to create a high sodium gradient to reabsorb water from the kidneys. In the early stages of the disease, these pets drink large amounts of water to keep up with their significant water losses. Often these pets will begin to show increased thirst and urination as a first symptom of these diseases. The inability to concentrate urine can be caused by the following.

- **Chronic renal disease:** Kidneys loose the ability to concentrate urine normally (i.e., chronic renal disease in the older cat).
- **Hormonal disease:** In specific diseases, a hormonal imbalance inhibits the kidney's abilities to concentrate urine normally. Some hormonal diseases are
  — hyperadrenocorticism (Cushing's disease; see Chapter 16); hypoadrenocorticism (Addison's disease; see Chapter 16); and diabetes mellitus (see Chapter 15).
- **Renal neoplasia:** Renal tumors (i.e., lymphoma, adenocarcinoma) can destroy normal renal tissue affecting the kidney's ability to concentrate urine.

Assessing Medullary Disease
The kidney's ability to concentrate urine is measured by an instrument called a **refractometer** (see Chapter 23). This instrument measures the specific gravity or the measure of

However, protein in the urine can also suggest an active bladder infection, since inflamed and infected bladder walls can leak protein. Presence of urinary blood, white blood cells, and bacteria can help differentiate between an active bladder infection and a true renal proteinuria.

Potassium
In normal functioning kidneys, potassium is excreted by a specialized cellular pump in the proximal tubules at the same time sodium is reabsorbed (see Figure 13.4).

As kidneys begin to fail, their ability to concentrate urine also fails. This produces a massive loss of fluids through the kidneys (called **diuresis**). So much fluid is lost that there can be a general dilution of electrolytes. This can produce low blood potassium (**hypokalemia**), especially in cats. Normal sodium and potassium levels produce electrical energy that stimulates normal muscle and neurological activity. With severely affected cats, potassium depletion can be so severe that they are unable to lift their neck into a normal position. This is called **ventroflexion** of the neck and is observed with

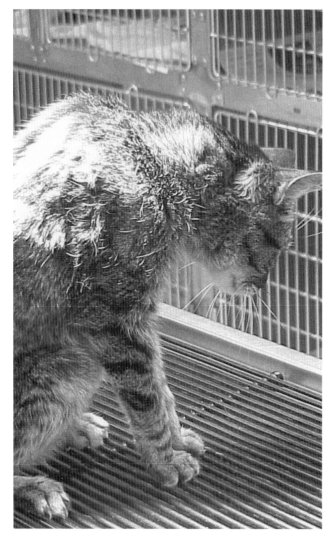

Figure 13.8. Image of a cat with ventroflexion of the neck. The cat is unable to lift its neck due to a profound hypokalemia.

the concentration of a fluid. The specific gravity of fluids is measured from 1.001 to above 1.045. The higher the number, the more concentrated the fluid. A urine specific gravity is the best assessment of the concentrating ability of the renal medulla and is a key **indicator in determining**

if renal disease is present. Normal values for urine are as follows.

- Canines: urine specific gravity (USG) >1.025
- Felines: USG >1.035

Assessing Pre-renal, Renal, and Post-Renal Azotemia

Azotemia is defined as the buildup of toxins within the bloodstream, which is defined as increases in the BUN and creatinine. It is necessary when assessing renal function to be able to differentiate between pre-renal, renal, and post-renal azotemia (see Table 13.1). Azotemia that is produced from a primary renal disease is caused by a kidney that can no longer filter out toxins or concentrate urine. Pre- and post-renal azotemia is caused by the body's inability to filter out toxins due to another systemic disease affecting glomerular filtration. In these syndromes, the animal is still severely azotemic but does not lose the ability to concentrate urine.

Pre-Renal Azotemia

Pre-renal azotemia is defined as an increase in blood kidney chemistry elevations due to a primary problem that decreases blood perfusion and glomerular filtration to the kidneys. The problem is not associated with kidney disease but is secondary due to the body's inability to adequately perfuse the kidneys. *The primary cause of pre-renal azotemia is dehydration.* In severe cases, dehydrated animals have decreased amounts of fluid in the blood. The animal cannot perfuse its body normally, and glomerular filtration decreases. In these animals

- the pet is azotemic (i.e., increased elevations in the creatinine and BUN);
- the urine specific gravity is high because the kidneys have not lost their ability to concentrate urine and the body is doing everything it can to conserve fluids; and
- the azotemia reverts to normal levels after hydration is restored.

Renal Azotemia

In renal azotemia there is an increase in blood kidney chemistry elevations due to a primary problem with the kidneys.

Table 13.1. Outline of azotemia.

Type of Azotemia	Urine Specific Gravity	Cause	Prognosis	Other Concerns
Pre-Renal	High	Dehydration	Kidney chemistry values usually return to normal when patient is rehydrated	
Azotemia	Dilute	Primary renal disease	Can be poor due to underlying renal disease	Hypokalemia Proteinuria
Post-renal azotemia	High (but can become dilute with long-term urinary obstruction)	Urinary obstruction (FLUTD)	Can be poor if obstruction is prolonged, which can produce primary renal disease	Hyperkalemia

The disease can either be glomerular or medullary or both. Up to 65–70% of the kidneys must be damaged before these elevations in BUN, creatinine, and phosphorus are seen, and chemistry elevations can be significant. The kidneys have lost the ability to concentrate urine, thus the urine specific gravity can be much lower than normal <1.015. It is extremely important to run a urinalysis to fully assess kidney function, since azotemia with diluted urine is the key to diagnosing primary renal disease. *With severe chronic renal disease, kidney enzymes may not revert to normal.*

Post-Renal Azotemia

In post-renal azotemia, there is a rise in kidney enzymes due to an obstruction of the outflow of urine distal to the kidneys. This causes a retrograde backflow of urine into the kidneys that then produces a back flow of toxins. The best example is a lower urinary tract obstruction (i.e., **feline lower urinary tract disease [FLUTD]**). Renal enzymes can be severely elevated; however, urine specific gravity tends to be high. Also with this acute obstruction, blood potassium levels can be very high and potentially life threatening. Generally, once the animal is unobstructed, and rehydrated on fluids, the azotemia can dissipate. However, the building retrograde urinary pressure can produce permanent kidney disease if the obstruction remains long enough.

The key to understanding these three syndromes is that all affected pets are ill, dehydrated, and may have a marked azotemia. However, only animals with affected kidneys (**renal azotemia**) have lost the ability to adequately concentrate their urine in times of severe dehydration, indicating a primary renal disease. The differentiation of these animals is made by the animal's inability to concentrate urine measured by the urine specific gravity.

Obtaining a Thorough History with Urogenital Disease

It is important to get a good history in an animal that may be presenting with moderate to severe renal disease. Pets can have a serious disease that presents with very mild medical complaints and can show virtually no physical symptoms. Some key questions when obtaining a medical history are presented next.

Is the Animal Young or Old?

Renal disease tends to be a middle- to older-age problem. However, kidney disease can occur in younger animals.

What Is the Breed of the Pet?

Some specific breeds can be more prone to kidney disease. Some of these breeds are as follows:

- Felines: Abyssinian and Persian
- Canines: bull terrier, Cairn terrier, German shepherd, and Sharpei

Has the Progression of the Disease Been Sudden or Chronic?

The length of progression can differentiate between chronic and acute renal disease, which can change the veterinarian's disease differential list, the diagnostic tests, and the potential treatment plan.

Has There Been a Sharp Increase in Water Consumption or Urination?

- Dramatic increases in water consumption (polydipsia) and urination (polyuria), especially over the past few days, weeks, and months, can suggest impaired renal function.
- Pets that cannot adequately concentrate urine must drink larger quantities of water to prevent dehydration.
- In felines, increased urination can be demonstrated by increased saturation of the litter box. Owners may report an increased incidence of heavy litter boxes that must be changed more often.

Has There Been a Decrease in Appetite?

- With acute disease, the rapid buildup of toxins can lead to rapid loss of appetite, depression, and vomiting.
- With chronic disease, the buildup of toxins can slowly wean the appetite.

Has There Been a Progressive Weight Loss?

Weight loss may be the chief medical complaint presented by the client. Weight loss of just 1–2 pounds in a 10-pound animal can represent 10–20% loss of body mass.

Is the Animal a Chronic Vomiter or Is Vomiting Occurring More Often?

With the chronic increase of toxins, vomiting can occur more readily because of hyperacidity of the stomach. The hormone, **gastrin,** which produces stomach acid, is eliminated in the kidneys. With kidney disease this hormone increases in the bloodstream. This can cause hyperacidity of the stomach, producing chronic vomiting.

Is the Animal Having Chronic Diarrhea?

Animals with renal disease can have a profound colitis because of the increased blood toxins and stress.

Has the Pet Been Acting Constipated?

This is an extremely important question for owners of male cats. Many early obstructed male cats will go to the litter box and strain, acting as if they are constipated. Most clients bring the pet in for constipation only to find that the male cat is obstructed.

Practice Tip: Potential "constipated" male cats should be handled as an emergency situation until the medical team can assess the pet fully.

Has the Pet Been Exposed to Toxins or Poisons?

In most temperate climates in fall and winter, there is increased risk of exposure to antifreeze. Ethylene glycol, a major component of antifreeze, is a very toxic chemical, which produces acute renal failure (see disease section).

Has the Animal Had Trouble Urinating?

Trouble urinating, including straining to urinate or vocalizing while urinating, can suggest lower urinary tract disease, or possibly an obstruction. It can also suggest prostatic disease (canines only).

Obtaining an Initial Assessment on a Patient with Renal Disease

Renal disease may not be easily diagnosed by medical history and physical examination. The pets may only show mild signs of weight loss, anorexia, and depression and still have significant chronic disease. Animals with acute renal disease can be severely affected, but may show only signs of life-threatening dehydration, vomiting, and diarrhea. Some key points to monitor when dealing with a possible renal patient follow.

- **Mentation:** Animals with acute renal disease can show severe depression and neurologic signs because of the rapid accumulation of toxins within the body. Animals can be depressed to comatose and can also have seizures or neurologic excitement due to the increased ammonia, which affects the central nervous system.
- **Hydration:** Dehydration with acute and chronic renal disease can be significant and potentially life threatening.
- **Oral Ulceration:** Animals with acute azotemia may have oral ulcerations and halitosis because of severe blood ammonia levels (see Figure 13.9).
- **Abdominal palpation:** (See below.)

Abdominal Palpation

One method used to gather information for an initial assessment is through palpation of the abdomen. Palpation should be accomplished with light pressure, checking for abdominal tenderness, organ enlargement, or other abdominal masses. When evaluating the abdomen during an initial assessment, special attention should be focused on evaluation of the bladder. With obstructive disease (FLUTD), the bladder may be very large and painful, and the pet may vocalize and act uncomfortable when the region is palpated. Extreme care should be used in palpating a large bladder, because rupture is possible. In some cases, it is sometimes hard to tell if an abnormal structure in the caudal abdomen is a mass or an enlarged bladder.

Although pets can have severe renal disease and be stable, the parameters presented in Table 13.2 should be monitored to help distinguish if the pet is in a life-threatening condition.

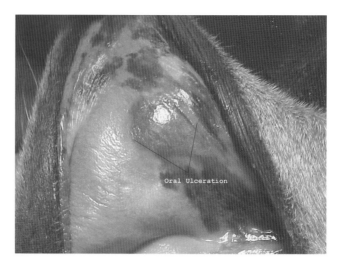

Figure 13.9. Image of an oral ulcer secondary to severe ammonia buildup in the blood (azotemia).

Table 13.2. Triage concerns in the renal patient.

Systems	Trouble Signs That Indicate an Emergency Situation
Mentation	Nonresponsive/comatose or seizures/ hyperexcitability
Fever	Hypothermia, temperatures <99° (secondary to severe metabolic upset)
	Possible fever (temperature >102°) secondary to infectious renal disease (i.e., leptospirosis)
Hydration	Severe dehydration >5–7%
Gum color	Injected (red)/tacky mucous membranes
CRT	CRT >2–3 seconds
Heart rate/pulse	Rate: Heart rates <80 bpm or >180–200 bpm
	Pulse: Change in pulse quality secondary to seizure and shock
	• Weak pulse
	• No pulse
	• Paradoxical
	• Pulse deficits

CRT, capillary refill time; bpm, beats per minute.

Urogenital Diagnostic Tests

Because renal disease can be a chronic subtle process and because elevations in kidney chemistry can be seen with other disease entities (dehydration, urinary obstruction), a full diagnostic workup may be indicated. An overview of these procedures follows.

Diagnostic Blood Work

Diagnostic blood tests help determine if there are elevations in kidney enzymes. Further changes in the complete blood count and chemistry may suggest infectious or other organ or hormonal diseases that could change medical and treatment options.

Urinalysis

Urinalysis (see Chapter 23) is one of the most important clinical tests in assessing renal function. Major components that can suggest renal disease are as follows.

- **Urine specific gravity:** Low urine specific gravity in the face of azotemia suggests primary renal disease.
- **Presence of protein in the urine:** Without the presence of a urinary tract infection the presence of protein in the urine may be suggestive of glomerular disease.
- **Sediment:** Cellular cytology may suggest the evidence of renal casts, white blood cells, urinary crystals, or abnormal cells, indicating disease of the bladder, kidneys, or reproductive organs (e.g., prostate).

> Practice Tip: It is important to note that urine samples that have been sitting out for long periods of time (refrigerated or at room temperature) can form artifactual calcium oxalate crystals. When receiving a sample from a client, the team member should obtain a brief history of how long ago the sample was collected and how it was stored.

Complete Blood Count

The complete blood count allows the veterinarian to assess the following parameters that can be associated with renal disease.

Changes in the Red Blood Cell Count

Increases in the red blood cell count can be generally associated with dehydration secondary to an acute or chronic renal syndrome. The pet is unable to adequately concentrate its urine; hence, the pet can easily dehydrate, increasing the amount of red blood cells in the blood in relation to its fluid component (see Chapter 21).

> **Key Points in Discussing the Need for a Blood and Urine Evaluation with the Client**
> - General blood work allows the veterinarian to determine if there are increases of toxins within the bloodstream that should normally be eliminated by the kidneys.
> - Increases in these toxins can suggest a decrease in the removal of these toxins (glomerular filtration).
> - A urinalysis allows the medical team to assess if the pet can concentrate urine normally, if there is protein in the urine (suggesting problems with the kidneys' ability to filter), and if there are changes in the cells of the urine that could suggest infection, neoplasia, or other kidney disease.
> - The urinalysis is a very important diagnostic tool in determining if increases in kidney toxins are secondary to renal disease or another systemic problem.

A decreased red blood cell population (**anemia**) can be secondary to chronic renal disease due to a lack of erythropoietin.

Elevations in the White Blood Cell Count

In infectious renal disease, there can be significant elevations of the white blood cell populations.

Blood Chemistry

As described above, elevations in creatinine, BUN, phosphorus, and changes in electrolytes can all aid in the diagnosis of potential azotemia.

Radiography

Abdominal x-rays can be very helpful in suggesting kidney disease. Some parameters examined are discussed next.

Kidney Size

Enlarged kidneys can be suggestive of acute renal disease, kidney neoplasia, or obstruction from renal stones (see Figure 13.10). Small and irregular-shaped kidneys may suggest chronic end-stage kidneys.

Presence of Urinary Stones

The presence of stones can suggest chronic infection and/or metabolic disease. There are many possible types of renal and bladder calculi and stones; *not all stones are visible on x-rays.*

Kidney Stones

Unlike humans, kidney stones (renolithiasis) are less common in pets. The presence of small to medium-sized stones may not always suggest severe pathology and may need only be monitored at regular intervals. Stones are not generally passed nor do they produce a serious health concern. If stones occur near the renal pelvis or urethra and become obstructive, surgery may be indicated (see Figure 13.11).

Bladder Stones

Bladder stones (urolithiasis) are a more common problem than renal calculi in dogs and cats. These stones can range from small to very large. They represent formation of dietary elements that precipitate out of the urine in response to urinary pH and infection. The stones have very rough, irritated surfaces that can house bacterial pathogens even while the pet is on antibiotics. Further stones can obstruct the lower urinary outflow tract producing a life-threatening condition (see Figure 13.12).

Ultrasound

Ultrasound imaging can allow visualization of the internal architecture of the kidneys and bladder. Furthermore, on ultrasound studies, images of bladder stones that may not able to seen on x-ray, as well as bladder tumors, renal tumors, and cysts, can be evaluated.

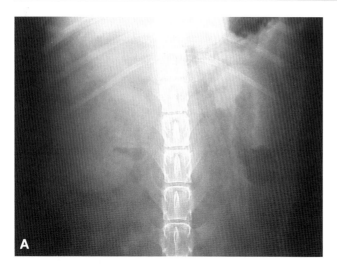
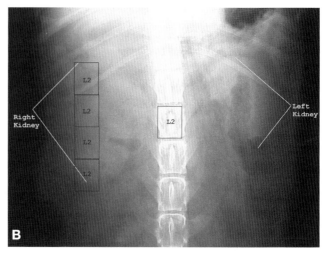

Figure 13.10. X-ray image of enlarged kidneys. Normal kidneys should be about 2–2.5 times the size of the second lumbar vertebra (a). In this radiograph, the right kidney is almost 4 times the length of the second lumbar vertebra (b).

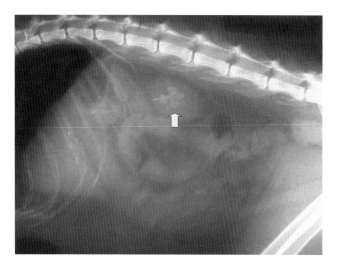

Figure 13.11. Image of large renal stones. These stones are large enough to become obstructive, producing an obstructed kidney that may require surgical removal.

Advanced Diagnostic Procedures

Urine Protein/Creatinine Ratio

The urine protein/creatinine ratio test is usually run when there is a persistent urine protein presence without evidence of urinary tract disease. Normally, the protein molecules are too large to pass through the glomerular filters. The smaller amino acid creatinine is released in the urine in large amounts. When there is glomerular damage, protein can leak through the filters, increasing the amount of protein in the urine and increasing the protein/creatinine ratio. Generally, the higher the ratio, the more severe the glomerular disease.

> **Key Points in Discussing the Need for a Radiographic and Ultrasonic Evaluation with the Client**
>
> A radiograph study is being recommended because of concerns regarding a urinary tract disease. The radiographs will allow the veterinarian to do the following.
>
> - Assess size and shape of the kidneys that may suggest acute or chronic disease.
> - Check for the presence of renal or bladder stones that may need surgical or medical treatment to help eliminate long-term problems. However, it is important to note that not all types of urinary stones will show up on plain film radiographs.
> - Check for external changes in kidney, bladder, and other organ architecture that could suggest infectious, cancerous, or other metabolic diseases.
>
> An abdominal ultrasound is being suggested to assess the internal architecture for changes that could suggest infectious, metabolic, and cancerous disease. Furthermore, ultrasound allows imaging of certain types of bladder stones and soft tissue masses that may not be visible on radiographs.

In-House Urine Protein Quantitation

As with the urine protein/creatinine ratio, there are in-house clinical diagnostics that are used as screening tests to detect minimal levels of albumen in the urine (i.e., ERD test). These tests are extremely sensitive and can help veterinarians monitor for changes in urine that could indicate early renal disease.

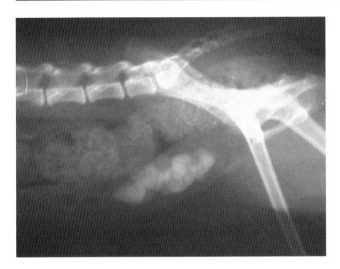

Figure 13.12. X-ray images of multiple bladder stones that may need to be surgically removed or nutritionally dissolved.

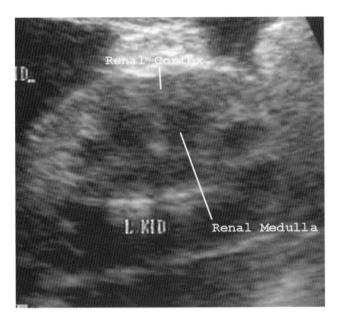

Figure 13.13. Ultrasound image of the left kidney in cross section. Notice the bright renal cortex above the darker renal medulla.

Urine Culture and Sensitivity

If a resistant pathogenic bacterium is suspected, a urine culture and sensitivity test may be run to determine what the pathogen is and what antibiotics would prove to be most effective. Urine culture can be run only on sterile urine samples taken from a catheter sample or a needle aspirate of the bladder (**cystocentesis**).

Blood Pressure Monitoring

Since high blood pressure (hypertension) can both occur secondarily to renal disease and make renal disease poten-

tially worse, monitoring blood pressure routinely will help screen for hypertension before secondary signs of the disease occur (e.g., retinal hemorrhage, cardiac enlargement, retinal detachment, etc.). (See below in the disease section.)

Ethylene Glycol Test

If antifreeze intoxication is suspected, an ethylene glycol test can be run in the hospital to detect ethylene glycol in the system for up to 8 hours.

Key Points in Discussing the Need For Advanced Diagnostics with the Client

- **Urine protein quantitation (urine protein/creatinine ratio or in-house diagnostic):** This diagnostic test is an early-detection clinical diagnostic for kidney disease used to quantitate the amount of protein leaking into the urine. In healthy kidneys, protein molecules are too large to pass through the glomerular filters. As the glomerular filters are damaged, protein can leak into the urine. The more protein in the urine, the more serious the kidney disease.
- **Urine culture and sensitivity:** A urine culture and sensitivity is being suggested to check the urine and urogenital system for possible pathogenic bacteria that could produce a kidney or bladder infection. The test identifies the bacterial component, as well as the antibiotics that will be effective against the infection.
- **Blood pressure monitoring:** A common secondary disease to kidney disease is high blood pressure or hypertension. Diseased kidneys that cannot adequately filter blood toxins at a normal level increase blood pressure to increase the speed the blood is moving and filtering through the kidneys. As the disease process worsens, the kidneys continue to raise blood pressure and eventually can produce hypertension. Since hypertension can lead to heart disease, a worsening of the existing kidney problems, and other serious problems, blood pressure is an important parameter to monitor in the pet with chronic kidney problems.
- **Ethylene glycol test:** This clinical diagnostic tests for the presence of ethylene glycol, a component of antifreeze, in the bloodstream. This chemical produces an acute kidney failure, which, if not detected and treated immediately, can produce life-threatening disease.

Diseases of the Urogenital System

Not all diseases are mentioned below, but the common diseases are discussed with the main goal being to understand and be able to explain to the client what the diseases are, how they can present, and what the overall short- and long-term concerns of each disease can be. Any discussion of overall diagnostic and treatment protocols should be discussed based on the recommendations of the doctor and the medical team. Please use the following information as a basis to discuss and educate the client, *but never to diagnose a patient.*

Acute Renal Disease

In acute renal disease, the kidney's glomerular filtration rate and renal concentration is decreased, producing a life-threatening renal azotemia and dehydration. Furthermore, the toxins present as a result depress appetite and water consumption, which dehydrates the pet and decreases nutrient intake. Finally, the acute buildup of toxins can act on the central nervous system, producing seizures and other neurologic signs.

Etiology
Causes of acute renal failure can be due to multiple diseases, discussed next.

Emergency Conditions
There are life-threatening emergency conditions that can acutely affect normal blood flow through the kidneys due to low blood pressure, blood loss, or massive dehydration. These syndromes can inhibit normal glomerular filtration and produce an acute renal shutdown.

When body temperatures increase above 106° Fahrenheit, the pet can enter a life-threatening syndrome, **heat stroke,** producing massive dehydration, poor blood flow, and metabolic disease. The resulting syndrome can stop glomerular filtration and shut down renal function and urine production (see Chapter 30).

Although there are many forms of **shock** (see Chapter 30), a shock situation can greatly decrease normal perfusion to renal tissue and lead to shutdown of glomerular filtration and urine production.

There are a number of **drugs** and **toxins** that can affect the kidneys and produce acute renal disease and failure.

Drugs that produce an acute renal failure are typically associated with overdose situations where the pet ingests a large quantity of the medication suddenly, or when the pet is placed on the wrong type of medication by an owner or client. Some examples of drugs that can produce acute renal failure are as follows.

- **Aminoglycoside antibiotics:** Systemic antibiotics such as amikacin or gentamycin can produce kidney toxicity.
- **Antifungal medication:** The antifungal amphotericin B can produce severe kidney disease.
- **Nonsteroidal anti-inflammatory drugs (NSAIDs):** Typically, the over-the-counter drug preparations (i.e., aspirin, Naprosyn, ibuprofen) given at inappropriate doses can damage renal tissue and potentially produce acute renal disease.

- **Chemotherapy drugs:** These potent drugs that are used in specific types of cancer can have serious secondary effects on other organ systems.

There are many potential toxins that can affect the kidneys acutely. Some are antifreeze (ethylene glycol—see below) and heavy metals (lead, mercury, arsenic).

Infectious Disease
There are a few bacterial infections (i.e., **leptospirosis**) or massive infections of the body (**sepsis**) that can acutely infect renal tissue, inhibiting glomerular filtration and urine production.

Systemic Disease
There are systemic diseases that can decrease renal perfusion and affect kidney tissue, disrupting normal function. Some examples of these conditions are

- hepatic disease,
- heart disease, and
- cancer.

Signalment
Acute renal disease can affect animals of any species, breed or sex.

Common Points in Medical History
With these syndromes, the pet's renal function is acutely impaired, producing a massive buildup of toxins in the blood. This produces an acutely ill, profoundly affected animal. Common medical complaints in this condition are

- vomiting,
- not eating,
- profound depression,
- history of seizures, and
- diarrhea.

Common Points on Initial Assessment
These affected pets can be severely ill and depressed from the increased toxin load. *However, since this disease has affected these animals so acutely, their body condition and weight are usually normal.* Key points to monitor during the initial assessment are as follows.

- **Hydration:** Pets can be moderate to life-threateningly dehydrated.
- **Oral cavity:** Some pets may have ulcers on the tongue, gums, and lips due to the high levels of ammonia, which causes burns of the oral cavity.
- **Abdominal palpation:** Due to acute onset of renal disease, the following changes may be noted:
  — Pain over the middle back region (kidney area)
  — Kidneys may be swollen and painful on palpation
  — Small bladder present, suggesting decreased urine production

- **Mentation:** The pet may be acutely depressed to severely comatose.
- **Neurologic:** Some pets may show focal to grand mal seizures and have altered vocal and behavior patterns.

Complications

If acute renal disease is not diagnosed and treated, the pet may develop acute renal failure, halting glomerular filtration, stopping urine production (**anuria**), and producing a life-threatening syndrome.

Diagnosis

Since acute renal failure can be caused by many possible diseases and syndromes, a thorough workup involving blood and urine diagnostics and abdominal imagery may be recommended.

Treatment

Treatment is focused on diagnosing and treating the underlying disease while treating and relieving the toxin load that is building up and allowing the kidneys to return to normal function. Some possible treatment options are discussed next.

Intravenous Fluids

Intravenous (IV) fluid therapy is strongly recommended to help increase glomerular filtration to help the kidneys push the toxins into the bloodstream (**diuresis**). Further, IV fluids help to rehydrate and maintain the patient.

> **Practice Tip**: It is extremely important to monitor urine output while acute renal failure patients are on large amounts of IV fluids. These patients can stop producing urine (anuria) and begin to build up fluids within the tissue and lung fields (pulmonary edema). *Anuria carries a very poor prognosis, and decreased urine production should be reported to the veterinarian when evident.*

Medications

Medications are focused on decreasing the amount of toxins the pet has to deal with and decreasing the nausea and vomiting secondary to renal disease. Some medications are discussed next.

- **Anti-emetics:** Drugs, such as metoclopramide and others, help reduce vomiting and can make the pet feel more comfortable, allowing them to eat.
- **Decreased acid producers:** Drugs, such as cimetidine and famotidine, help decrease stomach acid that builds up secondary to kidney disease.
- **Antibiotics:** Antibiotics may be indicated if a bacterial infection is suspected.
- **Phosphate binders:** These groups of oral medications, such as Amphogel, allow the binding of oral phosphorus

in the diet before it is absorbed by the body, thus decreasing the amount of work the kidneys do.

Diet

Low-protein diets, such as Hill's K/d, also help to decrease ingested proteins, decreasing the amount of ammonia produced from protein metabolism that must be removed by the kidneys.

Advanced Procedures

Typically, these procedures are done at critical care and university facilities. These procedures, discussed next, are not always options due to availability of equipment, prognosis of case, or financial constraints.

- **Dopamine administration:** Dopamine is administered when the kidneys shut down. The drug helps to increase kidney blood flow to help return urine formation. *If urine production decreases or stops, the pet's prognosis is grave.*
- **Peritoneal lavage:** Administration of specialized fluids directly into the abdomen can sometimes help decrease the toxin load. The fluid is then drained from the abdomen. This procedure may have to be performed regularly. *This suggests a poor to grave prognosis.*
- **Blood dialysis:** This process is the continuous filtering of toxins from the blood. It must be sustained many times per week with specialized machinery, usually done in a university setting.
- **Kidney transplants:** Kidney transplants have been done successfully in a university setting. Treatment can include long periods of hospitalization, blood dialysis, surgery, and long-term medications that cause immunosuppression.

Prevention

Keeping pets away from medication and drugs that can produce an acute renal disease can help prevent its occurrence.

> **Discussing Acute Renal Disease with the Client**
> - Acute renal disease can be caused by bacterial or systemic diseases, or the ingestion of toxins or poisons.
> - The syndrome causes an acute shutdown of the filtering abilities of the kidneys, causing a massive buildup of ammonia toxins within the body.
> - This rapid buildup can make the pet very ill, dehydrated, nauseous, and life-threateningly dehydrated.
> - The overall prognosis depends on what has caused the renal disease. However, if severe enough, the kidneys can shut down and stop producing urine. If this occurs, the pet's prognosis is poor.
> - Most animals will require hospitalization, intensive fluid therapy, and medications to begin treating the acute renal syndrome.

Antifreeze Poisoning

Although already discussed in the acute renal disease section, antifreeze intoxication is a specific renal toxin. Antifreeze is sweet tasting and will be consumed by dogs and cats when available. Most antifreeze contains a toxin called **ethylene glycol,** which is a severe renal toxin. The longer the toxin is in the body, the more damage is done. *If the animal is seen more than a few hours after ingestion takes place, there may be irreversible kidney disease and a life-threatening condition.*

Etiology

Antifreeze is absorbed into the body rapidly, causing severe metabolic upset. The toxin begins to crystallize in the bloodstream, especially within the kidneys, selectively destroying the tissue and causing acute and potential irreversible kidney disease (see Table 13.3).

Table 13.3.   Minimum lethal dose of antifreeze.

Canine	2–3 ml/kg
Feline	1.4 ml (1/5 of a teaspoon)/kg

Signalment

The disease can affect any dog and cat. This problem is seen generally in the colder months of the year when radiators are winterized.

Common Points in Medical History

As discussed with acute renal failure, medical complaints usually reveal animals that are rapidly affected and may be profoundly ill. Some medical complaints can be

- mild to severe depression,
- nausea,
- vomiting,
- inability to balance properly,
- tripping easily,
- altered vocalization, and
- acting strangely.

Common Points on Initial Assessment

Physical signs depend on the amount of toxin ingested and the duration since ingestion occurred. In early disease signs can be

- severe muscular tremors,
- tremor movements in the eyes (**nystagmus**),
- head tremors,
- increased thirst and urination,
- low body temperature,
- acting abnormally

— change in vocalization,
— acting blind,
— sudden aggression.

In late disease, signs can be

- severe kidney disease,
- decreased to no production of urine,
- coma,
- seizure, and
- death.

Complications

If not diagnosed and treated immediately, ethylene glycol intoxication can produce acute renal disease/failure and death.

Diagnostics

Clinical diagnostics for suspect antifreeze intoxication can be the following.

- **Complete blood count:** Changes observed in the complete blood count are elevations in red blood cell count and total protein secondary to severe dehydration.
- **Chemistry:** With ethylene glycol poisoning there can be significant elevations in the renal enzymes (BUN, creatinine, and phosphorus), as well as elevations in potassium and blood sugar.
- **Urinalysis:** Urinalysis can show a dilute urine (urine specific gravity <10.15), suggesting a renal azotemia. Further evidence of antifreeze intoxication is the presence of calcium oxalate crystals in the urine within 8 hours after intoxication.
- **Ethylene glycol test:** A positive ethylene glycol test within 6 hours after ingestion suggests the presence of the toxin in the bloodstream. After 6 hours after ingestion, the test can be negative.

Treatment

Treatment is dependent on history, diagnostic tests, and physical exam findings on presentation of the pet. However, it is important to note, especially in the feline, the longer the pet goes without treatment after ingestion, the worse the diagnosis. Some treatment options may be the following.

- **Hospitalization and fluid therapy:** It is extremely important to make sure the pet is on intravenous fluids to continue perfusion to the kidneys and stimulate urine formation.
- **Vomiting and gastric lavage:** If ingestion has just occurred, the goal is to induce emesis (vomiting), remove any remaining antifreeze in the intestinal system, and administer activated charcoal to deactivate any remaining toxin.
- **Medication:**
  — **4-methylpyrazole** inhibits the crystallization of ethylene glycol from the bloodstream. This drug must be

administered over 48 hours with the pet in the hospital. This drug is only effective in dogs.

— **Ethanol:** The use of 95% grain alcohol also inhibits the formation of the crystal from the blood. It is the only available treatment in cats and must be given intravenously over 2 days.

Monitoring

The pet will have to be monitored very carefully in the hospital for urine formation and changes in the blood chemistry to help the veterinarian determine the overall prognosis. *If kidney toxin blood levels begin to climb and urine production is not present in the first 24–48 hours, the prognosis is usually grave.*

Prevention

The key to prevention is to limit the availability of antifreeze or use antifreeze without the ethylene glycol component.

Discussing Ethylene Glycol Intoxication with the Client

- Most antifreeze contains a toxin called ethylene glycol. Once ingested, it is rapidly absorbed into the body and enters the bloodstream. The chemical begins to crystallize out of the blood as it enters the kidneys. The progressive crystallization destroys normal kidney tissue, producing an acute kidney failure.
- The failure can begin within hours after ingestion, and if not diagnosed and treatment begun, the prognosis is very poor.
- Cats are much more susceptible to the toxin.
- Clinical signs are depression (sometimes to coma level), vomiting, diarrhea, changes in attitude, seizures, and possibly death.
- Treatment can require days of hospitalization and medications; there may still be high risk of kidney shutdown and death.

Chronic Renal Disease

Chronic kidney disease is a slowly progressive destruction of kidney tissue. This causes renal toxins to build up in the bloodstream and makes the pet nauseous, anorexic, and dehydrated.

Etiology

The disease is a chronic destruction and breakdown of normal renal tissue secondary to age, inflammatory or infectious disease, or cancer. Physical signs occur as over 75% of the kidney tissue is slowly, progressively destroyed, inhibiting normal glomerular and medullary function.

Signalment

The disease can affect both dogs and cats, with higher incidence in older pets (mean age of onset is 9 years old). The Abyssinian and Persian cats, bull terrier, Cairn terrier, German shepherd, and Sharpei can have a genetic predisposition for kidney disease.

Complications

Without proper diagnosis and treatment, the pet can continue with chronic weight loss, vomiting, and anorexia. If toxins continue to rise unchecked, the pet can chronically waste and may enter a life-threatening state. Furthermore, secondarily, hypertension (high blood pressure) can be a significant concern (see below).

Common Points on Medical History

This disease can be slow and insidious in progression. Medical complaints can vary depending on how affected the kidneys are and how long the pet has dealt with chronic azotemia. If renal damage occurs slowly, animals can appear asymptomatic, with severe renal impairment. Some common medical complaints can be

- chronic weight loss, sometimes severe, with animals losing 30–40% of original weight;
- increased thirst and urination;
- chronic vomiting; and
- decreased appetite.

Common Points in Initial Assessment

These pets can show very few physical symptoms because they have adapted to the slow increase in azotemia and are still eating and acting normally. However, other pets may have acute episodes because of sudden dramatic rises in blood toxins. The following symptoms may be evident on initial assessment.

- Dehydration
- Weight loss and poor body condition
- Diarrhea and constipation
- Neurologic signs—seizure

Diagnostics

Since chronic renal disease can present with very mild to severe general medical symptoms (i.e., weight loss, vomiting, depression), a thorough workup, including blood work, urinalysis, radiology, and other diagnostics, may be recommended.

Treatment

Treatment of chronic renal disease can take several forms, depending on the severity of disease, physical symptoms of the pet, and how the owner elects to manage treatment at home. Treatment goals are broken into two categories: short-term goals and long-term goals.

Short-Term Goals

- **Fluid therapy:** Usually accomplished with intravenous fluids, the goal of fluid therapy is to help clear the toxins from the bloodstream by forcing kidneys to push out the toxins while rehydrating the pet **(diuresis).** This process is usually done in the hospital on intravenous fluids over a period of days.

- **Medication:** During severe episodes of kidney disease, the hormone gastrin, which produces stomach acid, stays high in the body, causing increased amounts of stomach acid. This can make the pet feel nauseous. By placing the animal on drug that decreases stomach acid, such as cimetidine, it may help stimulate the pet's appetite.

- **Correcting electrolyte abnormalities:** Restoring the normal levels of sodium, potassium, and chloride help to decrease lethargy, weakness, and anorexia.

Long-Term Goals
- **Subcutaneous fluids:** Once the kidneys have undergone diuresis, giving subcutaneous fluids under the skin at home every other day to a few times a week may allow the kidneys to maintain adequate hydration on detoxification.

- **Potassium supplementation:** Giving oral potassium supplements can keep the pet's electrolytes in balance and help maintain appetite.

- **Medications:** The pet may be placed on medications to help decrease nausea associated with toxin buildup and help bind phosphorus in the diet before it enters the body.

- **Erythropoietin supplementation:** This hormone, which is produced by the kidney, stimulates red blood cell production in the bone marrow. In advanced cases of chronic renal disease, this hormone helps stimulate red blood cell formation and prevent anemia.

Prevention

There is no way to prevent chronic renal disease. However, through routine blood and urine diagnostics in older animals and breeds that are more sensitive to renal disease, early diagnosis and treatment can help increase quality of life and life span of the pet.

Discussing Chronic Renal Disease with the Client
- Chronic renal disease is a chronic, progressive destruction of both kidneys.
- Physical symptoms of chronic vomiting, weight loss, and anorexia become evident as 66–75% of the kidney tissue is damaged.
- Blood and urine clinical diagnostics can help determine the extent of the kidney disease and help the veterinarian decide on effective treatment options.
- There is no cure for chronic renal disease. The goal of short-term and long-term treatment is to help maintain hydration, decrease toxin load on the body, and maintain appetite and quality of life.
- Hypertension can be a common secondary disease concern from chronic renal disease, and blood pressure should be routinely monitored.

Lower Urinary Tract Disease

Lower urinary tract disease is caused by a bacterial infection of the bladder and/or obstruction of the urinary outflow tract with urinary crystals, stones (**urolithes**), or debris. There are, overall, two forms of the disease that cause obstruction.

- **Primary bacterial bladder infections with secondary urolithiasis (predominant canine form):** The diseases occur as bacteria invade and irritate the bladder wall, which becomes inflamed and thickened. As this occurs, blood and protein begin to ooze from the bladder wall, serving as further nutrients for the bacteria and making the infection worse. As the infection continues, dietary components can crystallize in the urine. These crystals can further unite and form stones. It is these crystals and stones that obstruct the urethra (outflow tract of the bladder) and can cause an obstructed bladder.

- **With primary urolithiasis (predominant feline form):** The urinary outflow tract (urethra) obstructs with crystalline debris, mucus (mucous plugs), or stones that crystallize out of the urine due to the urinary environment and dietary components. These crystals obstruct the urinary outflow tract causing the bladder to swell and urine to backflow into the kidneys. This can severely decrease or permanently damage kidney function.

Etiology

There are predisposing factors for lower urinary tract disease.

- Conditions that keep the animal from urinating normally or fully, such as an infrequent cleaning of the litter box.
- Stress in the household, such as new pet.
- Dietary factors that change urinary pH or environment.
- Dietary factors high in a specific compound that precipitates out in the urine to form crystals.
- Insufficient water intake, which can also predispose to bladder infections and bladder stones.

There are many types of crystals that can precipitate out of the urine causing obstruction and disease. The most common ones are:

- **Struvite (magnesium ammonium phosphate)** crystals occur as the urine begins to have an alkaline pH (>7.0). The diet may have higher amounts of the mineral magnesium. The presence of the alkaline urine and the higher dietary magnesium level combines with normal urine components to form crystals.

- **Calcium oxalate crystals** are produced when there are high levels of calcium in the diet and the urine is acidic (pH <7.0). The stones are seen more in males than females. They are more common in Himalayan and Persian cat breeds and miniature schnauzers, Lhasa apso, and Yorkshire terriers dog breeds.

Signalment
Urinary obstruction can occur in both dogs and cats, affecting the male pet more commonly.

Complications
If not treated immediately, a blocked pet will develop severe accumulations of renal toxins, develop secondary renal disease, and enter acute renal failure and death.

Common Points on Medical History
The disease can start subtly with increases in urination, vocalization while urinating, urinating outside of the litter pan, and spraying urine (male or female cats). The urine can have a blood tinged or brown color. Occasionally, pets will come acutely obstructed, severely depressed, dehydrated, and vomit due to the acute azotemia. *Often feline patients will be brought in with the complaint of constipation because both female and male cats strain and posture to suggest issues with constipation.*

Common Points in Physical Examination
These pets are beginning to feel ill or can be severely depressed due to the buildup of toxins in the bloodstream. Clinical signs on initial assessment can be

- dehydration,
- vomiting,
- lateral/sternal recumbence,
- painful abdomen with a large bladder evident,
- vocalization while palpating abdomen,
- licking vaginal/penile region, and
- extended red, raw penis

Diagnosis
Diagnosis is made based on medical history, physical examination, and changes in the blood and urine clinical diagnostic tests.

Treatment
If urinary obstruction is evident, it should be considered a life-threatening emergency. The treatment is focused on both short- and long-term care.

Short-Term Care
Medical treatment consists of the following.

- Catheterization of the bladder with a urinary catheter allows normal flow of urine (usually done under sedation).
- Fluid therapy, either intravenous or subcutaneous, to allow proper rehydration of the pet and increase the outflow of urine.
- The use of antibiotics to help clear up the initial bladder infection, if present.
- If the catheter is removed and the pet re-obstructs, surgery may be needed to clear the obstruction (see below).

Surgical treatment consists of the following.

- **Felines—perineal urethrostomy/cystotomy:** In some cases in cats that have recurrent obstruction, a surgery to create a new opening above the penis is preformed. This procedure is called a **perineal urethrostomy**. It decreases the likelihood of reobstruction. Also if stones are present within the bladder, a surgery to remove these stones (**cystotomy**) may also be recommended.
- **Canines—cystotomy:** In general, bladder stones are surgically removed through a cystotomy.

Discussing Urinary Tract Disease and Urinary Obstruction with the Client

- Bladder infection can occur as urine sits for extended periods of time. The bacteria in the urine begin to reproduce and irritate the bladder wall; the bladder begins to leak protein and blood. The protein and blood acts as an excellent growth medium for the bacteria, making the bladder infection worse. The cells, debris, and protein can combine and obstruct the urinary outflow tract.
- Urinary crystals form as dietary components begin to crystallize out from the urine at a specific urinary pH. Crystals can occur primarily or as associated with urinary tract infection. Given enough time, crystals can form into urinary stones.
- Cellular and bacterial debris and crystals can obstruct the urinary outflow tract, making the pet unable to clear the toxins from its body. These toxins begin to backflow into the kidneys and back into the bloodstream. This produces an acute syndrome that can make the pet very ill and dehydrated.
- Urinary obstruction is a life-threatening emergency that, if not treated immediately, can produce a life-threatening syndrome within a very short period of time (<4–8 hours).
- In tomcats with a repeated history of obstruction, the veterinarian may suggest a surgical procedure called a **perineal urethrostomy (PU)**. This procedure creates a larger opening above the pet's penis. Although these sites can still obstruct, the larger opening decreases concern for obstruction.
- To help prevent re-formation of the urinary crystals or stones (i.e., struvite), it may be recommended that the pet go on a specific diet that changes the urinary pH and has decreased elements of the specific stone in the diet.
- The veterinarian may recommend routine recheck of the urine to help detect any changes that may precede crystal reformation.

Long-Term Care:

- **Diet:** Once the type of crystal or bladder stone (**uroliths**) has been identified, the pet should be placed on a prescription diet that alters the pH of the urine and has decreased dietary elements to help prevent reformation of crystals.
- **Urinalysis:** Once diagnosed and placed on a prescription diet, regular re-evaluation should be performed on urine for changes suggestive of bladder infection or crystal reoccurrence.

Prevention

Prevention is focused on diagnosing and treating urinary tract disease before a pet obstructs. If crystals or urolithes have been diagnosed, specific diets to help control pH and dietary components are available to help prevent stone reoccurrence.

Renal Secondary Hypertension

Hypertension is a chronic elevation of blood pressure causing a potentially severe systemic disease.

Etiology

In chronic renal disease, hypertension is an increase in systemic blood pressure caused by an increased production of renin–angiotensin due to decreased glomerular filtration in diseased kidneys. The activated angiotensin produces a significant vasoconstriction increasing systemic blood pressure. Hypertension can also occur secondarily to the following disease entities:

- diabetes mellitus (dog and cat),
- hyperadrenocorticism (dog mostly),
- hyperthyroidism (cat mostly),
- heart disease (cat mostly), and
- can also rarely occur as a primary disease

Signalment

Hypertension affects both dogs between 2 and 14 years of age (mean age of 8–9 years) and cats between 7 and 20 years of age (mean age of 15 years). There is no genetic or sex predisposition.

Common Points in Medical History

Hypertension can be a very subtle disease process; the chief medical complaint is that the pet may be slowing down or "getting older." Concerns of hypertension should occur with a history of chronic renal disease or any of the above-listed diseases. Some other medical complaints can be

- bumping into furniture and objects (acting blind),
- nose bleeds,
- weight loss, and
- exercise intolerance.

Table 13.4. Normal blood pressure levels.

Species	Systolic	Diastolic	Mean Arterial Pressure
Canine	<160 mm Hg	<95 mm Hg	117 mm Hg
Feline	<180 mm Hg	<120 mm Hg	140 mm Hg

Common Points on Initial Assessment

Hypertension can produce very subtle signs on initial assessment of the patient. Some concerns may be

- acute blindness,
- bleeding from the nose, and
- central nervous system disease (e.g., seizures, depression).

Complications

If hypertension is not detected and treated, it may produce displacement of the retina of the eye, producing acute blindness, heart disease and failure, and central nervous system signs.

Diagnostics

Clinical diagnostics for hypertension are completed with a Doppler or oscillation method to obtain systolic systemic pressure. Animals are said to have systemic hypertension when their blood pressure is above the values given in Table 13.4.

A persistent elevation in any of the three blood pressure categories is defined as hypertension.

Treatment

Treatment is focused on the following guidelines.

- **Identify and treat the underlying disorder:** Because hypertension commonly occurs as a secondary disease entity, identification of the primary disorder and treatment of the disease are necessary to help control blood pressure. The veterinarian may suggest getting a diagnostic baseline of blood work, urine, x-rays, and other tests to help rule out any primary disease.
- **Decreasing dietary sodium:** By decreasing salt content in the diet, it decreases the amount of fluid retained by the body, thus decreasing the amount of fluid the body must pass through the heart and blood supply.
- **Medications:** Medications are focused on decreasing systemic hypertension by inhibiting the renin–angiotensin system. These drugs inhibit the activation of renin in the kidney, which decreases the production of the vasoconstricting hormone angiotensin.

Prevention

The key to prevention of hypertension is early detection of high blood pressure in animals and identification of the underlying primary disease.

Discussing Secondary Renal Hypertension with the Client

- High blood pressure is an increase in constriction of peripheral blood vessels, which increases resistance in blood circulation in the body.
- Normal, healthy kidneys require 20% of the body's blood to flow through kidney filters every minute to maintain normal detoxification of the blood.
- To maintain glomerular filtration, the kidneys release a potent chemical that stimulates constriction of the blood vessels of the body, increasing blood pressure and blood velocity.
- As kidneys become diseased and there are fewer filters available in the kidney tissue, the kidney continues to secrete large amounts of hormone to maintain adequate circulation for filtration of the blood.
- Over time this process can elevate blood pressure to abnormally high levels, producing hypertension.
- Over time hypertension can produce blindness, seizures, and produce or worsen cardiac disease.
- Monitoring blood pressure routinely can help prevent serious life-limiting disease.
- If hypertension is diagnosed, medication can help control blood pressure.

CD-ROM 1 reviews material presented in this chapter. Please try the cases for Section 2 (Anatomy and Physiology—The Science behind the Diseases) *to help reinforce the information presented here.*

Chapter 14

Liver

Introduction

The liver is the largest gland in the body. It serves as a warehouse and production plant, producing most of the products essential for life. The liver functions in the following areas.

- **Storage:** The liver stores an extremely small sugar supply to use when the body needs quick energy. The sugar molecule called **glycogen** is transformed from glucose by the liver for storage. When the body is running low on sugar, the liver converts the glycogen back into sugar.
- **Detoxification of toxins:** There are heavy loads of toxins and bacteria brought to the liver from the gastrointestinal tract. Enzymes in the liver detoxify these toxins into inert waste products that are then excreted by the intestines and kidneys.
- **Formation of building blocks:** The liver takes amino acids and proteins, triglycerides (fat), and simple sugars from the intestine and uses them to produce necessary proteins and structures for the body. The liver can change these nutrients and then export them for:
  — **production:** milk, eggs,
  — **growth:** muscle, fat,
  — **maintenance:** skin, hair, clotting factors, blood protein, and
  — **reproduction.**

The liver is located behind the diaphragm in the cranial aspect of the abdomen. It sits cranial to the stomach, small intestine, pancreas, and spleen. The liver is covered in **peritoneum**, the same tissue that lines the abdomen. This tissue secretes a clear sterile fluid to prevent attachment of bacteria to help resist infection. The liver sits more on the right side of the abdomen and is divided into a number of lobes by fissures or separations within the tissue (see Figure 14.1). The lobes are divided into the

- left lateral lobe,
- left medial lobe,
- right lateral lobe,
- right medial lobe,
- quadrate lobe, and
- caudate lobes.

Within the liver architecture, there is a special indentation (**fossa**) within the right medial lobe that houses the gall bladder. The gall bladder serves as a collecting bag for the toxins excreted by the liver. Many of these toxins are pigments (i.e., bilirubin) that give the feces its color. The gall bladder empties through a duct known as the biliary tree into a common bile duct that empties into the duodenum. The common bile duct also shares ducts from the pancreatic ducts that secrete digestive enzymes that aid in digestion of food. Ingestion of food and water stimulates the release of the pancreatic enzymes and constriction of the gall bladder through the common bile duct.

The blood supply to the liver is a unique system to help keep the liver healthy while detoxifying the body. The major nutritional support for the liver is from the **hepatic artery**, a branch of the celiac artery, which supplies nutrition for the liver. The **hepatic vein** takes deoxygenated blood and nutrients away from the liver toward the heart, emptying into the caudal vena cava. However, another large venous system called the **portal vein** drains the stomach, small intestines, and colon, and helps to bring absorbed nutrients, toxins, and bacteria to the liver (see Figure 14.2). The portal vein is the only venous system in the body that does not have a matching arterial system with it.

The internal architecture of the liver is composed of one-cell-thick layers of **hepatocytes** that are surrounded by blood within a hepatic sinus on either side of the cell (see Figure 14.3).

The function of these cells is to absorb all toxins, bacteria, and nutrients that are in the portal blood supply. The nutrients are absorbed, changed into proteins, energy, and fats that the body can use, and then re-released into the blood supply to enter the general circulation through the caudal vena cava and the heart. The toxins and bacteria are detoxified and de-activated and then released into channels, called **canniculi,** running through the layers of hepatocytes. These canniculi then connect to the bile ductules, which lead to the gall bladder. The major waste material secreted is a chemical called **bilirubin**. Bilirubin is a breakdown pigment from blood. When the red blood cell becomes aged and fragile, the spleen destroys the red blood cells and harvests the hemoglobin inside. Hemoglobin is the part of the red blood cell that carries oxygen. The spleen removes iron molecules that are closely related to the hemoglobin and passes the rest of the molecule to the liver as bilirubin, a yellow waste pigment.

Within the hepatocytes are specific chemicals called enzymes that function to change or produce specific body pro-

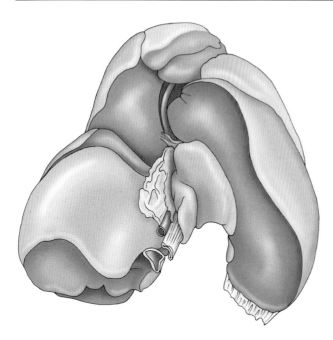

Figure 14.1.   Illustration of the canine liver.

teins, sugar, and fats or to detoxify toxic chemicals in the body.

Enzymes involved with protein metabolism are

- alanine aminotransferase (ALT),
- aspartate aminotransferase (AST),
- lactic dehydrogenase (LDH), and
- gamma-glutamyltransferase (GGT).

There are series of enzymes (called pathways) that deactivates toxins step by step. These enzyme pathways are

- glucoronidation enzymes, and
- cytochrome P_{450} enzymes.

These enzyme systems are responsible for deactivating many of the drugs that are used in veterinary medicine. Without these enzymes, even normal doses of antibiotics or other drug categories could become toxic to our body. Furthermore, felines lack the **glucoronidation enzymes;** this is why cats are much less able to handle ingestion of specific categories of drugs (i.e., nonsteroidal anti-inflammatory medication, or NSAIDs).

Hepatocytes also produce chemicals called **bile acids** that help emulsify fat within the small intestine. Eating stimulates bile acid production, and they empty through the gall bladder and into the common bile duct. As the gall bladder empties into the small intestine by the common bile duct, these chemicals are then released to help in the breakdown of fat. The bile acids are then rapidly reabsorbed by the small intestine.

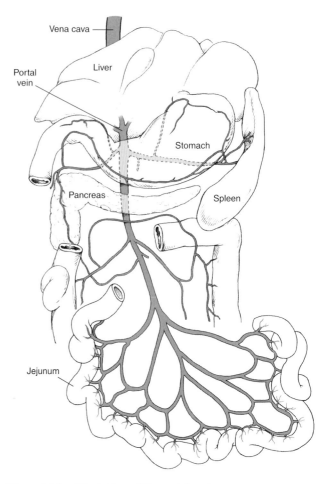

Figure 14.2.   Illustration of the portal system.

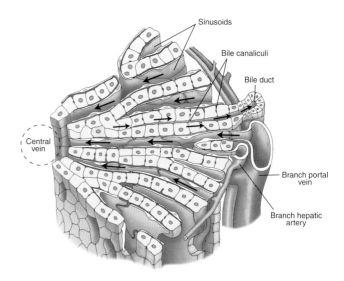

Figure 14.3.   Cross-section of the liver. Notice the branch of the portal vein bringing in nutrients, toxins, and microbes into the liver tissue. The hepatocytes absorb the nutrients and modify them for use by the body. The toxins and microbes are detoxified and then pushed into the bile canaliculi, which then accumulate in the gall bladder.

Clinical Expressions of Liver Disease

Because the liver functions on so many levels, liver disease can produce variable signs depending on the type of disease evident. As with other organ disease, liver malfunction can be acute or chronic, subtle or severe, and each form of the disease can be treated very differently. Disease categories are discussed next.

Infectious Liver Disease
The liver can be affected by viral, bacterial, fungal, and parasitic infection. The infection invades normal liver tissue, slowing or stopping the liver's ability to detoxify the body and produce building blocks. Some examples of infectious hepatic diseases are

- canine viral hepatitis,
- bacterial hepatitis,
- fungal hepatitis (e.g., coccidiomycosis), and
- parasitic hepatitis (e.g., liver flukes).

Inflammatory Disease
Inflammatory diseases are those functional diseases in which the liver is unable to breakdown the pigments and infection, producing an influx of white blood cells into hepatic tissue. The white blood cells invade through the healthy liver, causing damage and irritation. Inflammatory disease can be broken down into three categories, depending on the chronicity of the process.

- Acute hepatitis
- Chronic hepatitis
- End-stage liver disease—cirrhosis

Neoplasia
The liver is both the site of primary cancer and a common site of metastatic disease (see Figure 14.4). Although liver

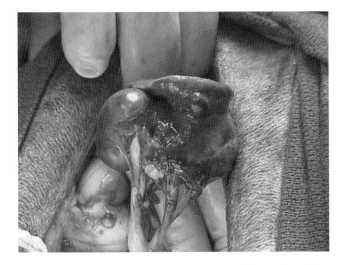

Figure 14.4. Abnormal diseased liver with evidence of neoplasia or metastasis.

masses can be benign, the liver can also be affected by malignant cancer. Some common primary liver tumors are

- hepatic adenocarcinoma,
- hepatic cholangioadenocarcinoma,
- lymphoma,
- mast cell tumor, and
- hemangiosarcoma.

Metabolic Disease
This form of liver disease occurs as inert proteinaceous material or fat builds up within the liver, destroying the normal architecture and function. Examples of metabolic liver disease are

- **amyloidosis** (protein), and
- **hepatic lipidosis** (fat).

Toxic Disease
Because the liver is the major shock organ in the dog and is a source of detoxification, severe toxins can affect normal liver metabolism and function.

Porto-Systemic (Porto-Caval) Shunts
The portal vein brings nutrients, toxins, and bacteria to the liver to be metabolized, used, and excreted. In some animals, small vessels, called **shunts**, can bypass the liver, moving blood directly into the caudal vena cava, heart, and central nervous system. The increased blood toxin load can produce severe neurological and systemic signs. Shunts can occur as a congenital defect or as an acquired disease and can occur within the liver (**intrahepatic**) or outside of the liver (**extrahepatic**) (see below).

Signs Specific to Liver Disease

Liver disease can show specific symptoms that can suggest liver dysfunction.

Jaundice
Jaundice refers to a buildup of yellow pigmented toxins within the skin, sclera of the eye, and gums of the animal (see Figure 14.5). This process occurs secondary to the buildup of bilirubin due to one of the following concerns:

- Inability of the liver to detoxify the waste products (i.e., **liver disease**)
- Obstruction of the gall bladder (i.e. **cholestatic disease**)
- Massive destruction of the red blood cells within the blood vessels of the body (e.g., **immune mediated hemolytic anemia**)

Ascites
Ascites refers to the buildup of a low protein–low cellularity abdominal fluid (**transudate** or a **modified transudate**). This can occur secondary to the following.

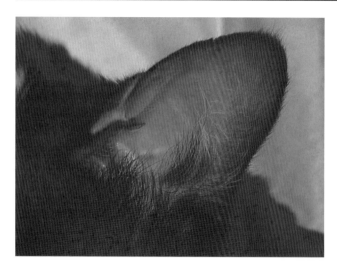

Figure 14.5.   Ear pinna are common sites to evaluate for jaundice.

- **Liver disease:** The liver produces a series of proteins (mainly **albumin**) that maintains vascular pressure within the vessel, which keeps fluid within the blood. With severe liver disease, blood protein levels decrease, allowing fluid pooling outside of the blood supply.
- **Right-sided heart disease:** When there is disease in the right heart, blood cannot flow properly, causing a backlog or congestion within the hepatic sinusoids. When this occurs, the liver begins to ooze fluid into the abdomen (ascites; see Chapter 12).

Hepatic Encephalopathy

Hepatic encephalopathy refers to a neurologic syndrome caused by the improper hepatic detoxification of toxins. The toxins build up within the bloodstream and directly affect the central nervous system. The syndrome commonly occurs 15–20 minutes after eating a meal because of the massive inflow of toxins associated with eating. Common neurologic signs can be

- seizures,
- disorientation,
- circling,
- head pressing,
- atypical behavior, and
- blindness.

Coagulopathy

A coagulopathy refers to a patient that has a decreased ability to clot blood. The liver produces specific proteins that help in clot formation. In severe liver disease and failure, the clotting proteins are not being manufactured at adequate levels. Animals can present with

- bruising,
- nose bleeds,
- rectal bleeding, and
- poor color.

Animals for which there are concerns of significant liver disease or failure must be monitored closely for spontaneous hemorrhage or bruising. When drawing blood from these pets, only smaller blood vessels (i.e., the cephalic—front arm) should be used. *A team member should never draw blood from the jugular vein in a pet with a potential coagulopathy because of the concern for continued bleeding from the larger jugular vessel.*

Obtaining a Thorough History with Hepatic Disease

Diagnosing hepatic disease based on physical examination can be very difficult. It becomes exceedingly important to get a good history in an animal that may be presenting with moderate to severe hepatic disease. Animals can have serious disease and present with very mild signs; they can be almost normal on physical examination. Some key questions when obtaining a medical history are presented next.

Is the Animal Young or Old?

Although liver disease tends to be evident in middle-aged to older animals, it does not have to be an old-animal problem. Some very young animals can have serious liver problems.

Is There Breed Specificity for Liver Disease?

Specific breeds can have underlying liver disease at different life stages. Although liver dysfunction can occur in any animal, the following breeds have a greater genetic disposition for hepatic problems.

- Beddlington terrier
- West Highland white terrier
- Skye terrier
- Doberman pinscher
- Yorkshire terrier
- Shar pei

Has the Progression of the Disease Been Sudden or Chronic?

The progression of the disease can differentiate between chronic and acute disease and potentially change the differential disease list, the diagnostic tests, and treatment by the veterinarian and medical team.

Has There Been a Sharp Increase in Water Consumption or Urination ?

As with renal disease, increased water consumption (polydipsia) and urination (polyuria) occur as the pet tries to excrete through diuresis the toxins in their body by increasing their water intake and urination. It is important to discuss if the changes have occurred over the last few days, weeks, or months. Furthermore, with cat owners, the most notable change may be that the litter box is more saturated or heavy.

Has There Been a Slowly or a Rapidly Decreasing Appetite?

With chronic disease, the loss of liver function and increased blood toxins can slowly suppress the appetite.

Has There Been a Progressive Weight Loss?

Weight loss may be the only symptom noted by the client. Weight loss of 1–2 pounds in a 10-pound animal represents 10–20% weight loss. It is very important to differentiate over what period of time this weight loss has occurred.

Acute significant weight loss in the cat can suggest an acute shutdown of the liver due to infiltration of fat into the liver tissue (**hepatic lipidosis**; see below). With **chronic liver disease**, there tends to be more severe chronic anorexia associated with a decreased liver function, producing physical symptoms such as a pendulous or pot-bellied abdomen and a poor hair coat.

Is the Animal a Chronic Vomiter or is Vomiting Occurring More Often?

With the chronic increase of toxins, vomiting can occur more readily.

Is the Animal Having Chronic Diarrhea?

Animals with liver disease can have a profound small bowel diarrhea because of lack of normal digestive enzymes that are produced by the liver (maldigestion syndrome; see Chapter 10). However, with enough toxins, large-colon diarrhea is also possible. Furthermore, gastrointestinal bleeding secondary to coagulopathies can produce digested blood (**melena**) from the small intestine and frank blood from the colon.

Has the Animal Been Exposed to Toxins or Poisons?

Although there are very few toxins that specifically destroy liver tissue, almost all toxins are eliminated by the liver and therefore can damage normal liver tissue. Some possible toxins to discuss with the owner are

- mushrooms, and
- acetaminophen (Tylenol).

Is the Patient on Any Long-Term Medications?

Patients on long-term medications can develop secondary liver disease. In many circumstances, these patients have routine blood work evaluated to make sure there is no evidence of liver issues. However, even with screening blood work, patients can develop serious liver dysfunction. Common drugs that can affect the liver are discussed next.

- **NSAIDs:** Drugs such as carprofen (Rimadyl) and other NSAIDs can have a chronic effect on liver function in some cases.

- **Anticonvulsants:** Medications such as phenobarbital can also affect liver function and produce liver damage.
- **Steroids:** Long-term steroid usage (such as prednisone, dexamethasone, triamcinolone) can have an effect on liver tissue.

What Is the Vaccination Status of the Patient?

Both adenovirus and leptospirosis can cause an infectious hepatitis. Determining vaccine status can help the medical team determine if the pet is at more risk due to a lapse in vaccination.

Have There Been Any Neurologic Signs or Disorders

Have there been any seizures, acting blind, changes in vocalization, etc., especially associated with eating? Because of limited detoxification of toxins and microbes associated with liver disease, neurologic symptoms can occur as a sharp increase in bloodborne toxins affect the central nervous system (hepatic encephalopathy; see below).

Has Your Pet Traveled in the Last 3–6 Months?

There are specific gastrointestinal parasites (i.e., flukes) that can migrate to the liver and destroy normal tissue. If there has been an extended travel history, the medical team should be informed to research any possible regional disease that could produce liver dysfunction.

Obtaining an Initial Assessment on a Patient with Hepatic Disease

As with renal disease, liver disease may not be easily diagnosed with physical examination. Pets may show just generic symptoms of weight loss, anorexia, vomiting, and or diarrhea. Specific signs such as **jaundice** and **ascites** may help indicate a hepatic dysfunction; however, these symptoms can also suggest other disease problems. Furthermore, there can be significant liver disease without jaundice or ascites. Some important observations to evaluate on the initial assessment follow.

- **Hydration:** Animals with an acute liver dysfunction can be extremely dehydrated due to the buildup to toxins producing dehydration and anorexia.
- **Poor, unkempt hair coat/distended pendulous abdomen:** The decreased production of proteins and other metabolic needs associated with chronic liver disease can chronically produce a poor hair coat, large distended abdomen from potential ascites, and abdominal muscle breakdown (see Figure 14.6).
- **Jaundice:** Yellowing of the mucous membranes or ear pinna (see above).
- **Bruising:** Obvious evidence of bruising on the abdomen or other parts of the body can suggest a problem with the animal's ability to clot blood. Small pinpoint hemorrhages are called **petechiation.** Large more geographic hemorrhages are called **ecchymosis** (see Figure 14.7).

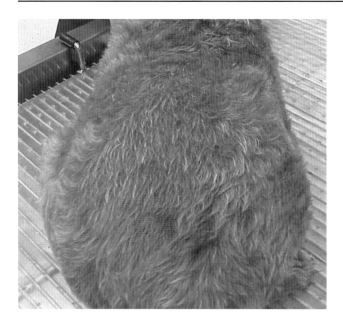

Figure 14.6. Schnauzer with a poor, unkempt hair coat and distended abdomen, possibly suggestive of liver disease.

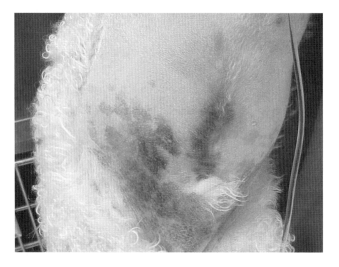

Figure 14.7. Spontaneous ecchymosis from an acute coagulopathy on the ventral abdomen.

Although pets can have severe hepatic disease and be stable, the following parameters should be monitored to help distinguish if the pet is in a life-threatening condition (see Table 14.1).

Hepatic Clinical Diagnostics

Because there are many potential forms of liver disease, blood work can be normal and there can still be significant disease. Blood work serves as a useful tool but must also be assessed along with history, physical examination, and other diagnostic aids. Some clinical diagnostics are discussed next.

Table 14.1. Triage concerns in the cardiology patient.

Systems	Trouble Signs That Indicate an Emergency Situation
Mentation	Nonresponsive/comatose/seizures
Fever	Hypothermia: Temperatures <99° (secondary to severe metabolic upset)
	Possible fever: Temperature >102° (secondary to infectious liver disease, i.e., bacterial hepatitis)
Hydration	Severe dehydration >5–7%
Gum color	Jaundice
Capillary refill time	CRT >2–3 seconds
Integument (skin)	Spontaneous bruising
Heart rate/pulse	Rate: Heart rates <80 bpm or >180–200 bpm
	Pulse: Change in pulse quality secondary to seizure and shock

Complete Blood Count
Red Blood Cells
- With chronic wasting disease, low red blood cell count may be present (**anemia**).
- Anemia is secondary to the lack of precursors for cellular material; with liver disease, the body does not have enough material to produce cellular components.
- Also, chronic liver disease can produce animals that are more prone to bleeding and hence there may be chronic blood loss and anemia.
  — Usually this type of bleeding problem is associated with lower total protein and lower platelet counts.
  — The animal should be carefully assessed for bruising.

White Blood Cells and Platelets
With infectious processes, elevation in white blood cells may be observed.

With certain forms of cancer (i.e., hepatic lymphoma), white blood cell elevations can be severe. White blood cells can have an extremely abnormal cytology, and populations can be very high. A blood smear is always suggested with sick animals to better assess cell morphology (red blood cells and white blood cells; see Chapter 21) as well as platelet numbers. With animals with coagulopathy, platelets counts are low.

Chemistry
Blood work on a routine chemistry panel can be extremely variable with chronic liver disease, portal-caval shunts, and neoplasia. *It is important to understand the difference between clinical diagnostics that assess liver damage and those that assess liver function.*

In acute liver disease with significant damage to liver cells, the internal enzymes with the hepatocytes leak out and increase dramatically in the bloodstream. *This suggests acute liver damage.*

However, with chronic disease, where only small

amounts of the liver may be affected day to day, the internal enzymes may be normal or low. In these cases, the veterinarian must assess clinical diagnostics that indicate liver function. These are chemicals that are produced by the liver normally. Chronic disease impairs liver function.

Indicators of Liver Damage

These enzymes increase in the bloodstream as normal hepatocytes are damaged acutely. These enzymes suggest an acute or ongoing large-scale injury to the liver.

Alanine Aminotransferase

Alanine aminotransferase (ALT or SGPT) is an intrahepatic enzyme that is responsible for the conversion of 2-oxoglutarate to pyruvate and glutamate. Increased levels of the enzyme in the blood occur when there are alterations in the lipid membrane of the hepatocytes, secondary to injury, inflammation, or infection within the liver. ALT can also be elevated secondary to

- trauma (i.e., hit by car),
- anticonvulsants (i.e., phenobarbital), and
- steroids.

Aspartate Aminotransferase

Aspartate aminotransferase (AST or SGOT) is an intracellular enzyme in all cells, but is predominantly in larger concentration in muscle and liver cells. AST can be elevated in muscle disease or disease that affects muscle acutely, such as

- trauma, and
- seizure.

AST is also present in red blood cells, thus massive red blood cell destruction (immune-mediated hemolytic anemia) can also increase AST levels.

Alkaline Phosphatase

Alkaline phosphatase refers to a large number of intracellular enzymes that are present within the liver, intestine, bone, kidneys, and placenta. *On most chemistry panels, alkaline phosphatase levels represent all alkaline phosphatase sources of the body.* The liver form has high levels within the hepatocytes and the canniculi. It is a very helpful indicator of bile stasis or gall bladder obstruction and can also be seen with liver disease and other hormonal diseases (i.e., hyperadrenocorticism; see Chapter 27).

Gamma-Glutamyl Transferase

Gamma-glutamyl transferase (GGT) is an intracellular enzyme responsible for clearing a specific chemical group from a larger molecule. All cells contain GGT; however, renal epithelial, bile duct, and hepatic cells contain the highest activity. Elevations can be represented with decreased bile flow (cholestasis), especially in felines. GGT is more of a liver enzyme indicator in large animals.

Indicators of Liver Function

These chemicals are normally produced by the liver. As the liver becomes damaged, production of these enzymes can be altered. Although alterations in liver function can occur with acute disease, these indicators are very important in differentiating chronic liver dysfunction where liver enzymes can be normal.

Total Protein/Albumin

The liver produces albumin, which is a small protein used for carrying other compounds and minerals throughout the blood. Decreases in albumin can represent a **functional** problem with the liver. Decreases in albumin can suggest liver disease; however, decreased albumin can also be seen with

- internal bleeding,
- hormonal disease,
- renal disease—glomerular disease,
- intestinal disease, and
- certain types of cancer.

Blood Urea Nitrogen

The liver unites two ammonia molecules together to form blood urea nitrogen (BUN). This toxin is then removed from

---

Discussing Clinical Diagnostics with the Client

- The doctor has recommended general blood work to determine if there is liver damage, suggestions of liver dysfunction, or other changes in the body to suggest infection, inflammation, or other organ disease.
- The basic blood work evaluates the level of intracellular liver enzymes in the bloodstream. The more cellular liver damage in an acute disease process, the higher these enzymes levels register. With acute disease, these values can change significantly because of acute damage to liver tissue.
- In chronic disease, in which only small amounts of the liver are affected day to day, the internal liver enzymes may be low to normal. However, the chronic damage may have greatly affected the overall function of the liver. To better evaluate if the liver is functioning normally, the doctor may suggest liver function tests.
- One common liver function test is **paired bile acids.** Bile acids are normally produced by the liver to help emulsify fat in the diet. Once secreted and used, they are readily absorbed by the liver. This test evaluates the animal's ability to secrete and reabsorb bile acids in a fasted animal. Pets with chronic liver disease will have mildly high bile acids prior to feeding and exceedingly high bile acids 1–2 hours after a meal. This observation suggests liver dysfunction and potential serious disease.

the body through the kidneys. With decreased liver function, BUN levels can be low.

Bilirubin

The normal liver deactivates this toxin produced from red blood cell destruction and pushes it into the intestinal system through the bile ducts and gall bladder. With certain forms of liver disease or gall bladder disease, the pigment is not properly deactivated by the liver and builds up in the bloodstream and the tissue. Elevations of total bilirubin can suggest **functional liver disease**. However, disease that causes massive destruction of the red blood cells can also raise bilirubin levels.

Bile Acids

As described earlier, bile acids are secreted to help emulsify fat when an animal eats. In liver disease, bile acids are not properly reabsorbed. Clinically, to test for bile acids, an animal is fasted for 12 hours, then a baseline level of bile acids is drawn. The animal is then fed, and 2 hours later another level is collected. In normal animals, the acid level in the fasted sample is very low, and the postprandial sample is only slightly more elevated because a normal liver reabsorbs the bile acids quickly. In an animal with liver dysfunction, prefeeding (**preprandial**) bile acids are high and postfeeding (**postprandial**) bile acids are even higher.

Radiology

As with renal disease, changes in liver size can be suggestive of disease. **Hepatomegally** refers to generalized liver enlargement, which can suggest acute disease, abscess, or possibly cancer (see Figure 14.8). Smaller livers can suggest chronic liver disease or a portal-caval shunt. Finally, gall bladder stones (**choleliths**) are small, radio-dense stones near or within the liver parenchyma. Often these stones are unobstructive and can be happenstance findings.

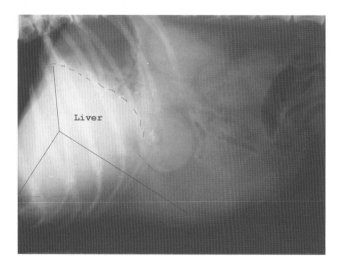

Figure 14.8. X-ray showing a liver extending beyond the edge of the rib cage. This suggests pathologic enlargement or hepatomegally.

Ultrasound

Abdominal ultrasounds can suggest changes within the internal tissue of the liver. Focal masses, focal abscesses, and diffuse disease can be visualized. Ultrasound cannot diagnose the type of liver disease but can define how much of the liver is affected and if the disease is focal (i.e., a mass) or diffuse (see Figure 14.9). Ultrasound-guided biopsy fine-needle aspirate can be very helpful and may be necessary in diagnosis of the type of disease.

Exploratory/Laparoscopic Surgery

On occasion, the abdomen does need to be explored and larger wedge tissue biopsies or liver lobe removal may be needed.

Discussing Imaging and Biopsy Diagnostics with the Client

- An **abdominal radiograph** will help the veterinarian assess the liver region for changes in liver size and liver margins suggestive of acute or chronic disease. Furthermore, the veterinarian can assess for the presence of gall bladder stones (cholelithiasis).

- An **abdominal ultrasound** will allow the veterinarian to assess the internal architecture of the liver tissue to differentiate the difference between focal disease (i.e., tumor, abscess, or nodule) and diffuse disease. Also, the gall bladder, the bile ducts, and gall bladder wall can be imaged for changes secondary to disease. The ultrasound cannot diagnose the type of liver disease, but it can help obtain fine-needle aspirates or core samples to help the veterinarian obtain a diagnosis.

- **Exploratory/laparoscopic procedures** may be needed. On occasion, when larger samples of the liver are needed for diagnosis or when a mass is detected, an exploratory surgery may be recommended. Under anesthesia and through an abdominal incision, the abdomen is explored and tissue for biopsy taken.

Diseases of the Hepatic System

Although not all diseases are mentioned below, the common diseases are discussed. The main goal of this section is to understand and be able to explain to the client what the diseases are, how they can present themselves, and what can be the overall short- and long-term concerns of each disease. Any discussion of overall diagnostic and treatment protocols should be discussed based on the recommendations of the doctor and the medical team. Please use the following information as a basis to discuss and educate the client, *but never to diagnose a patient.*

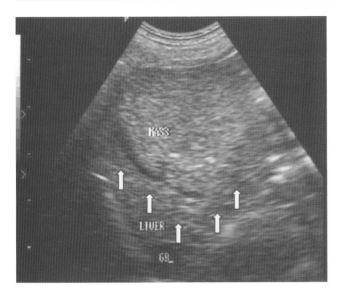

Figure 14.9. Liver (outlined by line) with a focal mass evident within the tissue (outlined by white arrows).

Acute Liver Disease

Acute (rapid) liver disease occurs because of a sudden loss of liver function due to a severe metabolic, toxic, or infectious cause. The disease comes on rapidly and makes the pet very ill.

Etiology

Acute hepatic disease is caused by sudden injury to the cells of the liver. The disease tends to affect dogs more than cats. There are no breed or sex predilections. Acute hepatic disease can be caused by the following:

- **Shock:** Any pet that becomes unable to maintain the demands placed on its body enters a shocky state. Altered blood flow, toxins and/or increased bacterial toxins associated with shock can produce an acute liver disease. Some examples of types of shock that can produce secondary liver disease are heat stroke or massive bacterial infection (sepsis) (see Chapter 30).
- **Obstruction:** Patients can become acutely ill from primary obstruction of the bile ducts and gall bladder. The obstruction causes a backflow of bile toxins back into the blood, causing an acute depression and illness. Obstruction can occur secondary to severe pancreatitis (see Chapter 15), cancer or tumors of the bile ducts, and gall stones (rare).
- **Infectious agents:** Infectious agents (i.e., infectious hepatitis virus or leptospirosis), can cause a massive infection and inflammation of the liver, producing an acute disease/failure syndrome.
- **Drugs/toxins:** Overdose or reaction to ingested drugs and toxins can cause acute liver damage and cell death (**necrosis**). Examples of types of toxins and drug over-

doses that can cause these reactions are anticonvulsants (i.e., phenobarbital), NSAIDS, antimicrobials (i.e., tetracyclines), specific types of mushrooms, heavy metals, and other toxins.

Signalment

Acute liver disease can affect animals of any species, breed, or sex.

Common Points in Medical History

With these syndromes, the patient's hepatic function is acutely impaired, producing an inability to detoxify chemicals and microbes and exposing the body to a high level of toxins. This produces an acutely ill, profoundly affected animal. Common medical complaints in this condition are

- vomiting,
- anorexia,
- profound depression,
- diarrhea, and
- possible neurological signs, such as
  — seizure,
  — coma,
  — dementia, and
  — blindness.

Common Points on Initial Assessment

These affected pets can be severely ill and depressed from the increased toxin load. However, since this disease has affected these animals so acutely, their body condition and weight are usually normal. Key points on the initial assessment are presented next.

- **Jaundice:** Yellowing of the mucous membranes (i.e., gums, rectum, penis, whites of the eye) or skin can suggest an acute buildup of toxins in the bloodstream that is secondarily building up in the tissue.
- **Hydration:** Pets can be moderate to life-threateningly dehydrated.
- **Mentation:** The pet may be acutely depressed to severely comatose.
- **Neurologic symptoms:** Some pets may have grand mal seizures, act blind, comatose, and have altered vocal and behavior patterns.

Complications

If acute hepatic disease is not diagnosed and treated, the patient may develop acute life-threatening dehydration, profound neurologic depression, bleeding problems, shock, and death.

Clinical Diagnostics

Since acute liver disease and failure can be caused by many possible diseases and syndromes, a thorough workup involving blood and urine diagnostics, abdominal imaging, and liver fine-needle aspirate/surgical biopsy may be recommended.

Treatment

Treatment is focused on providing fluid support, diuresis, and reducing toxin and microbial lode in the patient. Treatment protocols may include the following.

- **Fluids:** Fluid therapy is used to help rehydrate the pet while diluting the toxins within the body (**diuresis**).
- **Antibiotics:** Antibiotics are often used to help the body reduce the increased bacterial load absorbed from the small intestine, which the liver normally detoxifies.
- **Antiemetics:** Drugs that help decrease vomiting and nausea caused by secondary upsets to the gastrointestinal tract are often used.
- **Stomach acid blockers:** These drugs help decrease stomach acidity and decrease nausea.
- **Lactulose:** This drug helps decrease ammonia in the small intestinal system, which would normally be absorbed and detoxified by the liver.
- **Fresh whole blood or plasma:** Infusions may need to be given to help transfuse blood-clotting factors normally produced by the liver.

Discussing Acute Hepatic Disease with the Client
- Acute liver disease is a severe disease with sudden onset caused by many possible bacterial, toxic, obstructive, or systemic diseases.
- The syndrome causes an inability of the liver to detoxify chemical and bacterial toxins from the body.
- The resulting rapid buildup can make the pet very ill, dehydrated, and nauseous.
- The overall prognosis is dependent on what has caused the hepatic disease. However, if severe enough, the pet can have problems clotting blood and may begin to bleed spontaneously. This carries an extremely poor prognosis.
- Most animals will require hospitalization, intensive fluid therapy, and medications to begin treating the acute liver syndrome.

Prevention

To help prevent acute renal disease, the patient's exposure to potential toxins and poisons should be limited, and the animal should be regularly vaccinated for adenovirus and leptospirosis (in endemic areas).

Chronic Active Hepatitis

Chronic active liver disease occurs secondary to a slowly progressive buildup of fibrosis and inflammation within the liver tissue at the microscopic level. The disease can have acute flare-ups because the liver can have decreased ability to detoxify poisons and chemicals.

Etiology

Chronic liver disease is caused by many possible factors.

- **Infectious agents:** Infectious hepatitis virus (adenovirus) can cause chronic liver disease.
- **Drugs:** Chronic exposure to long-term anticonvulsants (i.e., phenobarbital), steroids, and antimicrobials can produce chronic damage of the liver.
- **Toxins:** Chronic exposure to heavy metals (such as copper) can lead to a chronic inflammation and damage to the liver.
- **Immune-mediated causes:** In these cases, the immune system attacks the liver due to chronic inflammation and disease. The white blood cells respond by entering and going through healthy liver tissue to the inflamed and infected sites. Over time, this can produce severe inflammation and fibrosis through the entire liver.

Signalment

Chronic active hepatitis is a common syndrome in the older dog. The disease tends to affect dogs more than cats, with females being more affected. The mean age of onset is 6 years old. Common breeds affected are Bedlington terrier, Doberman pinscher, cocker spaniel, Labrador retriever.

Common Points on Medical History

This disease can be slow and insidious on progression. Medical complaints can vary depending on how much of the liver is affected and how long the patient has dealt with the chronic buildup of toxins. *If the damage has been done slowly, animals may appear asymptomatic with severe liver impairment.* Some common medical complaints can be

- chronic weight loss, sometimes severe, with animals losing 30–40% of original weight;
- increased thirst and urination;
- chronic vomiting; and
- decreased appetite.

Common Points on Initial Assessment

These patients can show very few physical symptoms because they have adapted to the chronic disease. However, other pets may have acute episodes, such as blood toxins becoming too high to tolerate. The following symptoms may be evident on initial assessment:

- Dehydration
- Jaundice
- Fluid accumulations in the abdomen (ascites*)*
- Weight loss/poor body condition
- Diarrhea/constipation
- Neurologic signs: seizure, acute blindness, changes in behavior

Clinical Diagnostics

Because chronic liver disease can be caused by several diseases, a thorough clinical diagnostic workup, including blood work, urinalysis, abdominal imaging and hepatic biopsy, may be recommended.

Treatment

Treatment is focused on providing fluid support, diuresis, and reducing toxin and microbial load in the patient. Treatment protocols may include the following.

- **Fluids:** Fluid therapy is used to help rehydrate the pet while diluting the toxins within the body (diuresis).
- **Lactulose:** This drug helps to decrease ammonia in the small intestinal system that would normally be absorbed and detoxified by the liver.
- **Antibiotics:** Antibiotics are often used to help the body reduce the increased bacterial lode absorbed from the small intestine that the liver normally detoxifies.
- **L-Adenosyl methionine (SAM-E):** This is a nutrient supplement that helps reduce hepatic inflammation and toxic injury to hepatocytes.
- **Immunosuppressant drugs:** This drug category is used in different forms of inflammatory liver disease to help decrease the inflammatory response of the body and decrease white blood cell invasion of the liver.
- **Urosidiol:** This drug helps deactivate toxic bile acids produced by the liver into a less dangerous form.

Prevention

There is no way to prevent chronic hepatic disease. Routine blood and urine diagnostics in older animals and breeds that are more sensitive to liver disease can help diagnose and treat liver disease, potentially increasing the patient's quality of life.

Discussing Chronic Hepatic Disease with the Client

- Chronic liver disease is a slowly progressing and damaging disease. The syndrome causes an inability of the liver to detoxify the body, causing a massive buildup of toxins and microbes.
- Animals can have sudden acute episodes as the pet becomes overwhelmed with chemicals and bacteria that are normally detoxified by the liver.
- Physical symptoms are chronic weight and muscle mass loss, poor hair coat, increased thirst and urination, and potentially a yellowing of the skin, gums, and whites of the eyes (jaundice).
- Diagnosis of liver disease may require general blood work, urinalysis, abdominal imaging, and biopsy. *Routine liver enzymes may be normal since the destruction to normal liver tissue is a slow process taking months to years.*
- The overall prognosis depends on what has caused the hepatic disease. However, if severe enough, the pet can have problems clotting blood and may begin to bleed spontaneously. This carries an extremely poor prognosis.
- Most animals will require hospitalization, intensive fluid therapy, and medications to begin treating the acute flare-ups of the chronic liver syndrome.

Congenital Porto-Systemic Shunt

In the congenital porto-systemic shunt (PSS, or porto-caval shunt) disease process, toxins that are normally metabolized by the liver, bypass the organ and go directly into the general circulation and central nervous system, causing severe metabolic and neurologic reactions. It is important to note the PSS can be an acquired disease secondary to chronic liver disease. The congenital form will be discussed.

Etiology

As animals with PSS are developing in utero, the pet's blood is detoxified by the maternal liver. Because the animal's liver is not needed to detoxify blood coming in from its portal system, a small vessel, called the **ductus venosus,** connects the portal vein to the caudal vena cava bypassing the liver (see Figure 14.10).

Normally, this vessel closes down shortly after birth. In patients affected by porto-caval shunts, the vessel remains open and takes blood from the intestinal tract around the liver and sends it directly into systemic circulation. This blood is full of bacterial and chemical toxins that are normally inactivated by the liver. These toxins enter the central nervous system and begin causing neurologic signs.

Signalment

PSS is more common in dogs than in cats. Congenital shunts are seen in animals between 6–24 months of age. There is no sexual predilection for this disease. Breeds that are more susceptible to porto-caval shunts are Yorkshire terriers and miniature schnauzers.

Common Points in Medical History

With congenital PSS, most affected animals seem small and do not grow well. These pets tend to have poor body scores and poor hair coats because of decreased liver production of necessary proteins and amino acids. Other common medical complaints are generally associated with hepatic encephalopathy and seen more often 20 minutes after the pet is fed. These complaints include

- drooling (especially in cats),
- behavior changes,
- visual deficits (blindness),
- circling,
- seizures,
- head pressing, and
- comas.

Common Points on Initial Assessment

Often these pets can present during or after a seizure episode. The pet may seem small for its age with a poor or immature hair coat and poor muscle development.

Complications

If not diagnosed and treated, animals affected with PSS will continue to be chronic poor doers with worsening neurologic signs.

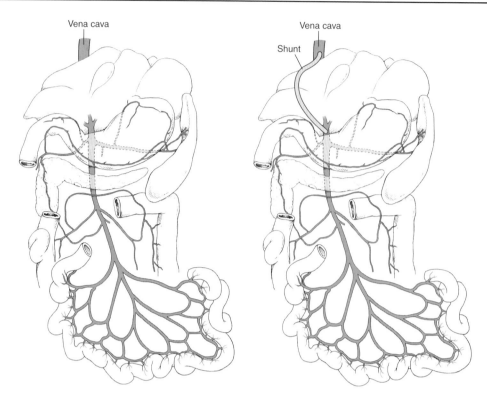

Figure 14.10. The illustration on the left shows normal blood flow from the portal vein into the liver. The image on the right illustrates what compromises a shunt, in which the majority of blood moves around the liver and into the vena cava from the portal vein.

Diagnosis

A workup for possible PSS can include blood work (especially bile acids), urinalysis, and advanced abdominal imaging.

Treatment

Treatment is based on the location of the shunt (intrahepatic versus extrahepatic) and the severity of the disease noted. Treatment options can include the following.

- **Intravenous fluids/hospitalization:** With severely affected animals, the patient may require hospitalization, monitoring, intravenous fluids, and diagnostics to monitor the pet.
- **Medications:** Medications depend on the signs with which the pet presents and can be focused on decreasing the amount of ammonia produced from the intestinal digestion, helping decrease bacteria and bacterial toxins within the intestine, and preventing or treating systemic disease.
- **Diet:** Diet can aid in decreasing the amounts of ammonia and fat the liver has to deal with, thus decreasing the toxin load.
- **Surgery:** Especially with extrahepatic shunts, the goal of surgery is to carefully close down the shunt and redirect blood flow back to the liver. Care must be taken to slowly redirect blood flow so as not to produce liver hypertension. On occasion, multiple surgeries or specialized sur-

gical implants are used to slowly reduce blood flow through a shunt over time.

Prevention

There is no way to prevent PSS.

Discussing Porto-Systemic Shunt with the Client
- A porto-systemic shunt is typically a congenital abnormality in which a small congenital vessel shifts incoming blood from the intestines around the liver and into general circulation.
- In affected pets, the chemical- and microbe-laden blood from the intestines does not go through the liver to be detoxified.
- The toxins enter the general circulation and have a direct effect on the body and central nervous system.
- These pets start out as smaller poor doers because their liver production has been so severely affected. Furthermore, these pets may show neurologic signs, such as seizures, blindness, and attitude change because the toxins directly affect the central nervous system. These signs are closely associated after feeding due to the inflow of increased toxins from the intestine.

Hepatic Lipidosis

Hepatic lipidosis is a severe metabolic disease of the liver, mainly affecting cats, in which the liver becomes infiltrated with large amounts of body fat, shutting down the liver, and leading to a buildup of hepatic toxins in the bloodstream.

Etiology

Hepatic lipidosis is a massive shunting of fat into the liver that is so severe that the liver is unable to function on a microscopic level (see Figure 14.11). Hepatic lipidosis can be a primary problem or secondary to some other disease entity. *The primary causative factor is anorexia (not eating), causing a massive mobilization of fat to the liver. In cats this can occur with as little as 2 days of anorexia.* This can be caused by

- stress and changes in the environment,
- intestinal disease (inflammatory bowel disease; see Chapter 10), and
- other organ and infectious diseases that produce a sustained anorexia.

Signalment

The disease affects cats from 1 to 16 years of age (mean age of 8 years). Obesity can be a predisposing factor. This possibly can occur more frequently in female cats.

Common Points on Medical History

These pets present with a history of massive short-term weight loss (i.e., 3–4 pounds in 2–3 weeks in a 16-pound cat), anorexia, depression, and possible neurologic symptoms (i.e., seizures).

Common Points on Initial Assessment

Pets present acutely depressed, weak, and dehydrated. Other clinical signs of the disease are

- not eating (can be as little as 2–3 days),
- jaundice (yellowing of gums, whites of eyes, skin, etc.),
- vomiting,
- loss of muscle mass,
- neurologic disease (acting blind, seizuring, head pressing, circling).

Complications

If not diagnosed and treated, these patients can enter acute liver disease and failure, which can be life threatening.

Diagnosis

A workup for possible hepatic lipidosis shunt can include blood work, urinalysis, advanced abdominal imaging, and possible liver biopsy.

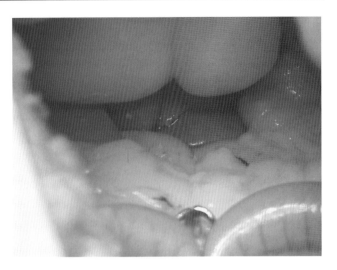

Figure 14.11. Liver affected by the hepatic lipidosis. Note the mottled appearance of the liver and the large amounts of fat evident in the abdomen.

Treatment

Treatment for this disease is focused on the following.

- **Treating the underlying disease:** The veterinarian may suggest further clinical diagnostics (i.e., liver and intestinal biopsy) to help diagnose a primary disorder.
- **Fluid therapy:** Fluid therapy (usually intravenous fluids) is recommended to help rehydrate and diurese the patient.
- **Antibiotics:** Antibiotics may be used if there is a suspicion of infection. Also, they can help the liver deactivate bacterial pathogens normally destroyed by liver action.
- **Lactulose:** Lactulose is a drug that aids in breaking down ammonia buildup in the intestine. The liver normally breaks down the ammonia.
- **Diet and feeding tubes:** The most important treatment is to keep the patient eating so that eventually the liver can metabolize the fat and remove it from the affected tissue. To maintain adequate energy needed, the veterinarian may suggest a **long-term feeding tube (i.e., stomach tube)**. This will allow the medical team or the client to feed the pet daily while the patient may be too sick to want to eat. These tubes can stay in for months if needed.

Prevention

Keeping cats within normal weight recommendations and preventing obesity can decrease the concerns of hepatic lipidosis.

Discussing Hepatic Lipidosis with the Client

- Hepatic lipidosis is a metabolic disease in the cat in which large amounts of fat are shunted into the liver in response to a stress or an underlying systemic disease.
- The normal response to decreasing blood sugar is to move fat into the liver to be modified into sugar. With hepatic lipidosis, large amounts of fat move into the liver, completely infiltrate the tissue, and shut down the liver.
- The disease occurs secondary to other organ and intestinal disease that produces anorexia in the pet for more then 2 days.
- Once the liver is completely infiltrated with fat, it looses the ability to detoxify chemicals and microbes in the body, and the pet becomes very ill, dehydrated, nauseous, and jaundiced.
- Obese animals are more predisposed to hepatic lipidosis than leaner pets.

CD-ROM 1 reviews material presented in this chapter. Please try the cases for Section 2 (Anatomy and Physiology— The Science behind the Diseases) *to help reinforce the information presented here.*

Chapter 15

Exocrine and Endocrine Pancreas

The pancreas is a white/pink organ separated into two distinct lobes. The right lobe lies parallel to a section of the duodenum extending from the middle part of the right kidney to the pyloric region of the stomach. The left lobe lies parallel to the greater curvature of the stomach (perpendicular to the duodenum) (see Figure 15.1).

The pancreas has two ducts that empty liver and pancreatic contents into the duodenum. Both ducts enter the duodenum through a small opening called the **duodenal papilla.** The ducts are the **accessory pancreatic duct,** the main duct of the pancreas (dog), and the **pancreatic duct,** a smaller, less-evident duct that is sometimes absent in the dog.

The pancreas works both as an exocrine and endocrine organ. **Exocrine glands** discharge their secretions outwardly through a duct. Their secretions control many important body functions (i.e., salivary glands, sweat glands, mammary glands, etc.). The exocrine pancreas secretes the digestive enzymes **lipase** and **amylase** through the pancreatic duct into the duodenum to aid in the breakdown of foodstuffs. Amylase breaks large sugar molecules into smaller single-unit sugars. Lipase helps breaks down fat into free fatty acids and triglycerides for absorption by the intestine. Lipase and amylase are produced in response to ingestion of food and water and increased production of hydrochloric acid by the stomach. Both enzymes are critical to the digestive process.

Endocrine glands secrete hormones or other chemicals directly into the bloodstream and influence metabolism and other body processes (i.e., pituitary, thyroid, sex organs, etc.). The pancreas produces insulin and glucagon, which help maintain normal blood sugar levels. Insulin and glucagon are produced by specialized cells within a region of the pancreas called the **islets of Langerhans** (see Figure 15.2).

Exocrine Disease of the Pancreas

Acute or chronic inflammatory condition of the pancreas (**pancreatitis**) causes leakage of pancreatic enzymes to the pancreas and surrounding tissue. This produces an inflammatory change so severe that the pancreas can become secondarily infected, producing abcessation. Furthermore, inflammation can obstruct the common bile duct, producing gall bladder obstruction and secondary liver disease. The inflammation and secondary infection can be severe enough to produce systemic inflammation affecting the liver and the kidney and possibly producing a severe whole-body infection (**sepsis**). As discussed below, pancreatitis can produce acutely ill patients with severe vomiting, diarrhea, and anorexia due to the severity of the systemic inflammation and possible infection.

Exocrine exhaustion (exocrine pancreatic insufficiency, or EPI) occurs when the pancreatic cells are unable to produce normal lipase and amylase enzyme levels because of congenital disease or damage secondary to inflammation and infection (see Figure 15.3).

These pets cannot digest food properly and a maldigestion/malabsorption syndrome results. Physical symptoms of EPI include severe small bowel diarrhea (see Chapter 10), weight loss, and abnormal voracious appetite. There are two forms of the disease.

- **Primary disease:** This **juvenile idiopathic** form is a congenital disease that occurs in young dogs from a lack of sufficient production of lipase and amylase in the pancreas. The cause of the disease is unknown.
- **Secondary disease:** A condition secondary to chronic relapsing pancreatitis produces massive scarring and loss of normal pancreatic tissue.

Lastly, **pancreatic cancer (adenoma/adenocarcinoma)** can be destructive to normal tissue, causing inflammation, necrosis, and changes in pancreatic function. Symptoms tend to mimic an acute severe pancreatitis but may be more chronic and longer in duration. Typical types of pancreatic tumors are pancreatic adenoma and adenocarcinoma.

Obtaining a History for Exocrine Disease of the Pancreas

As with other organ syndromes, diseases of the exocrine pancreas have specific questions to ask to help the medical team delineate if pancreatic disease may be evident.

What Is the Age of the Animal?

In general EPI is seen in younger animals. Pancreatitis can occur in middle-aged to older animals.

Is There Breed Specificity?

Specific breeds can be more predisposed to pancreatic exocrine disease. These breeds are as follows.

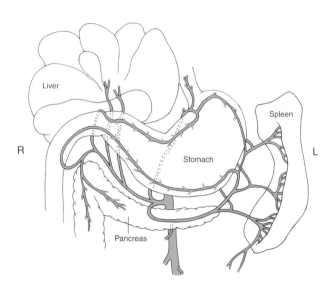

Figure 15.1. Illustration of normal pancreas, stomach, liver, and spleen.

- For EPI, German shepherds are more predisposed.
- For pancreatitis, breeds of concerns are
  — miniature schnauzer
  — miniature pinscher
  — cocker spaniel
  — Siamese cat

Is There a Previous History of Disease?

Animals with a history of pancreatitis can have reoccurrences even when on controlled bland diets. The resulting episodes of pancreatitis can be much more severe.

What Has the Animal's Body Condition Been in the Last Few Months to Years?

- **Has the pet been chronically thin?** With EPI, there is improper digestion of food because of **malabsorption/ maldigestion**. The animal cannot maintain body weight and is very thin.
- **Has the pet been chronically obese?** Obesity can make the animal more predisposed to pancreatitis.

Is There Diarrhea and What Type of Diarrhea Is Present?

- Small bowel diarrhea (cow patty) suggests EPI because the pet cannot absorb nutrients through the small intestine.
- Colitis and/or small bowel diarrhea is caused by generalized inflammation. The inflammation can affect either the large or small bowel.

How Is the Pet's Appetite?

With EPI the animal cannot eat enough (polyphagia). These animals are ravenous because they cannot absorb enough nutrients. These pets may also try to eat abnormal or unusual things (i.e., their own feces, rocks, bones, etc.). With **pancreatitis** animals have decreased to no appetite due to vomiting and nausea.

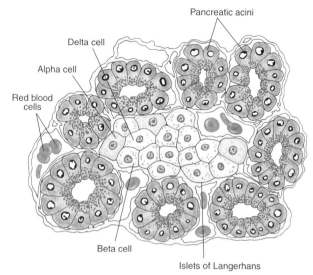

Figure 15.2. The pancreatic acini are responsible for producing digestive enzymes that empty into their central lumen and empty into the intestinal systems via the pancreatic ducts (exocrine functions). The islet of Langerhans cells are responsible for producing insulin and other hormones that enter the bloodstream and control blood sugar in the body (endocrine glands).

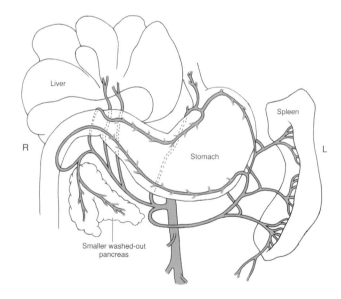

Figure 15.3. Image of an exhausted pancreatic region. Note the smaller, scarred pancreatic tissue.

Is the Animal a Chronic Vomiter?

With pancreatitis, pets can vomit due to inflammation and toxin buildup.

Does the Pet's Diet Change Rapidly or Does the Pet Get into Abnormal Things?

Animals that have rapid changes in diets or eat table food or trash are much more prone to inflammation in the pancreas, setting up pancreatitis.

Initial Assessment of Pets with Exocrine Disease of the Pancreas

Most animals with pancreatic disease can show mild to severe signs. Signs vary dramatically depending on whether they have EPI or pancreatitis. Key elements to observe in the initial assessment of these syndromes are as follows:

- **EPI:** These animals are suffering from a severe malabsorption/maldigestion syndrome. The pets are usually bright, alert, and responsive; however, the body condition is usually severely thin to skeletal. Their hair coat is poor, with dry skin evident due to decreased nutrient uptake. The pet will have decreased muscle as it converts muscle protein into energy. Finally, these pets will have a profuse cow patty diarrhea.
- **Pancreatitis:** These animals tend to be quiet, alert, and range from responsive to depressed. Patients can have normal to extremely painful abdomens, which are sensitive to palpation. Depending on the amounts of vomiting and diarrhea present, pets can be mildly to severely dehydrated. Furthermore, if there is obstruction of the pancreatic and gall bladder ducts secondary to inflammation and swelling, jaundice may be present.
- **Pancreatic tumors:** Tumors in the pancreas can closely mimic pancreatitis. Patients may have symptoms of chronic vomiting and diarrhea, abdominal tenderness, dehydration, and depression.

Although pets with exocrine pancreatic disease can be stable (i.e., EPI), the following parameters should be monitored to help distinguish if the pet is in a life-threatening condition, especially with a severe pancreatitis (see Table 15.1).

Exocrine Pancreatic Clinical Diagnostics

As with liver disease, blood work is a large part of the diagnostic protocol; however, with chronic inflammatory disease, *baseline blood work may not indicate the severity of the syndrome.* Some clinical diagnostics are discussed below.

Complete Blood Count

Changes in the complete blood count can vary depending on the disease entities and the acuteness or chronicity of the syndrome itself. For EPI, there is no overall change in complete blood count.

The blood counts for pancreatitis vary depending upon whether the disease is acute or chronic.

- **With acute disease:** The red blood cell count can be increased due to dehydration. The white blood cell count can be increased due to infection and inflammation. **Furthermore, it is important to check peripheral blood smears for immature neutrophils (bands) to detect acute inflammatory or infectious changes in the white blood cell population (see Chapter 21).**
- **With chronic disease:** The complete blood count can be normal.

Table 15.1. Triage concerns in the exocrine pancreatic patient.

Systems	Trouble Signs That Indicate an Emergency Situation
Mentation	Nonresponsive/comatose/seizures
Fever	Hypothermia: (Temperatures less than 99°) suggestive of massive shock secondary to severe pancreatitis. Fever: (Temperature >104°) secondary to infection or inflammation of the pancreas
Hydration	Severe dehydration >5–7%
Gum color	Jaundice
Capillary refill time	CRT >2–3 seconds
Abdomen	Pain, tensing or groaning on light palpation
Heart rate/pulse	Rate: Heart rates <80 bpm or >180–200 bpm Pulse: Change in pulse quality secondary to pain or shock.

In pancreatic tumors chronic (nonregenerative) anemia may be noted due to the progressive nature of the disease that consumes normal red blood cell precursors that are necessary to produce normal red blood cells (anemia of chronic disease).

Chemistry

Just as with the complete blood count, blood chemistry work can vary dramatically. With **pancreatic insufficiency,** chemistry results are generally within normal listed parameters.

The blood chemistry results for pancreatitis may vary in the canine and the feline.

- **In the canine:** Amylase and lipase can be elevated in the acute disease as the inflammation and infection of the pancreas causes leakage of the enzymes into the tissue and into the bloodstream, producing higher blood enzyme levels. In chronic disease, there can be significant pancreatic inflammation and infection, but since there is slow, progressive damage to the tissue, *blood enzyme levels can be normal.*
- **In the feline:** Lipase and amylase levels can be completely normal even with severe or chronic disease.

With pancreatic tumor, prolonged elevations of lipase and amylase can be observed due to increased production of the tumor mass within the pancreatic tissue.

Trypsin-Like Immunoassay

In the canine, a trypsin-like immunoassay (TLI) is a blood test that allows the medical team to assess the levels of trypsin, a proteolytic enzyme, in the body. Trypsin activity is directly linked to pancreatic function as follows:

- Increased TLI levels are suggestive of chronic pancreatitis or pancreatic cancer.

- Decreased TLI levels are a key diagnostic indicator of decreased pancreatic function or exocrine pancreatic insufficiency.

Discussing Clinical Diagnostics with the Client
- The doctor has recommended general blood work to evaluate if there are changes that suggest pancreatic disease, inflammation, infection, or other organ disease.
- The basic blood work evaluates the level of intracellular pancreatic enzymes in the bloodstream. The more pancreatic cellular damage in an acute disease process, the higher these enzymes levels go. In the canine with acute disease, these values can change significantly because of significant damage to pancreatic tissue.
- In chronic disease, in which only small amounts of the pancreas is affected day to day, the internal enzymes may be low to normal. However, the chronic damage may have greatly affected the overall function of the organ. To better determine if the pancreas is functioning normally, the doctor may suggest a trypsin-like immunoassay (TLI).
- A TLI is a blood test that analyzes pancreatic activation of the enzyme trypsin; thus a TLI is a pancreatic function test and helps the veterinarian delineate an inability of the pancreas to produce digestive enzyme for the intestinal tract.

Radiology
Changes in the pancreatic region are hard to appreciate with radiographs. Some diagnostic changes can be seen, such as enlargement of the pancreas due to inflammation and secondary infections.

Ultrasound
Ultrasound studies of the pancreatic region are very helpful in diagnosing pancreatic disease, abscess, or neoplasia.

Discussing Imaging and Biopsy Diagnostics with the Client
- An **abdominal radiograph** will help the veterinarian assess the pancreatic region, other organs, and intestines to suggest disease syndromes.
- An **abdominal ultrasound** will allow the veterinarian to assess the internal architecture of the pancreas and differentiate between focal disease (i.e., pancreatitis, pancreatic tumor, etc.) and diffuse disease. The ultrasound cannot diagnose the type of pancreatic disease, but it can help obtain fine-needle aspirates or core samples to help the veterinarian obtain a diagnosis.

Ultrasound-guided fine-needle aspirates are extremely helpful in differentiating the type of pancreatic disease.

Diseases of the Exocrine Pancreas

Although not all diseases of the pancreas are mentioned below, the common diseases are discussed, with the main goal being to understand and be able to explain to the client what the diseases are, how they can be present, and what can be the overall short- and long-term concerns of each disease. Any discussion of overall diagnostic and treatment protocols should be discussed based on the recommendations from the doctor and the medical team. Please use the following information to discuss the treatment and educate the client, *but never to diagnose a patient.*

Pancreatitis
When the pancreas becomes inflamed, the digestive enzymes produced from the pancreas leak out of damaged cells and begin to digest pancreatic tissue. The inflammatory change causes systemic inflammation affecting the intestine, liver, and kidneys. The secretion of digestive enzymes is stimulated by food and water or by increased gastric acid.

Etiology
There are many theories for the cause of pancreatitis; however, it has been shown to be associated with

- rapid changes in diet,
- eating garbage,
- eating unusual food (table scraps), and
- taking certain types of medications (especially steroids).

These changes produce an inflammation of the pancreatic tissue, which allows the digestive enzymes to leak out and begin autodigestion of the surrounding tissue. The inflammation that is produced can affect other organs of the body and possibly lead to pancreatic abcessation. *Pancreatitis can reoccur in an animal's life. It can become more severe, causing chronic damage and destruction to the pancreas.*

Signalment
Pancreatitis occurs in both dogs and cats. It is more common in miniature schnauzer, miniature pinscher, and cocker spaniel dog breeds and the Siamese cat breed. It is more common in females than males.

Common Points in Medical History
In acute syndromes, pets can be severely affected, producing depression and gastrointestinal signs. Chronic disease can produce a much more subtle entity, showing mild to moderate gastrointestinal signs, weight loss, anorexia, and other organ disease. Common medical complaints in this condition are, in acute disease,

- lethargy/depression,
- not eating,
- vomiting (often severe), and
- watery diarrhea (sometimes bloody).

Complaints in chronic disease are

- chronic vomiting (1–2 times per day or less),
- anorexic or a "finicky" appetite,
- decreased energy, and
- secondary diabetes mellitus.

Common Points on Initial Assessment
Physical signs on initial assessment depend on the onset and severity of disease. For acute disease, some common elements that should be focused on during the initial assessment are as follows.

- **Dehydration:** Mild to severe dehydration may be noted, depending on the amount of vomiting and diarrhea evident.
- **Tender abdomen:** More noticeable in canines, pets may tense due to pain on light palpation of the abdomen.
- **Walking hunched:** Patients with severe abdominal pain can have an altered gait—walking hunched to the point that some owners will consider this back pain.
- **Jaundice:** Yellowing of the gums, whites of the eyes, and other mucous membranes with pancreatitis suggest that there is obstruction of the gall bladder and bile ducts secondary to severe pancreatic swelling and inflammation. This is a sign of a severe pancreatitis and, if noted, should be discussed with the veterinarian immediately.

Animals with chronic pancreatitis may present without severe changes on initial assessment. The pet may have a poor body condition from chronic disease; however, other body systems may be within normal limits.

Complications
If untreated, acute pancreatitis can cause severe dehydration, infection of the abdomen (**peritonitis**), and liver and kidney disease and can be life threatening. Successive episodes of pancreatitis can result in diabetes mellitus.

Clinical Diagnostics
Since acute and chronic pancreatitis can be a very subtle disease at times, a thorough workup involving blood work and abdominal imaging may be recommended.

Treatment
Treatment of pancreatitis depends on the acuteness and severity of disease and the species of the patient.

In the canine with acute disease treatment focuses on the following.

- **Keeping food and water away from the animal—nothing per os (NPO):** Eating and drinking can cause continued production of pancreatic enzymes, making the inflammation worse. While the animal is being treated for this disease in a *hospital setting,* food and water are generally not started again until vomiting and pancreatic enzyme levels decrease.
- **Fluids:** Fluid therapy, usually in a hospital setting, is used to maintain hydration, diurese toxins and inflammatory by-products, and maintain nutrition while the pancreas is allowed to heal.
- **Drugs that decrease acid production:** Drugs such as famotidine help to decrease stomach acid, which stimulates pancreatic secretions.
- **Antibiotics:** Drugs that help treat secondary infection caused by pancreatitis may be administered.
- **Surgery:** In rare instances, with severe inflammation or abcessation of the pancreas and obstruction of common bile ducts, some animals may require surgery to transplant the common bile duct to another location within the intestine, lavage the abdomen, and drain a pancreatic abscess.

In the feline with acute disease treatment focuses on the following.

- **Force feeding:** Unlike treating canine pancreatitis, the feline patient must continue to eat a high-fiber bland diet (such as Science diet W/d, etc.) to help prevent hepatic lipidosis.
- **Fluids:** Fluid therapy, usually in a hospital setting, is used to maintain hydration, diurese toxins and inflammatory by-products, and maintain nutrition.

Discussing Pancreatitis with the Client
- The pancreas is an organ lying between the stomach and small intestine that produces digestive enzymes to help break down food and water. It secretes the digestive enzymes into the intestines by the pancreatic duct.
- When there are rapid changes in the diet, the pancreas can become inflamed, and the digestive enzymes can leak into the pancreas causing digestion of the pancreatic tissue and systemic inflammation.
- The inflamed pancreas produces severe vomiting, diarrhea, not eating, depression, and a tender abdomen.
- With severely acute disease, the inflammation can produce a massive infection and abcessation of the pancreas, liver, and/or kidney disease.
- In some cases, chronic pancreatitis can produce weight loss, poor body condition, chronic vomiting, and diabetes mellitus.
- Pancreatitis can occur with rapid changes in diet, obesity, and getting into abnormal dietary elements (i.e., trash, table food, etc.).

- **Drugs that decrease acid production:** Drugs such as famotidine help decrease stomach acid and stimulate appetite.

Prevention

The occurrence of pancreatitis can be decreased by preventing obesity in the pet, making very slow transitions in diet change, and avoiding table scraps and foods high in fat.

Exocrine Pancreatic Insufficiency

EPI is caused by a decreasing production of the digestive enzymes produced by the pancreas.

Etiology

The pancreas secretes the digestive enzymes lipase and amylase, which aid in the digestion of sugars and fats. Due to congenital disease or chronic inflammatory pancreatic disease, the pancreas loses the ability to produce the necessary digestive enzymes to break down food and water.

Signalment

The disease can affect both dogs and cats; however, it is rare in cats. In German shepherds the disease has been reported to be hereditary, affecting primarily younger dogs. The disease can also be associated with animals that have chronic pancreatitis.

Common Points in Medical History

These pets present as happy and energetic, with history of severe cow patty diarrhea (small intestine diarrhea), ravenous appetite, and an inability to maintain normal weight. Furthermore, the pet may have a history of increased flatulence as well as an aberrant appetite (i.e., eating feces, rocks, etc.).

Common Points on Initial Assessment

Affected animals are generally stable, bright, alert, and responsive. Furthermore, the symptoms on initial assessment may be as follows.

- **Body score:** The patient may be thin to emaciated with generalized poor muscle mass.
- **Gastrointestinal signs:** The patient may have chronic watery to cow patty diarrhea (not responsive to medication), severe flatulence (gas), and increased intestinal sounds (**borborgymi**).

Complications

If not diagnosed and treated, the pet will continue having profuse diarrhea, weight loss, and dietary problems.

Clinical Diagnostics

Since pancreatic exocrine insufficiency can mimic gastrointestinal and other organ disease, a thorough workup is recommended. Common clinical testing may include blood work, including TLI, fecal examination, and abdominal imaging.

Treatment

With affected pets, the addition of a powdered enzyme, called Pancreazyme, sprinkled on the food prior to feeding will begin the digestion process and replace the lipase and amylase that is not being produced.

Prevention

Preventing reoccurrences of chronic pancreatitis (see above) may help prevent progressive damage to the pancreas that may set up pancreatic exocrine insufficiency.

Discussing Exocrine Pancreatic Insufficiency with the Client

- The pancreas is an organ that lies between the stomach and small intestine that produces digestive enzymes to help break down food. It secretes the digestive enzymes into the intestines by the pancreatic duct.
- In this disease, the pancreas loses the ability to produce the digestive enzymes to break down normal dietary elements.
- Because the pet cannot properly digest and absorb food, the patient has heavy, foul-odor cow patty diarrhea, weight loss, and ravenous appetite.
- This disease can occur congenitally or secondary to severe chronic inflammatory disease of the pancreas (i.e., pancreatitis).
- Once diagnosed, the disease can be controlled by the addition of topical enzymes to the diet.

Disease of the Endocrine Pancreas

Disease entities of the endocrine pancreas focus largely on the production of insulin by the islets of Langerhans (see Figure 15.2). The islet cells of Langerhans produce two hormones in response to blood sugar.

- **Insulin** is secreted in response to increasing blood sugar to stimulate **uptake of glucose by the cells.** Without insulin present, there is no way for the cells of the body to utilize sugar. Furthermore, insulin stimulates the production of glycogen in the liver and fat deposition in the body.
- **Glucagon** is secreted in response to decreasing amounts of blood sugar to stimulate the liver to increase blood sugar levels by converting glycogen to glucose. Glucagon also breaks up fat for the production of sugar (**gluconeogenesis**).

The most common disease entity produced by the endocrine pancreas is **diabetes mellitus**, which occurs when insulin production is not sufficient to adequately control normal blood sugar levels. In the absence of insulin, the body must clear excess blood sugar by excretion through the urine.

As blood glucose increases to extremely high levels, the body metabolizes excess sugar by converting sugar to **acetone,** a ketone. Acetone is a toxin that acidifies the blood, making the pet anorexic, ill, and weak. The condition is called **ketoacidosis** and can produce a life-threatening condition. Diabetes can occur because of exhaustion of the islet cells secondary to disease, cancer, and chronic obesity. Some diseases that can cause diabetes are hyperadrenocorticism (Cushing's disease; see Chapter 16), chronic pancreatitis, hyperthyroidism (see Chapter 16), and a long-term drug therapy (i.e., progesterone, estrogens).

A less-common disease of the endocrine pancreas is a tumor of the endocrine islet of Langerhans, called an **insulinoma.** These tumors are usually benign microscopic or encapsulated tumors within the pancreatic mass that are metabolically active. These tumors can overproduce insulin, causing a severe decrease in blood sugar that continues to produce insulin even with decreased blood sugar levels. The tumors can be localized or diffuse. Due to the rare occurrence of this disease, the discussion of insulinoma will be limited to dealing with acute hypoglycemia in emergency conditions (see Chapter 30).

Obtaining a History for Endocrine Disease of the Pancreas

As with exocrine syndromes, diseases of the endocrine pancreas have specific questions to ask to help the medical team determine if pancreatic disease may be evident.

Is the Animal Young or Old?

Endocrine pancreatic diseases are typically more common in middle-aged to older animals.

Is There a Chronic History of Other Systemic Diseases?

Animals with a long-term history of pancreatitis/pancreatic abcessation and other systemic disease are at higher risk for diabetes.

Has There Been an Acute Weight Loss and Loss of Body Condition?

Body cells cannot internalize glucose without insulin, and the body responds to the cellular need by increasing fat and muscle utilization, further increasing blood sugar and producing a significant weight loss and emaciation.

How Is the Pet's Appetite?

Animals can have normal to ravenous appetites. However, **ketoacidotic** animals can have decreased to no appetite due to increasing toxins (i.e., acetone) in the bloodstream.

Is the Animal Drinking and Urinating More?

This is usually a key symptom for the beginning of diabetes. The pet consumes more water to excrete the excess sugar into the urine. As the patient drinks more, urinary output increases.

Is the Patient on Any Long-Term Oral and Injectable Medication?

Certain long-term medications (i.e., steroids, diethylstilbesterol, etc.) make the patient more prone to chronic high blood sugar (**hyperglycemia**) and predispose it to diabetes.

Initial Assessment of Pets with Endocrine Disease of the Pancreas

Physical symptoms can vary dramatically, depending on the patient's diabetes status (i.e., uncomplicated vs. ketoacidotic; see below). Key elements to observe in the initial assessment of these syndromes are presented next.

Physical Condition

Canines can be thin but have a pot-bellied appearance because of muscle wasting and fat utilization. Cats can be thin with moderate to severe weight loss. The patient's hair coat can be poor with oily skin due to inappropriate nutrient utilization.

Mentation

Animals can tend to act normally, but with ketoacidosis can be severely depressed and lethargic.

Cataracts

Diabetic animals are more prone to cataract formation due to prolonged hyperglycemia (see Figure 15.4).

Neurologic

Cats with long-term diabetes can develop an abnormal gait in which the pet begins to walk on its hind end, dropping its full weight from its toes, and walking on the back of its hock. This is a called **plantigrade gait** and is secondary to prolonged low blood sugar in the cells of the long nerves (sciatic nerve) of the leg, producing a decrease in nerve function (see Figure 15.5). When noted, this is highly suggestive of diabetes.

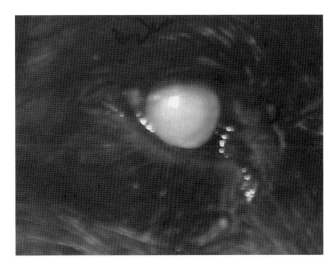

Figure 15.4. Note the early cataract formation in this eye secondary to hyperglycemia from diabetes mellitus.

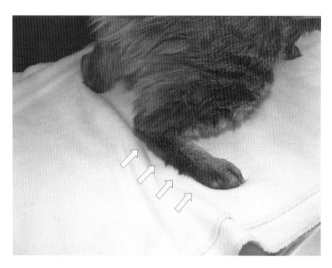

Figure 15.5. In this image the feline has dropped its weight from bearing weight on its toes to bearing weight on the caudal aspect of the tarsus (ankle; white arrows).

Endocrine Pancreatic Clinical Diagnostics
Clinical diagnostics for diabetic patients are largely based on blood and urine testing.

Complete Blood Count
Typically in diabetic animals there are no overall changes in complete blood count.

Chemistry
Blood Sugar
The most notable change in the chemistry is a persistent **hyperglycemia** (high blood sugar). *It is important to note that there can be moderate elevations in blood sugar with stress.* Animals that come into the hospital can have moderately high blood sugar just because of the change of environment. In general, the following glucose level may be associated with stress:

- **Canines:** Glucose <200 mg/dl can be secondary to stress.
- **Felines:** Glucose <300 mg/dl can be secondary to stress.

If a pet presents with a questionable elevation in blood sugar, either repeat a blood sugar later or check a urinalysis. This can help distinguish stress from diabetes.

Liver Enzymes
With chronic diabetes, mild to moderate elevations in liver enzymes (i.e., alanine transferase, aspartate transferase) can be observed. Furthermore, due to increases in fat metabolism, the blood cholesterol level elevations can be observed, and the serum of the blood can have a white coloration from increased fat (**lipemia**).

Urinalysis
A urinalysis is key in the diagnosis and maintenance of the diabetic patient. The evidence of glucose in the urine can support the finding of hyperglycemia in the diagnosis of di-

abetes. Another concern is the presence of ketones (acetone) in the uncontrolled diabetic, suggestive of a ketoacidotic diabetic (see below). Furthermore, bacterial bladder infections can occur because of the higher levels of sugar in the urine, increasing bacterial growth in the urine (see Chapter 13).

Fructosamine Levels
Fructosamine is another type of blood sugar that is metabolized in the body at a slower rate. A fructosamine level allows the veterinarian to determine how the patient is metabolizing sugar over the past 7–10 days. Significantly elevated fructosamine levels can suggest decreased control of blood sugar. Low levels may suggest too little release of glucose in the body, suggesting potential for life-threatening hypoglycemia.

Discussing Clinical Diagnostics with the Client
- The doctor has recommended general blood work to evaluate the potential for diabetes mellitus or other organ or hormonal diseases that could be affecting your pet.
- The veterinarian will be evaluating the blood and urinalysis for evidence of increased blood sugar levels suggesting early to severe diabetes.
- Furthermore, the pet's urinalysis will be evaluated for the presence of a toxin called acetone, which suggests severe diabetes that may require more significant care.
- If the pet is diagnosed with diabetes and treatment is initiated, continued diagnostic monitoring of blood and urine may be needed until the pet has stabilized on insulin therapy.

Diabetes and ketoacidotic diabetic crises are discussed next. The main goal is to understand and be able to explain to the client what the diseases are, how they can present themselves, and what can be the overall short- and long-term concerns of each disease. Any discussion of overall diagnostic and treatment protocols should be discussed based on the recommendations of the doctor and the medical team. Please use the following information as a basis to discuss and educate the client, *but never to diagnose a patient.*

Diabetes Mellitus (Uncomplicated)
Diabetes mellitus is a lack of insulin production or decreased responsiveness to insulin in the body. This produces an inability of the cells of the body to uptake and use insulin as an energy source. Diabetics are more prone to infection and disease and must be monitored more closely than other animals.

Etiology
The disease can occur as a primary syndrome or occur secondarily to other systemic disease (i.e., chronic pancreatitis, hyperadrenocorticism, chronic obesity, etc.).

Signalment

Diabetes can occur in canines or felines between the ages of 4–14 years (canine) and 8–13 years (felines). In dogs, the female is more susceptible, whereas in cats the male is more sensitive to the disease. The following breeds of canines are at more risk.

- Keeshond
- Puli
- Miniature pinscher
- Cairn terrier
- Poodle
- Dachshund
- Miniature schnauzer
- Beagle

For felines there is no breed specificity.

Common Points on Medical History

In uncomplicated early diabetes, the client may notice a mild to moderate weight loss, increased thirst and urination, and changes in the hair coat and abdomen.

Common Points on Initial Assessment

Physical symptoms observed during initial assessment can vary depending on the severity and duration of onset of the diabetes. Physical signs can consist of

- a poor body condition with increased muscle loss;
- a poor hair coat;
- a chronically bloated abdomen;
- lethargy/depression;
- chronic vomiting;
- neurologic signs—in cats walking flat on back legs to the level of the ankle (plantograde stance); and
- ocular changes—early cataract formation/bluing of the corneas

Short-Term Complications

If diabetes goes untreated or is improperly treated, animals can have chronic weight loss, poor condition, or, due to severe **hyperglycemia,** can become **ketoacidotic** (see below).

Clinical Diagnostics

As described above, the diagnosis of diabetes is based on the clinical blood work and urinalysis.

Treatment

Treatment is focused on long-term diet and medical treatment of the patient. Medical control of diabetes can be a slow and protracted process, relying on a great deal of owner compliance and medical care. Owners need to understand that medical treatment of the diabetic is a life-long process that will change the long-term care of their pet. Medical treatment of diabetes focuses on the following.

- **Insulin therapy:** Injectable insulin is the main therapy for controlling the diabetes. The type of insulin is chosen based on its duration of effect on the animal. In canines, insulin-N (NPH) is typically used twice a day. In felines, PZI insulin is generally recommended 1–2 times a day. In most management cases, insulin is given subcutaneously by the owner.
- **Diet:** The pet can burn its carbohydrates on a slower schedule, making the insulin more effective by feeding diets high in fiber and low in rapidly burned carbohydrates. Generally 40–50% of the diet is given in the morning with the initial insulin injection, and the remainder is given 12 hours later with the second insulin shot (if a second shot is needed).
- **Monitoring glucose:** To help make sure the animal is on an adequate level of insulin that helps control the diabetes but does not leave the pet **hypoglycemic,** blood or urine glucose levels are monitored.
- **Blood glucose levels in the hospital:** These levels are generally monitored in hospital by taking routine fructosamine levels or by doing a glucose curve. A blood glucose curve monitors blood sugar levels over the course of a 12- to 24-hour period. These tests may need to be repeated a number of times until the proper level of insulin is found to control the patient's blood sugar.
- **Blood glucose levels at home:** In some cases, glucose monitoring is done at home by the owner by taking small amounts of blood from the pinna or other region of the body.

Prevention

Keeping pets lean and reducing concerns that may lead to chronic pancreatitis (see above) may help decrease the potential for diabetes.

Long-Term Complications

In treating the diabetic animal, there are many possible complications that can occur secondarily. The major concerns are:

- **Infection:** Diabetic animals are less effective at fighting off infection and at healing. These pets tend to be more fragile and must be closely monitored while treating any type of skin or systemic infection.
- **Hypoglycemia:** The brain and the muscles depend on glucose for normal activity. If too much insulin is given to a pet or the pet receives its normal amount of insulin and does not eat properly, the pet can become hypoglycemic. Signs of hypoglycemia can include
  — depression,
  — decreased activity,
  — weakness,
  — shaking,
  — unresponsiveness,
  — seizure, and
  — death

Communication with the Owner

Owners must understand the concerns and physical symptoms of hypoglycemia and what to do if their pet starts showing its signs. Sending take-home instructions or a medical release can help the owner understand and identify this potentially life-threatening syndrome.

Sample Take Home Information for the Client
Please contact us immediately

1. if your animal begins to act *weak, depressed, is not eating, or is seizuring or shaking,* it may suggest a low level of sugar due to too much insulin;
2. if your pet is not eating and you have given the normal dose of insulin;
3. if you have given the wrong dose of insulin or you are not sure how much insulin your pet has received; and
4. if your pet is depressed, vomiting, and listless.

If you are concerned, place a small amount of honey or Karo syrup across tongue. *Never squirt directly back into the mouth as this could cause aspiration into the lungs.*

Discussing Diabetes Mellitus (Uncomplicated) with the Client
- Diabetes mellitus is a lack of insulin production or nonresponsiveness to insulin in the body.
- Without insulin, the cells cannot utilize sugar, and the body increases fat and muscle breakdown in response to a decrease of sugar within the cells.
- This produces an excessively high blood sugar that the pet must eliminate through the urine. To push this large molecule into the urine, the patient must drink large amounts of water and urinate large volumes.
- Early signs of diabetes are increased thirst and urination, weight loss, an unkempt hair coat, and loss of muscle tone.
- Once diagnosed, diabetes is controlled with medication and diet.
- Typically, diabetics will require medication and monitoring for life.

Ketoacidotic Diabetes

Ketoacidosis occurs when glucose levels are high for prolonged periods and the body begins turning the glucose into ketones. The presence of ketones produces a metabolic acidosis, making the pet ill and depressed.

The animal's clinical signs can be

- depressed to obtund,
- dehydration,

- vomiting,
- diarrhea,
- anorexia, and
- weakness.

Treatment

These pets can be so severely ill that, if not treated, they can become life threatened. Treatment generally requires hospitalization and fluid therapy, focusing on lowering the body's glucose levels and removing ketones from the body. Treatment components can be a follows.

- **IV fluids:** Fluids are used to help to rehydrate the patient, help control acidosis, and flush the toxins from the body.
- **Short-acting insulin therapy:** The pet is given a dose of short-term insulin (Humilin R) every 1–3 hours until the blood sugar and ketone levels return to normal, which can take 24–48 or more hours.
- **Hospitalization and monitoring:** The patient must be closely monitored to assess the pet's blood glucose and urine ketone levels, while making sure the pet does not enter a hypoglycemic state.

Discussing Long-Term Treatment and Potential Complications with the Client
- Managing the diabetic patient is a life-long commitment to monitoring diet, blood and urine sugar, and changes in the pet's health.
- Treatment can involve daily to twice daily injections of insulin and monitoring the pet's diet closely.
- The diabetic patient is more fragile, being much more susceptible to infection and disease. Pets must be more closely monitored for chronic systemic and skin infections.
- While treating diabetes with insulin therapy, the pet may have periods of hypoglycemia or low blood sugar. These pets can get severely weak, disoriented, and could potentially become comatose and die. Therefore, the patient must always be monitored for clinical signs of low blood sugar.
- If the pet is not well and has very high blood sugar, the patient may change its glucose into a toxin called ketones. These toxins acidify the blood and make the pet extremely weak, nauseous, and potentially life threatened.
- If there are any concerns or changes in the health status of the pet, medical attention should be sought immediately.

CD-ROM 1 reviews material presented in this chapter. Please try the cases for Section 2 (Anatomy and Physiology—The Science behind the Diseases) *to help reinforce the information presented here.*

Chapter 16

Thyroid Gland

The thyroid glands are a set of paired dark red glands on either side of the trachea, sitting lateral and ventral to the trachea. There can be tremendous variation between location and numbers of variations of glands depending on the animal. The more proximal edge of the thyroid begins close to the distal laryngeal region and ends at the fifth tracheal ring (see Figure 16.1).

The thyroid glands are responsible for the production of the **thyroxin** hormone that sets the **basal metabolic rate (BMR).** The BMR regulates the level at which cells burn energy and turnover. The hormone is released with ebb and flow patterns throughout the day to produce a sustained effect. Animals with decreased production (**hypothyroid**) do not burn energy fully or turn over cells in a normal time period. These animals have a poor hair coat due to decreased hair turnover, can be chronically obese, can seek out warmth even in hot environments, and can have decreased energy. Animals with increased production (**hyperthyroid**) produce energy at too rapid a rate. These animals are chronically thin with a history of weight loss, chronic vomiting, increased appetites (**polyphagia**), and can have explosive/hyperactive energy.

There are two categories of diseases that can affect thyroid function; diseases that produce a low thyroid state (**hypothyroidism**) and diseases that produce a hyperactive thyroid condition (**hyperthyroidism**). The diseases that produce hypothyroidism are broken into the following categories.

- **Idiopathic thyroid gland atrophy:** The normal thyroid tissue is replaced over time with fat tissue. The cause of disease is unknown.
- **Immune-mediated disease:** Immune-mediated thyroiditis is an inflammatory disease in which the white blood cells of the body attack the thyroid cells as foreign bacteria. The white blood cells functionally destroy the thyroid-producing cell and cause a decreased production of thyroid hormone.
- **Pituitary neoplasia:** The pituitary is a small gland in the brain that regulates the release of hormones from other glands of the body (see Chapter 17). A pituitary tumor, which occurs rarely, destroys the pituitary's ability to release the **thyroid-stimulating hormone**. Without this hormone, no thyroxin can be produced.

In hyperthyroid animals, a thyroid tumor of the gland itself produces an overproduction of thyroid hormone. This disease is most commonly seen in cats, where small, microscopic tumors within the thyroid gland lead to an overproduction of hormone. This is a common syndrome in older felines, with 97% of the tumors being benign and only 3% chance of a malignant thyroid adenocarcinoma. In canines, the disease is rare, but thyroid tumors have a much higher chance of malignancy.

Obtaining a History for Animals Affected by Thyroid Disease

Thyroid disease can manifest itself with very nonspecific signs. Many times thyroid disease is found secondarily when running general blood work. Some questions to focus on when thyroid disease is suspected are presented next.

What Is the Age of the Patient?
Thyroid disease tends to affect middle-aged to older animals. The disease can come on very slowly, and its full effect may not be fully observed by the owner.

What Is the Breed of the Pet?
There are some specific breeds that are more prone to thyroid disease; however, any breed can be susceptible to thyroid dysfunction.

With **hypothyroidism**, the susceptible breeds are the

- airedale,
- boxer,
- cocker spaniel,
- dachshund,
- Doberman pinscher,
- golden retriever,
- Great Dane,
- Irish setter,
- miniature schnauzer,
- old English sheepdog,
- Pomeranian,
- poodle, and
- Shetland sheepdog.

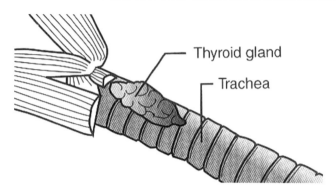

Figure 16.1. Illustration of the thyroid gland sitting on the trachea.(Image courtesy of *Clinical Anatomy and Physiology for Veterinary Technicians.* Colville, T., and Bassert, J. Mosby, Philadelphia, PA 2002. Used with permission of Elsevier publishing.)

With **hyperthyroidism** there is no breed predilection; however, the disease is mostly observed in cats.

What Is the Pet's Energy Level?
In general, because BMR is affected, the pet's energy may also be altered. Some general patterns are listed here.

- **Hypothyroid:** The animal may be lethargic and have decreased energy. With low-thyroid animals, their BMR decreases their available energy.
- **Hyperthyroid:** These patients may be hyperactive, with explosive energy. The animal burns energy at an explosive rate, producing so much energy that the patient acts hyperactive. These animals cannot consume enough food to maintain their needs. Some animals may have aggressive behavior changes.

Is There an Overall Problem with Weight?
Pets may have chronic weight change because the BMR is accelerated or slowed. Some basic patterns of weight change may be as follows.

- **Obesity:** Hypothyroid animals will not burn energy normally. Their energy intake goes into storage and is not rapidly turned over.
- **Leanness:** Hyperthyroid animals will burn energy so rapidly that most animals cannot keep muscle and fat stored in their body. In some cases animals can have severe weight loss, *which may be the only physical symptom evident.*

Has the Animal Been Shedding Excessively?
With both hyper- and hypothyroid animals, their coat does not turn over properly. Usually, both conditions produce severe excessive year-round shedding that occurs regardless of season.

Is the Animal a Chronic Vomiter or Regurgitator?
Hyperthyroid animals may eat so rapidly that they are prone to chronic vomiting. **Hypothyroid** animals may rarely develop a **megaesophagus** (see Chapter 10). The abnormal dilated esophagus cannot properly propel food into the stomach, causing chronic regurgitation.

Does Your Pet Have a Tragic Expression?
Some hypothyroid animals can have a sullen or tragic expression. This is secondary to improper turnover of skin, producing thickened facial skin folds that make the eyes appear down turned.

Does the Pet Have a History of Chronic Ear Infections?
Low-thyroid animals may have chronic, sustained ear infections, secondary to decreased skin turnover and skin immunity.

Does the Animal Have a History of Reproduction Problems?
Rarely, low-thyroid animals may have decreased ability to produce sperm and eggs, ovulate properly, have normal conception, and maintain pregnancy. Generally, this is observed only in animals with severely low thyroid.

Key Points on Assessing a Patient with Thyroid Disease

Animals may have severe thyroid disease and not all physical signs are present. Some patients may be diagnosed with thyroid dysfunction secondary to routine blood work. The thyroid glands affect many of the body's systems, including the **skin, cardiac, neuromuscular, intestinal, reproductive,** and **ocular systems.** It is important to try to get an accurate history and monitor for potential minor changes upon initial assessment, which may suggest thyroid dysfunction. Some key points to observe on initial assessment are discussed next.

Changes in the Pet's General Appearance
Most animals with thyroid disease have poor hair coats with a lackluster appearance that appears unkempt.

- **Hyperthyroid animals** have very thin coats, which tend to be oily to dry. These pets can be chronic shedders. Furthermore, these patients may have chronic weight loss with poor muscle quality and muscle atrophy.
- **Hypothyroid animals** also show severe shedding, with potentially poor hair coat and with a symmetrical hair loss over the sides of the abdomen (**symmetrical flank alopecia**). There can be increased pigmentation of the skin, dry or oily skin, and thickening areas of skin. The animal may seem to have low energy, a tragic facial expression, and is more prone to skin and allergy problems.

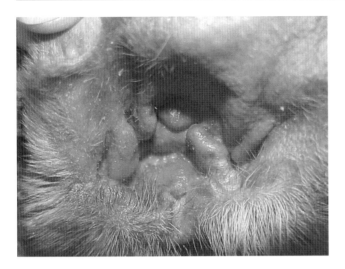

Figure 16.2. Chronically infected and inflamed ear can be secondary to low thyroid disease.

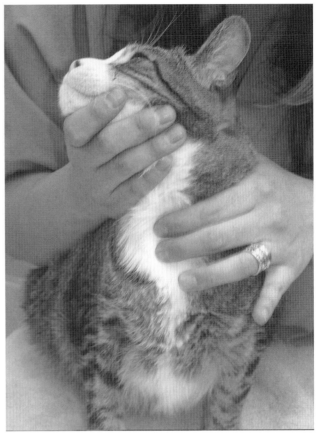

Figure 16.3. Image of proper approach to palpating an enlarged thyroid gland.

Ears
Low-thyroid patients may have chronic ear infections with red inflamed ears (see Figure 16.2).

Heart Rate
Because the BMR is affected, heart rate may also change. Although not always noted with animals that have thyroid dysfunction, if abnormality is observed, it should be documented and discussed with the medical team. General changes in heart rate can be as follows:

- **Bradycardia** (heart rates <80 beats/minute) can occasionally be noted in hypothyroid patients.
- **Tachycardia** (heart rates >200 beats/minute) can be observed in hyperthyroid cats. In extreme cases, the rapid heart rate can make the heart prone to cardiac arrhythmias and murmurs.

Thyroid Gland Enlargement
Most hyperthyroid animals have palpable thyroid glands on one or both sides.

To evaluate for thyroid enlargement perform the following examination.

- Flex the neck to one side, and then place a finger down the ridge of the jugular groove on the other side.
- A small nodelike mass can be palpated above the jugular groove if the gland is enlarged.
- Repeat on other side.
- This should be done three to four times per second to make sure the gland can be palpated (see Figure 16.3).

If an enlarged thyroid gland is palpable, it is abnormal, and the finding should be reported to the medical team. Most animals with a palpably large thyroid gland will either be hyperthyroid or turn hyperthyroid within the next 6 months.

Neuromuscular Changes
Although rare, animals may have facial nerve paralysis. Some animals may present with an inability to blink, move their ears, or have increased drooling due to decreased lip tone. This is due to decreased facial nerve function that innervates the muscle. This process has been linked to hypothyroidism. This disease is most commonly seen in the cocker spaniel.

Keratoconjunctivitis Sicca
Keratoconjunctivitis sicca (KCS), or dry eye, can be a secondary problem to hypothyroid patients. Patients with red, inflamed eyes, chronic purulent discharge, and decreased tear production (determined by using the **Schirmer tear test**) should be evaluated for hypothyroid disease (see Chapter 20; see Figure 16.4).

Emergency concerns are rare when dealing with thyroid dysfunction; even severely affected animals are usually stable. If there are concerns of stability based on the team member's triage assessment (see Chapter 6), the medical team should be notified and the pet evaluated further for other conditions.

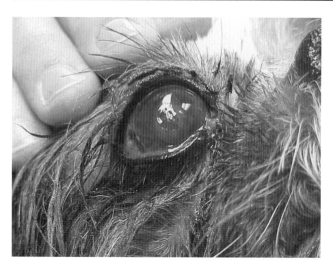

Figure 16.4. Image of red irritated eye with corneal ulcer that can occur secondary to chronic dry eyes. Animals with KCS should have their thyroid levels evaluated.

Clinical Diagnostic Testing for Evaluating Thyroid Function

The diagnosis of thyroid disease is determined by blood tests, which largely evaluate primary thyroid hormone levels and secondary changes in the organ function occurring from thyroid dysfunction. Some possible clinical diagnostics follow.

Chemistry

- With a **hyperthyroid patient**, there can be changes in liver enzymes. Increased alanine transferase (ALT) levels have been reported secondary to increased metabolism and energy turnover. Less commonly, there can be elevations in alkaline phosphotase, blood urea nitrogen, glucose, phosphorus, and bilirubin.
- With the **hypothyroid patient,** elevations in blood cholesterol levels can be observed due to alterations in metabolism secondary to a lowered BMR.

Evaluating Thyroid Level

There are many different tests to evaluate changes in thyroid production. Depending on the age and species of the pet, the concerns of the medical team, and the symptoms observed, monitoring of the following hormone levels may be recommended.

- **Total T_4:** A total T_4 represents that total amount of active thyroid and inactive thyroid hormone in the bloodstream. Abnormal elevations can suggest hyperthyroidism, whereas deficiency can suggest hypothyroidism. However, chronic organ or infectious disease can suppress thyroid production. This condition, called **euthyroid sick,** occurs as the patient mobilizes its nutritional reserves to

fight off a chronic problem while not being able to keep up with normal thyroid production.

- **Free T_4 done by equilibrium dialysis:** This test is a measure of the active free hormone in the bloodstream. Early thyroid dysfunction may cause changes in these levels before total T_4 is affected.
- **T_3 Level:** The T_3 level is a precursor to the active T_4 hormone. Decreases in this hormone can sometimes indicate a hypothyroid state.
- **T_3/T_4/thyroglobulin autoantibodies:** These diagnostics test for the presence of antibodies against thyroid hormone and thyroid precursor hormone in the body. It is the key test for **immune-mediated thryoiditis**.

Discussing Clinical Diagnostics for Thyroid Dysfunction with the Client

- Blood work has been suggested to detect if your pet has evidence of thyroid dysfunction.
- Furthermore, other clinical diagnostics (i.e., complete blood count and chemistry) will help evaluate if there is evidence of other underlying hormonal, organ, infectious, or inflammatory disease that may be secondarily suppressing normal thyroid production.
- If thyroid levels appear normal but there is suggestion of early disease based on history or physical examination, there are tests that evaluate the concentration of active free thyroid hormone and thyroid precursor hormones in the bloodstream. In some cases these hormone levels will show early changes in concentration before total thyroid hormone levels are affected.

Diseases of the Thyroid Gland

Although not all diseases are mentioned below, the common diseases are discussed with the main goal being to understand and to be able to explain to the client what the diseases are, how they can present themselves, and what can be the overall short- and long-term concerns. Any discussion of overall diagnostic and treatment protocols should be discussed based on the recommendations of the doctor and the medical team. Please use the following information as a guideline to discuss and educate the client, *but never to diagnose a patient*.

Hyperthyroidism

Hyperthyroidism is an overproduction of thyroid hormone from the thyroid glands. The hormone, **thyroxine,** helps control the rate with which cells burn energy in the body (BMR). When an animal is hyperthyroid, there is too much thyroxine in the body, and the rate with which cells burn energy and turn over is greatly accelerated.

Etiology

Hyperthyroidism is caused by microscopic masses within the thyroid gland that overproduce thyroxine. In cats 97% of these tumors are benign and do not metastasize. In dogs, the percentage of malignancy is higher.

Signalment

This disease is common in older cats (usually more than 8 years of age). The disease is rare in dogs. There is no sex or breed predilection.

Common Points in Medical History

Owners can report a variety of medical complaints with a hyperthyroid patient. The most common is **weight loss,** which can be mild to severe. Other common symptoms can be the following.

- **Increased appetite (ravenous):** Pets with an increased BMR can have increased energy needs producing an increased to ravenous appetite.
- **Increased thirst and urination:** Due to increased metabolic rate and turnover of cells, patients tend to drink more water and secondarily urinate more.
- **Explosive energy (hyperactive):** Patients can have explosive energy bordering on hyperactivity due to the increased BMR.
- **Shedding and hair loss:** Cells are turned over at an accelerated rate, which produces constant year-round shedding.
- **Behavior changes:** With increased energy output, patients may develop behavior changes; the most common is aggression.
- **Gastrointestinal signs—vomiting and diarrhea:** Secondary to increased metabolic turnover and ravenous intake of the diet, pets may develop chronic vomiting and diarrhea.

Common Points on Initial Assessment

Affected animals are generally stable, bright, alert, and responsive. They may show the following symptoms on initial assessment:

- Thin to emaciated
- Generalized poor muscle mass
- Tachycardia
- Poor hair coat
- Palpable thyroid gland (see above)

Complications

If left untreated, hyperthyroidism may cause hypertension, heart disease, liver disease, kidney disease, retinal detachment, and death.

Clinical Diagnostics

As described above, hyperthyroidism is diagnosed by blood work. Typically a total/free T_4 can be very helpful in suggesting hyperthyroidism.

Treatment

There are three basic treatment options for this disease. Treatment is based on the animal's condition, the severity and concerns of the disease, and the medical options available to the medical team.

Medication

Medications, such as methimazole, are an antithyroid compound that blocks thyroid hormone formation. This medication is usually the first course of medication prior to surgical or radiation treatments to help the patient normalize thyroid levels. Methimazole can also be the primary treatment choice; however, the medication would need to be maintained for life, and thyroid and organ function would need to be monitored regularly.

Surgical Removal of the Thyroid Gland

Thyroidectomy, or surgical removal of the thyroid gland, removes the affected thyroid gland or glands from the pet's neck. If both glands need to be removed, the procedure could make the patient **hypothyroid** and may require the pet to be supplemented with thyroid medication. The surgery may also affect a smaller gland near the thyroid gland, called the **parathyroid** gland, which controls the level of calcium within the bloodstream.

Radioactive Iodine Therapy

Thyroxine is composed largely of iodine molecules. Eighty percent of the iodine in the body is stored within the thyroid glands. By injecting a radioactive isotope of iodine into the

---

Discussing Hyperthyroidism (Feline) with the Client

- The thyroid gland sits in the middle of the neck of most animals and secretes a hormone called thyroxin.
- Thyroxin regulates at what rate the cells burn energy; this is called the **basal metabolic rate.**
- In the large majority of hyperthyroid feline patients, there is an overproduction of thyroid hormone due to microscopic benign tumors within the thyroid gland.
- Due to their increased energy utilization, these pets can show many different symptoms. The most common is weight loss; however, pets can also show increased appetite, hyperactivity, shedding, and changes in personality.
- Hyperthyroidism can usually be detected with routine blood work and controlled with medical or surgical care.
- If hyperthyroidism is not diagnosed and treated, patients can develop serious secondary disease, such as hypertension, heart disease, blindness, and organ disease.

body, it can selectively destroy the thyroid tissue without affecting other tissues in the body. Generally, the pet will have to be in isolation for a few days to a few weeks while the treatment is completed. Isolation interval varies from state to state.

Prevention
There is no known way to prevent hyperthyroidism from occurring. However, through routine clinical diagnostic screening of the senior patient, the disease can be picked up in its early stages, minimizing severe systemic affects of the disease

Hypothyroidism
Hypothyroidism is an underproduction of thyroid gland from pituitary or idiopathic/immune-mediated disease of the thyroid (see above).

Signalment
The disease is most common in middle-aged to older dogs and very rare in cats. The common canine breeds are the

- airedale,
- golden retriever,
- boxer,
- great Dane,
- cocker spaniel,
- Irish setter,
- dachshund,
- miniature schnauzer,
- Doberman pinscher,
- old English sheep dog,
- Pomeranian
- poodle, and
- Shetland sheep dog.

Common Points in Medical History
Often the diagnosis of hypothyroidism is found in routine diagnostic blood work. Owners may be unaware of any medical changes in the pet that may suggest low thyroid. However, the following observations should be discussed with owners.

- **Chronic obesity:** Hypothyroid animals are generally obese, even with significant dietary restrictions.
- **Chronic skin/shedding issues:** Hypothyroid patients have decreased turnover of hair and skin cells. Many patients will present with a focal symmetrical hair loss on both sides of the abdomen (**flank alopecia**). The pet can have chronic year-round shedding problems. Furthermore, patients may present with chronic ear and skin infections as the normal healthy skin barrier cannot be adequately maintained.
- **Decreased energy:** Patients with decreased BMRs may have low energy and seem more lethargic.
- **Animal becomes heat seeking:** Due to decreasing BMR, pets may be unable to maintain normal internal warmth and may seek warm areas even in hot environments.

- **Reproductive issues:** Hypothyroid patients may not have enough energy to maintain normal reproductive cycles. These pets tend to have decreased sperm production, ovulation, abnormal heat cycles, and have problems with normal fertilization and maintenance of pregnancy.

Common Points on Initial Assessment
The chronic hypothyroid patient may show very few physical signs on initial assessment. The concern of low thyroid may be associated with older animals with poor skin, ears, allergy, and obesity issues.

Complications
If left untreated, hypothyroidism may cause chronic skin, obesity, and hair coat issues.

Clinical Diagnostics
As described above, hypothyroidism is diagnosed by blood work. Typically, a total/free T_4 test can be very helpful in suggesting hypothyroidism.

Treatment
Treatment is medical supplementation of thyroid hormone called thyroxine. This medication is given once or twice a day for the rest of the pet's life. Thyroid levels must be checked throughout the pet's life because the need for supplementation can change as the pet ages.

Prevention
There is no known way to prevent hypothyroidism. However, through routine clinical diagnostic screening of the senior patient, the disease can be picked up in its early stages, minimizing severe systemic affects of the disease.

Discussing Hypothyroidism (Canine) with the Client
- The thyroid gland sits in the middle of the neck of most animals and secretes a hormone called thyroxin.
- Thyroxin regulates at what rate the cells burn energy; this is called the **basal metabolic rate.**
- In the large majority of hypothyroid canine patients, there is an underproduction of thyroid hormone.
- Due to their decreased energy utilization, the pets can show many different symptoms. The most common is chronic obesity; however, pets can also show chronic shedding, ear and skin infections, and reproductive problems.
- Hypothyroidism can usually be detected with routine blood work and controlled with medication.

CD-ROM 1 reviews material presented in this chapter. Please try the cases for Section 2 (Anatomy and Physiology—The Science behind the Diseases) to help reinforce the information presented here.

Chapter 17

Adrenal Gland

The adrenal glands are organs that control chronic and acute stress in the body by regulating blood pressure, heart rate, bronchodilatation, electrolyte balance, and emergency blood sugar levels. The adrenal glands are small peanut-shaped glands that sit cranial to both left and right kidney (see Figure 17.1).

The gland is composed of two distinctive and separate tissues, and each part has a different function.

The **adrenal cortex** is the outer tissue layer responsible for producing different types of steroids for maintenance of blood sugar, electrolytes, and sex steroid production. The cortex has three distinct levels and compromises 75% of the entire gland. It comprises three distinct tissue layers.

- **Zona granulosa:** This is the outermost area of the cortex, which is responsible for producing a steroid hormone called **aldosterone**, also called a **mineralocorticoid.**
- **Zona fasciculata:** This layer is the inner region of the adrenal cortex that produces a prednisone-like steroid called **cortisol.**
- **Zona reticularis:** The zona reticularis is the inner region of the adrenal cortex that produces a prednisone-like steroid called **cortisol.**

The **adrenal medulla** is the section of tissue in the middle of the gland that is responsible for producing **epinephrine** to assist the body in times of crisis or life and death concerns (**fight or flight**). Epinephrine has the following effects on the body:

- Increases heart rate
- Increases blood vessel constriction, thus increases blood pressure
- Dilates bronchial airways
- Decreases intestinal secretion and movement
- Dilates the eyes

In general, the adrenal gland serves the body in three functions to aid in normal maintenance and response to stress: cortisol production, adrenal–mineralocorticoid production, and epinephrine production.

Adrenal Cortisol Production

Cortisol is produced by the adrenal cortex to take protein and fat and turn them into glucose in times of low blood sugar. The process is controlled by a small gland in the brain called the **pituitary gland**, also called the master gland. When the brain senses low blood sugar, the pituitary gland releases a hormone called adrenocorticotropic hormone (**ACTH**) to stimulate the adrenal gland to produce cortisol. ACTH is released into the bloodstream until it encounters specific protein receptors in the adrenal cortex to stimulate the release of cortisol. Cortisol is then released into the bloodstream to stimulate the breakdown of protein and fat into sugar. As cortisol levels rise in the body, the pituitary decreases the amount of ACTH release. *This is called a negative feedback loop* (see Figure 17.2).

Adrenal Mineralocorticoid Production

The adrenal cortex also produces a mineralocorticoid called **aldosterone** that is responsible for the reabsorption of sodium and expulsion of potassium in the proximal convoluted tubules in the kidney. Without this hormone, the renal medulla is unable to maintain the high sodium gradient and cannot concentrate urine. (see Chapter 13). *This hormone, above all other adrenal hormones, is needed for normal handling of stress and body maintenance. Without sufficient levels of this hormone, an animal can get into a life-threatening crisis.* Aldosterone is necessary for the following.

- It is necessary for maintenance of the sodium/potassium balance within the body. Sodium is the electrolyte found in highest concentrations in the serum and extracellularly in the body. Potassium is found in the highest concentrations inside the cell.
- When the body needs to produce an electrical rhythm to produce muscular contraction, nerve depolarization, heart contraction, and millions of other muscular and neurologic activity, sodium is pumped intracellularly at the same time potassium is pumped extracellularly. This movement of electrolytes across the cell membrane produces an electrical potential (see Figure 17.3).
- When the normal sodium and potassium levels are affected, the body has a more difficult time producing the normal electrical activity, and the pet becomes weakened, with muscle fasciculations and abnormally slow heart rhythms. Severely affected animals can arrive in shock and life threatened. This syndrome is called an **Addisonian crisis** (see below).

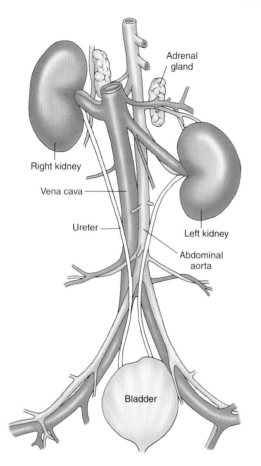

Figure 17.1. Illustration of the normal position of the adrenal gland in the body.

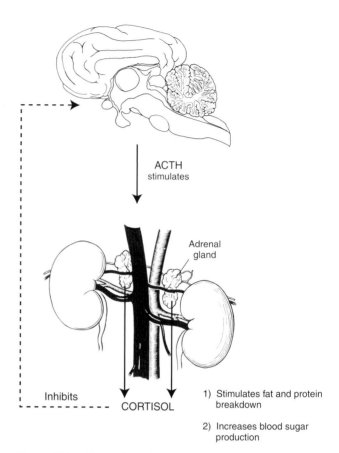

Figure 17.2. Illustration of normal release of ACTH to stimulate the release of cortisol. Cortisol then stimulates production of blood sugar from fats and muscle, while also decreasing the production of ACTH. This type of model is called a **negative feedback loop.**

Adrenal–Epinephrine Production

Epinephrine is closely associated with the sympathetic nervous system, a division of the autonomic nervous system of the body. Epinephrine is produced when an animal is threatened, making the animal ready to stand and fight or to run (**flight or fight response**). This reaction produces the following changes in the body:

- Quick bursts of speed
- Increased heart rate
- Increased blood pressure
- Bronchodilatation to increase airflow into the lungs
- Stopping intestinal movement and salivation
- Dilation of the eyes

Hyperadrenocorticism

There are three overall manifestations of adrenal disease commonly seen in general practice. The first is **hyperadrenocorticism (Cushing's disease)**, which is an overproduction of cortisol caused by a primary adrenal or pituitary disease. There are three overall forms of the disease.

- **Pituitary-dependent hyperadrenocorticism (PDH):** This disease syndrome is produced by microscopic pituitary tumors that overproduce ACTH, stimulating the adrenal glands to constantly produce cortisol. These tumors do not respond to negative feedback of increasing amounts of cortisol. If the tumors within the pituitary become enlarged, neurologic disease may (rarely) be seen (i.e., seizures, etc.) (see Figure 17.4).
- **Adrenal tumor–neoplasia:** A less common event is a tumor of the adrenal cortex, which can produce excessive amounts of cortisol. In this syndrome, one adrenal gland is usually affected. The high levels of cortisol and the secondary increase of glucose produces a significant negative feedback on pituitary. Because there is decreased ACTH, the other adrenal gland is usually small and atrophied (see Figure 17.5).
- **Iatrogenic cause:** Animals on a long-term dose of oral or injectable steroids (i.e., prednisone) can mimic the physical symptoms and conditions caused by the pituitary and adrenal forms of this disease. In this syndrome, both adrenal glands are small and atrophied due to decreased

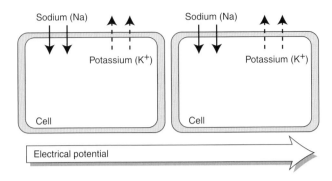

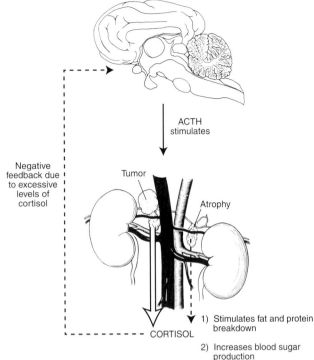

Figure 17.3.   Illustration of sodium/potassium exchange that occurs within the cell to produce an electrical wave. These electrical waves are key in normal neurological, cardiovascular, and muscular actions. Without proper levels of sodium and potassium, the patient is severely weakened.

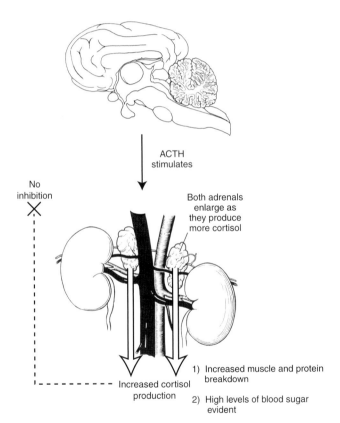

Figure 17.5.   With a tumor of the adrenal cortex, the affected gland overproduces cortisol, irrespective of the ACTH level of the body. The increasing blood sugar levels decrease ACTH production, causing a secondary atrophy of the unaffected adrenal gland.

Figure 17.4.   Illustration of pituitary-dependent hyperadrenocorticism. In this disease, both adrenal glands enlarge secondary to chronic pituitary ACTH stimulation. The pituitary tumors do not respond to the increasing levels of blood sugar; increased ACTH continues to produce cortisol.

The second form of adrenal disease is **hypoadrenocorticism (Addison's disease),** which is a decreased production of aldosterone. With this disease, the lack of aldosterone inhibits the body's ability to retain sodium and expel potassium. Addison's disease can be produced by the following disease syndromes.

- **Idiopathic (immune-mediated) hypoadrenocorticism:** This syndrome is caused by a generalized systemic inflammatory disease of unknown cause that destroys the cortex of the adrenal gland.
- **Granulomatous disease:** Granulomatous disease is the destruction of the adrenal cortex by a chronic infectious or inflammatory product that produces a microscopic granulomatous reaction within tissue.
- **Neoplasia:** Cancer of other tissue (i.e., adrenal medulla) can destroy normal adrenal cortical tissue.

The third and final syndrome is cancer of the adrenal medulla (i.e., epinephrine-producing tissue). This rare type of cancer is called a **pheochromocytoma.** This adrenaline-producing tumor can produce severe hypertension, rapid heart rates, weakness, and eventually death.

ACTH production. This occurs because of negative feedback on the pituitary from the steroidal medications administered. This form of the disease can sometimes be corrected with a slow withdrawal of oral steroids.

Obtaining a Medical History for Adrenal Disease

Diagnosing adrenal disease based on medical history and physical examination can be very difficult. It becomes exceedingly important to get a complete history on an animal that may be presenting with moderate to severe adrenal disease. Patients can have serious disease and present with very mild signs and can be almost normal on physical examination. Some basic questions for the client are presented next.

How Old Is the Pet?

Adrenal disease is not necessarily a problem of old age in animals. However, adrenal dysfunction tends to be observed in older animals.

Is There Breed Specificity for Adrenal Disease?

Although adrenal dysfunction can occur in any breed, there are some breeds more sensitive to adrenal disease.

- **Hyperadrenocorticism (Cushing's disease):** Canine breeds that are more susceptible are poodles, dachshunds, Boston terriers, boxers, and beagles. There is no breed sensitivity in the cat.
- **Hypoadrenocorticism (Addison's disease):** Canine breeds that are more susceptible are the great Dane, rotteweiler, Portuguese water dog, standard poodle, West Highland white terrier, and the Wheaton terrier. There is no breed sensitivity in the cat.

Has the Progression of the Disease Been Sudden or Chronic?

Most adrenal disease is chronic in nature. However, with hypoadrenocorticism, there are acute manifestations called an **Addisonian crisis** (see below). The body is unable to maintain a normal sodium and potassium balance, and the pet enters a crisis state.

Has There Been a Sharp Increase in Water Consumption (Polydipsia) or Urination (Polyuria)?

With hyperadrenocorticism, there can be a sharp increase in water consumption and urine output, especially over the past few days, weeks, and months. In felines, this may be noted as increased saturation in the litter box. This increase in thirst and urination is due to the steroid's affect on the renal medulla (see Chapter 13).

Does the Animal Shake, Have Muscle Tremors, or Act Weak?

Animals with abnormal electrolyte levels may produce severe muscle weakness, shaking, and tremors.

Has There Been a History of Vomiting and Diarrhea?

Hypoadrenocorticism patients can have periodic and episodic vomiting and diarrhea.

Table 17.1. Triage concerns in the adrenal patient—Addisonian crisis.

Systems	Trouble Signs That Indicate an Emergency Situation
Mentation	Nonresponsive/comatose
Fever	Temp <99° (due to shock, DIC, coma)
Hydration	Dehydration >5–7%
Gum color	Pink to pale pink (poor perfusion)
Capillary refill time (CRT)	CRT >2–3 seconds
Heart rate/pulse	Rate: Heart rate <80 bpm Pulse: Pulses can have normal to decreased quality depending on whether the pet is in shock.

Has the Animal Been on Oral Steroidal Medication (Prednisone)?

- **Hyperadrenocorticism:** Chronic steroid usage over months to years can produce iatrogenic hyperadrenocorticism (see above).
- **Hypoadrenocorticism:** Animals that have been on oral steroids and that have been removed from the medication too quickly can produce an Addisonian crisis situation. The prednisone naturally inhibits the body's production of cortisol. If the patient is removed from the steroid too rapidly, the body does not have enough time to restart adequate production, and the patient can enter an Addisonian crisis (see below).

Initial Assessment of Pets with Adrenal Disease

Most animals with adrenal disease can show a variety of symptoms. The patient may have no overall medical complaints or may be severely affected (see Table 17.1).

Hypoadrenocorticism

In hypoadrenocorticism (Addison's disease), except for animals in severe crisis, animals may show little to no physical symptoms of disease. The owner may bring the pet in with a history of lethargy, depression, gastrointestinal signs, and or muscle tremors.

Mentation

Patients can be depressed to comatose and can be sternally to laterally recumbent.

Symptoms

- **Cardiovascular symptoms:** Animals can be severely bradycardic with heart rates less than 60–80 beats per minute. Pulses can vary depending on how severely affected the pet is.
- **Musculoskeletal symptoms:** Pets may occasionally have muscle tremors or spasms from electrolyte abnormalities.

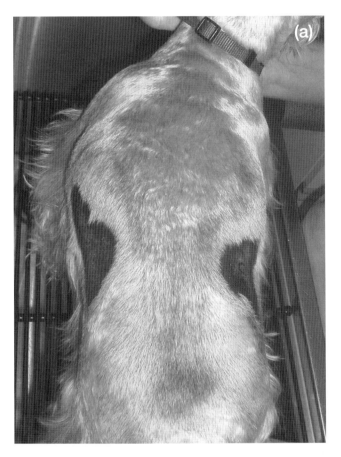

- **Dehydration**: These pets can be moderately to severe dehydrated due to improper reabsorption of sodium, leading to a decreased ability of the kidneys to concentrate their urine.

With hyperadrenocorticism, symptoms are generally mild, with the chief complaints being changes in the skin and muscle, increased thirst, and increased urination. With hyperadrenocorticism, there tends to be more severe protein and fat breakdown. This produces moderate to severe muscle loss and changes in the hair coat and skin (see Figure 17.6). There are some common notable changes.

- **Pendulous abdomen:** The abdominal muscle becomes weakened and thinned, making the animal appear potbellied.
- **Flank alopecia:** The hair coat of a hyperadrenocorticism dog can show severe symmetrical bilateral hair loss in the flank region over the dorsal and lateral hips. It is important to note that this hair coat change can be observed with other hormonal diseases, too (i.e., hypothyroidism, diabetes mellitus) (see Figure 17.6).
- **Increased pigmentation of the skin:** Often these pets will have increased regions of pigmentation, thinning of the skin (fragility), and changes in appearance of the skin due to increased protein turnover and chronic affects of steroids.

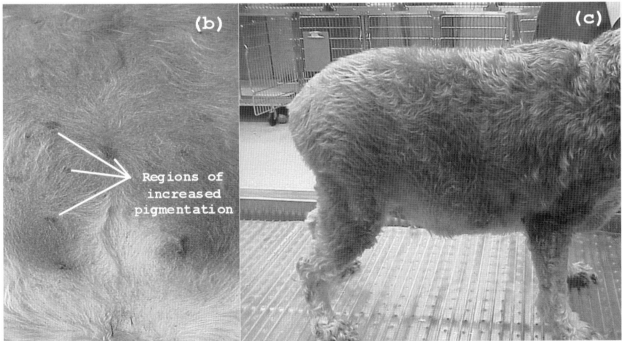

Figure 17.6. Image of changes in the skin and hair coat that could be suggestive of hyperadrenocorticism. The first image shows bilateral hair loss (**flank** alopecia), which can be observed with patients suffering from hormonal disease (a). Note the thinning hair coat and areas of pigmentation on the ventral abdomen (b). Finally, observe the poor hair coat and large pendulous abdomen (c).

Clinical Diagnostics of the Adrenal System

Testing for adrenal dysfunction can be a complicated process, requiring advanced blood and imaging diagnostics. Each hospital team has its own diagnostic protocols for each type of adrenal disease depending on the concern regarding the syndrome present.

Hyperadrenocorticism

For hyperadrenocorticism, it is very difficult to diagnose most forms of Cushing's disease with baseline blood work. *Although indications of adrenal hormonal disease can be suggested*, diagnosis of this disease based solely on baseline blood work is difficult. Advanced blood work and imaging diagnostics are needed to diagnose Cushing's disease and differentiate between primary pituitary and adrenal disease (see Table 17.2). Some common clinical diagnostic results for adrenal dysfunction are discussed next.

Routine Diagnostics
Complete Blood Count
The complete blood count can be essentially normal. However, on occasion, a **stress leukogram** can be seen. A stress leukogram is noted by

- a slight increase in the white blood cell count,
- an increased neutrophil count, and
- a decreased lymphocyte count.

Chemistry
Results from blood work for a routine chemistry panel can be extremely variable. There is no absolute baseline test for adrenal disease on routine chemistries. There are some observable changes, however.

- **Alkaline phosphatase:** This refers to a large number of intracellular enzymes that are present within the liver, intestine, bone, kidneys, and placenta. Alkaline phosphatase can be elevated with liver disease, gall bladder obstruction, and other types of organ and systemic illness. However, increases in alkaline phosphatase are also associated with liver tissue chronically exposed to long-term steroids (i.e., cortisol, prednisone, etc.).
- **Cholesterol:** Increased cholesterol can be seen with Cushing's disease due to increased fat breakdown into sugar.
- **Blood sugar:** Animals with chronically high levels of cortisol can be **hyperglycemic.** Blood sugar in nondiabetic animals can range from 200 to 300 mg/dl. If an animal is chronically hyperglycemic long enough, diabetes can occur.

Urinalysis
With Cushing's disease, the ability of the kidneys to concentrate urine can be affected. Animals are usually **hyposthenuric**, with urine specific gravities less than 1.015. The effect is caused by the steroids producing an electrolyte washout in the renal medulla (see Chapter 13).

Radiology
Abdominal radiographs are used to assess organ enlargement (i.e., hepatomegally) or potential adrenal masses associated with Cushing's disease.

Advanced Diagnostics
Although there are multiple clinical diagnostics available, there is no one correct diagnostic path to indicate Cushing's disease (see Table 17.2). Some clinical tests that may be recommended are discussed next.

Urine Cortisol/Creatinine Ratio
In animals with Cushing's disease, the excess cortisol is excreted by the kidneys, increasing the amount of cortisol in comparison to the normal levels of creatinine in the urine. By obtaining a urine sample at home and submitting it to the lab, a simple test for increased cortisol levels in the body can be assessed.

Increased levels of cortisol raise the cortisol/creatinine ratio greater than 1. A normal urine cortisol/creatinine ratio rules out Cushing's disease; however, an elevated ratio does not absolutely identify it. Elevated levels of cortisol can be seen with other systemic disease (e.g., liver disease, neoplasia, other hormonal diseases, etc.). Thus, this test is used primarily as a prescreening test to rule out hyperadrenocorticism.

ACTH Stimulation Test
Follow the following procedure for an ACTH Stimulation test.

- In a 12-hour-fasted dog, a blood sample is taken for a prestimulation cortisol level.
- Then ACTH (pituitary hormone) is given, either intramuscularly or intravenously, depending on the form of ACTH.
- One or 2 hours later (depending on the ACTH form), a poststimulation cortisol level is obtained.

Hyperadrenocortical patients show a significant elevation of cortisol levels (far above normal response to ACTH) after stimulation of the adrenal gland due to hypertrophic adrenal glands. Although this disease is helpful in suggesting hyperadrenocorticism, this does not distinguish it from pituitary-dependent Cushing's disease or from an adrenal tumor.

Low-Dose Dexamethasone Suppression Test
Follow the following procedure for a low-dose dexamethasone suppression test.

- In a fasted animal, a blood cortisol level is drawn.
- A low dose of dexamethasone is injected intravenously.
- Six and 8 hours after injection, additional blood cortisol levels are drawn.

The normal animal will suppress its cortisol levels by half the pre-cortisol level amount 6–8 hours after the initial dexamethasone injection. This is caused by the dexamethasone reducing the ACTH production in the pituitary and secondarily reducing the cortisol production.

In the hyperadrenocortical animal, there is no suppression of the cortisol after 8 hours.

- With **pituitary disease**, the small pituitary tumors will not decrease ACTH levels when faced with increasing cortisol or cortisol-like drugs.
- With **adrenal tumors,** there is no decrease in cortisol production when faced with decreasing ACTH levels.

This test is an excellent screening for Cushing's disease. However, it does not differentiate between pituitary and adrenal Cushing's disease.

High-Dose Dexamethasone Suppression Test
This test can be completed after the low-dose dexamethasone suppression test to differentiate from adrenal or pituitary forms of Cushing's disease.

Follow the following procedure for a low-dose dexamethasone suppression test.

- In a fasted animal, a blood cortisol level is drawn.
- A high dosage of dexamethasone is injected intravenously.

The decision tree in Table 17.2 is designed to give team members an idea of what some of the clinical diagnostic protocols may be in order to help confirm or rule out hyperadrenocorticism. This diagram is not meant for the team member to help diagnose the disease, but to understand the complexity of testing to help discuss diagnostic options with the client.

- Six and 8 hours after injection, additional blood cortisol levels are drawn.

With **pituitary-dependent Cushing's disease** most pituitary tumors will decrease the ACTH level in the face of higher dexamethasone levels. The decreased ACTH decreases cortisol, and the animal suppresses cortisol.

In an **adrenal tumor form** of Cushing's disease, three out four tumors will not suppress cortisol in the face of higher dexamethasone levels.

Ultrasound

Once hyperadrenocorticism is suspected through routine clinical diagnostics or a Cushing's screening test (i.e., ACTH response test), abdominal ultrasound imaging can help confirm bilaterally enlarged adrenal glands. Ultrasound can help detect the following.

- **Pituitary-dependent disease:** With this form of the disease, an abdominal ultrasound can help confirm enlargement (1–2 times normal size) of both adrenal glands due to increased ACTH production from the pituitary gland.
- **Adrenal tumor:** With this form of the disease, an abdominal ultrasound can help assess if there is moderate enlargement of one adrenal gland and atrophy of the second gland secondary to negative feedback of increasing cortisol levels and decreasing ACTH levels.
- **Pheochromocytoma:** With a pheochromocytoma, an epinephrine-producing tumor of the adrenal medulla, an abdominal ultrasound can reveal a moderate to severe enlargement of one adrenal gland. The other gland is usually a normal size.

Discussing Clinical Diagnostics for Hyperadrenocorticism with the Client
- The veterinarian is recommending initial baseline blood and urinalysis diagnostics to help evaluate your pet for Cushing's disease, which is an overproduction of steroids from the adrenal gland.
- Although baseline blood and urine will not absolutely confirm if Cushing's disease is evident, the diagnostics will help indicate if further testing is needed to confirm the disease. Furthermore, the blood and urine will allow the veterinarian to assess other organ and hormonal disease that could occur secondary to Cushing's disease (i.e., diabetes mellitus).
- If Cushing's disease is suspected, advanced blood work and abdominal imaging may be suggested.
- The proper form of the disease must be diagnosed in order for an appropriate treatment protocol to be recommended.

Hypoadrenocorticism (Addison's Disease)

Primary Addison's disease is more easily diagnosed with routine blood and urine diagnostics. Observable changes in baseline diagnostics can be as follows.

Chemistry

With primary Addison's disease, blood electrolytes are out of balance.

- The patient has decreased levels of sodium and increased concentration of potassium.
- The electrolyte balance is described in a sodium/potassium ratio.
- The normal ratio is more than 25:1 (Na/K); when the ratio of Na/K is less than 23:1, Addison's disease is suspected.

Urinalysis

The ability of the kidneys to concentrate urine is affected due to the decreased sodium in the renal medulla (see Chapter 13). Animals are usually hyposthenuric with a urine specific gravity of less than 1.015.

ACTH Stimulation Test

With animals that may have a questionable sodium/potassium ratio, an ACTH response test is recommended to evaluate the adrenal gland's response to ACTH.

The normal response produces a measurable moderate rise in blood cortisol 2 hours after ACTH administration. In the hypoadrenocortical patient, there is poor response to cortisol levels after stimulation.

Discussing Clinical Diagnostics for Hypoadrenocorticism with the Client
- The veterinarian is recommending initial baseline blood and urinalysis diagnostics to help evaluate your pet for Addison's disease, which is lack of production of steroids from the adrenal gland.
- The veterinarian will evaluate changes in the urine and the blood electrolytes (i.e., sodium and potassium) that could suggest an imbalance in the normal regulation of sodium and expulsion of potassium from the body.
- If Addison's disease is suspected, advanced blood work may be recommended.

Diseases of the Adrenal Gland

Although not all diseases are mentioned below, the common diseases are discussed, with the main goal being to understand and to be able to explain to the client what the diseases are, how they can present themselves, and what the overall short- and long-term concerns are for each disease. Any discussion of overall diagnostic and treatment protocols should be discussed based on the recommendations of the doctor and the medical team. Please use the following information as a basis to discuss and educate the client, *but never to diagnose a patient.*

Hyperadrenocorticism (Cushing's Disease)
Cushing's disease is a hormonal imbalance from overproduction of a prednisone-like steroid, called **cortisol**, in the adrenal glands of the body. Cortisol is normally produced in times of stress to break down protein (muscle) and fat to produce sugar. The release of cortisol is controlled by another hormone, called **ACTH**, from the pituitary.

Etiology
As discussed earlier in this chapter, there are three forms of hyperadrenocorticism.

- **Pituitary-dependent form:** This is the most common form of the disease. In this form, there is an overproduction of pituitary ACTH from microscopic tumors within the pituitary. This causes an overproduction of steroid from *both* adrenal glands.
- **Adrenal-dependent form:** This is a cancerous process in one adrenal gland, causing it to enlarge and overproduce cortisol. The other adrenal gland is atrophied.
- **Iatrogenic form:** This disease is produced in animals on long-term oral or injectable steroids (i.e., prednisone). These patients have been on medications for months to years, and the chronic levels of oral and injectable steroids begin to produce signs of Cushing's disease.

Signalment
The disease is commonly seen in older dogs of both sexes. The breeds with higher prevalence are poodles, dachshunds, Boston terriers, boxers, and beagles. This disease is rare in cats.

Common Points in Medical History
Owners can report a variety of medical complaints with a Cushing's disease patient. *The most common is increased thirst and urination.* Other symptoms can be

- hair loss/alopecia,
- decreased energy,
- increased panting,
- muscle loss, and
- neurologic signs—seizures (rare).

Common Points on Initial Assessment
Affected animals are generally stable, bright, alert, and responsive, but may show the following symptoms on initial assessment:

- Pendulous (hanging) abdomen
- Hair loss, especially over the top of the backbone
- Whole-body generalized muscular wasting
- Increased regions of pigmentation on skin

Complications
Due to chronic hyperglycemia, diabetes mellitus can occur if Cushing's disease is not treated. Furthermore, the chronic release of cortisol can also trigger chronic hypertension or high blood pressure. Patients, even those under control for Cushing's disease, should have their blood pressure routinely monitored.

Diagnosis
As outlined above, clinical diagnostics for Cushing's disease can involve baseline diagnostic blood and urine tests, advanced clinical blood and urine diagnostics, radiography, and abdominal ultrasound.

Treatment
Treatment is based on the presentation of the animal and the type of Cushing's disease evident. In general, overall treatment guidelines are as follows:

- **Pituitary-dependent hyperadrenocorticism:** With pituitary-dependent disease, patients are generally placed on medication that is focused on stopping steroid production in the adrenal glands. These medications are generally needed for the life of the pet. These patients must be closely monitored at regular intervals for normal adrenal function, diabetes, liver disease, and hypertension.

> **Discussing Hyperadrenocorticism with the Client**
> - Each pet has two adrenal glands that sit in front of the kidneys. Their function is to produce adrenaline and specific steroids for emergency situations.
> - Cortisol is produced from the adrenal gland to take muscle and protein and produce sugar. It is stimulated by the hormone ACTH, produced by the pituitary gland of the brain. ACTH is stimulated in response to stress or low blood sugar.
> - Hyperadrenocorticism (Cushing's disease) is an overproduction of the hormone cortisol.
> - The disease is caused by either changes in the pituitary or the adrenal gland itself. The disease can also be associated with the administration of long-term oral or injectable steroids.
> - Initial signs of the disease are increased thirst and urination due to the chronic exposure to prednisone-like steroids.
> - Over time this chronic breakdown of muscle and fat leaves the pet pot-bellied, with a poor hair coat and chronic changes and irritations in the skin.
> - If not diagnosed and properly treated, the pet can have secondary liver disease, diabetes mellitus, chronic skin and urinary tract infections, and high blood pressure (hypertension).

- **Adrenal-dependent hyperadrenocorticism:** With adrenal tumors, a removal of the affected adrenal gland is recommended.
- **Iatrogenic Cushing's disease:** In these patients, to prevent an Addisonian crisis (see below) prednisone medication is slowly reduced over time until the patient is completely weaned off prednisone.

Prevention

There is no way to prevent hyperadrenocorticism. However, through routine wellness blood work and urinalysis of the middle-aged to older pet, Cushing's disease can be detected in its early stages.

Hypoadrenocorticism (Addison's Disease)

Addison's disease is a lack of production of the hormone **aldosterone**. Aldosterone is produced to aid in the reabsorption of sodium and expulsion of potassium from the kidneys.

Etiology

There are several potential causes that can damage the normal adrenal tissue that produces aldosterone.

- **Immune-mediated disease:** The body sends white blood cells to destroy the adrenal gland itself. The cause of this process is unknown.
- **Granulomatous disease:** Infectious diseases produce chronic infection within a specific organ or tissue. In this case, the disease occurs within adrenal tissue, the gland itself can be injured. Fungal infections (i.e., valley fever) can produce these long-standing granulomatous diseases.
- **Overdose of Lysodren medication:** Animals that are treated for Cushing's disease with a medication called Lysodren (Op'DDD) can develop significant destruction of the adrenal cortex.
- **Cancer:** A metastasis from tumor types somewhere else in the body can grow into the adrenal gland.
- **Too rapid a withdrawal of long-term prednisone therapy:** A too-rapid withdrawal of long-term steroidal medication can produce an Addisonian crisis. Patients must be taken off steroid medication slowly to allow the body enough time to restimulate its normal cortisol production. Animals removed too quickly will not resume normal cortisol and aldosterone production and can enter a crisis situation.

Signalment

Addison's disease affects dogs from 1 to 12 years of age and cats from 1 to 9 years of age. Female canines are more predisposed to this syndrome, whereas there is no sex predilection in the cat. Common canine breeds affected by hypoadrenocorticism are standard poodles, great Dane, Portuguese water dogs, West Highland white terriers, and Wheaton terriers.

There is no reported breed predilection in felines.

Common Points in Medical History

Unless the patient has a severe Addisonian crisis, most Addisonian patients may have very mild medical complaints. These can be

- lethargy,
- weakness,
- chronic vomiting/regurgitation (episodic),
- weight loss, and
- increased thirst and urination.

Common Points on Initial Assessment

Animals that are not in an acute crisis may appear normal on initial assessment. Animals in an Addisonian crisis can have the following symptoms:

- Lethargy to sternal recumbence to lateral recumbence
- Slow heart rate (usually less than 60–80 beats per minute)
- Chronic diarrhea
- Increased thirst/urination
- Collapse
- Muscle tremors
- Black tarry stools

Complications

If primary Addison's disease is not diagnosed and treated, patients can enter a life-threatening Addisonian crisis, which leads to hypovolemic shock (see Chapter 30) and, potentially, death.

Diagnosis

As outlined above, clinical diagnostics for hypoadrenocorticism can involve baseline diagnostic blood work and urine and advanced clinical blood diagnostics (i.e., ACTH response test).

Treatment

Treatment is dependent on the presentation and history of the patient.

- **Addisonian crisis:** These animals generally need to be admitted to the hospital for fluid therapy and medication to help rebalance their sodium and potassium levels. These pets may be in shock and severely life-threatened states.
- **Chronic primary Addison's disease:** These animals are stable but will require life-long daily medications or monthly injections to replace the aldosterone and possibly the cortisol not produced by the adrenal glands.

Prevention

There is no way to prevent hypoadrenocorticism. However, through routine wellness blood work and urinalysis of the middle-aged to older pet, Addison's disease can be detected in its early stages, and if treated successfully, it can prevent a life-threatening crisis.

Discussing Primary Hypoadrenocorticism with the Client

- Each pet has two adrenal glands that sit in front of the kidneys. Their function is to produce adrenaline and specific steroids for times of emergency need.

- One such steroid hormone is aldosterone; it is produced in the adrenal gland to stimulate the reabsorption of sodium and expulsion of potassium in the kidney.

- These electrolytes are responsible for producing the body's electric current that produces muscle movement, heart contraction, neuron function, and other necessary body functions.

- Without normal levels of aldosterone and cortisol, the pet cannot respond to stress. These patients can become weak and lethargic (sometimes comatose), have abnormally slow heart rhythms, muscle spasms, low blood pressure, and may collapse.

- If not diagnosed and treated, the pet may enter a crisis situation.

CD-ROM 1 reviews material presented in this chapter. Please try the cases for Section 2 (Anatomy and Physiology—The Science behind the Diseases) *to help reinforce the information presented here.*

Chapter 18

Reproduction

Surgical sterilization, breeding animals, and neonate care can be a large part of the medical team's responsibilities in a busy general practice. It is important to have a good working knowledge of the reproductive system to be able to discuss the importance of sterilization and health concerns of both the male and female pet with the client.

The Female Reproductive Tract

The female reproductive tract comprises

- **reproductive organ:** ovaries;
- **female duct system:** oviducts, uterus, and cervix; and
- **external genitalia:** vagina and vulva.

The **ovaries** are the primary reproductive organ that produces the female gametes (**ova**), as well as the female hormones **progesterone** and **estrogen** (see Figure 18.1).

When the pet is in heat (**estrus**), the maturing ova begin to produce a hormone called estrogen. Increasing estrogen levels are responsible for the physical signs of estrus: swollen, enlarged vulva, attractiveness to the male, a willingness to stand for mounting, and a bloody vaginal discharge. Once the ova have matured, one to several eggs are released into the oviducts and uterus where fertilization takes place. After conception, the embryos implant in the uterine wall and mature through a normal pregnancy cycle. The ovaries are then responsible for producing a hormone called **progesterone,** which helps to maintain the pet's pregnancy.

The Male Reproductive Tract

The male reproductive system consists of

- **reproductive organ:** testes;
- **male duct system:** the epididymis and spermatic cords; and
- **external genitalia:** the penis.

The testicles (see Figure 18.2) are the primary organ of reproduction, producing the male gametes (the **sperm**) and testosterone, the male sex hormone.

In mammals, testes are carried outside the body cavity; they develop behind the kidneys in the fetus, and then descend into the scrotum through the inguinal canal. Normally,

the testicles descend by birth, but they can remain in the inguinal or abdominal region for 6–12 months. Animals without normally descended testicles are called **cryptorchid,** which is a **heritable condition.** If left unresolved, the increased body temperature of the inguinal canal or abdominal cavity can make the testicles more likely to become cancerous in later life. These animals can show normal sexual interest but tend to be infertile.

When the pet reaches puberty, the testicles begin to produce sperm. The early sperm then move into the epididymis where they mature and are stored. During sexual contact, the sperm move through the spermatic ducts into the penis for ejaculation.

The male also has accessory sex glands, which produce secretions for transport and maintenance of the sperm. In the canine, the most important secondary sex gland is the **prostate gland.** This single gland is located around and along the urethra just behind the excretory ducts of the vesicular gland, producing a small amount of fluids for the ejaculate and producing necessary electrolytes to help sperm motility and fertility.

The penis is the external genitalia that encompass a route for both the reproductive and urinary systems. Different species have variations of the penis to help maximize delivery of the sperm.

In the canine, there are two overall specializations.

- **Glans penis:** The glans penis is the region of specialization located in the middle of the penis. It will swell like a balloon prior to and during sexual contact. It prevents premature separation from the female during coitus and increases the chances of fertilization.
- **Os penis:** The male penis contains a bone called the os penis. It is a common site of urinary obstruction secondary to stone formation.

In intact male cats, the feline penis has barbs on the distal surface of the penis; the barbs are there only under the influence of testosterone.

The Reproductive Cycle

Puberty is defined as the age at which a female has a first heat cycle with an ovulation or the age at which the male can produce fertile sperm. The age of puberty varies.

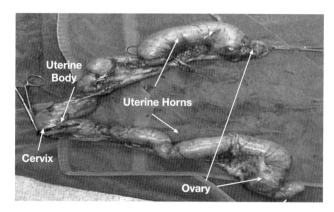

Figure 18.1. Image of an enlarged uterus secondary to infection. Note the normal anatomy of the ovaries and oviducts (encased in the fatty pedicle), the uterine horns, and the uterine body.

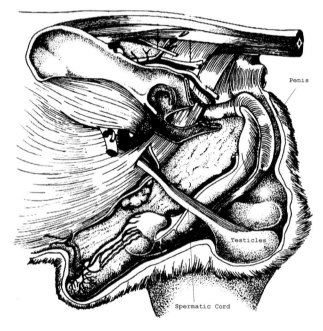

Figure 18.2. Illustration of the male reproductive system. (Image courtesy of *Anatomy of Domestic Animals*, 7th Edition. Pasquini, Chris, and Pasquini, Susan. Sudz Publishing, Pilot Point, TX 1989. Used with permission from Sudz Publishing.)

- **Canine puberty** can range from 4 to 6 months in small dogs and up to 6–8 months in larger dogs.
- **Feline puberty** generally occurs by 4–6 months of age.

The **estrus** or **heat cycle** is defined as the period prior to ovulation and is denoted by the physical signs of heat (i.e., standing to be mounted, interest in the male, vaginal swelling, and discharge).

- **In the canine:** The canine generally comes into heat every 4–6 months, and the length of the heat cycle is 9–30 days.

- **In the feline:** The female will come into heat every 3–4 months for 3–4 weeks at a time.

Most species are spontaneous ovulators, which means there is no one specific event that stimulates ovulation. However, cats and ferrets are **induced ovulators.** These animals will go into heat and become sexually active, but will not ovulate unless sexual contact occurs. The sexual act stimulates a neuroendocrine response that stimulates ovulation. This greatly increases chances of conception with just one sexual encounter.

Species have also developed variations in sexual contact (coitus) to help increase the chance of conception. In dogs, the male will mount, enter, and rotate around the female so they are standing back to back. At this point the animal is said to be "tied" and is unable to separate from the female. It will take at least 20–30 minutes for the tie to break and before the pets are able to separate.

Practice Note: Reproductive behavior of the cat and dog can seem abnormal or strange to new pet owners. These clients may call with very serious concerns about their pet's normal sexual behaviors and anatomy. Some common examples follow.

Example I The owner calls to inform the medical team that their female cat is acting extremely strangely, vocalizing, rolling on the ground, attacking the owner's feet, and then running away. The cat may also be very temperamental. This may suggest normal symptoms of feline estrus.

Example II The owner calls and informs the medical team that they are concerned that their new puppy has a mass on its penis or they are afraid that the pet got bit or stung on its penis. This may suggest the pup has become excited and has inflated its glans penis. In a few minutes, the swelling tends to go away.

Example III An owner calls to inform you that their male and female canines are stuck together and they cannot get separated. Although this is a normal part of coitus, new owners can become very concerned about "tied" pets. Furthermore, owners should be instructed not to try to physically separate these animals.

Although these concerns could suggest other, more serious problems, it is important to discuss with new owners normal sexual habits of intact pups and kittens before they enter puberty.

Pregnancy and Labor

Average pregnancy lengths are as follows.

- Canine: 60–63 days
- Feline: 60 days

The term of expected pregnancy is calculated from the first day of conception. However, because canines may breed on a daily basis, the pregnancy due date can vary up to 5–7 days.

The fetuses mature within the uterus, each in its own placenta. In the first two trimesters of pregnancy (40–46 days), the fetuses mature, specialize, and grow with very little outward changes in the mother. In the last trimester, the pet begins to show signs of pregnancy, which include

- enlargement and engorgement of the mammary tract,
- abdominal distention, and
- behavior changes (late pregnancy); nesting.

As the female canine prepares to enter labor, her progesterone (the hormone of pregnancy) begins to decrease 24–48 hours prior to the initiation of labor. When this occurs, the female's body temperature will drop .5° 24 hours prior to the initiation of labor. If the owner takes the dog's temperature at the same time every day and notices a .5° decrease in temperature, it suggests labor may start within 24–48 hours.

In the dog, there are two phases of labor. The first phase of labor can be seen as early as a day or two before full labor. Common physical symptoms of this phase are

- excitement,
- nest building,
- anxiety,
- decreased appetite,
- vomiting, and
- restlessness.

These signs are caused by changes in the hormone patterns in the animal's body. *This phase can last for a very long time, and the animal can prolong this period indefinitely if she feels nervous or unsure of her environment.*

The second phase of labor starts with the first abdominal contraction. Once this phase begins, the animal is in full labor and there is no way to stop this process. Once abdominal pushing begins,

- if it is the patient's first litter, she should produce a first puppy or kitten within 4 hours and average one kitten or puppy every other hour; and
- if the animal has already had its first litter, she should produce her first offspring within 2 hours and average one kitten or puppy every other hour.

Patients that exceed these time parameters can suggest a problem pregnancy or **dystocia.** These pets should be evaluated by a veterinarian immediately.

All fetuses have an individual placenta around them. Many owners will become concerned when they note one placenta or extra membrane ruptures and the puppies do not quickly pass. Overall, one placenta can rupture and the remaining pups can be very stable. Furthermore, 40% of all canine and feline fetuses are born normally in the breach position. This is a very important point to reinforce with the owner since a breach presentation can suggest a problem with a human pregnancy. Finally, the normal placental pigments are black and green, and this does not suggest problems with the pregnancy.

Discussing Labor with the Client—Key Points

A pet can maintain the first stage of labor indefinitely. Once early signs of labor are displayed, new breeders want to be with the pet continuously from the first signs of nesting until the animals are born. It is important for the client to understand that most times even the most devoted animal wants to be alone during labor. Suggest that the clients make the pet comfortable in her nest and check on her occasionally (i.e., every 30–60 minutes).

Have the clients monitor for the first contraction, which will signal the second stage of labor. Once this occurs the pet should be monitored as follows:

- Females that are having their first litter should have their first pup within 4 hours.
- Females that have had litters before should have a kitten or pup within 2 hours.
- Then, from there the female should have one newborn every 2 hours on average. Females may have two offspring initially and then wait 2–3 hours for another. But on average one should come every 2 hours.

Finally, and most importantly, let the mother handle the newborns.

- Many owners want to help the newborns by breaking the placenta and handling the newborn animal for the mother.
- Unless there is some problem with the mother cleaning the newborn and breaking the placenta themselves, allow nature to take its course. This allows
  —strengthening of the maternal bond,
  —decreases chance of maternal rejection, and
  —prevents bite or injury of owner from protective mother.

Once the newborn is cleaned off and inspected by the mother, the neonate should be allowed to nurse. The female's first milk is a thicker, waxy secretion called **colostrum**. It contains maternal antibodies to help the animal's resistance to disease in the first 5 weeks of life. The mother should be current on vaccinations and have lived in her whelping environment for the last trimester of her pregnancy to make sure she has adequate immunity in her colostrum.

Owners should be encouraged to contact the medical team or local veterinary emergency hospital with any concerns during this process.

Neonate Care

Proper neonatal care and environment are essential for the proper health and growth of the pets. The female should be exposed to the whelping area a few days to a few weeks prior to labor. This allows the pet to get comfortable and relaxed in her whelping environment and, thus, be less likely to try to move the newborns after birth. The area should be clean and free from electrical outlets, hard surfaces where newborns can be crushed, or plants. If the area is portable and light, it makes it easy to clean and dry every few days. A good example is a child's new plastic play pool, which can then be disposed of after 6–8 weeks of use.

Newborn puppies and kittens have very little fat reserves to help them maintain normal body temperature. Their area should be kept at a constant temperature range from 90–95° Fahrenheit (see Figure 18.3). A heat lamp above the whelping area is highly recommended. This will allow the center of the area to be slightly warmer than the outer region; if the newborns are too warm they can lie on the outer area to be cooler. If a safe heat lamp is not available, warm water blankets or warm water bottles (filled with warm bath water) underneath the blankets can help maintain environmental temperature. Although more labor intensive, these systems are safer than heating pads. *Newborns are unable to move away from an uncomfortable heat source and a heating pad can cause pain and severe burns to the skin.*

New pups and kittens should eat 5–8 times per day, sleep, and have normal stool and urine. Newborns in a comfortable environment should sleep on their sides without signs of shivering or piling on each other for warmth. They all should be nursing contently without too much crying. It is recommended that each animal be weighed and identified with a marker (i.e., a spot of colored nail polish works well). This will allow the client to keep track of the daily weight of the newborns. Basic weight guidelines for the neonate are as follows:

- Newborns should gain weight every day or at least maintain weight.
- They should double their birth weight in the first 10 days and then double that weight again by day 20.
- By day 10–14, the pets' eyes should be opening up and they should be more mobile.

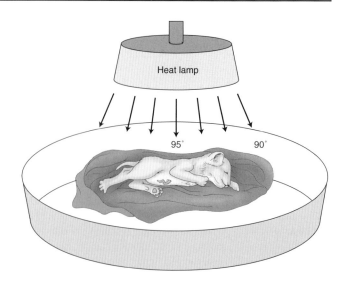

Figure 18.3.   An illustration of an environmental setup for a neonate. Their area should be kept at a constant temperature range from 90 to 95° Fahrenheit.

- By 21–28 days, they should be more active and possibly ready to start another diet, such as milk replacer or soft canned puppy food. Start any dietary supplement at this time slowly, because it can change the stool.
- By day 35–42, pups or kittens should begin weaning onto dry or canned food and are ready for their first vaccines and check of the stool for parasites.

Signs of Neonate Problems
- Newborns will not nurse or cannot suckle.
- Newborns try to nurse but do not seem to get enough nutrition. They cry excessively.
- Newborns do not gain weight daily or do not double weight by day 10.
- Newborns are sleeping on top of each other, shivering and moving very slowly.
- Newborns have a liquid diarrhea.
- Milk keeps appearing at nostrils while newborn is suckling, and the newborn is not growing well or acting right.

Wellness for Pregnant Animals

Creating a preventative wellness plan for a pregnant animal that outlines recommendations for monitoring and care can be an invaluable resource to the client. Some possible recommendations for a wellness program are discussed next.

Prebreeding
All perspective breeding animals should have a prebreeding exam.

The exam should evaluate the pet for chronic or low-lying disease that may affect the pet's ability to become pregnant and maintain pregnancy. Depending on the breeding situation, this may require full blood work to evaluate body and organ function and to test for infectious diseases.

In canines that are used primarily for breeding, a blood test for the infectious disease brucellosis may be required. Brucellosis is a sexually transmitted disease producing infertility in the male and abortion and fetal death in the female. Furthermore, felines should be tested for feline leukemia and feline immunodeficiency virus prior to breeding to prevent spread of the diseases to the newborn kittens.

The exam should identify any congenital disease that may potentially discourage the owner from breeding the pet. Some examples of concern regarding congenital disease are

- hip dysplasia (see Chapter 8),
- luxating patella (see Chapter 8),
- a propensity for demodectic mange (see Chapter 19),
- history of cryptorchid males in the family line, and
- pets with jaw length abnormalities.

During the exam all vaccines should be updated. Vaccines may have a small chance of affecting the developing embryo or producing a systemic reaction; vaccinations are not generally recommended in the pregnant animal. All female patients should be brought up to date on vaccines for all regional infectious diseases to help promote a strong immunity for their newborns.

Pregnancy Interval
Medications
Specific medications should be avoided in the pregnant animal. Some medications (i.e., steroids) can lead to early abortion, whereas others may produce side effects in the neonates. *All medications (prescribed and over the counter) should be discussed with the veterinarian.*

Physical Examination
The schedule for examinations may vary from doctor to doctor, but in general the following schedule is suggested.

- **Day 21–24: Ultrasound detection of pregnancy.** Although not always a required exam, an ultrasound exam can pick up early fetal heart beats in puppies and kittens. This exam is recommended for animals that have had a previous problem with conception.
- **Day 25–30: A thorough physical exam.** An exam can evaluate the mother for any early signs of disease and further help detect a dilated enlarged uterus.
- **Day 55: X-rays of the abdomen.** At this time, an x-ray is safe for the mother and may be used to determine fetal size and number. Generally, two views of the abdomen are recommended to get a close estimate of the number of newborns expected, as well as to get an estimation of fetus size (see Figure 18.4). This is also an excellent time to go over the stages of labor, neonate care, and what to expect and what should be monitored with the client.

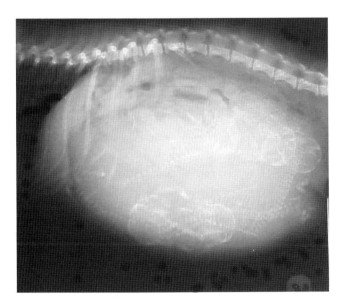
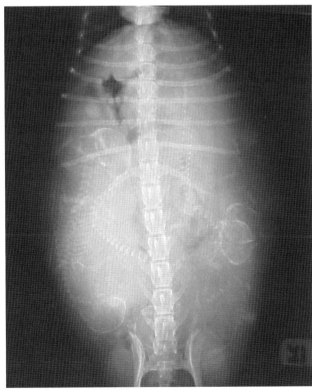

Figure 18.4. An x-ray image of the abdomen of a pregnant canine. At day 55, the fetal skeletons can be imaged, a number of pups can be estimated, and the fetuses can be evaluated for size in relation to pelvic canal width to indicate if there may a dystocia.

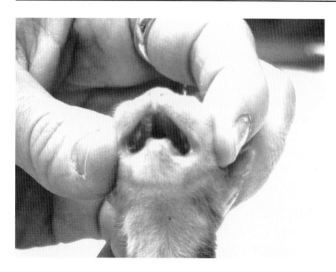

Figure 18.5. Image of a complete cleft palate, a congenital opening from the roof of the mouth and the nasal cavity.

Newborn Interval
Medications
There are many medications that can have significant levels of drug buildup in the milk and affect the newborn animals. While the female is lactating, *all medications should be discussed with the veterinarian.*

Physical Examination

- **Day 1—After pregnancy:** The mom and newborns should all be examined and their health status should be checked. Each neonate should be examined for congenital abnormalities, such as cleft palate, limb abnormalities, etc. (see Figure 18.5). Also, all pups should be weighed and identified so that the clients can continue to monitor weight in the next 10 days.
- **Day 3–4:** Tails and dewclaws should be removed from newborn pups if needed.
- **Day 10:** All newborns should be rechecked to evaluate their weight, which should be a 100% increase above the birth weight. Any problems or concerns about mother and newborn animals should be discussed with the client.
- **Day 20:** Recheck all newborns and make sure there is a 100% increase in weight from day 10. Any problems or concerns should be discussed with the client about mother and newborn animals.
- **Day 42:** Puppy or kitten fecal evaluations and first vaccines.

Obtaining a Medical History for Reproductive Disease

Reproductive problems usually fall into two categories: reproductive failure and pregnancy problems and primary disease of the reproductive system. Reproductive disease and pregnancy problems focus on the diagnosis of infertility in the pet. Because almost any chronic disease can produce reproductive failure, a systemic approach in the evaluation of all the patient's systems must be taken by the veterinarian. Many veterinarians will have specific, thorough questionnaires that may help delineate the failure in reproduction. This chapter will not focus on reproductive failure and pregnancy issues.

Primary reproductive disease refers to problems within the urogenital system. These diseases can occur secondary to pregnancy, the age of the animal, and if the animal remains intact in its later life. The following questions aid in obtaining a thorough history in patients with reproductive disease.

- **What is the age of the animal?** Reproductive disease tends to affect middle-aged to older animals. However, there are some forms of vaginitis or vulvitis that can be seen in young pets.
- **Is the pet spayed or neutered, and if so when was this done?** Late-spayed and neutered animals can still have significant tumors and disease of the reproductive tract. Some owners may not know if the animal has been spayed or neutered (i.e., animals are adoptions or strays).
- **When was the last heat cycle in the female dog?** Chronic infections or full-blown infections of the uterus (pyometra) can be seen 1–2 months after the last heat cycle. Furthermore, lack of a heat cycle can suggest hormonal imbalance, such as thyroid disease, liver disease, and kidney disease.
- **Is the pet straining to urinate or dripping urine?** This can be a sign of prostate disease (male) or a urinary tract disease.
- **Is the pet dripping blood from its penis or vagina?** Male dogs with prostate disease, pets with urinary obstruction, or patients with a vaginal or a bladder tumor can also drip blood.
- **When, if ever, was your pet last bred?** Animals who have been multiply bred can be open to sexually transmitted disease: that is, brucellosis (canine), transitional venereal tumor (TVT), feline immunodeficiency virus, or feline leukemia virus.
- **Is the animal still showing signs of heat or acting like they are constantly in heat?** This can suggest ovarian or uterine disease, infection, or cancer.
- **Is the animal having a progressive vaginal discharge?** Any vaginal discharge in an intact or spayed female is abnormal and should be discussed with the veterinarian.
- **What is the reproductive history of the pet?** Finding out a full history of breeding and pregnancy is important to determine if the pet has had past problems becoming pregnant or if it has had a history of abortion or dystocia.
- **Does the vulva show a progressive swelling or mass?** Small to large vegetative or round masses can suggest a tumor, polyp, or overproduction of the normal tissue of the vagina.

- **Is there any coughing, sneezing, diarrhea, vomiting, increased thirst (polyuria), or polydipsia (C/S/V/D/ PU/PD)?** Other systemic signs may help you discriminate whether the reproductive concerns are a primary reproductive disease or secondary to other systemic illness. Furthermore, animals with **pyometra** (massive infection of the uterus) often show vomiting, anorexia and increased thirst.

Initial Assessment of Pets with Reproductive Disease

Depending on the type of disease and the sex of the patient, reproductive illness can show a variety of symptoms. It is important for the team member to closely monitor these patients because some reproductive diseases (i.e., pyometra) can produce potential life-threatening states (see Table 18.1). Key elements to observe in the initial assessment of these syndromes are as follows.

- **Fever:** Fever can suggest an infectious or metabolic disease affecting the reproductive or mammary system in the female. Fever may also suggest inflammation, infection, or cancer of the prostate in the male.
- **Muscle spasm/rigidity:** Certain reproductive disorders (i.e., **eclampsia**, see below) can produce severe muscular spasms and rigidity in lactating female dogs. Some patients may be so rigid they have a sawhorse-like stance (see Figure 18.8 in the eclampsia section).
- **Weakness/dehydration:** This may suggest a systemic illness stemming from the reproductive system (i.e., pyometra).
- **Discharge from the reproductive organs:** Drainage or discharge can suggest normal physiology, infection, inflammation, and cancer. Any obvious external discharge should be collected by cotton swab or in a sterile collection vial in case the sample is needed for clinical diagnostics.
- **Swelling, heat, or pain from the mammary tract:** This can suggest an infection (**mastitis**) or cancer of the mammary glands (see Figure 18.9 in the mastitis section).

Clinical Diagnostics of the Reproductive System

The core of clinical diagnostics for reproductive disease is baseline blood work, urinalysis, cytology, radiology, and possibly ultrasonic examination. Although clinical outcomes may vary depending on medical diseases, a general overview of reproductive diagnostics follows.

Complete Blood Count

The complete blood count may be normal; however, with concerns of infection (i.e., pyometra) there can be sharp elevations in the white blood cell population secondary to infection.

Table 18.1. Triage concerns in the reproductive patient.

Systems	Trouble Signs That Indicate an Emergency Situation
Mentation	Nonresponsive/comatose
Fever	Temp <99° (due to shock, DIC, coma) or Temp >104° secondary to infection or muscular tremors
Hydration	Dehydration >5–7%
Gum color	Pink to pale pink (poor perfusion)
Capillary refill time (CRT)	CRT >2–3 seconds
Heart rate/pulse	Rate: Heart rates <80 bpm (eclampsia) or >200 bpm (early shock) Pulse: Pulses can have normal to decreased quality dependent if the pet is in shock.
Muscular activity	Animal is having uncontrolled muscular tremors and spasms.
Vulvar/penile discharge	Evidence of purulent (pus), sanguineous (blood), or serosanguineous (serum and blood) discharge

Chemistry
There is no clinical diagnostic assay for reproductive organs available. Unlike human medicine where assays have become available (i.e., PSA for prostate disease), the chemistry does not rule in or out reproductive disease. However, with eclampsia (see below), significant **hypocalcemia** (low body calcium) can be observed.

Urinalysis
Urinalysis helps to differentiate diseases of the reproductive organs with that of the lower urinary tract. Urine samples obtained by cystocentesis and catheter can help distinguish changes in the urine that are occurring in the bladder and kidney versus through the urethra and reproductive organs.

Cytology
Cytological evaluation of vulvar or penile discharge can aid in the diagnosis of reproductive disease.

Radiology
Abdominal radiographs are evaluated for changes in the internal reproductive organs or pregnancy. Furthermore, with concerns of possible mammary tumors, radiographic evaluation of the thorax (**metastasis protocol**; see Chapter 25) may be recommended to evaluate the lung fields for obvious metastatic tumors.

Ultrasound
Abdominal ultrasound is an excellent resource for evaluating reproductive organs for pregnancy, infection, or cancer. In specific cases, fine needle aspirates or biopsy can be completed in conjunction with an ultrasound examination.

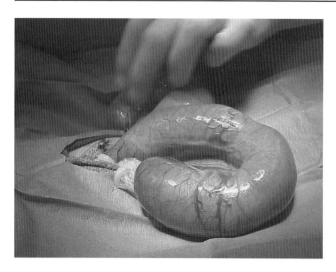

Figure 18.6. Image of a pyometra. This uterus is severely infected and filled with purulent (pus) debris. If not treated, the infection may cause erosion of the uterine wall and spillage of the infectious debris into the abdomen. This can set up a massive infection of the abdomen (peritonitis) and a potential life-threatening condition.

Diseases of the Reproductive System

Although not all diseases are mentioned below, the common reproductive diseases are discussed with the focus being to understand and explain to the client what the diseases are, how they can present themselves, and what can be the short- and long-term concerns of each disease. Any discussion of overall diagnostic and treatment protocols should be discussed based upon the recommendations from the doctor and the medical team. The following information is a basis to discuss and educate the client, *but never a tool to diagnose a patient.*

Pyometra

A pyometra is a severe overwhelming infection of the uterus of a female intact dog. As a female pet goes in and out of heat cycles over years, low-grade infections of the uterine lining may occur (**endometritis**). Eventually, the uterus can become overwhelmed with the infection and can fill with purulent debris (pus), acting much like a human appendicitis (see Figure 18.6). The uterus may become so infected and enlarged that it can rupture, causing a massive and life-threatening infection of the abdomen, **peritonitis**.

Signalment

Pyometra is typically seen in both older intact female dogs and cats, but it can occur in young animals (2–3 years of age), as well.

Etiology

Pyometra is caused by chronic infection of the uterus that eventually produces a massive infection, filling the uterus

with pus and debris. On occasion in spayed females, infection of the remaining uterine stump can occur, causing signs similar to a full-blown pyometra; this is called a **stump-pyometra** infection.

Common Points in Medical History

A pyometra is a severe whole-body infection (**sepsis**) producing moderately to severely ill patients that are depressed, listless, anorexic, vomiting, and have increased thirst. Symptoms can appear acutely.

Common Points on Initial Assessment

Affected animals can be severely ill, dehydrated, and depressed. There is commonly vulvar swelling, with purulent vaginal discharge that can have a severe fetid odor. Animals can have significant fevers (>104.5° Fahrenheit). Furthermore, the patient's abdomen may be distended and painful.

Complications

If not aggressively treated, pyometra can rupture through the uterus, producing a massive peritonitis and potentially death.

Diagnosis

The diagnosis of pyometra is based on medical history, physical signs, and the following possible changes in clinical diagnostics.

- **Complete blood count:** In most cases, patients will have a significant rise in white blood cells, suggesting a massive infection. If a blood smear is made (see Chapter 21), increased band neutrophils may be observed, suggesting an acute massive infection.
- **Cytology:** Degenerate neutrophils and bacteria can be observed on cytology of the vaginal discharge.
- **Radiographs:** Abdominal radiographs can show a large distended mass craniodorsal to the bladder (see Figure 18.7).

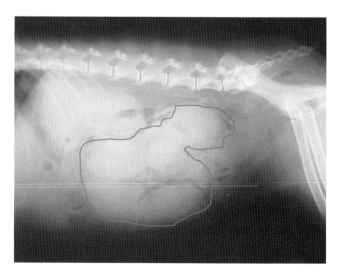

Figure 18.7. Radiographic image of a pyometra. Notice the large soft-tissue density in the caudal abdomen.

- **Ultrasound:** Abdominal ultrasound can reveal an enlarged or distended fluid-filled uterus suggestive of infection.

Treatment

The goal of treatment is to resolve the uterine infection or to surgically remove the infected uterus while supporting the pet with medications and fluids for the massive bacterial infection. With severe pyometra, surgery is usually recommended due to the concern of uterine perforation and peritonitis.

Prevention

A complete ovariohysterectomy at a young age helps prevent pyometra.

Discussing Pyometra with the Client

- A pyometra is an overwhelming infection of the uterus whereby the uterus fills with purulent debris and pus.
- Much like human appendicitis, the chronically infected uterus can rupture and can spill the infection into the abdomen, producing a life-threatening infection of the abdomen (peritonitis).
- Pyometra is common in older intact female pets. The hormone interactions that are produced in the normal heat cycle can set up a chronic reoccurring infection in the uterus. As the pet ages, the infection can become overwhelming and produce a pyometra.
- Diagnosis of a pyometra can be focused on routine blood work, cytology of vaginal discharge, and abdominal imaging.
- With severe bacterial infection and concern of uterine rupture, treatment may be focused on fluid support, medication, and surgical removal of the infected uterus.
- Although similar to a spay surgery, pyometra surgery removes a much larger infected uterus and ovaries from the abdomen. The surgery is much longer and more complicated, and the uterus must be handled very carefully so as not to produce a rupture.
- If the pyometra is severe and the pet ruptures the uterus, the resulting infection can make the pet very ill and life threatened.
- *The best way to prevent pyometra is to spay the female pet while young.*

Eclampsia

Eclampsia, or **postparturient hypocalcemia,** is a serious condition affecting the canine shortly after pregnancy. When the female begins to produce milk (**lactation**), the body's stores of calcium drop quickly. Calcium is needed by almost every cell in the body to control cellular activity, aid in muscular contraction, help heart function, and aid nerve conduction, as well as other body functions. With the demands of lactation, the calcium levels fall so rapidly that the patient cannot compensate, and the muscular, cardiac, and neurologic systems are severely affected.

Signalment

The disease is more common in small breed dogs and is more predominant in the animal's pregnancy with its first litter. The disease is rare in cats.

Etiology

Eclampsia is caused by an increased demand on body calcium for lactation. Large litter size, improper diet, and improper calcium supplementation after birth can cause the pet's body to be unable to keep up with its calcium needs.

Common Points in Medical History

Symptoms come on acutely and the owners will report the following:

- Restlessness
- Nervousness
- Whining
- Walking stiffly

Common Points in Initial Assessment

Pets can be severely affected and can present with the following signs:

- Muscular tremors
- Walking stiffly (see Figure 18.8)
- Seizure-like activity
- Rapid respiratory rates
- Convulsions
- High body temperature (secondary to muscular spasms)

Complications

Eclampsia can produce a life-threatening syndrome of muscle spasms, irregular heart rhythms, and high body temperatures if not diagnosed and treated.

Diagnosis

The diagnosis is based on history, physical signs, and evidence of a low blood calcium level in the blood chemistry panel.

Treatment

Pets can be severely affected and often require hospitalization, intravenous fluids, and calcium supplementation. The newborns are generally weaned and placed on milk replacer because of the concern of continued hypocalcemia.

Prevention

There is no way to predict if a female pet will become eclamptic. However, small pets with larger litters should be

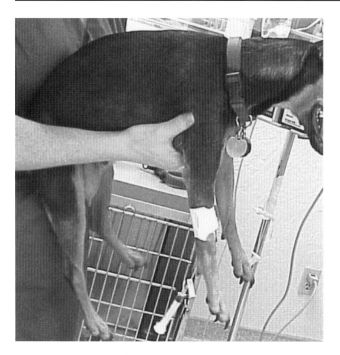

Figure 18.8. Image of a female dog with eclampsia. Notice the rigid limbs and sawhorse position evident. This patient is unable to have normal muscle contraction and is rigid and stiff.

monitored carefully. Supplementation with calcium after birth in early lactation can help blood calcium levels. However, it may be recommended that the patient be spayed if severe eclamptic episodes occur.

Mastitis

Mastitis is the inflammation or infection of the mammary chain in dogs and cats. Mastitis is caused by infectious bacteria entering the gland ascending from the teat, a topical injury to the mammary chain, or from bloodborne infections of the body.

Signalment

Infections are typically associated with female dogs and cats after birth when animals are lactating.

Etiology

The cause of mastitis is a bacterial infection or a general inflammation of the mammary gland. If the infection is severe enough, it can cause a life-threatening whole-body infection (sepsis).

Common Points in Medical History

Affected animals can act sore and sensitive to touch or lifting from the ventral abdomen. Pets may be anorexic, depressed, and lethargic because of infection. Owners may report that the puppies or kittens are not nursing well and are constantly hungry.

Common Observations in Initial Assessment

These patients present with mammary glands of variable size and swelling and firmness affecting one gland to the entire chain or both chains. There can be evidence of bloody, purulent (pus), or fetid discharge from the mammary masses. The chains can be painful or hot to the touch. Pets may also have mild to moderate fevers (see Figure 18.9).

Discussing Eclampsia with the Client
- Eclampsia is a metabolic disease of the lactating female generally in the first 2 weeks after pregnancy.
- The disease is caused by the increasing demand of calcium for the milk.
- Calcium is an element needed by the body for muscular contraction, heart movement, electrical conduction of nerves and many other normal body functions.
- With excessively low calcium levels, the body cannot maintain normal function and pets become severely stiff, can have muscle spasms and seizures, and have elevated body temperature secondary to prolonged muscular activity.
- Diagnostic blood work does indicate low blood calcium levels and aids in the diagnosis of eclampsia.
- If not diagnosed and aggressively treated, affected animals can become life threatened, shocky, and die.
- If eclampsia is severe, the newborns may need to be weaned to prevent this episode from occurring again in this lactation.
- Females with larger litters, especially small pets, should be carefully monitored and potentially supplemented with calcium in early lactation.

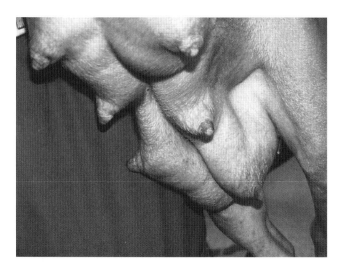

Figure 18.9. Image of hot, swollen, painful mammary glands secondary to mastitis

Complications

Mastitis can greatly affect milk production and normal nutrition, health, and weight gain in the newborn if not diagnosed and treated. Severe mastitis can produce abcessation of the mammary gland, loss of a gland or mammary chain, and possible whole-body infection (sepsis).

Diagnosis

Diagnosis of mastitis is based upon history, physical examination, elevations in the white blood cell count suggestive of infection, and cytology of the milk.

Treatment

Treatment can vary depending on one gland or multiple glands being affected. The goal of treatment is to stop milk production in the affected glands while controlling and eliminating the infection.

Isolating the infected mammary glands or chain is necessary to prevent the newborns' access to the affected glands. In many cases the pet may need to have the affected mammary glands wrapped (i.e., with a T-shirt) to prevent the newborns from nursing on the infected gland. With severe infection, the pups or kittens may have to be weaned early and placed on milk replacer. The lack of nursing will stop lactation in those chains.

Discussing Mastitis with the Client

- Mastitis is a localized infection of one mammary gland, one mammary chain, or both chains.
- The disease is caused by bacteria invading the localized gland, trauma to the mammary chain, or from a whole-body infection.
- The infection sours and infects the milk, so that newborns will not suckle from the infected glands. The newborns will try to suckle and not be able to get adequate nutrition, begin to cry and act hungry, and eventually loose weight and energy.
- Affected pets can be depressed, lethargic, and anorexic. They may be very sensitive to touch on the abdomen. The glands can also be very painful, swollen, and hot to the touch.
- Diagnosis of mastitis is based on history, physical exam, and changes in the milk and blood that can suggest infection.
- Treatment is focused on isolating the infected gland from the newborns and treating the infection. In severe cases, the newborns may need to be weaned and placed on milk replacer.
- If not diagnosed, newborns can become weak, loose body mass, and can die. The female can have severe infection and abcessation of the mammary chain and can have a severe life-threatening bacterial infection.

The infection is controlled by placing the patient on antibiotics and hot packing the mammary gland once to twice a day. With more severe sepsis, the patient may need to be admitted to the hospital for fluid support, intravenous antibiotics, and monitoring.

Prevention

There is no known way to prevent mastitis. Careful monitoring of the female pet and the mammary chain, and preventing injury, can help detect and treat mastitis before it becomes a severe sepsis.

Canine/Feline Mammary Tumors

Mammary tumors are benign or malignant growths of the mammary tissue and the tubular epithelium. Malignant adenocarcinomas of the mammary chain can be fast growing, metastasize to the body rapidly, and are life threatening.

Signalment

Mammary tumors are generally observed in intact female pets more than 5 years of age. However, less commonly, mammary tumors have been reported in spayed females and male pets.

Etiology

The causes of mammary masses are unknown but generally linked to chronic stimulation of the mammary chain associated with the pet's heat cycle. **Masses can be benign or malignant.** Malignant mammary tumors do metastasize rapidly, typically going into the local lymph nodes and then into the lung fields, although mammary tumors can also metastasize to other tissue (liver, spleen, kidneys, etc.).

Common Points in Medical History

Owners will usually present the pet with a concern of a focal swelling on the chest or abdomen. Masses can range from pea-sized to a large grapefruit. The tumor can be producing a bloody/purulent (pus) discharge and may be painful on palpation. In more severely affected animals, the owner may discuss concerns of weight loss, decreased energy, and cough.

Common Observations in Initial Assessment

Pets will present with a focal mass in the mammary chain. Other symptoms can be

- weight loss,
- poor body mass,
- chronic cough, and
- enlarged lymph nodes.

Complications

If not diagnosed, malignant mammary tumors can metastasize to the lungs and chest and produce a life-threatening cancer.

Diagnosis

Diagnosis is based on physical presence of the tumor, clinical diagnostics, fine-needle aspirate or surgical biopsy of the mass. Some possible recommended diagnostics follow.

- **Complete blood count/chemistry:** Although blood work is beneficial to evaluate the pet for surgical risk, underlying disease, or infection, *there is no blood test available for the detection of mammary cancer.*
- **Radiographs—metastasis screen:** Radiographic evaluation of the chest for obvious tumors within the lung fields is strongly recommended to evaluate for potential metastasis (see Chapter 25). If tumor masses are observable, systemic cancer is already evident, and the patient is a significant anesthetic risk.

Fine-Needle Aspirate versus Surgical Biopsy

Fine-needle aspirate of the mass can suggest benign versus malignant tissue. However, fine-needle aspirates sample only hundreds of cells out of millions. If an area of the mass aspirated does not show a malignant region, this could produce a false-negative test.

The presence of a mammary tumor can warrant the recommendation of excision and histopathology. *It is extremely important for the mass to be evaluated and its margins examined.* If the mass is malignant, the mass should be completely removed, along with one-quarter inch of normal tissue around it. Although this does reduce the chance of regrowth, it does not eliminate the possibility, and the region should be continued to be monitored.

Discussing Mammary Tumors with the Client
- Mammary tumors are a concern in intact older female patients.
- Although masses can be benign, there is a high percentage that can be malignant and metastasize to the lungs and the body.
- Once detected, the patient should be evaluated with clinical blood work and urinalysis to evaluate the pet for other infectious, metabolic and organ disease, as well as evaluating the pet for anesthetic risk.
- The veterinarian may also recommend chest radiographs to evaluate the chest for obvious metastatic masses to the lungs. If lung masses are visibly present, it can make the prognosis of survival poor and make the patient a poor anesthetic risk.
- Once surgically removed, the masses should be sent in for histopathology to evaluate the mass and determine if the surgical margins are clean of any malignant tissue. Although a clean margin of a malignant tumor carries a better prognosis, it does not eliminate the possibility of tumor regrowth or metastasis.

Treatment

The presence of a mammary mass warrants surgical removal and biopsy. A **mastectomy** is a removal of a section of the mammary chain. The surgical procedure requires that the area of affected mammary chain, the teats overlying the gland, and a large area around the affected tissue is taken. This may remove a large area of tissue overlaying the abdomen. Once removed, the subcutaneous layer and skin are closed. If there is a large area of tissue removed, a plastic drain may be placed within the incision to allow the surgical site to drain debris as the body heals (see Figure 18.10).

Chemotherapy or radiation therapy may be available depending on the type of tumor and its location.

Prevention

The best way to prevent mammary tumors is to spay the female patient before its first heat cycle (less than 6 months of age). It has been shown that pets spayed before their first heat have eight times less chance of developing mammary tumors than an intact female. Females spayed before 2 years of age have four times less change of developing mammary tumors.

Prostate Disease

The prostate is a secondary sex organ located behind the bladder that secretes fluid into the ejaculate for nutrition and protection of the sperm. In males with exposure to chronic testosterone, the prostate can enlarge, become infected, or possibly become cancerous over the pet's lifetime (see Figure 18.11).

Signalment

Enlargement of the prostate is seen in male dogs between 1 and 16 years of age, with mean age of 7–11 years. It occurs only in the male and seems to occur more commonly in Doberman pinschers.

Etiology

There are many causes of prostatic enlargement in dogs and cats. Some causes can be as follows.

- **Infections:** Bacterial infections and abcessation can occur as bacteria ascend the urethra from the penis or descend from a urinary tract infection. Once seated, a painful systemic infection can occur. Chronic fungal or granulomatous prostatis is rare.
- **Cancer:** Male dogs can have prostatic adenocarcinoma occur. This tumor can spread to the regional lymph nodes, lungs, and skeleton.
- **Benign enlargement:** The prostate will enlarge due to chronic stimulation of testosterone.

Common Points on Medical History

Patients present with a concern of inappropriate urination, pain while urinating, the presence of blood or pus dripping from the penis, and possibly pain while rising or going up or down stairs.

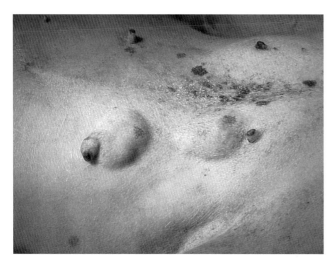

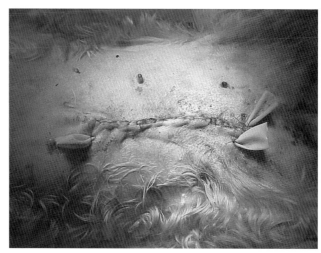

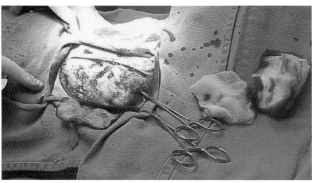

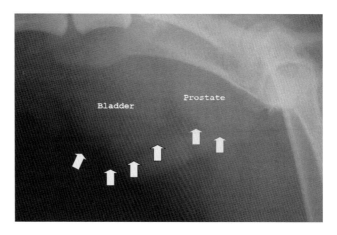

Figure 18.10. Images of a surgical mastectomy. Note how large an incision is needed to remove these two smaller nodules. With this procedure, the masses, the skin, the teats, and large amounts of tissue are removed and submitted for biopsy.

Common Observations in Initial Assessment
Clinical signs of prostatic disease can be

- frank blood or purulent debris (pus) from the penis,
- fever,
- depression, and
- having trouble defecating.

Complications
If not diagnosed and treated, infectious or benign enlarge-ment produce continued signs, discomfort, and potential persistent infection. If prostatic adenocarcinoma is present, the disease can metastasize to lymph nodes and other organ systems. This progression may still occur with treatment.

Diagnosis
Diagnosis of prostatic disease can be made through the fol-lowing possible diagnostics.

- **Rectal palpation:** Rectal palpation to check for prostate size and sensitivity can aid in the diagnosis of prostatic disease.
- **Blood work:** Changes in routine blood work can suggest changes in the prostate. Increases in the white blood cell population can indicate whole-body infection or inflam-mation stemming from prostatic disease. *There is no PSA testing available for animals.*

Figure 18.11. Image of an enlarged prostate (lightly shaded arrows) caudal to the bladder (white arrows).

- **Urinalysis:** Urinalysis can suggest blood, protein, and cells that may support a prostatic disease.
- **Radiographs:** Caudal abdominal radiographs can suggest enlargement of the prostate caudal dorsal to the bladder. Radiographic prostatic enlargement cannot differentiate between infection, inflammation, or cancer of the prostate.
- **Ultrasound:** Abdominal ultrasound can help evaluate prostatic size and shape and ultrasonic fine-needle aspi-rates can be taken to determine the disease process.

Treatment

Treatment is based on the type of disease evident.

- **Neutering:** Chronic testosterone stimulation can produce inflammation and irritation of the prostate. By removing the testicles and decreasing testosterone levels, prostatic swelling can decrease. This can be curative for benign prostatic enlargement.
- **Medications:** Antibiotics can help in reducing infected enlarged prostates.
- **Surgery:** With adenocarcinoma of the prostate, surgical excision is possible.

Prevention

The likelihood of prostatic disease can be decreased by neutering young male pets.

Discussing Prostate Disease with the Client
- Disease of the prostate is common in middle-aged to older adult male dogs.
- Prostatic disease can be infectious, cancerous, or secondary to chronic testosterone stimulation.
- Physical symptoms of disease are inappropriate urination, dripping blood/pus, pain or discomfort while urinating, and occasionally pain getting up and down.
- The veterinarian may recommend blood work, urinalysis, radiographs, and abdominal ultrasound exam to evaluate the prostate for changes suggestive of disease.
- Depending on the type of disease, prostate problems can usually be controlled with neutering the male pet and medication. Occasionally with prostatic cancer more in-depth procedures may need to be recommended.

CD-ROM 1 reviews material presented in this chapter. Please try the cases for Section 2 (Anatomy and Physiology—The Science behind the Diseases) *to help reinforce the information presented here.*

Chapter 19

Integument

Introduction

This chapter will focus on skin diseases, with an emphasis on diagnostic approaches, an overview of treatment options, and client education. The anatomy and physiology of the skin will be discussed in the disease section of this chapter and will be limited to changes in the skin architecture. Because skin is one of the first organ systems affected in many systemic diseases, the medical team must pay close attention to medical history, initial assessment, and clinical diagnostics to help the veterinarian determine if there is a primary or secondary disease state occurring. Some examples of diseases that can affect the skin but that are not primary skin diseases are

- nutritional disease/deficiency,
- chronic infectious disease,
- intestinal parasitism,
- kidney disease,
- liver disease,
- hormonal disease, and
- cancer.

Some of these skin diseases (i.e., ringworm and sarcoptic mange) can be zoonotic, thus causing infection in humans. Although the diseases produced are usually not serious, they can cause discomfort, itching, and irritation. These infections can be picked up when the spores of the fungi or the skin mite come in contact with the skin. Furthermore, some animals with ringworm can be chronic carriers and may not show any physical symptoms. Any patient with hair loss, flaking of the skin, or itchy (**pruritic**) skin should also be treated as a potential suspect. If a zoonotic disease is suspected, gloves should be worn when handling the pet, and the team member should wash well after contact. *Most importantly, when discussing the potential diseases with the owners, make them aware of the zoonotic concerns, and document this discussion in the chart.*

Obtaining a History in Patients with Skin Disease

A great deal of the diagnosis depends on a strong history gained through physical examination and appropriate diagnostic testing. With chronic skin disease, patients may have seen a number of veterinarians and been placed on many treatments, which can include injectable and oral medications, food trials, and topical treatments. When encountering a new patient with chronic skin problems, it is essential to get a full and detailed history. Some medical teams have developed a dermatologic questionnaire that can be given to clients before the appointment time and filled out at home. These questionnaires help start the diagnostic process. These questions are presented next.

When Did the First Signs Occur?
Documenting when signs first occurred in the patient's life can give the veterinarian an understanding of how chronic this problem is.

What Other Treatment Has the Pet Had?
The owner should be encouraged to bring in all previous medication or records that relate to past treatments. Furthermore, the client should be questioned about how effective each treatment was in controlling or eliminating the physical symptoms.

Does Your Pet Have a Reoccurrence of Skin Problems Seasonally?
Seasonal skin changes can suggest an allergenic problem when the grass and weed pollens may be at highest levels in the environment.

Does the Pet Stay Mainly Inside or Outside?
Outside pets have more exposure to vegetation and soils. Inside animals have more exposure to detergents and topical cleaners on floors, carpets, furniture, and to house dust mites. Changes in these environments could suggest the beginning of a topical allergy or new sensitivity (i.e., rug shampoos, new grass/trees, lawn treatments, etc.).

Does Your Pet Have Problems with Fleas and Ticks?
Chronic tick or flea infestation and other ectoparasites can produce skin problems and irritations.

Have There Been Changes in Topical Medications Used on Your Pet?
Changes in hair and coat products (i.e., shampoos, conditioners, topical medications, topical oils, etc.) can produce dry skin, irritation, and itchiness (**pruritus**).

What Diet Has Your Pet Been on and For How Long?
Food allergies can stem from long-term dietary exposure. Getting a history of what types of diets and for how long the animal has been on them can help the veterinarian determine if food sensitivity may be present.

Is Your Pet on Any Dietary Supplements?
Certain types of dietary supplements can produce changes in the skin and other body systems.

Has Your Pet Shown Any Signs of Systemic Disease?
Coughing, sneezing, vomiting, diarrhea, increased thirst, and increased urination can suggest other systemic and hormonal diseases that may secondarily affect the integument.

Has There Been a History of Weight Change or Chronic Obesity?
History of significant weight loss (more than 5%) in a short period could suggest other systemic or hormonal disease. Further, chronic obesity may suggest other hormonal diseases (i.e., canine hypothyroidism)

Are There Any Other Animals in the Household?
Are the other animals present in the household healthy? Other pets with similar symptoms may suggest a potential infectious or parasitic disease.

Physical Changes in the Hair Coat Noticeable on Initial Assessment

The key to understanding and explaining dermatologic conditions is that the same physical symptoms can be evident in many different types of skin disease. Common symptoms are presented here.

- **Erythema:** Redness of the skin secondary to inflammation, infection, or allergy. The redness can be localized or generalized, depending on the condition (see Figure 19.1).
- **Pruritus:** Pruritus is generalized itchiness secondary to infection, allergy, topical irritation, and inflammation. Pruritus can be localized to a specific region (i.e., head and ears) or generalized all over the body. Severe pruritus can make the animal scratch so severely that the patient can damage the hair coat and skin (see Figure 19.2).
- **Alopecia:** Hair loss can be a primary concern from hormonal and nutritional disease or secondary to pruritus (see Figure 19.3).
- **Pustules:** Pustules can occur due to bacterial, parasitic, or fungal infection but can also be due to immune-mediated skin conditions (see Figure 19.4).
- **Excoriation:** Excoriations occur when the skin is damaged into its deeper layers, producing a red, inflamed, moist lesion. Excoriation is secondary to pruritus and secondary to allergy, infection, or topical irritation (see Figure 19.5).

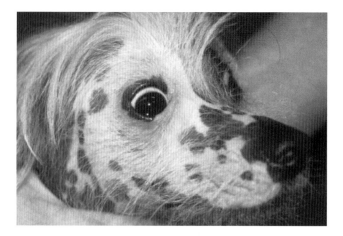

Figure 19.1. Image of a patient affected with an erythema of the skin around the eye. Although the redness cannot be shown, the moist, irritated skin around the eye should be noted.

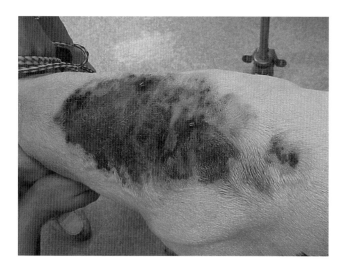

Figure 19.2. Image of a large hot spot-like lesion on the dorsal neck. This was created by severe pruritus secondary to allergies.

- **Hyperpigmentation:** With chronic pruritus, hormonal conditions, and skin damage, the affected region can start having increased amounts of pigment in response to the chronic irritation (see Figure 19.6).
- **Seborrhea:** Seborrhea is characterized by a defect in keratinization (skin formation) with increased scaling with or without excessive greasiness of the skin and coat and often secondary inflammation. There are two types of seborrhea: dry (**seborrhea sicca**) and oily (**seborrhea oleosa**). In most animals, seborrhea is not a disease but a symptom of many possible diseases. Common diseases that cause seborrhea are allergies, infection, parasites, nutritional imbalances, or hormonal disease. Topical antiseborrheic products can be keratolytic (help remove scales) and/or keratoplastic (help normalize keratinization and decrease scale and skin oil production) (see Figure 19.7).

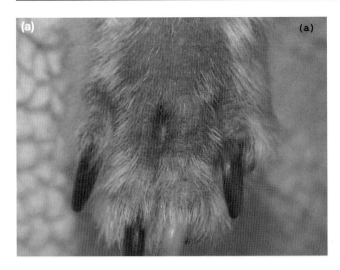

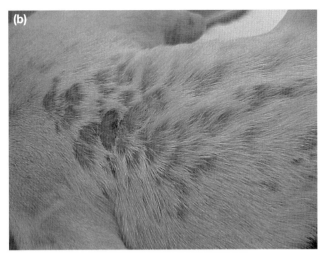

Figure 19.3. Image of focal alopecia on the dorsum of a paw (a) and over the dorsal neck (b).

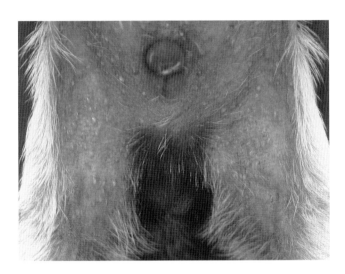

Figure 19.4. Image of pustules within the inguinal region due to bacterial infection.

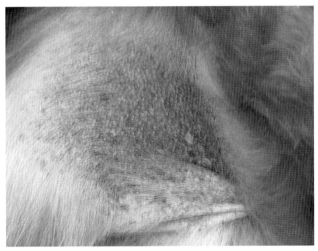

Figure 19.6. Image of hyperpigmentation of the skin in the inguinal area secondary to chronic irritation.

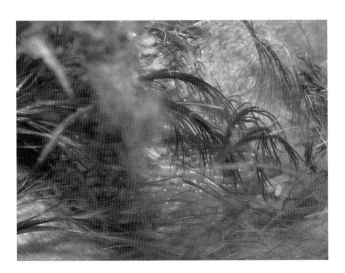

Figure 19.5. Image of ulceration and excoriation of the skin with a secondary maggot infestation.

When performing an initial assessment, the entire hair coat of the animal should be evaluated for change. It is important to assess where the changes in the hair coat are occurring most often.

The underarms of the forearm (axilla) and inguinal region should be evaluated because they are areas of wear and can show redness (**erythema**), itchiness (**pruritus**), and hair loss (**alopecia**) before there are changes to the entire hair coat. Furthermore, the region where the hair coat meets the skin margins (**mucocutaneous junctions**) should be evaluated. Examples of mucocutaneous junctions are the nail bed, lips, around the eye, the nasal planum, and areas around the genitals. These areas may be the first to see ulcers or irritations from immune-mediated disease, sunburn, topical skin irritants, and other sources.

Emergency concerns are rare when dealing with skin disease; even severely affected animals are usually stable. If there are concerns of stability based on the team mem-

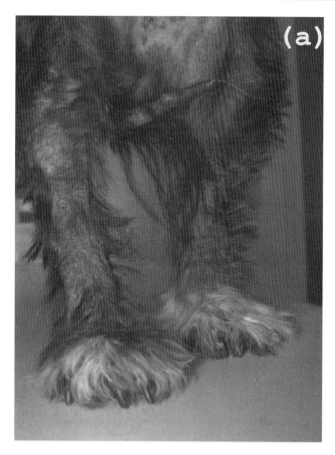

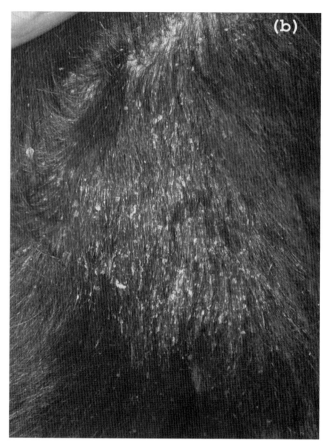

Figure 19.7.   Image of oily seborrhea affecting the forelimb of a patient (a). Image of dry seborrhea affecting the skin and coat of another patient (b).

ber's triage assessment (see Chapter 6), the medical team should be notified and the pet evaluated further for other conditions.

Diagnostics for Skin Problems

Although general blood work (i.e., chemistry and thyroid levels) is important in evaluating skin conditions, there are specific dermatologic diagnostic tests that help the medical team identify the primary cause of disease. An overview of the in-hospital clinical diagnostics is discussed next.

Skin Scrapings

A skin scraping should be performed on all pruritic animals. Animals presenting with weeping or moist lesions, crusts, excoriation, erythematous or alopecic areas, papules or pustules should also have skin scraping performed. A properly performed skin scraping may aid in the diagnosis of Demodectic and Sarcoptic mange, and less commonly, identify cheyletiella mites (see below). Bacteria, yeast, and various inflammatory cells may also be present on a skin scrape but are best diagnosed and evaluated by skin cytology methods. Skin scrapes should be repeated any time there is development of new lesions, lesions that do not resolve with treatment, or when evaluating of response to treatment.

Procedure—Performing a Skin Scraping

1. For a skin scraping you will need a pair of clippers with a #10 blade, a dulled scalpel blade (#10 or #11, whichever you are more comfortable with), mineral oil, and several microscope slides and coverslips (see Figure 19.8a).

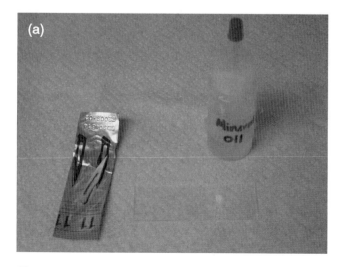

Figure 19.8(a).

2. Place a drop of mineral oil on the slide (see Figure 19.8b).

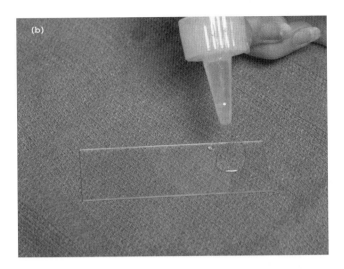

Figure 19.8(b).

3. Choose a spot at the edge of an alopecic area or clip an area of hair over the skin lesions with a #10 blade (clipping is optional). Do not scrub the area (see Figure 19.8c).

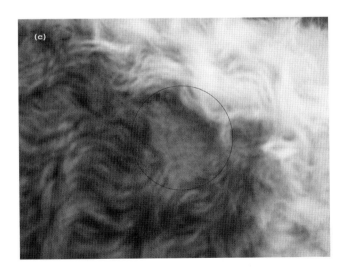

Figure 19.8(c).

4. Dip the end of the scalpel blade into the oil. Hold the scalpel blade at a 90-degree angle to the skin while pinching the portion of the skin you are going to scrape between your thumb and forefinger. Scrape the skin with short strokes between your finger until there is a reddening and a small amount of blood forms on the surface of the skin (see Figure 19.8d).

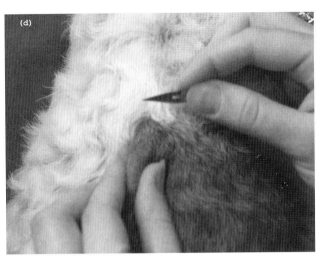

Figure 19.8(d).

5. Transfer the material from the scalpel blade to the mineral oil on the prepared slide. Pinching the skin throughout the scraping process will help express mites from the hair follicles (see Figure 19.8e).

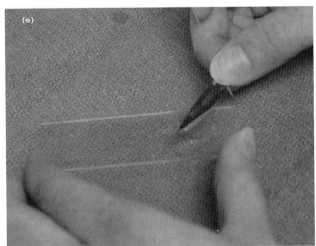

Figure 19.8(e).

6. The slide is then placed on the microscope and evaluated at low (4×) power to evaluate the slide for possible parasites (see Figure 19.8f, see Flowchart 19.1, p. 256).

Black Light

Some species of infectious fungal pathogens (**dermatophytes**) will light up or fluoresce in the presence of a black light. Fluorescing can suggest a fungal infection; however, if the area does not light up, *a fungal infection could still be present*. Additionally, false-positive fluorescence tests can occur with topical medication or other types of infection.

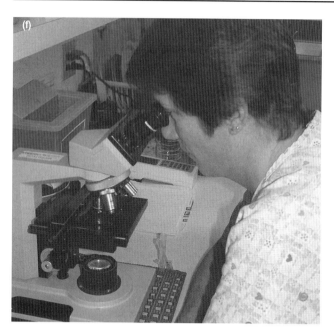

Figure 19.8(f).

Discussing a Skin Scraping with the Client
- The veterinarian is recommending a skin scrape to evaluate the skin for possible parasitic infection.
- A suspect region of hair loss, irritation, or infection is isolated and scraped with a scalpel blade until the region begins to bleed.
- The scraped skin debris is then placed on a microscope slide and evaluated for skin parasites.
- Evidence of a specific skin mite is diagnostic for a parasitic infection. A negative skin scrape does not rule out a mite infection because not all skin mites are easily obtained.
- Multiple scrapings may be required, and on occasion some animals are treated for skin mites based on physical changes in the skin.

Fungal Culture
Fungal culture is used to help detect and identify dermatophyte (ringworm) infection. The cultures use a special medium that grows fungal pathogens over a 2–4 week interval.

Procedure—Performing a Fungal Culture
A fungal culture is used to isolate and define the infectious fungal pathogen. Once the sample is collected and plated, it can take *up to 4 weeks* to adequately grow the dermatophyte for identification.

To properly culture for dermatophyte/fungal infection, the team member will follow this process.

1. You will need a clean disposable tooth brush and DTM or other dermatophyte agar (see Figure 19.9a).

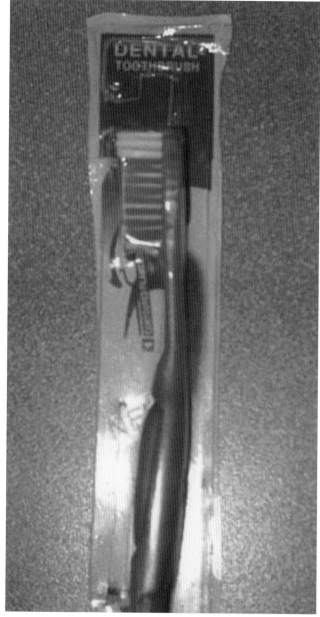

Figure 19.9(a).

2. Brush the entire area of concern at the skin level with the toothbrush (see Figure 19.9b).
3. The DTM agar is opened, and the toothbrush is placed on both sides of the agar (see Figure 19.9c).
4. The agar is then sealed, labeled with the patient's name and the date, and then stored in a dark place. The agar is checked every day for growth and color change. Dermatophytes will change the agar to red (see Figure 19.9d).

Positive dermatophyte pathogens are noted as **white or brown colonies** that change the agar color to red as they grow. Contaminants are usually **gray, black, or green in**

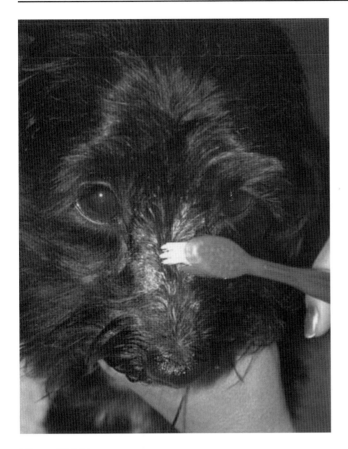

Figure 19.9(b).

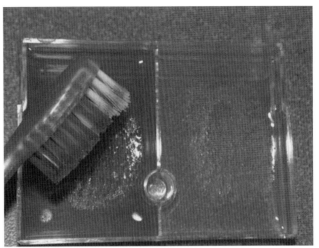

Figure 19.9(c).

colony and then lifted and pressed onto a slide and stained with **Lactophenol Cotton Blue** dye. The slide is then examined under high power for hyphae and fruiting fungal bodies (**macroconidia**) (see Flowchart 19.2, p. 257).

Skin Cytology

With concerns of bacterial and fungal skin infection, skin cytology can be an extremely helpful tool in identifying causative agents that produce signs of pruritus, alopecia,

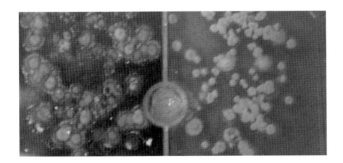

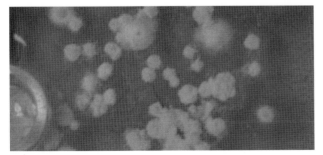

Figure 19.9(d).

color, and the agar color change does not occur for several days after the development of the colonies. Once a possible pathogen is isolated, samples of the colony are collected using clear Scotch Tape®. The tape is pressed onto the

Discussing Fungal Culture with the Client
The veterinarian has recommended fungal black light test and culture to determine if the patient is affected by a fungal pathogen.

- **Black light evaluation:** Certain types of ringworm (fungal) infections will fluoresce when a black light is shone over the affected region of the skin. Although a positive test strongly suggests ringworm, a negative evaluation does not rule out the fungal infection because some strains of fungus do not fluoresce under a black light. Furthermore, false-positive results can occur.
- **Fungal culture:** If ringworm is suspected, the veterinarian can sample affected hair and dander around the lesion and place it on a special culture media. If the culture grows organisms and there is a red coloration in the agar below the colonies, then a fungal infection is suspected. It takes up to 2–4 weeks to produce a positive culture.

If fungal pathogens are detected, the veterinarian may suggest specific shampoos and medications that will selectively destroy the fungal infection.

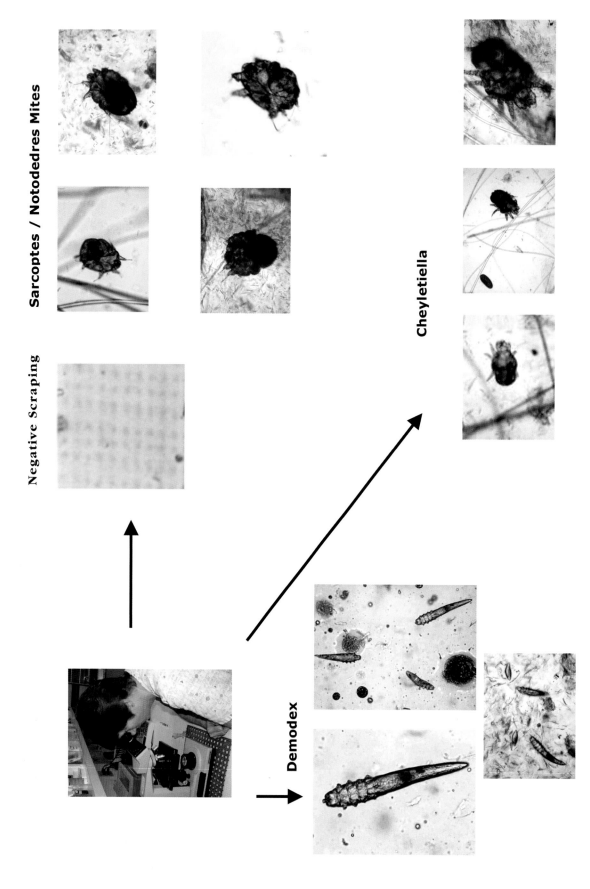

Sarcoptes / Notodedres Mites

Negative Scraping

Cheyletiella

Demodex

Flowchart 19.1. Outcome of Microscopic Examination of Skin Scraping. (Compliments of Heska Corporation, 3760 Rocky Mountain Avenue, Loveland, CO 80538)

Positive macroconidia / fungal spores from white colonies with agar color change

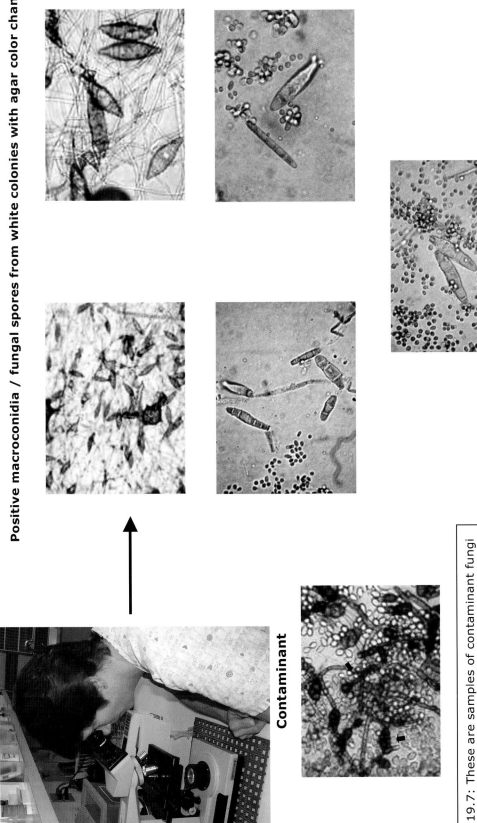

Contaminant

19.7: These are samples of contaminant fungi from the gray colonies above. These colonies did not change the agar color for 3-4 days after the colonies grew. Note the different hyphae and fruiting bodies as compared to the pathogenic fungi.

Flowchart 19.2. Outcome of Microscopic Examination—Positive Macroconidia/Fungal Spores. (Compliments of Heska Corporation, 3760 Rocky Mountain Avenue, Loveland, CO 80538)

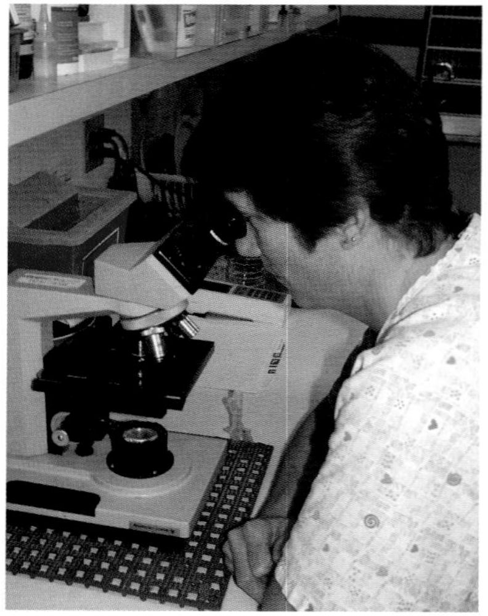

Malasezzia & Cocci

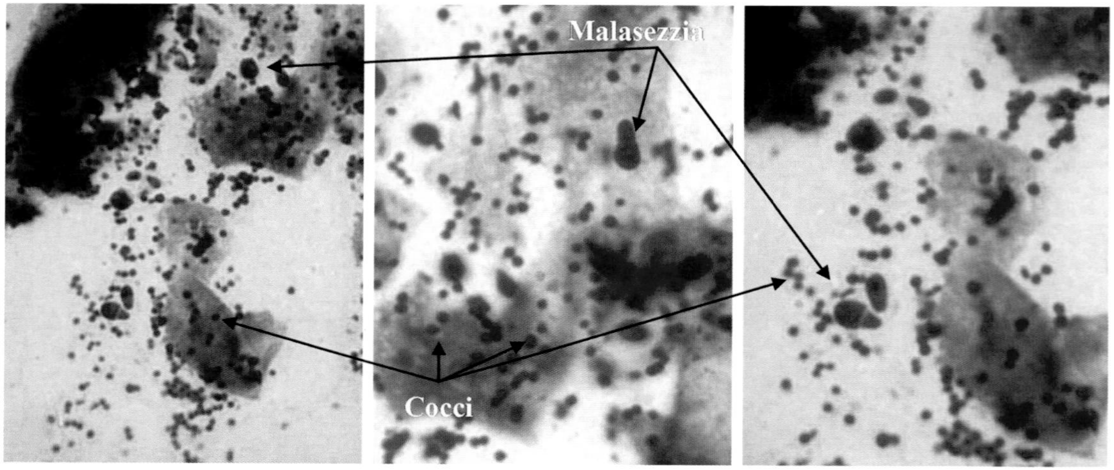

Malasezzia

Cocci

Fig 8: Images of a combination of bacterial (small round cocci) and Malasezzia (peanut shaped yeast organisms) colonizing epithelial cells.

Bacteria

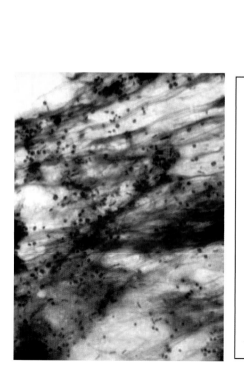

Fig 9: Bacterial cocci in streaming neutrophilic debris.

Flowchart 19.3a. Outcome of Microscopic Examination—Pathogens Malasezzia.
(Compliments of Heska Corporation, 3760 Rocky Mountain Avenue, Loveland, CO 80538)

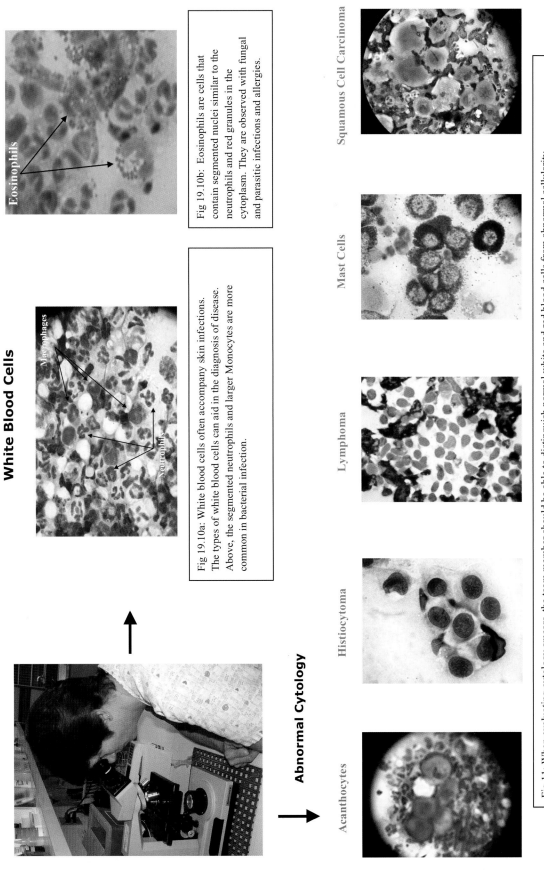

White Blood Cells

Eosinophils

Fig 19.10b: Eosinophils are cells that contain segmented nuclei similar to the neutrophils and red granules in the cytoplasm. They are observed with fungal and parasitic infections and allergies.

Macrophages

Neutrophils

Fig 19.10a: White blood cells often accompany skin infections. The types of white blood cells can aid in the diagnosis of disease. Above, the segmented neutrophils and larger Monocytes are more common in bacterial infection.

Abnormal Cytology

Squamous Cell Carcinoma

Mast Cells

Lymphoma

Histiocytoma

Acanthocytes

Fig 11: When evaluating cytology smears, the team member should be able to distinguish normal white and red blood cells from abnormal cellularity. Abnormal cell types can help the veterinarian identify possible autoimmune skin disease or cancer. Any observed abnormal cytology should be discussed with the veterinarian and possibly submitted for pathology review.

Flowchart 19.3b. Outcome of Microscopic Examination—White Blood Cells.
(Compliments of Heska Corporation, 3760 Rocky Mountain Avenue, Loveland, CO 80538)

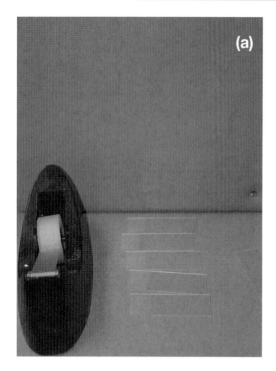
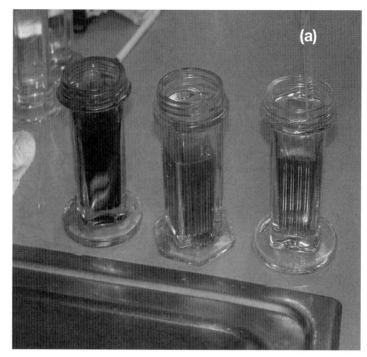

Figure 19.10(a).

erythema, scaling, and rash. There are many excellent ways to evaluate skin cytology.

Performing Skin Cytology

There are many methods of performing skin cytology, depending on the type of lesion evident. No matter which method is used, the key is to try to identify cells and organisms that can be suggestive of the cause of infection.

Scotch Tape Preparation

The Scotch Tape procedure is helpful in identifying fungal and bacterial components in moist, red, and raw regions of skin where active infection is occurring.

1. To perform a Scotch Tape cytology, the team member will need Scotch Tape, slides, and a staining system (i.e., New Methylene Blue, tricolor, Gram stain, etc.) (see Figure 19.10a).
2. The Scotch Tape is applied to the regions of concern on the patient, and a light pressure is applied to the length of the tape (see Figure 19.10b).
3. The tape is then applied to a clean slide, sticky side down, and light pressure is again applied to the slide. The tape is then removed (see Figure 19.10c).
4. The slide is dried and examined under the high-power oil objective (100×) for abnormal cell types and infectious pathogens (see Figures 19.10d and e).

Direct Smear

Direct smears are used when lesions produce a liquid discharge, which can be clear, purulent (pus), or bloody in nature. To perform the smear, the following procedure is used.

1. The team member will need slides, stain, and a syringe to obtain the liquid sample (see Figure 19.11a).
2. The team member then aspirates fluid and cells from the lesion with a syringe (see Figure 19.11b).
3. The content of the syringe is then applied to the middle of the slide. At a ninety-degree angle another slide is placed on top of the original slide. The slides are then drawn away from each other in a single motion, smearing the cell and debris over the original slide (see Figure 19.11c).
4. The team member then heat fixes and stains the slide using a preferred staining system (see Figure 19.11d).
5. The microscope slide is then evaluated for fungal hyphae, bacteria, and abnormal cellularity.

Impression Smear

Impression smears are obtained when there is a lesion that is moist or producing a clear, purulent, or hemorrhagic discharge. These lesions are open and draining such that infectious agents and cells may be apparent at the surface of the skin. To perform the smear the following procedure is used.

1. The team member will need slides and stain to obtain a sample of debris and discharge from the lesion (see Figure 19.12a).
2. The slides are placed directly onto the lesion and a slight pressure is applied to the area to increase production of the exudate from the region (see Figure 19.12b).
3. The slide is heat fixed and stained using a preferred staining system (see Figure 19.11d).
4. The microscope slide is then evaluated for fungal spores, fungal hyphae, bacteria, and abnormal cellularity.

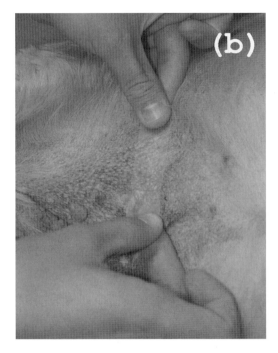

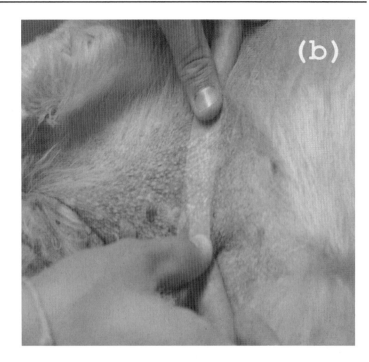

Figure 19.10(b).

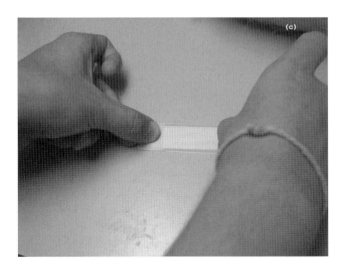

Figure 19.10(c).

Swab Method: The Cotton Swab Method

A cotton swab is used to obtain crusts and debris from regions where a direct or impression smear is not possible (i.e., ear canal, interdigital region, skin fold, etc.). To perform this cytology the following procedure is used.

1. The team member will need cotton swabs, slides, and stain to obtain a sample of debris and discharge from the lesion (see Figure 19.13a).
2. The swabs are placed directly onto the lesion and exudate and debris is collected. The applicator swab with debris is then rolled with a slight pressure onto the slide (see Figure 19.13b).

3. The slide is heat fixed and stained using a preferred staining system (see Figure 19.11d).
4. The microscope slide is then evaluated for fungal spores, fungal hyphae, bacteria, and abnormal cellularity.

Fine-Needle Aspirate

A fine-needle aspirate is performed to obtain cell and fluid aspirates of masses and lesions that are involved within or below the skin. The fine-needle aspirate samples a few hundred cells out of millions, and although it can be very helpful in suggesting the cause of the mass or lesion, a *negative fine-needle aspirate cannot rule out malignancy.* To perform a fine needle aspirate the following procedure should be used.

1. The team member will need a syringe, surgical prep, clippers, slides, and stain to obtain a sample of debris and discharge from the lesion (see Figure 19.14a).
2. The region is generally shaved and cleaned with surgical prep to minimize contamination of the site. The region is held by the thumb and pointer finger, and a syringe and needle is placed through the mass in a sewing machine-like motion to obtain cell samples (see Figure 19.14b).
3. The content of the syringe is then applied to the middle of the slide. At a ninety-degree angle another slide is placed on top of the original slide. The slides are then drawn away from each other in a single motion, smearing the cell and debris over the original slide (see Figure 19.14c).
4. The slide is heat fixed and stained using a preferred staining system (see Figure 19.11d).

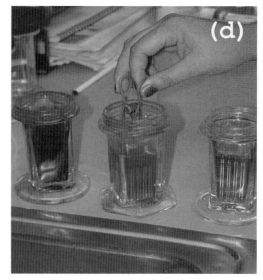

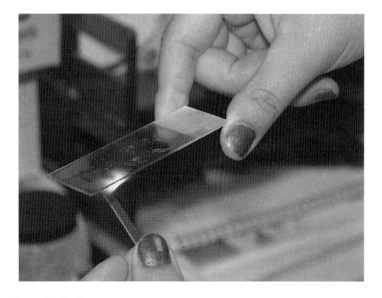

Figure 19.10(d).

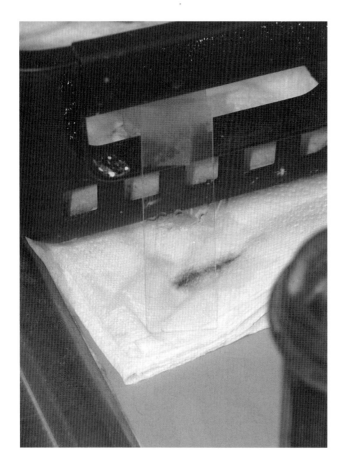

Figure 19.10(e).

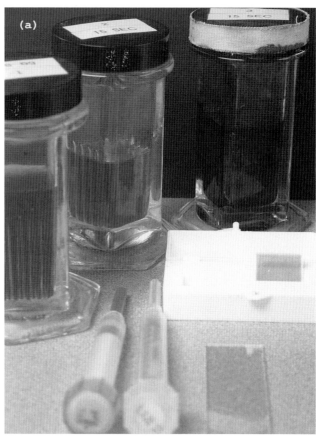

Figure 19.11(a).

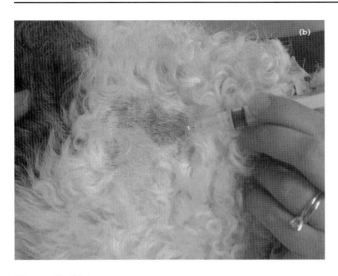

Figure 19.11(b).

5. The microscope slide is then evaluated for fungal spores, fungal hyphae, bacteria, and abnormal cellularity.

(See Flowchart 19.3a and 19.3b, pp. 258 and 259.)

Discussing Skin Cytology with the Client
- The veterinarian is recommending a skin cytology to help identify bacterial or fungal pathogens or abnormal cell types that may be causing the skin disease.
- Depending on the type of lesion, the medical team may obtain cells using a catheter, direct contact onto a slide, or a cotton swab.
- By examining these cells with a special stain under a microscope, the veterinarian can evaluate the cause of the skin problems.
- If abnormal cell types are identified, the veterinarian may recommend submitting the slides for a review by a pathologist.

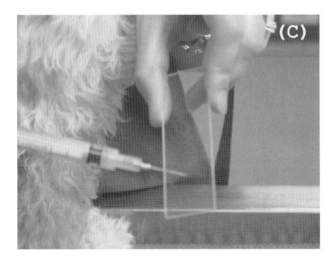
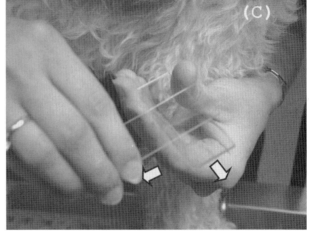

Figure 19.11(c).

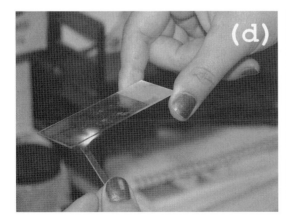
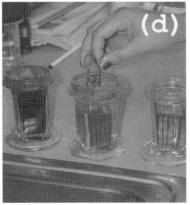
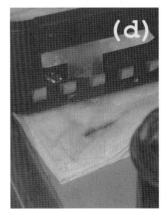

Figure 19.11(d).

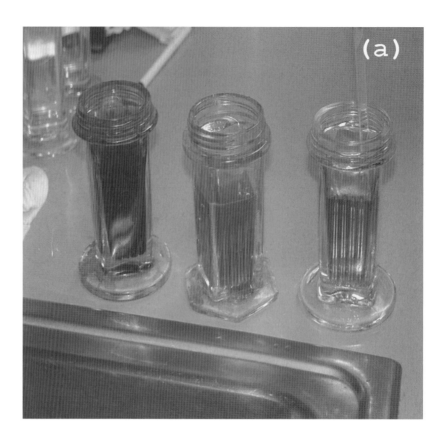

Figure 19.12(a).

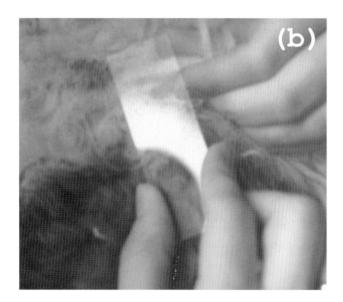

Figure 19.12(b).

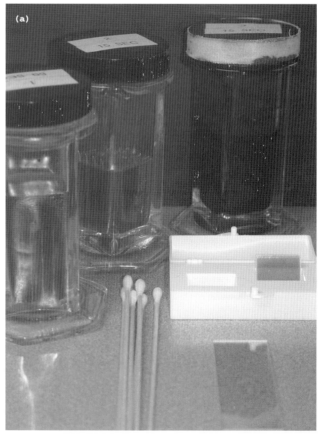

Figure 19.13(a).

264

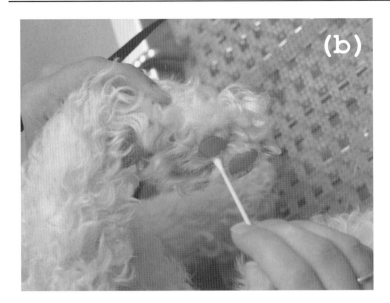

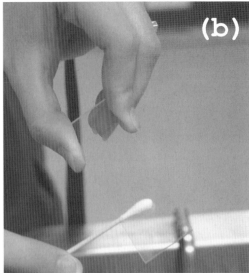

Figure 19.13(b).

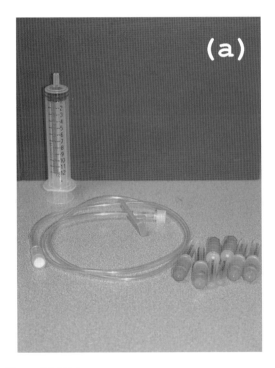

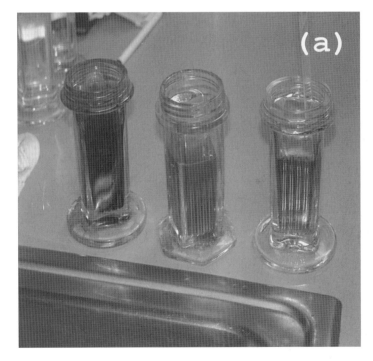

Figure 19.14(a).

Advanced Diagnostic Procedures

Skin Biopsy

Taking a small skin biopsy of the full thickness of the skin with a specialized blade can allow veterinarians to more specifically identify what types of diseases may be affecting the pet's skin. The procedure is done with light to no sedation and a small local block at the biopsy site. The tissue is placed in formalin and sent into the reference lab for histopathology.

Skin Allergy Testing

In a manner very similar to that which occurs in human medicine, the animal is tested for specific allergens to inhalant allergies. Once the types of irritants are known, a vaccine can be made to try to help desensitize the pet to the specific allergens.

Blood Allergy Testing

It is also possible to draw samples of blood to help detect to what allergens the patient is sensitive. From the results of

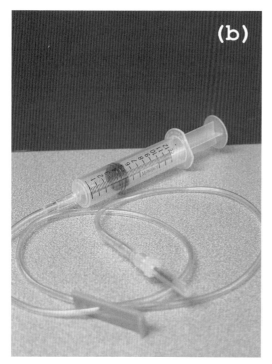

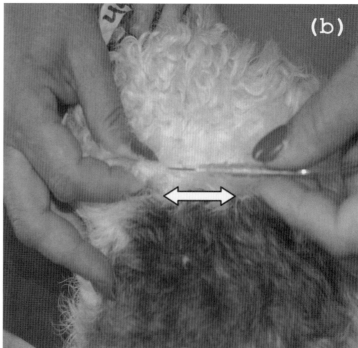

Figure 19.14(b).

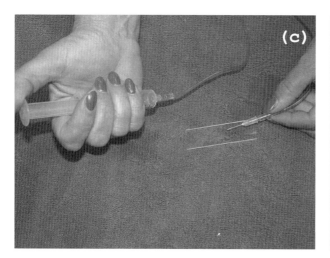

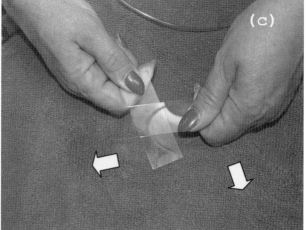

Figure 19.14(c).

blood allergy testing, desensitization vaccines can be produced. Blood allergy testing can be less specific than skin testing, producing less reliable results.

Blood Chemistry Panels

Blood work can help detect if there are changes in the blood suggestive of chronic infectious, organ (i.e., liver or kidney), inflammatory, or hormonal diseases that can cause the skin problems. Furthermore, thyroid blood work can evaluate if the patient has a thyroid abnormality (see Chapter 16).

Diseases of the Integumentary System

Although not all diseases are mentioned below, the common diseases are discussed, with the goal being to understand and explain to the client what the diseases are, how they can present themselves, and what can be the overall short-and long-term concerns of each disease. Any discussion of overall diagnostic and treatment protocols should be discussed based on the recommendations of the doctor and the medical team. Please use the following information as a guideline to discuss and educate the client, *but never to diagnose a patient.* Changes in the skin due to hormonal disease (i.e., thyroid, adrenal, and pancreatic diseases) are discussed in the related chapters.

Allergies

Allergies are one of the most frustrating non-life-threatening illnesses the patient and client may have to face. Allergies are an allergic response to components of diet, inhalant allergens, fleas, and topical irritants. Successful treatments vary from patient to patient and can involve dietary trials, medications, and desensitization vaccinations.

Signalment

Allergies can occur in both dogs and cats of any age, sex, or breed. There is a genetic component. Allergies can begin at any age; however, the younger the animal begins showing signs, the worse the pet's allergies may be. *Allergies tend to worsen as the animal ages.*

Etiology

Typically, the pet is not sensitive to just one type of allergen. The animal is usually allergic to a large number of irritants and begins to show physical symptoms with increased exposure. There are four basic components of allergies.

The most common cause of allergies is called **atopy.** Atopic animals have allergies to airborne material, such as pollen, dust, mites, cat dander, and ragweed. These allergens lie in the hair coat and are absorbed through the skin (**transdermally**) to produce an allergic response.

The second common type of allergies is **food allergies.** This is an allergy to some component of the diet, such as corn, poultry, beef, pork, the cereal fillers, and other components. Most diets contain some similar dietary elements. An animal that becomes allergic to corn, cereal fillers, or some other dietary component will show sensitivity to most commercial diets since they contain similar products.

Another major type of allergies is **flea allergy**. This is an allergy to a single fleabite. The animal does not need to be infested with fleas to have this allergy. One single bite can cause red, inflamed skin, heavy itching, and discomfort.

Lastly, **contact allergies** to a specific chemical or plant can cause redness and discomfort when the animal's skin is exposed to the irritant.

Common Points in Medical History

As discussed previously in this chapter, obtaining a specific detailed history of previous treatments and the animal's response is very important for successful diagnosis and treatment. Common points in medical history are

- reoccurring pruritus, erythema, and hair loss that occurs seasonally (i.e., fall and spring) or year-round;
- chronic ear infections;
- chewing and licking between the toes;
- pustules or rashes; and
- excessive shedding.

Common Observations in Initial Assessment

All skin disease can have very similar signs. Common symptoms may be

- itching/scratching (often severe),
- redness of the skin,
- licking of the paws,
- chewing between the toes,
- red-hot, inflamed draining areas in the skin (hot spots),
- discharge of the eyes and nose (occasionally),
- pustules or rashes,
- areas of hair loss, and
- dry flaky skin.

Complications

If not diagnosed and treated, the pet can be significantly affected with chronic skin infections, severe pruritus, and hair loss.

Diagnosis

As discussed previously, a full diagnostic workup can involve skin scrapes, fungal cultures, blood work, hypoallergenic diet trials, and allergy testing.

Treatment

There is no absolute cure for allergies. The goal of treating allergies is to control the symptoms with the appropriate medication. Medical options in treating pets with seasonal and year-round itching are as follows.

- **Antihistamines:** Antihistamines, such as diphenhydramine, chlorpheniramine, or hydroxyzine, can be moderately to extremely effective at controlling the itchiness associated with allergies. These drugs are extremely safe and can be used as needed without worrying about stopping or starting medication. Antihistamines sometimes do cause drowsiness. They work well with skin vitamins to further help control the symptoms associated with allergies. The only drawback is that not all antihistamines work with all animals; sometimes two or three different types of antihistamines must be used before one is found that is effective.

- **Essential fatty acids (EFA):** EFA supplements help to minimize the effects of inflammation and scratching, which damage the hair coat. These capsules work synergistically with antihistamines.

- **Steroids:** Steroids (i.e., prednisone) are extremely effective at decreasing the redness and irritation associated with systemic allergies. There are short-acting steroids, such as prednisone, that last for a few days to a week. There is also longer-term medication, such as triamcinolone or beta-methasone, that can last for weeks at a time. *However, steroids have immediate side effects of increased thirst, urination. and appetite, and if used over the long term can affect liver and adrenal function.*

- **Cyclosporine:** The use of the immunosuppressant cyclosporine has helped reduce allergic symptoms in many patients that have been refractory to other treatment options. Cyclosporine therapy comes as oral medication that is given 1–2/day; at this time the expense of the drug can be a limiting factor for some clients, and the effects of long-term therapy are uncertain.

Discussing Allergies with the Client

- Allergies are a chronic, recurring potentially incurable non-life-threatening disease.
- Pets can have allergies to inhalant allergens, food, fleas, and topical products.
- Unlike humans, animals will begin to itch, scratch, lose hair, and have reddening of the skin in response to exposure.
- Allergies are a sum total of multiple allergens and the animal will begin to show signs when exposed to a significant number of allergens. The more allergens exposed, the worse the physical signs may be.
- Allergies can be seasonal (i.e., spring and fall) or can be year-round.
- Allergies can get worse as the pet ages.
- Diagnosis of allergies depends on physical signs, medical history, and outcome of skin and blood diagnostic testing.
- Treatment can be a combination of medication, diet, and desensitization serum. *There is no one specific treatment for an allergy patient; treatment can vary from animal to animal, even with animals in the same litter.*

- **Food trial:** A food trial removes any potential food allergens from the patient's diet to see if any signs of allergies become less severe. A new diet is chosen based on the patient's existing diet. The goal is to choose a protein and vegetable source that the animal has never been exposed to, such as fish and potato, lamb and rice, or venison and rice. A diet trial takes 8–12 weeks to see if there is any change in allergy signs. *The pet must be on that diet and water only; any other diet or treat during a food trial will make the test inaccurate.*

- **Allergy testing/desensitization vaccines:** The goal of allergy testing is to determine what environmental allergens the animal is sensitive to so that a serum can be produced to help desensitize the patient. The serum is relatively safe and produces natural immunity to the allergies. *It takes months to years to produce adequate immunity.* The allergy serum does not always produce a complete or partial resolution of allergies.

Prevention
There is no known way to prevent allergy issues in the pet.

Demodecosis (Demodectic Mange)
Demodecosis is a parasitic mite infection of the hair follicle.

Signalment
Most common forms of the disease are seen in young animals from 3 to 6 months of age. There are no sexual or breed predilections. When the disease is seen in adult animals, it may suggest a genetic predisposition to demodex infections or an underlying disease that is challenging the normal immune system. *Animals that are genetically sensitive to demodectic mange can pass on this sensitivity to their offspring; therefore, these animals are discouraged from reproducing. Additionally, animals treated chronically with steroids are immunosuppressed and prone to development of demodecosis.*

Etiology
Canine demodectic mange is a parasitic infection of a skin mite in the hair follicles of the pet. The mite is normally present in the pet's skin, but when overwhelming numbers of mites occur, the patient can show symptoms (see Figure 19.15). Demodectic mange is noninfectious and noncontagious to humans or other animals.

Common Points on Medical History
Generally, demodectic mange produces a mild to moderate pruritic localized to generalized infection in young pets.

Common Observations in Initial Assessment
Common physical symptoms are

- areas of hair loss (localized to general),
- redness of the skin,
- itchiness,

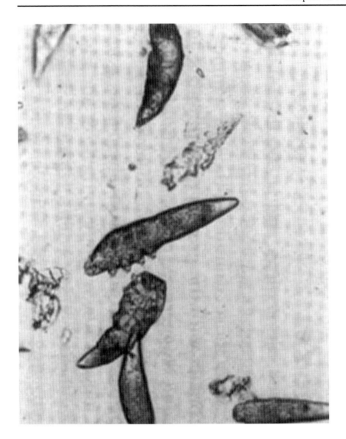

Figure 19.15. Image of adult demodectic mange mite as seen on a skin scrape.

- areas of the skin that begin to ooze pus and debris (secondary bacterial infection), and
- scaling and dry flaky skin.

Complications

If not diagnosed and treated, demodectic mange can produce generalized whole-body erythema, alopecia, and pruritus.

Diagnosis

Diagnosis of the mite is based upon finding the mite on a microscopic examination of a skin scraping. If the pet is an older animal with generalized demodex infection, other clinical diagnostics (i.e., complete blood count, chemistry, thyroid panel, and infectious disease screenings) may be suggested to make sure there is no underlying disease that may be challenging the pet's immune system.

Treatment

Demodectic mange can be treated with topical salves, whole-body dips, or oral medications to help eliminate the active infection. While under treatment, repeated skin scrapes will be necessary to see how the animal is responding to treatment.

Prevention

Because there is genetic sensitivity for demodectic mange, treatment is focused on preventing susceptible adult animals from reproducing. Furthermore, chronic steroid therapy should be avoided.

> **Discussing Demodectic Mange with the Client**
> - Demodectic mange is a skin mite infection of the hair follicle. The demodectic mite lives on all cats and dogs in low numbers but does not usually produce physical symptoms.
> - Young pets are more prone to localized systemic infection producing hair loss, reddening of the skin, rash, and itchiness.
> - On occasion, adult pets may have a genetic sensitivity to a mite infection and show physical signs when stressed. This sensitivity is genetically based and can be passed to a pet's progeny.
> - This infection is not contagious or infectious to humans or other animals.
> - Diagnosis is largely made by observation of the mite in a skin scrape.
> - Treatment can be a combination of medication, medicated dips, and topical ointments.

Sarcoptic Mange (Scabies)

Sarcoptic mange is a parasitic infection with a skin mite in the epidermal skin layers. The infection produces a severe, intensely pruritic skin disorder as the mite burrows through the deeper skin layers. *Sarcoptic mange has a high incidence of infection to other animals or humans through direct contact; care must be taken when handling affected pets.*

Signalment

The mite can affect both dogs and cats, but outdoor roaming animals or animals in multi-pet households are at more risk.

Etiology

Sarcoptic mange, also called red mange or scabies, is caused by the transmission of the *Sarcoptes scabei* mite from an already infected animal (see Figure 19.16).

Common Points on Medical History

Sarcoptic mange produces a severely pruritic pet with regions of alopecia, rashes, and scaling.

Common Observations in Initial Assessment

Common physical symptoms are

- areas of hair loss (localized to general),
- redness of the skin (severe),
- itchiness,
- areas of the skin that begin to ooze pus and debris (secondary bacterial infection),
- scaling and dry flaky skin, and
- generalized enlargement of all external lymph nodes.

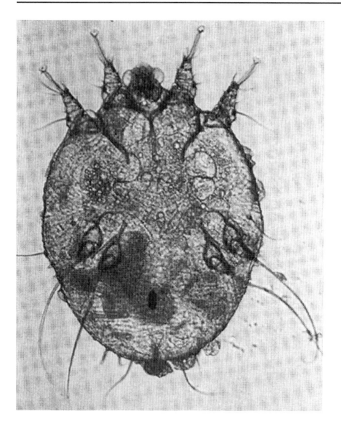

Figure 19.16. Image of adult sarcoptic mange mite as seen on a skin scrape.

Complications

If not diagnosed and treated, sarcoptic mange can produce severe hair loss and skin damage and can be infectious to other animals and humans.

Diagnosis

Diagnosis is based on medical history, physical signs, skin scraping, and response to treatment. Unlike demodex infection, sarcoptic mange is sometimes hard to find on multiple skin scrapings. *A negative skin scrape does not rule out sarcoptic mange.* Furthermore, on occasion, a **fecal flotation** may show mite eggs or adult mites evident in the feces. In some cases, responding to a treatment protocol for sarcoptic mange may be definitive enough to provide a diagnosis.

Treatment

Treatment generally involves oral, topical, or injectable medication to eliminate the infection, oral antibiotics to help decrease secondary bacterial infection, and oral and topical medication to decrease pruritus. *Furthermore, all dogs that have contact with the patient should also be treated.*

Dermatomycosis (Ringworm)

Ringworm is a cutaneous fungal infection affecting the regions of the hair, nails, and the superficial layers of the skin. *Ringworm has a high incidence of infection to other animals*

Discussing Sarcoptic Mange with the Client
- Sarcoptic mange is a skin mite infection of the deeper skin layers.
- The sarcoptic mange mite produces a severe whole-body infection, hair loss, itchiness, and red, irritated skin.
- *Sarcoptes* mites are highly infectious to other animals and humans, and care should be taken when handling pets infected with them.
- Diagnosis of sarcoptic mange is based on history, physical examination, and skin scraping. Because the skin mite lives deeper in the skin tissue, a negative skin scraping does not rule out an infection.
- On occasion a fecal examination will reveal mite eggs or adult skin mites.
- Treatment is based on topical and oral medications to help eliminate the mite and any secondary bacterial infection and to control itchiness and scaling.
- The pet may have to go through weeks of treatment until the infection is cleared.

and humans through direct contact; care must be taken when handling affected pets.

Etiology

Ringworm is a skin fungal infection caused by *Microsporum canis, M. gypseum,* and *Trychophyton mentagrophytes.* These skin fungal agents (**dermatophytes**) exist in moist, warm environments and are introduced to a break in the skin. Animals that are immunocompromised or on medications that produce immunosuppression are more likely to be affected.

Signalment

Ringworm can affect dogs and cats of any age; however, it is more common in younger animals. In the cat, long-haired breeds are also more commonly affected.

Common Points on Medical History

Affected animals present with small- to moderate-sized regions of hair loss and dry, flaky skin with moderate levels of pruritus.

Common Observations on Initial Assessment

Some pets may have no physical symptoms of disease; cats are often carriers of the disease without any physical signs. The fungus can exist below the hairline, and it can still be infectious. However, classic symptoms can be

- circular regions of hair loss,
- poor hair coat,
- scales,
- erythema,
- areas of hyperpigmentation, and
- pruritus.

Complications

If not diagnosed and treated, ringworm can produce a chronic skin infection that can affect other animals and humans.

Diagnosis

Diagnosis is based on medical history, physical examination, and the following clinical diagnostic methods.

- **Black light evaluation:** Some dermatophytes will fluoresce under a black light. A positive test strongly suggests ringworm, a negative test does not eliminate the possibility, and false-positive tests can occur.
- **Dermatophyte culture:** The affected region is scrubbed with a clean, unused toothbrush and the scraping is then applied to the dermatophyte culture. If fungal dermatophytes are present, the agar will grow the fungus and change to a specific color, usually red. Impression smears can then be sampled from the agar, and microscopic identification can help diagnose the dermatophytes.

Treatment

Treatment is based on topical medicated shampoos, topical antifungal ointments, and oral antifungal medications. Fungal cultures are repeated at 2- to 4-week intervals. The patient may need to be treated for weeks to months until the pet has had two negative dermatophyte cultures.

Prevention

By limiting exposure to wet and dank environments and stray animals, ringworm infections can be reduced.

Discussing Ringworm with the Client

- Ringworm is a fungal infection of the skin.
- It produces dry, scaly regions with hair loss and moderate alopecia.
- It is spread by contact with the fungus from the environment or other infected animals through a break in the skin layer.
- Ringworm is potentially infectious to humans and other animals, and caution should be used when handling pets that are infected.
- Diagnosis is based on identification of the fungal organism on a cultured media.
- Treatment is focused on long-term oral and topical medications until there are two successive negative fungal cultures.

CD-ROM 1 reviews material presented in this chapter. Please try the cases for Section 2 (Anatomy and Physiology—The Science behind the Diseases) *to help reinforce the information presented here.*

Chapter 20

Eyes and Ears

In this section, the anatomy, physiology, physical examination, diagnostic testing, and diseases of the eyes and ears will be discussed. A discussion of the oral cavity has already been presented in Chapter 9.

The Eye

The eye consists of three ocular walls of tissue (**tunic**). The outer tunic consists of the thick fibrous scleral wall, normally opaque, which consists of the white portion of the eye, and the clear outermost section of the eye, the **cornea**. The second tunic of the eye consists of the vascular layer, the **uveal coat** of the eye, which supplies nutrients and oxygen. The cranial aspect of the uvea contains the **iris**; the caudal aspect of the uvea contains the blood supply to the retina. The third ocular tunic consists of the neural tissue containing the **retina** and optic nerve (see Figure 20.1).

The eye has three ocular cavities:

1. The **anterior chamber** occupies the space cranial to the lens; it is filled with aqueous fluid that helps to maintain the shape and nutrition of the cranial aspect of the eye.
2. The **posterior chamber** lies between the caudal aspect of the iris and the cranial aspect of the lens.
3. The **vitreous chamber** lies between the caudal aspect of the lens and the retina. This chamber has a special type of fluid called **vitreous,** which further supports the shape and health of the eye.

The outer fibrous tunic allows the attachment of the extraocular muscles to control the movement of the eye; the lids and third eyelids to protect the eye; the lacrimal gland and gland of the third eyelid to lubricate the eye; the glands of the lids to protect the cornea, and the skin around the eye (**conjunctiva**) to protect the entire globe.

The eye may be considered to function like a camera; rays of light coming in from an object being viewed travel to the cornea where they enter the eye. The lens focuses the light on the retina and optic nerve, which communicates with the brain, bringing images into the cerebrum for conscious response.

The cells of the retina that process light into an electrical signal are called **photoreceptors.** There are two types of cells: the **rod cells,** which process light in the dim and dark environments, and the **cone cells,** which process bright light and colors. In general, domestic animals have poor color vision and better vision in dim light and darkness because they have more rod cells in the retina.

The light level is analyzed, and the iris of the eye is opened or closed by a reflex pathway of the optic nerve. If there is low light or darkness, the iris opens up, increasing the amount of light entering the eye. If the environment is bright, the iris constricts, decreasing the level of light reaching the retina. This is called the **pupillary light response (PLR)**. Both irides will respond to a bright light perceived by one iris. If a light shines into one iris and it constricts, we call this a **direct PLR**. If a light shines into one iris and the opposite constricts as well, it is called an **consensual PLR**. If a direct or indirect PLR is absent in a pet, it can suggest disease of the eye, optic nerve, or a part of the central nervous system. Furthermore, in times of ocular pain (i.e., corneal ulceration), the iris of the affected eye can be constricted. *Any changes in pupil response should be brought to the attention of the medical team immediately* (see Figure 20.2).

The **lens** is located behind the iris and is supported by fibrous ligaments within the eye. The tension on these ligaments can be changed by muscle activity altering the focal length of the lens, allowing the eye to switch focus from the far to the near field. This process is called **accommodation**. In general, domestic animals have poor accommodation capabilities.

The lens should appear clear. A true opacity of the lens is called a **cataract** (see Figure 20.3). However, normal ageing of the lens in animals produces a chronic thickening that is perceived as a bluing of the lens. This process is called **lenticular sclerosis** and is not a cataract formation.

The aqueous fluid in the anterior chamber should be clear. Aqueous fluid is constantly being formed and leaves the eye in small drainage angles near the iris. Aqueous fluid in the anterior chamber maintains the pressure within the eye. Abnormalities in the aqueous fluid circulation may result in elevated pressure in the eye, producing a disease called **glaucoma.**

The **cornea** is made up of a series of cellular layers. The cornea should be clear, free of blood vessels or pigment. Sensory nerves in the anterior cornea make the tissue very sensitive to irritation (see Figure 20.4).

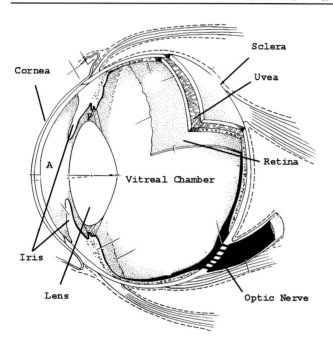

Figure 20.1.   Cross section of the eye. Image courtesy of *Anatomy of Domestic Animals*, 7th Edition. Pasquini, Chris, and Pasquini, Susan. Sudz Publishing, Pilot Point, TX 1989. Used with permission from Sudz Publishing.
A = Anterior chamber

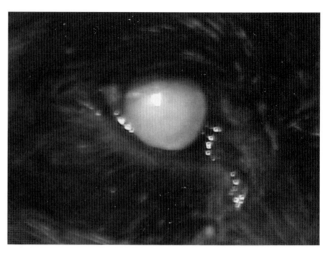

Figure 20.3.   A cataract is a complete thickening of the lens until no light or images can pass into the posterior chamber and be visualized by the retina. Reprinted with permission from Jeffrey Bowersox, DVM ACVO, Veterinary Specialty Center of Delaware, 1212 E. Newport Pike, Wilmington, DE 19804.

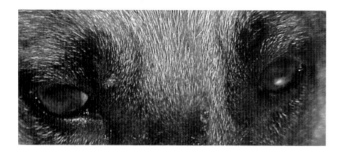

Figure 20.2.   Notice the left iris is constricted smaller than the right. Especially with a trauma case, this can suggest concussion or CNS damage.

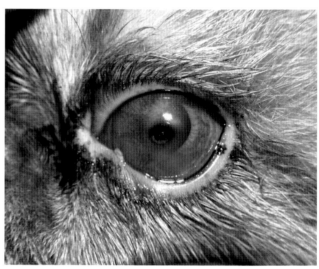

Figure 20.4.   In this picture note the corneal edema around the central lesion in the eye. Reprinted with permission from Jeffrey Bowersox, DVM ACVO, Veterinary Specialty Center of Delaware, 1212 E. Newport Pike, Wilmington, DE 19804.

Obtaining a History in Patients with Ocular Disease

In a general practice, the majority of ocular disease is presented as an acute problem. Ocular problems can be secondary to other systemic diseases, such as allergies and infectious, organ, and metabolic disease. When obtaining a general history, the same basic guidelines should be used as outlined in Chapter 5. However, some key ocular questions are discussed next.

Does the Eye Seem To Be Sensitive to the Light?
Animals with ocular disease can have sensitivity to bright lights. These patients may squint or move the affected eye away from a bright light source.

Is There Ocular or Nasal Discharge or Debris Evident?
The evidence of bloody to purulent discharge (pus) can suggest infection, trauma, or a foreign body.

Is the Pet Rubbing the Eye with Their Paw or on the Ground?
Chronic irritation can stimulate the pet to try to rub and scratch at the eye. This can produce further damage to the eye and cornea and may need to be corrected with an Elizabethan collar.

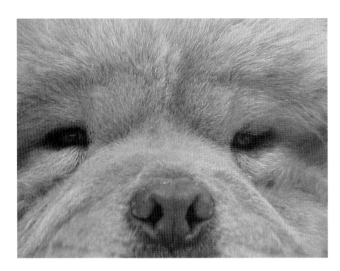 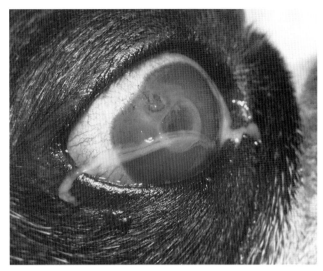

Figure 20.5. Image on the left of a chow with entropion. Notice how the upper lids are in direct contact with the eye. Image on the right of a severe corneal ulceration with edema. With this type of injury, it is impossible to assess the internal anatomy of the eye. Reprinted with permission from Jeffrey Bowersox, DVM ACVO, Veterinary Specialty Center of Delaware, 1212 E. Newport Pike, Wilmington, DE 19804.

Does the Eye Itself Seem To Be Enlarged?

An enlarged eye indicates chronic alterations in intraocular pressure (i.e., glaucoma).

Has There Been a Color Change to the Iris of the Eye?

Due to internal infection of the eye (**uveitis**) or certain tumor types (i.e., **melanoma**), part of or the entire iris may appear to have a color change. However, in some cases, color change can be normal.

Physical Changes to the Eye on Initial Assessment

When evaluating an animal on an initial assessment, some very simple observation of the eyes can tell you a great deal about the vision and overall health of the animal.

Can You Visualize the Eyes?

Many animals have a great deal of redundancy of skin around the face, causing abnormal turning in of the eyelids. This is called **entropion.** Chronic irritation of the cornea by hair follicles of the eyelids can result in chronic inflammation of the cornea, pain, and visual alterations (see Figure 20.5).

Are There Changes to the White of the Eye?

The white of the eye (sclera and the overlying tissue, the conjunctiva) may become red and the blood vessels become congested due to infection, inflammation, or metabolic disease of the eye and surrounding tissue (see Figure 20.6). The white of the eye can also appear yellow with jaundice from liver and blood disease.

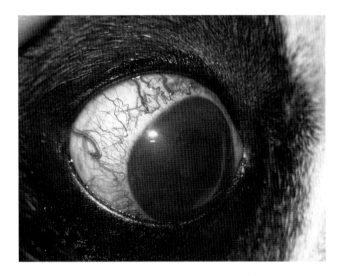

Figure 20.6. Image of a red, inflamed conjunctivitis. Reprinted with permission from Jeffrey Bowersox, DVM ACVO, Veterinary Specialty Center of Delaware, 1212 E. Newport Pike, Wilmington, DE 19804.

Are the Irides Responsive to Light and Are the Pupils the Same Size?

Iris should constrict evenly and quickly to a bright light. Irides that are uneven (**anisocoria**) or nonresponsive can suggest the following (see Figure 20.2):

- Concussion/CNS trauma
- Blindness
- Internal disease/infection of eye
- Corneal injury/ulcer

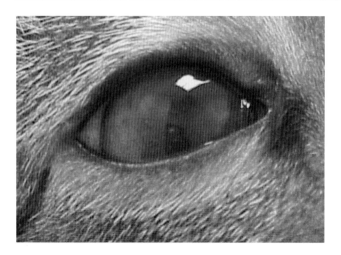

Figure 20.7. Image of blood in the anterior chamber of an eye. Reprinted with permission from Jeffrey Bowersox, DVM ACVO, Veterinary Specialty Center of Delaware, 1212 E. Newport Pike, Wilmington, DE 19804.

Is the Aqueous Fluid in the Anterior Chamber Clear?
Evidence of blood (**hyphema**) can suggest trauma or a bleeding problem (see Figure 20.7). Cloudiness in the aqueous fluid suggests intraocular inflammation.

Do the Eyes Seem Less Shiny, Sunken, Dull, and Are the Third Eyelids Elevated?
Eyes that change appearance, becoming less shiny, sunken, and dull, with an elevated third eyelid, can be a sign of dehydration. There are large fat pads behind the eye that keep the eyelid in a normal position in the skull. As animals become dehydrated, the fat pads lose moisture and shrink, making the eye sink back into the socket. As this occurs, the third eyelid elevates upward and the eyes sink backward.

Diagnostics of the Eye

As with most body systems, the eye has individual diagnostics that allow us to determine disease and the condition of the eye. However, ocular examination and diagnostics must be done carefully and when indicated. The ocular diagnostic tests are listed next.

- **Schirmer tear test:** This test checks for normal tear production in an eye. The Schirmer test strips are longitudinal thin lengths of filter paper. By placing the paper within the eyelid, the veterinarian can evaluate the amount of tears being produced over a 1-minute interval. Decreased tear production can suggest chronic dry eyes (**keratoconjunctiva sicca**; see below).
- **Fluorescein stain:** This test evaluates intact corneal epithelium; that is, it checks for ulcerations or scratches to the cornea. The fluorescein stain is a water-soluble stain that covers the eye and fluoresces under a black light. The superficial part of the cornea is waterproof; the deeper

layers are not. Thus, if there is a scratch or irritation to the cornea, the dye will adhere to the deeper layers and fluoresce under the black light.
- **Schiotz tonometry:** The tonometer measures the normal pressure within the eye itself. In order for the test to be completed, *the eye cannot have any corneal ulceration or scratches present because the tonometer itself must be placed onto the eye.* The eye must also be topically anesthetized with a short-acting topical anesthesia.
- **Electronic tonometry:** An electronic tonometer also measures the normal pressure within the eye itself. The eye must be topically anesthetized with a short-acting topical anesthesia. When used properly, the electronic tonometers (i.e., Tonopen) can produce accurate quantitative intraocular pressures.
- **Fundic examination:** A fundic examination refers to a full examination of the retina and the optic nerve by the veterinarian. Generally, a short-term topical drug is used to dilate the iris so the entire eye can be viewed.

Discussing Clinical Diagnostics for the Ocular System with the Client
The veterinarian has suggested specific diagnostics to help assess the eye for primary ocular disease. These tests help identify specific conditions that may require medication, blood work, or surgical care.

- **Fluorescein stain:** This test allows the veterinarian to assess if there are corneal scratches or ulcerations that are not visible with the naked eye. The superficial layer of the cornea is waterproof, the deeper layers are not. This water-based stain will attach to any exposed deeper area of the cornea and fluoresce under a black light.
- **Schirmer tear test:** The Schirmer tear test determines the amount of tears produced per minute by the tear glands of the eye. The veterinarian is suggesting this test to assess if the pet has chronic dry eye. Tear production of less than 20 mm tears per minute is suggestive of dry eye problems.
- **Tonometry:** This test allows the veterinarian to determine the internal pressure inside the eye. Increased ocular pressure can suggest serious underlying disease that could cause blindness, pain, and sensitivity.
- **Fundic examination:** In some cases where the entire retina needs to be examined, the veterinarian will suggest a complete retinal examination and will need to use short-term eyedrops to dilate the iris and examine the entire retinal region.

Ocular Diseases

Although not all diseases are mentioned below, the common diseases are discussed with the main goal being to understand and to be able to explain to the client what the diseases are, how they can present themselves, and what can be the short- and long-term concerns of each disease. Any discussion of overall diagnostic and treatment protocols should be based on the recommendations of the doctor. Please use the following information as a guideline to discuss and educate the client, *but never to diagnose a patient.*

Protruding Third Eyelid (Cherry Eye)
Cherry eye refers to the swelling and inflammation of the gland on the back side of the third eyelid, producing a protrusion and elevation.

Signalment
This syndrome is common in the dog, but rarer in the cat. Breeds predisposed to cherry eye are the

- cocker spaniel,
- bulldog,
- beagle,
- bloodhound,
- Lhasa apso,
- Shih Tzu, and
- Burmese and Persian cat breeds

Cause of Disease
Cherry eye is a congenital condition due to the weak attachment of the gland of the third eyelid.

Common Points in Medical History
The chief complaint is a red, irritated eye with a noticeable swelling in the medial aspect of the eye. There may also be a history of clear or purulent (pus) debris.

Common Observations on Initial Examination
Common changes in the affected eyes are as follows:

- Red inflamed painful eyes
- Swollen membranes around the eyes
- Clear to heavy purulent discharge evident
- Eyes closed in normal to bright light
- Protruding, swollen third eyelid (see Figure 20.8)
- Increased tearing of the eye (**epiphora**)

Complications
Unless linked to an another primary underlying disease of the eye, elevation of the third eyelid may not produce any significant ocular disease and could present as a simple cosmetic change to the face.

Diagnosis
Because cherry eye can be linked to other ocular diseases, it may be recommended that the affected eye be checked for corneal ulcerations or irritations, for chronic dry eye, or increased ocular pressure, depending on how the pet presents at the time of physical exam. This will allow a better assess-

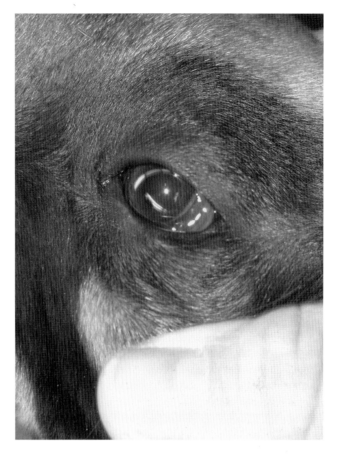

Figure 20.8. Image of a protruding, inflamed third eyelid. Reprinted with permission from Jeffrey Bowersox, DVM ACVO, Veterinary Specialty Center of Delaware, 1212 E. Newport Pike, Wilmington, DE 19804.

ment of the eye and the treatment options. Some diagnostics may be a

- Schirmer tear test,
- Ocular corneal staining, and
- Ocular pressure readings.

Treatment
Treatment is based on the presentation of the animal and the severity of the disease noted. Some treatment options are discussed next.

- **Medications:** Medications are focused on decreasing inflammation of the third eyelid with topical medication. Topical medication may reduce the swelling of the third eyelid but the eyelid may also require surgical treatment.
- **Elizabethan collar:** If the pet is rubbing at the eyes, an Elizabethan collar or buster collar may be suggested to prevent further injury to the eyes.
- **Surgery:** In many cases, the patient may need an elective surgical procedure. The procedure is **tacking of the third eyelid**, in which the third eyelid itself is sutured back into

place with a single suture, anchoring the eyelid to the lower orbital bone.

Prevention
There is no known way to prevent elevation of the third eyelid.

Discussing Elevation of the Third Eyelid with the Client

- All domestic animals have a triangular third eyelid that sits in the inner aspect of the eye to help produce tears and protective antibodies for the eye.
- When the gland of the third eyelid becomes inflamed and swollen, the third eyelid itself becomes visible in the corner of the patient's eye.
- It is common in younger animals, especially in the cocker spaniel, bulldog, beagle, bloodhound, Lhasa apso, Shih Tzu, and Burmese dog breeds and Persian cat breed.
- Diagnosis is based on medical history, physical signs, and diagnostic tests to help rule out other ocular and systemic disease.
- Treatment can be a combination of medical and surgical options.

Conjunctivitis

Conjunctivitis is defined as a redness, swelling, and inflammation of the tissue lining the eyelids and around the eye. Conjunctivitis can be acute or chronic in nature and can have an abnormal ocular discharge.

Signalment
Conjunctivitis is common in both dogs and cats of any age.

Etiology
There are many causes of conjunctivitis in dogs and cats. The disease can be a primary or secondary disorder. Some causes can be

- bacterial or viral infection that may be linked with an upper respiratory infection (**herpes virus, chlamydia**, etc.),
- infectious disease/upper respiratory infection,
- allergic reaction,
- foreign body (e.g., branch, spine, cactus, etc.),
- a mass or a topical irritant, and
- chronic dry eye.

Common Points in Medical History
The pet is generally brought in with the chief complaint of red, irritated eyes, with swelling of the skin around the eyes (conjunctiva), and clear to purulent (pus) discharge. With secondary conjunctivitis, there may be other systemic signs also noted (i.e., sneezing, coughing, hives, pruritus, etc.).

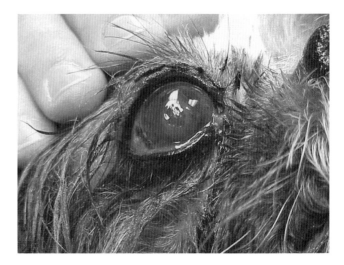

Figure 20.9. Image of a red, inflamed eye with swelling of the skin around the eye (conjunctivitis). There is also a central corneal ulcer. Reprinted with permission from Jeffrey Bowersox, DVM ACVO, Veterinary Specialty Center of Delaware, 1212 E. Newport Pike, Wilmington, DE 19804.

Common Observations on Initial Examination
Common changes in the affected eyes are

- red, inflamed eyes (see Figure 20.9),
- swelling of the conjunctiva,
- ocular discharge, and
- rubbing or scratching at or around the eyes.

Complications
If not diagnosed and properly treated, conjunctivitis can produce chronic ocular irritation, corneal ulceration, pigmentation, and loss of vision.

Diagnosis
Because conjunctivitis can be a primary or secondary disease, clinical diagnostics can include the following.

- **Viral serology:** Testing for specific antibodies against potential chronic infections (i.e., feline leukemia [Felv], feline immunodeficiency virus [FIV], herpes virus, etc.) may be indicated with chronic nonresponsive conjunctivitis in felines.
- **Infectious disease titer screens:** As with viral serology, testing for regional bacterial and fungal infections may also be recommended when faced with a persistent conjunctivitis.
- **Schirmer tear test:** The tear test is a key diagnostic to rule out chronic dry eyes (keratoconjunctivitis sicca or KCS) that may be producing secondary ocular disease.
- **Ocular corneal staining:** Staining is also necessary to help rule out corneal ulceration producing secondary disease. When treating conjunctivitis, ruling out corneal ulceration is important for proper choices of medical treatment.

- **Ocular pressures:** With chronically irritated red eyes, ocular pressures may be indicated.
- **Conjunctival cytology:** With concerns of specific infections (i.e., distemper virus), the veterinarian may obtain cell samples of the conjunctiva. These cytology samples can be sent into a reference lab and evaluated for changes in the cellular architecture suggestive of disease.

Treatment

Treatment is based on the presentation of the animal and the severity of the disease noted. Specific treatment options may be as follows.

- **Medications:** Medications are focused on decreasing conjunctival inflammation or infection around the eye. Medications can vary depending on the cause of the disease.
- **Sedatives/anti-inflammatories:** Depending on how irritated the eye is and how painful the eye may be, the veterinarian may suggest sedatives or anti-inflammatory medication.
- **Elizabethan collar:** If the patient is rubbing at the eyes, an Elizabethan collar or buster collar may be suggested to prevent further injury to the eyes.

Prevention

By monitoring, diagnosing, and properly treating primary disease that can produce secondary ocular disease, conjunctivitis may be prevented.

Discussing Elevation of the Conjunctiva with the Client

- The conjunctiva is the skin that lines the inner eyelid and eye within the eyelids.
- Conjunctivitis is an inflammation or infection of these tissues producing swelling, redness, and possibly ocular discharge.
- Conjunctivitis can occur as a primary allergenic, infectious, or irritation process, or can occur secondary to other ocular and infectious diseases.
- Diagnosis is based on medical history, physical signs, and diagnostic tests to help rule out other ocular and systemic disease.
- Treatment is focused on treating the conjunctivitis and any other underlying disease process.

Keratoconjunctivitis Sicca (KCS)

KCS (dry eyes) is defined as a lack of normal tear production in the eye, producing irritation of the outer segment of the eye, inflammation of the cornea, and chronic mucoid discharge.

Signalment

KCS is common in dogs and rare in cats. It can affect dogs at different ages; however, it has been reported commonly in cocker spaniels, bulldogs, West Highland white terriers, Lhasa apsos, and Shih Tzus. Some reports suggest female dogs may be more predisposed.

Cause of Disease

There can be many causes of KCS in dogs. Some causes can be

- chronic inflammation of the tear glands of the eye (chronic adenitis),
- congenital dry eye,
- drug related—increased sensitivity to sulfa-containing antibiotics
  — Tribrissen
  — Primor
- secondary to removal of the third eyelid.

Common Points in Medical History

The pet is generally brought in with the chief complaint of chronic red, irritated eyes, with swelling of the skin around the eyes (conjunctiva), and mucoid (pus) discharge.

Common Observations on Initial Examination

Common changes in the affected eyes are

- red inflamed eyes (see Figure 20.9),
- abnormal mucoid ocular discharge,
- rubbing or scratching at or around eyes,
- corneal pigmentation, vascularization, or ulceration, and
- elevation of the third eyelid.

Complications

If KCS is not diagnosed and properly treated, the patient may develop secondary chronic conjunctivitis, corneal ulceration, corneal pigmentation, and decreased visualization.

Diagnosis

Because this can be a primary or secondary disease, clinical diagnostics for conjunctivitis can include the following.

- **Schirmer tear test:** The tear test is a key diagnostic to rule out chronic dry eyes (KCS) that may be producing secondary ocular disease.
- **Ocular corneal staining:** Staining is also necessary to help rule out corneal ulceration. When treating conjunctivitis, ruling out corneal ulceration is important for proper choices of medical treatment.
- **Ocular pressures:** With chronically irritated red eyes, ocular pressures may be indicated.

Treatment

Treatment is largely focused on increasing tear production, supplying tear replacement, controlling infection, and reducing inflammation. Medication may need to be administered for the life of the pet.

Prevention
There is no known prevention for KCS.

Discussing Keratoconjunctivitis Sicca (KCS) with the Client

- Keratoconjunctivitis sicca (KCS) is a chronic lack of normal tear production of the eye.
- Due to decreased tear production, the eyes have chronic conjunctivitis, corneal irritation and ulceration, pigmentation of the cornea, and loss of vision.
- KCS can be associated with chronic ocular irritation and long-term use of certain ocular and systemic drugs and is prevalent in the following breeds:
  —Cocker spaniels
  —Bulldogs
  —West Highland white terriers
  —Lhasa apso
  —Shih Tzu
- KCS is diagnosed based on medical history, physical exam, and decreased tear production as measured by the Schirmer tear test.
- The goal of treatment is to implement medications to increase tear production, decrease ocular inflammation and irritation, and decrease pain.
- Medication may need to be administered for the life of the patient.

Corneal Injuries

The cornea is the most superficial clear layer protecting the eye. It contains about 7–11 cell layers in thickness, and the innermost membrane (**Descemet's membrane**) functions to remove fluid from the cornea to maintain its clarity.

Signalment
Corneal injury can happen in any age or breed of dog or cat.

Cause of Disease
The disease can be a primary or secondary disorder; some causes are chronic dry eyes, a bite or fight, infection within the cornea, foreign material in the eye, chronic hair and skin touching the eye (**entropion**), dysfunction within the cornea, glaucoma, and other causes.

Common Points in Medical History
Corneal disease is often uncomfortable for the patient, with the chief complaint being patients with their eyelids closed (especially to bright light [**photophobia**]) and abnormal ocular discharge.

Common Observations on Initial Examination
Common changes in the affected eyes are

- red, inflamed eyes,
- cloudiness of cornea,

- small fixed pupil,
- visible break or irritation in the cornea (see Figure 20.5),
- possible foreign body evident in cornea, and
- evidence of blood vessels invading from cornea of eye.

Complications
If not diagnosed and treated, corneal ulcers may become deeper and can perforate.

Diagnosis
Primary diagnosis of corneal ulceration is made by the observation of the ulcer with corneal stain. Even with an obvious ulceration, staining can help distinguish the depth of the ulceration as well as other ulcers that may not be visible without stain. Furthermore, since ulceration can be a primary or secondary disease, other clinical diagnostics can include the following.

- **Viral serology:** Testing for specific antibodies against potential chronic infections (i.e., Felv, FIV, herpes virus, etc.) may be indicated with chronic nonresponsive conjunctivitis and ulceration.
- **Infectious disease titer screens:** As with viral serology, testing for regional bacterial and fungal infections may also be recommended when faced with a chronic ulceration.
- **Schirmer tear test:** The tear test is a key diagnostic to rule out chronic dry eyes that may be producing secondary ocular disease.

Treatment
Treatment is based on the presentation of the animal and the severity of the disease noted. Some treatment components are presented next.

Medications
- Medications are focused on decreasing conjunctival and ocular inflammation (either topically or systemically) or infection around the eye while keeping the eye lubricated. Furthermore, medications to dilate the pupil may also be suggested if the eye seems painful and the pupil fixed and small.
- *Caution must be used in treating corneal ulceration with ophthalmic steroidal medication* (i.e., triple antibiotic with hydrocortisone, bacitracin/neomycin/polymyxin B with hydrocortisone, etc.). This type of medication slows the healing of corneal ulcers and can actually cause more damage.
- **Sedatives/tranquilizers:** Depending on how irritated the eye is and how much pain the pet may feel, sedation or tranquilizers may be suggested.

If your pet is rubbing at its eyes, an Elizabethan collar or buster collar may be suggested to prevent further injury to the eyes.

Discussing Corneal Ulceration with the Client

- The cornea is a thin, superficial clear layer protecting the eye. The cornea also actively pumps moisture out to maintain its normal clarity.
- When the cornea is damaged by physical trauma or disease, the eye becomes red and irritated and the conjunctiva becomes swollen and inflamed. The iris may also constrict secondary to ocular pain. Furthermore, the cornea may also begin to be cloudy and grayish because its abilities to remove fluid and maintain clarity have been impaired.
- The diagnosis of corneal ulceration is based on positive identification of the ulcer with fluorescein stain. Since corneal ulceration can occur secondary to other ocular disease, the veterinarian may suggest other clinical and ocular diagnostics.
- Treatment is generally focused on medical management of the eye to maintain lubrication, reduce infection and inflammation, and control pain. In severe ulceration, the veterinarian may suggest surgical treatment to promote healing.

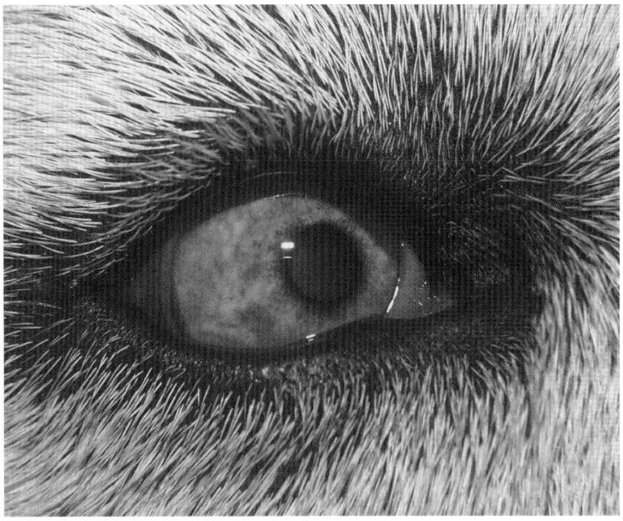

Figure 20.10. Image of an eye affected with uveitis. Notice the cellular infiltrate and constricted pupils. Reprinted with permission from Jeffrey Bowersox, DVM ACVO, Veterinary Specialty Center of Delaware, 1212 E. Newport Pike, Wilmington, DE 19804.

Uveitis

Uveitis is an inflammation of the uveal coat of the eye; the anterior uveal coat is the iris and the posterior uveal coat is the blood vessels supplying the blood to the retina.

Signalment

Uveitis can occur in any species at any age.

Etiology

Uveitis is an immune-mediated inflammation of the eye. Severe cases can alter intraocular structures, resulting in excessive scar tissue and tissue adhesion that may alter the normal function of the eye.

Infectious Disease

There are many bacterial, fungal, and viral diseases that can set up an ocular inflammation. Examples of these types of disease are

- feline leukemia virus FELV,
- feline infectious peritonitis (FIP),
- feline immunodeficiency virus (FIV),
- coccidioidomycosis,
- blastomycosis, and
- ehrlichiosis.

Other examples include the following.

- **Immune-mediated disease:** Alterations of the lens with cataract formation and other metabolic disturbances in the eye can produce an immune-mediated inflammation of the eye itself.

- **Trauma:** Blunt or traumatic injury, toxin, or irritation can set up chronic inflammatory change within the eye.
- **Neoplasia:** Masses or tumors within the eyes can cause uveitis.

Common Points in Medical History

The chief complaint is chronic red, irritated eyes, with swelling of the conjunctiva and purulent (pus) discharge. The eyes may be very sensitive to light and held closed. The patient may also be in pain and sensitive to touch around the eyes. Some owners will also suggest that there may be a change in eye color, which is secondary to the presence of white blood cells and cellular debris within the anterior chamber.

Common Observations on Initial Examination

Common changes in the affected eyes are the following:

- Red, inflamed painful eyes
- Swollen membranes around the eyes
- Clear to heavy purulent discharge evident
- Sensitivity to light (photophobia)
- Rubbing or scratching at or around eyes
- Cloudiness to the cornea and anterior chamber
- Constricted pupils (see Figure 20.10)
- Blood or cellular precipitates evident within the eye

Complications

If not diagnosed and treated, uveitis can block normal drainage of aqueous and vitreous humor and produce an increasing intraocular pressure leading to glaucoma and blindness.

Diagnosis

Because there are many possible systemic diseases that can cause uveitis, systemic and ocular diagnostics are often recommended. Some of these diagnostics tests are listed here.

- **Baseline blood clinical diagnostics (i.e., complete blood count and chemistry):** This clinical diagnostic tool evaluates the body for signs of systemic infection and metabolic or organ disease that may produce a secondary uveitis.
- **Viral serology:** Viral testing for Felv, FIV, and other chronic systemic diseases can help identify a potential primary cause of disease.
- **Infectious disease titer screens:** Testing for specific disease in the geographical area that could be linked to chronic infections in the eyes may be suggested (i.e. coccidioidomycosis, ehrlichiosis, histoplasmosis, blastomycosis, etc.).
- **Ocular pressures:** Ocular pressures are strongly recommended to monitor the eyes for possible secondary glaucoma.

Treatment

Treatment is focused on medication that decreases inflammation or infection in the eye while also treating any underlying systemic cause of the uveitis. Medications can vary depending on the cause of the disease.

Discussing Uveitis with the Client
- Uveitis is an infection or inflammation of the inner aspect of the eye.
- The disease can occur as a primary problem from trauma, irritant, or topical solution and sets up a moderate to severe inflammation. Uveitis can also occur secondarily to other systemic infectious disease.
- Common signs of uveitis are red, inflamed eyes that are sensitive to light with possible clear or mucopurulent discharge. The eyes can be painful to touch, the pupils may be constricted secondary to ocular pain, and vision may be affected because of the pet's sensitivity to light.
- Diagnosis is based on ocular examination and clinical diagnostics, as well as systemic blood work to help define the cause.
- Treatment is focused on medically treating the infections and inflammation of the eye and treating the primary systemic disease if evident.
- The patient must be closely monitored while being treated because of the concerns that the infection may affect the normal drainage of intraocular fluid, increasing intraocular pressure and potentially producing glaucoma and blindness.

Prevention

Diagnosing and treating a primary disease before uveitis can occur can help prevention of the disease.

Glaucoma

Glaucoma is a disease of the neural tissue involving the optic nerve and the retina. The major precipitating cause of glaucoma is an increase in intraocular pressure. Normal ocular pressure in dogs and cats is approximately 15–25 mm Hg, as measured by tonometry.

Etiology

The eye produces a fluid called **aqueous humor,** which is produced in a region behind the iris called the **ciliary body.** Aqueous fluid is produced at a constant rate and therefore must drain from the eye at a constant rate in order for intraocular pressure to be normal. Aqueous fluid normally leaves the eye through drainage angles located between the cornea and the root of the iris. If the drainage angle is abnormal because of congenital anatomical defects or becomes blocked with inflammatory cells, blood, or fibrin, intraocular pressure will elevate to abnormal levels. Glaucoma can come on acutely and affect either one or both eyes. Underlying causes of glaucoma are

- congenital abnormal development of the drainage angle,
- inflammation within the eye (**uveitis**),
- luxation of the lens from its normal position, and
- trauma to the eye causing blood in the eye (**hyphema**).

Signalment

The disease is possible in both dogs and cats, but rarer in cats. The disease typically affects dogs 4–9 years of age. Breeds with a predilection for primary glaucoma are the

- artic breeds (husky, malamute),
- Bouvier,
- basset hound,
- chow chow,
- shar-pei, and
- spaniel breeds (American and English cocker, Welsh springer).

Common Points in Medical History

The chief point is severe red, irritated eyes (conjunctivitis). There is acute pain and sensitivity to light. The patient may be acutely blind. Finally, with chronic disease, the eye itself may be enlarged (see Figure 20.11).

Common Observations on Initial Examination

Common changes in the affected eyes are

- an eye that is sensitive to light,
- a painful eye,
- a red, inflamed eye,
- a clear discharge from eye,

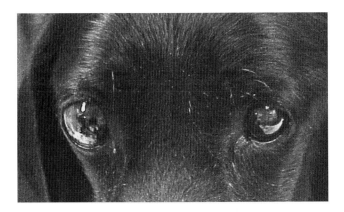

Figure 20.11. Image of a right eye affected with glaucoma. This eye is swollen, painful, and blind. Reprinted with permission from Jeffrey Bowersox, DVM ACVO, Veterinary Specialty Center of Delaware, 1212 E. Newport Pike, Wilmington, DE 19804.

- an eye (itself) that begins to look swollen and enlarged,
- a chronically inflamed eye, and
- cloudiness to the cornea.

Complications

If not diagnosed and treated quickly, glaucoma can produce permanent damage to the eye because acute glaucoma can rapidly progress to permanent visual loss.

Diagnosis

The diagnosis of glaucoma is based on increased intraocular pressure (more than 25 mm hg) as observed by Schiotz or digital tonometry (i.e., Tonopen). Because glaucoma can occur from other disease entities, the veterinarian may suggest other diagnostics to assess if there are any other ocular or systemic diseases that may predispose the eyes. Some of these diagnostics tests can be the following.

- **Baseline blood clinical diagnostics (i.e., complete blood count and chemistry):** This clinical diagnostic tool evaluates the body for signs of systemic infection and metabolic or organ disease that may produce uveitis.
- **Viral serology:** Viral testing for Felv, FIV, and other chronic systemic diseases can help identify a potential primary cause of disease.
- **Infectious disease titer screens:** Testing for specific disease in the geographical area that could be linked to chronic infections in the eyes may be suggested (i.e., valley fever, tick fever, histoplasmosis, blastomycosis, etc.).
- **Schirmer tear test:** The tear test will evaluate the eyes for an accompanying dry eye condition, which would also need to be treated.
- **Ocular corneal staining:** Staining detects ulceration in the cornea that can occur secondary to glaucoma. Corneal staining is also necessary to make sure that it is safe to use Shiotz tonometry to evaluate ocular pressures.

Discussing Glaucoma with the Client

- The eye produces a thick viscous liquid that helps maintain the shape and gives nutrition to the internal structures of the eye.
- This liquid medium is produced by small glands located behind the iris and is eliminated through small pores also located near the iris.
- If at any time there is a decrease in drainage of this liquid media, the ocular pressures can increase.
- If pressures are more than 25 mm Hg, the retina and nervous tissue within the eye can become damaged or destroyed.
- Glaucoma is more common in canines between 4 and 9 years of age. The following breeds are more susceptible to the disease:
  —Artic breeds (husky, malamute, etc.)
  —Bouvier
  —Bassett hound
  —Chow chow
  —Shar-pei
  —Spaniel breeds (American and English cocker, Welsh springer)
- The patient presents with red, irritated eyes that may be painful to touch. The pet may squint or show pain in normal room light or daylight. The eyes themselves may appear swollen.
- Diagnosis is based upon ocular pressures measured by a manual or electronic Tonometer. Other blood work may be recommended if the veterinarian is concerned about other ocular or systemic disease that could produce a secondary glaucoma
- Treatment is based on how severe and acute the onset of disease occurs. In acute cases, treatment is focused on medication and support. With chronic care, surgical options for the eye may also be discussed.
- Without treatment, the pet can become blind and have a severely painful eye.
- Many of these cases may need a referral to a veterinary ophthalmologist for more in-depth medical and surgical treatment options.

Treatment

Because acute glaucoma can rapidly progress to permanent visual loss, initial treatment by veterinarians is aimed at reducing intraocular pressure with oral and intravenous medications. Glaucoma cases may need to be referred to a veterinary ophthalmologist early in the onset of the disease for more specific medical and surgical treatment.

With acute glaucoma treatment goals are as follows.

- **Hospitalization and fluids:** The patient may need to be admitted into the hospital for monitoring intraocular pressure and the administration of intravenous and topical medication to help begin decreasing intraocular pressure.

- **Medications:** Both topical and systemic medications are used to aid in the decrease of pressure within the eye.
- **Treating the underlying disease:** If there is the presence of an underlying cause for the glaucoma (e.g., lens luxation, chronic infection inside the eye, etc.), the primary disease must also be treated and controlled.

With chronic glaucoma treatment goals are as follows.

- **Treating the underlying disease:** See the discussion above.
- **Medications:** Medications are both topical and systemic and will aid in the decrease of pressure and pain within the eye.
- **Surgery:** With blind, painful eyes, an eye **enucleation** (removal) or a prosthetic implant may be suggested.

Prevention
Monitoring ocular pressures in breeds that are predisposed to glaucoma and monitoring patients with underlying disease that could produce glaucoma can prevent the disease.

Entropion
Entropion is an abnormal turning of the lid with resultant irritation of the cornea by hair and lashes. Over time, chronic irritation and ocular pain make the affected animal very uncomfortable.

Signalment
Entropion is commonly seen in dogs and cats, especially those breeds with short noses and excessive skin folds. It has been reported in puppies as young as 2–6 weeks old (especially chow chow and shar-pei), but usually affects animals less than 1 year of age. It also occurs secondary to chronic infection around the eye (conjunctivitis/uveitis). Common breeds affected are the

- shar-pei,
- chow chow,
- spaniels,
- retrievers,
- English bulldog,
- pug,
- Pekingese,
- mastiff,
- Saint Bernard, and
- Newfoundland.

Etiology
Entropion is generally caused by a congenital predisposition in facial conformation producing an excess and redundancy of skin and facial folds on the head and eyes. In some cases, entropion can occur secondary to chronically inflamed and irritated eyes (**spastic entropion**).

Common Points in Medical History
The chief complaint is irritated eyes with excessive tearing.

Common Observations on Initial Examination
Common changes in the affected eyes (see Figure 20.5) are

- increased tearing of the eyes (**epiphora**),
- red, inflamed eyes,
- chronic mucoid discharge from eyes,
- cloudiness of cornea, and
- visible pigmentation in the cornea.

Complications
If not diagnosed and corrected, entropion can produce chronic irritation, ulceration, and pigmentation that may lead to pain and discomfort as well as decreased vision.

Diagnosis
The disease is generally diagnosed with evidence of conjunctivitis, corneal ulceration, and the presence of repetitive skin folds irritating and touching the cornea. However, since this disease could be caused by other causes, the veterinarian may suggest the following diagnostic tests:

Discussing Entropion with the Client
- Entropion is an abnormal turning of the lid with resultant irritation of the cornea by hair and lashes.
- Entropion is commonly seen in dogs and cats, especially in those breeds with short noses and excessive skin folds. The following common breeds are affected:
  —Shar-pei
  —Chow chow
  —Spaniels
  —Retrievers
  —English bulldogs
  —Pugs
  —Pekingese
  —Mastiffs
  —Saint Bernard
  —Newfoundland
- Clinical signs include red, irritated eyes with heavy clear to purulent discharge (pus) and increased tearing. The eyes themselves may be hard to visualize due to swelling of the skin around the eyes and hair touching and irritating the cornea.
- Treatment usually entails surgical procedures that temporarily or permanently tack up the extra skin around the eyes to prevent hair touching and irritating the cornea.
- If entropion is not diagnosed and treated, the chronic irritation can produce corneal ulceration, pigmentation, and, rarely, blindness.

- Diagnostic blood work
- Schirmer tear test
- Ocular corneal staining
- Conjunctival smear/biopsy

Treatment
Treatment is based on the presentation of the animal and the severity of the disease noted.

- **Medications:** Medications are focused on decreasing conjunctival and ocular inflammation (caused secondarily by the skin irritation) while keeping the eye lubricated. Medications can vary depending on the type of secondary disease present (e.g., conjunctivitis, corneal ulceration).
- **Surgery:** If the eyes are persistently irritated from invasion of the excess skin, temporary or permanent surgical repair may be recommended depending on the age of the pet and the severity of the condition.

Prevention
Early monitoring of susceptible breeds as puppies for obvious entropion can help decrease and prevent chronic corneal irritation and minimize damage and sight impairment.

The Ear

The ears have two functions; they receive auditory stimuli and maintain equilibrium and balance (see Figure 20.12). The ear is divided into two parts: the external and internal aspects of the ear.

- The external ear anatomy consists of the earflap (**pinna**) and the canal that leads from the eardrum outward (**external acoustic meatus**). These structures function as a funnel-like receptacle that collects sound vibrations and focuses them toward the inner ear.
- The inner ear structures, housed within the bony skull, are composed of the **middle and inner ear,** which functions to transmit and convert the sound vibrations into nerve impulses; they also act as a receptors for equilibrium.

In a general practice, the majority of otic disease is presented as an inflammatory external ear problem (**otitis**). In severe cases, the patient may present with balance and deafness issues. Otitis externa may be associated with bacterial, fungal, yeast, or parasitic infections (ear mites). Otitis can be made worse with other systemic problems, such as allergies, hormonal disease (i.e. hypothyroidism), and localized masses and tumors (i.e., polyps). Narrowing of the external ear canal, hair growing in the ear canal, and a pendulous floppy ear pinna may be associated with inadequate air circulation in the ear and may predispose the patient to an infection.

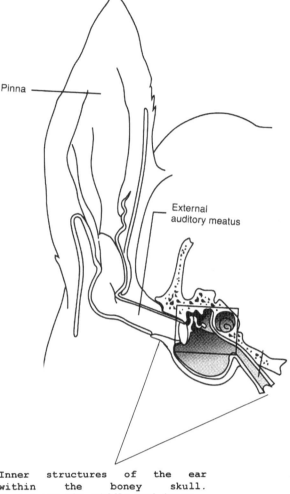

Pinna

External auditory meatus

```
Inner   structures   of   the   ear
within   the   boney   skull.
Comprising the middle and inner
ear canals.
```

Figure 20.12. Illustration of the architecture of the ear. Reprinted with permission from Jeffrey Bowersox, DVM ACVO, Veterinary Specialty Center of Delaware, 1212 E. Newport Pike, Wilmington, DE 19804.

Obtaining a History in Patients with Otic Disease

Key questions to ask when obtaining a history from a patient with ear disease are presented next.

Does the Pet Have a History of Chronic Ear Infections?
As previously discussed with skin allergies (see Chapter 19), it is important to know how often ear infections occur and what was used to treat the ear in the past.

Does the Pet Scratch and Chew Elsewhere, or Does the Patient Have a History of Skin Allergies?
Animals with chronic skin allergies can also have flare ups of ear infections. These patients may also need systemic medication for allergies to help reduce whole-body inflammation and pruritus.

Is the Canine Patient Being Treated for Hypothyroidism?

Low-thyroid animals can be more predisposed to ear infections.

Is the Animal a Swimmer?

Pets that swim frequently can predispose themselves to chronic ear infections.

Does the Animal Have a Long Pendulous Pinna That Covers the Opening of the External Ear Canal?

Animals that have longer pinna that fully cover the ear canal may be more prone to ear infections due to decreased oxygen concentration in the deeper ear.

Does the Pet Have Exposure to Strays and Other Animals?

Pets with exposure to other animals and strays have increased risk of contracting ear mites.

Physical Changes to the Ear on Initial Assessment

When evaluating an animal on an initial assessment, some very simple observation of the ears can tell you a great deal about ear infections and the overall health of the animal. These factors are as follows.

- **Is there debris, odor, or purulent discharge evident in the ear canal?** Does the ear canal seem swollen and inflamed (see Figure 20.13)? Does the ear canal appear to be narrowed?
- **Is there unusual pigment or bruising to the earflap?** Yellowing of the earflap (jaundice) can be seen with liver disease or autoimmune hemolytic anemia (see Figure 20.14). Bruising on the earflap and on other parts of the body can suggest a problem with the pet's ability to clot blood.
- **Does the pet have a head tilt?** Animals with severe inner ear infections will sometimes preset with significant head tilts to the left or right side. The direction of the tilt can suggest which ear is affected.
- **Does the pet have a balance problem, rapid side-to-side eye movement, or act as if it cannot balance itself?** Inner ear disease can present with severe loss of balance, rapid eye movements (**nystagmus**), and uncoordination so severe that the pet may almost seem as if it is seizuring. However, it is important to note that loss of balance can also be related to central nervous system disease as well.

Diagnostics of Ear Disease

As with the eye, there are specific ear diagnostic tests to help identify the cause of the problem. However, it is important to note that because the ear is also apart of the integu-

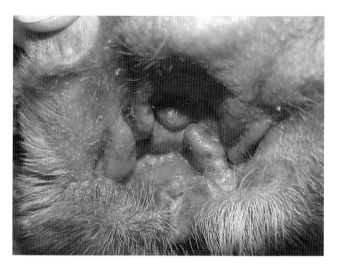

Figure 20.13. Image of an infected ear canal. Note the severe swelling of the canal itself.

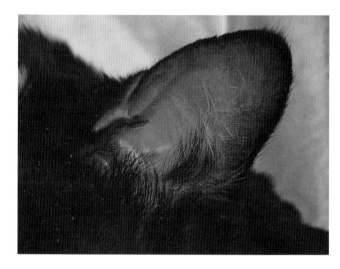

Figure 20.14. Image of a yellow ear flap. This pigmentation can suggest liver or an autoimmune disease.

mentary system, other diseases can set up a secondary otitis. Furthermore, some patients may be in pain and may need sedation or a short-acting anesthetic in order to perform a thorough ear examination. Some potential diagnostic tests may be as follows.

- **Ear cytology:** A clinical diagnostic test for acute/chronic ear disease is an ear cytology using tri-color/Diff-Quik stain. Cytology can show bacterial and fungal pathogens, as well as the presence of white blood cells.
- **Ear mite cytology:** Similar to ear cytology, the debris from the ear is placed on a slide containing mineral oil. If ear mites are present, the mite and its eggs may be observed.

- **Culture and sensitivity:** When chronic bacterial infection is suspected, the bacteria can be cultured and an effective antibiotic can be indicated.
- **Diagnostic blood work:** When concerns of systemic disease causing changes to the skin and ear canal are suspected, diagnostic blood work might be suggested:
  — Complete blood count
  — Chemistry panel
  — Thyroid level
  — Viral serology (Felv/FIV)
  — Infectious screens (fungal)

Discussing Clinical Diagnostics for the Ears with the Client

- **Ear cytology:** By taking an ear swab and examining it under the microscope, the veterinarian can observe if the infection is caused by yeast, bacteria, or if it is a mixed infection. This will aid in the choice of medication for treatment.
- **Ear mite cytology:** By examining the debris in mineral oil under magnification, the veterinarian can observe if adult ear mites or ear mite eggs are evident.
- **Culture and sensitivity:** With chronic severe ear infections, the debris can be cultured to find out exactly what type of bacterial component is evident and determine to what types of antibiotics the bacteria are sensitive.
- **Diagnostic blood work:** Since ear infections can occur secondary to other systemic diseases, general blood work, thyroid levels ,and infectious diseases titers may be suggested.

Diseases of the Ear

Ear Infections (Otitis)

Typically, ear infections are inflammations and/or infections of the external ear canal by bacteria or fungus. These infections (**otitis externa**) are generally the most common and benign. More rarely, infections of the inner ear canal (**otitis media** or **otitis interna**) can be much more serious because the infection can begin to affect balance.

Signalment

Ear infections can affect both cats and dogs of any age. However, dogs with long earflaps are more predisposed to infections. Some species with this type of ear anatomy are cocker spaniels, springer spaniels, golden retrievers, terriers, and poodles. There is no age or sexual predilection.

Etiology

The disease is caused by a chronic buildup of waxy debris and bacteria that cause a progressive inflammation within the ear canal. As the infection becomes more chronic, the ear canal's cartilage can become chronically infected, swelling shut and calcifying into bone. As the ear canal begins to close, infection continues at a more rapid rate, infecting the inner ear. Otitis can occur secondary to masses and polyps within the inner ear or from a bloodborne infection (rarely).

Common Points in Medical History

Patients will present with a history of shaking the head, rubbing at their ears, malodor coming from the ears, ear sensitivity, and observable debris within the ear canal.

Common Observations on Initial Examination

Physical symptoms depend on the type of ear infection, its chronicity, and severity of infection. Common signs may be as follows.

Physical Signs of Otitis Externa

- Ears red and inflamed
- Scratching of the ears
- Tilting of the head
- Pain and sensitivity around the ear
- Odor and debris in the ear canal

Physical Signs of Inner or Middle Ear Infection (Otitis Media/Interna)

- Shaking of the head
- Smell noted from the ears
- Ears red and inflamed
- Tilting of the head
- Pain and sensitivity around the ear
- Problems walking/uncoordination
- Vomiting/nausea
- Inability to eat properly
- Rapid movement of the eyes back and forth (**nystagmus**)
- Elevation of the third eyelid

Complications

If not diagnosed and treated, an outer ear infection (otitis externa) can become a chronic severe infection that enters the middle and inner ear drum, causing problems with the animal's ability to balance and hear.

Diagnosis

As discussed above, clinical diagnostics for the ear can involve cytology, culture and sensitivity, and possibly systemic blood work. The clinical tests depend on how the patient presents, the appearance of the ear canals based on preliminary examination, and past history of ear infections.

Treatment

Treatment is focused on destroying the infection present in the ear and returning the ear to proper health. It may be necessary to continue treating the ear infection until all signs of infection have been gone for 2–3 weeks. *Stopping treatment too early can set up bacterial resistance to antibiotics and produce a severe chronic ear infection.* Some possible treatment options are discussed next.

- **Medications:** With mild ear infections, ear-cleaning liquid and topical medication may be suggested. Systemic antibiotics are also possible given the evidence of severe infection.
- **Surgical ear flush/otoscopy:** With chronic infection or evidence of deeper infection, an ear flushing and inner ear exam under anesthesia can be extremely beneficial. This will allow the veterinarian to examine the deeper ear canal for foreign material, polyps or masses, or possible punctures to the inner eardrum, while also allowing a cleaning of the ears with large quantities of antiseptic solutions.
- **Surgical repair to the ear canal and opening of the inner ear drum:** This procedure is generally done only in severe infection of ear cartilage with closing of the ear canal and infection of the inner ear and bony labyrinth. This surgical resection of the ear canal and opening of the inner ear to allow drainage and removal of infected material may be the only way to resolve a severe chronic infection.

Prevention

Routine cleaning of the pet's ears and monitoring for changes in odor and debris can help prevent or detect early infection before a more serious long-term problem can occur.

> **Discussing Bacterial or Fungal Otitis with the Client**
> - Ear infections are inflammation of the outer ear canal, middle ear, or the inner eardrum and bone caused primarily by bacteria or fungus.
> - In most cases, infections are mild and of the outer ear canal, producing discharge and odor from the ear, sensitivity, and redness.
> - In severe cases, ear infections can infect the cartilage and bone of the ear, producing chronic inflamed ears that may not easily respond to medication. Furthermore, the pet may also have deafness and balance problems.
> - Diagnosis of ear infections is based on cytology of the ear debris, culture and sensitivity, and possibly general blood work, if a systemic cause of the disease is suspected.
> - Treatment is based on topical and systemic medications. In very sensitive or chronically infected ears, surgical options to flush and clean the ear may need to be explored.
> - If not treated, severe chronic ear infections can occur, producing early deafness, balance problems, and severe infections that may require surgery.

Ear Mite Infection (Otitis)

Ear mite infections are inflammations of the outer ear canal caused by the ear mite *Otodectes cynotis.*

Etiology

Ear mite infection is common in young puppies and kittens or outside cats. There is no age, breed, or sexual predilection. *The disease is spread by direct contact from animal to animal and is very contagious.*

Cause of Disease

The disease is caused by the ear mite *Otodectes cynotis.*

Common Points in Medical History

Patients will present with a history of shaking the head, rubbing at their ears, malodor coming from the ears, ear sensitivity, scratching at the ears, self-traumatizing the head and ear regions, and observable debris within the ear canal.

Common Observations on Initial Examination

Physical symptoms of an ear mite infection are

- shaking of the head,
- smell noted from the ears,
- ears red and inflamed,
- black to red flaky debris evident in ears,
- tilting of the head,
- scabbing and hair loss on head and ear region, and
- pain and sensitivity around the ear.

Complications

If not diagnosed and treated, ear mite infection can produce a chronic irritated outer ear infection that is infectious to other animals in the household.

> **Discussing Ear Mite Otitis with the Client**
> - Ear mite infections are caused by a microscopic mite, *Otodectes cynotis.*
> - In most cases, infections are mild and of the outer ear canal, producing discharge and odor from the ear, sensitivity, and redness.
> - Ear mites are contagious to other animals.
> - Diagnosis of ear infections is based on observing mites and/or their eggs upon an ear mite cytology.
> - Treatment is based on topical and systemic medications.
> - If not treated, the patient will develop severe chronic ear infections that can be infective to other animals.

Diagnosis
Ear mite cytology is usually suggested to observe the ear mite and its eggs.

Treatment
Treatment is focused on topical or systemic medication that kills the ear mites and cleaning of the ear. Repeat treatment to prevent reinfection may be necessary, as well as treating all pets within the household.

Aural Hematoma
An **aural hematoma** is an accumulation of blood between the cartilage of the earflap and the skin causing a firm, enlarging pocket of fluid to build. As the pocket progresses, the earflap becomes more engorged and painful.

Signalment
Aural hematomas can affect dogs and cats of any age.

Cause of Disease
The cause of the formation of the aural hematoma is due to the pet's shaking its head vigorously until blood vessels within the earflap begin to ooze and blood accumulates. Causes of head shaking are an ear infection, allergies, a bite or sting near or on the ear, or a small mass or polyp within the ear canal.

Common Points in Medical History
Patients will present with a swelling evident on the ear pinna and may also present with shaking the head, rubbing at their ears, malodor coming from the ears, ear sensitivity, and observable debris within the ear canal.

Common Observations on Initial Examination
Physical symptoms or an aural hematoma can be

- earflap becoming enlarged, swollen, and painful (see Figure 20.15),
- shaking the head and ears,
- head tilt toward affected ear,
- rubbing ear on ground or scratching ear, and
- smell or odor coming from the ear.

Complications
Once the hematoma is created, blood will continue to fill the area until the region is lanced and repaired. *Without any form of treatment, the earflap can be chronically painful and change its normal appearance.*

Diagnosis
Because this disease is possibly produced from an underlying infection, cytology, culture and sensitivity, and systemic blood work may be recommended.

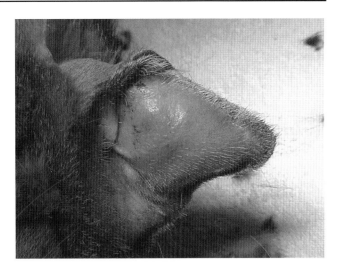

Figure 20.15.   Image of an aural hematoma. The swelling of the pinna is filled with blood secondary to the pet shaking its head and causing capillary bleeding.

Discussing Aural Hematomas with the Client
- An aural hematoma is a collection of blood within the ear flap.
- Normally, the ear flap is closely associated with the cartilage of the ear, and as the pet shakes its head, small capillaries below the ear flap can begin to bleed and ooze. As this process continues, a pocket of blood can form.
- Aural hematomas usually occur secondary to ear infections, ear masses and polyps, and pruritis.
- Diagnosis of the cause of the hematoma can include ear cytology, culture and sensitivity, and general blood work.
- Treatment is focused on draining the hematoma, usually surgically, and placing sutures or a drain to help prevent the blood clot from reforming. Once drained, the pet can be placed on medication to help control the cause of head shaking and itchiness.
- Aural hematomas can occur elsewhere on the pinna or on the other ear as well.
- If not treated, the hematoma can enlarge, affecting the entire pinna, become painful, and cause a permanent cosmetic change to the ear.

Treatment
The goal of treatment is to drain the hematoma and control the cause of the head shaking and pruritus. There are many different techniques used to lance and drain the hematoma.

Some techniques that have been used are

- repetitive drainage of the hematoma in the awake animal,
- surgical drainage and placement of a Penrose drain/teat canula, and
- surgical drainage and placement of full-thickness sutures to form granulomas that helps prevent reformation of the hematoma.

Please be aware, however, that hematomas can occur on other parts of the same earflap and on the other ear at any time.

A surgical ear flushing may also be recommended at the time of hematoma surgery to help decrease the amount of debris and infection occurring in the ear. Finally, topical and systemic medication can be used to help control/cure the underlying cause of the hematoma.

Prevention
Early detection and control of ear infections, polyps, and masses can prevent head shaking and pruritis.

CD-ROM 1 reviews material presented in this chapter. Please try the cases for Section 2 (Anatomy and Physiology— The Science behind the Diseases) *to help reinforce the information presented here.*

Section 3

Clinical Diagnostics—
The Science behind the Diagnostics

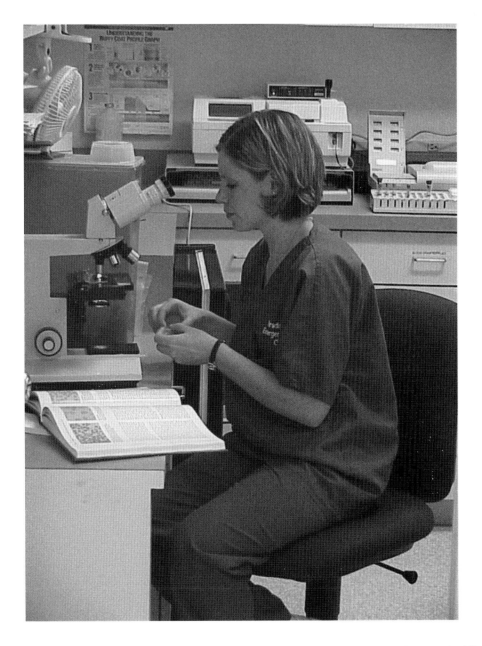

The goal of this section is to understand how each diagnostic test is performed and what each test's significance is. A team member should not only know how to perform a given diagnostic but also understand why the test is being evaluated and what other samples may need to be collected if there are abnormalities detected.

Chapter 21

Complete Blood Count

The complete blood count (CBC) examines the blood for changes in the red and white blood cell count, platelet count, blood parasites, and changes in cell morphology that can suggest underlying diseases. A CBC is an integral part of a routine minimum database or metabolic health screen. It's components are

- a packed cell volume (PCV)/total protein,
- red blood cell count,
- white blood cell count,
- a platelet count, and
  blood film evaluation (**differential**).

Depending on the hospital, the CBC can be done in-house or sent out to a veterinary diagnostic laboratory. The in-hospital instruments can be very accurate in obtaining blood cell counts; however, the hospital team members should be comfortable in evaluating PCV, total protein, and a differential blood film. All team members need to become proficient in evaluating acute changes in blood cell morphology that can help the medical team understand diseases affecting a patient. Furthermore, all team members should be able to discuss why the CBC is being recommended and be able to explain the type of information it gives the veterinarian.

Obtaining and Handling the Blood Sample: The Purple-Topped Tube

1. Once collected from a peripheral vein, the blood is placed into an EDTA (ethylene diamine tetraacetic acid). At least 1 cc of blood is needed in most cases.
2. The tube should be gently inverted 5–10 times to mix the anticoagulant thoroughly with the blood. This tube prevents blood clotting and allows a CBC to be performed.
3. Check the tubes. On initial blood collection, the blood tubes should also be checked. Changes in the EDTA tube can suggest disease or artifacts that can affect the CBC. The tube should be checked for the following.
   - **Amount:** If the tube cannot be completely filled, at least 1 cc of fresh blood should be added to a standard purple-topped tube. If there is not enough blood, the EDTA fluid can dilute the sample and decrease all blood parameters.
   - **Blood clots:** Although a blood clot is not suggestive of pathology, a blood clot occurs if the blood sample took too long to collect or if the tube was not adequately mixed. The presence of a clot will not allow an accurate determination of the platelet number and red blood cell count (PCV).
   - **Agglutination:** When mixing the purple-topped tube, it is important to check to see if the red cells precipitate out like snow in a snow globe. This can be suggestive of a severe disease process, **immune-mediated hemolytic anemia.** In this disease process, the red blood cells adhere (agglutinate) to each other because the patient's immune system is responding to their red blood cells as if they were a foreign substance. Once stuck together, the red blood cells are removed by cells in the spleen and destroyed. *If there is a concern of agglutination, the veterinarian should be notified immediately* (see Figure 21.1).

Sample Preparation and Evaluation

There are three components to the complete blood count. They are the

- PCV/total protein,
- white and red blood cell count, and
- differential slide cytology.

Each test is an important key to evaluating the overall health of the patient. Although it is the veterinarian's responsibility to evaluate and interpret changes in the blood work, the medical team members should have an understanding of what each test evaluates and the possible diseases the abnormalities suggest. This will allow the team member to alert the veterinarian when there are significant changes, better monitor the patient, and more effectively communicate the importance of the diagnostic tests to the client.

Packed Cell Volume (PCV/Total Protein)
The PCV is the most reliable measurement of the red blood cell level in a patient: It is the percentage of red blood cells present in a peripheral blood sample. It allows qualitative evaluation of any change in the volume of red blood cells in whole blood that could suggest a disease process (see Figure 21.2). Many blood cell counters do a calculated hematocrit (HCT), which is an evaluation of red blood cell concentration that is a calculated measurement based on the total red

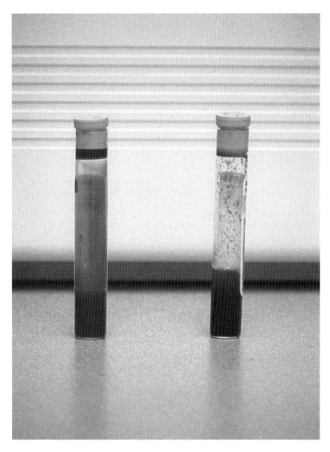

Figure 21.1.   The image shows two purple-topped tubes. The one on the left is normal blood. The one on the right shows agglutination. This pattern, which looks like snow in a snow globe, suggests the white blood cells are attacking the red blood cells as foreign bacteria. This suggests an immune-mediated hemolytic anemia.

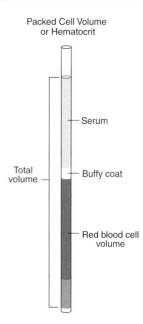

Figure 21.2.   Normal hematocrit. In this illustration, the hematocrit is spun down and separated into the red blood cell volume, the buffy coat, and the serum.

blood cell count and the size of the red blood cells. In an ill patient, abnormalities in the red and white blood cells can affect the PCV, making the measurement incorrect by a few percentage points.

The procedure for obtaining a PCV and total protein is as follows.

1. Whole blood from an EDTA or heparin tube is placed into a **microhematocrit tube**. The tube is sealed with clay.
2. The tube is placed in a centrifuge and spun for 5 minutes at high speed. The centrifuge should maintain a constant high speed to prevent artifactual changes in the cells.
3. While spinning, the blood separates into columns of red blood cells, white blood cells, and plasma.
4. The tube is placed on a hematocrit card reader, and the top of the plasma column and bottom of the red blood cell column are lined up with the card. The red blood cell level is then read and recorded as a percentage.
5. The white layer just above the red blood cells, the **buffy coat,** is small (usually <1%) and represents the white

blood cells and platelets. Significant increases or decreases in this level should be recorded.
6. The layer above the buffy coat is the **plasma** (or fluid component of the blood); it should be opaque and straw-colored. Changes in color should be recorded in the record.
7. The tube is then broken above the buffy coat layer and the plasma is placed on a refractometer. The sample is examined and the total protein is measured. This result is then recorded in the chart.

Normal Measurements
In Table 21.1, normal values of the PCV/total protein are listed. These reference ranges can vary depending on the lab or instrument used. The values are meant only as a reference, and any concerns regarding these measurements *must always be discussed with the veterinarian.*

Abnormalities in Packed Cell Volume
Changes in the PCV can suggest serious disease in the patient. Any significant changes should be discussed with the veterinarian immediately. The significance of overall changes is discussed next.

Low Packed Cell Volume(Red Blood Cell Concentration)
Decreases in the red blood cell concentration suggest disease or maybe an artifact. A low PCV can be caused from the following.

- **Dilution:** If the blood sample is too small, the EDTA in the tube can dilute the PCV. In this case, other parameters

Table 21.1. Normal hematocrit values.

Measurement	Normal
Hematocrit	Canine: 35–55%
	Feline: 26–46%
Buffy coat (qualitative measurement)	Should always be evident, but generally less than 1% of column.
Serum	Clear to light straw color.
Total protein	5.5–7.5 mg/dl

(i.e., white blood cells and platelets) are also usually low. If there is concern for dilution, a new sample should be drawn and tested.

- **Blood clot:** A blood clot in the EDTA tube lowers the amount of red blood cells available to be measured by the PCV. If a clot is suspected, a new sample should be drawn and tested.
- **Increased destruction of red blood cells:** If the patient is destroying red blood cells at an increased rate due to an immune-mediated disease (i.e., **immune-mediated hemolytic anemia)**, the PCV will be low. Furthermore, there may be agglutination present in the EDTA tube; the plasma should be hemolyzed (see below).
- **Blood loss:** When a patient is actively bleeding, the PCV will be low. With severe blood loss, there can also be a low total protein and low platelet count evident (see below).
- **Anemia of chronic disease:** In patients suffering from severe chronic disease (i.e., renal, liver, or infectious diseases), the animal may become increasingly anemic as the disease progresses. This is usually a mild anemia.

Increased PCV (Red Blood Cell Concentration)
Increases in the PCV generally suggest **dehydration**. As the patient's hydration status becomes more challenged, the amount of fluid in the blood decreases, increasing the percentage of red blood cells in the PCV. *The more significant the dehydration, the higher the PCV.* Dehydration also causes elevation in the total protein.

Qualitative Abnormalities in the Plasma
Serum color can change significantly with metabolic and immune-mediated diseases, difficulty with venipuncture, and feeding. *It is extremely important to note changes in the plasma because they can suggest disease conditions, as well as affect other chemical measurements in the chemistry profile (see Chapter 22).* Common changes in the plasma are discussed next.

- **Red: Hemolysis,** or increased red blood cell destruction, is seen with diseases that disrupt or lyse red blood cells (i.e., immune-mediated hemolytic anemia) or seen secondary to a difficult blood draw where increased move-

ment of the patient or excessive aspiration pressure of the syringe has artifactually produced hemolysis. If hemolysis is noted, the EDTA tube should be checked for agglutination.

- **Yellow: Jaundice** indicates an increased concentration of **bilirubin** in the plasma. Bilirubin is a breakdown pigment of hemoglobin from the red blood cell. Jaundice can occur when there is marked red blood cell breakdown in the vessels or removal of red blood cells by the macrophages in the spleen and liver (i.e., immune-mediated hemolytic anemia) or decreased clearance of bilirubin by the liver. If jaundice is caused by red blood cell breakdown, there should be anemia with either hemolysis or agglutination noted in the EDTA tube.
- **White: Lipemia** indicates high fat content in the plasma. It is often seen in animals that have just eaten a fatty meal that causes an increase in the fat (lipid) content in the plasma. It can also be associated with specific diseases affecting fat metabolism (i.e., diabetes mellitus, hyperadrenocorticism, pancreatitis, liver disease, hyperlipidemia, hypercholesterolemia). *Lipemia can affect many parameters in the chemistry and should be noted in the record.*

Abnormalities with Total Protein
Although many diseases can affect total protein concentration, it is important to understand overall changes in protein can suggest serious disease. Overall changes in protein concentration should be correlated with changes in the animal's overall health (see Table 21.2).

Abnormalities in the Buffy Coat
The buffy coat is the layer of cells just above the red blood cell column that corresponds to the white blood cells and platelets. The buffy coat layer is normally less than 1% of the total blood column. Changes in the buffy coat can suggest serious disease processes (see Table 21.3).

The Complete Blood Cell Count

With newer, less expensive technologies, complete red blood cell, white blood cell, and platelet counts can be obtained with an automatic cell counter in the hospital or by submitting a sample to an outside laboratory. Most instruments offer reliable evaluation of cell populations in most disease processes. Because of the availability of affordable cell counters, most hospitals do not spend the time or money educating their staff on performing manual blood cell counts. The manual techniques are time consuming, expensive, and must be practiced regularly for accuracy.

However, no cell counter can evaluate changes in blood cell morphology that can assist in characterizing acute infections, blood parasites, sepsis, cancer, and metabolic diseases. *It is essential that every technical team member be able to perform a blood cell differential count and identify changes in red blood cell, white blood cell, and platelet morphology. These observable changes may be the only indica-*

Table 21.2. An overview of changes in total protein.

Measurement	Possible Cause
Increased total protein Total protein >7.5 mg/dl	• In general, increases in total protein concentration are seen with dehydration. Similar to the increase in the hematocrit, the protein concentration is higher in blood with a lower fluid volume. • It is important to note that chronic infectious, inflammatory, and neoplastic disease can also cause increases in total protein concentration.
Decreased total protein Total protein <5.0 mg/dl, with decrease in hematocrit	• When decreased total protein concentration and decreased PCV are seen in acute disease conditions, the main concern is external blood loss. When the animal is actively bleeding, protein will follow the red blood cells out of the vessels. • It is important to note that chronic infectious, inflammatory, and neoplastic diseases can also cause decreases in both measurements.
Decreased total protein Total protein <5.0 mg/dl with normal hematocrit.	• Decreased total protein concentration with a normal red blood cell population can suggest diseases associated with decreased absorption of protein (gastrointestinal disease), decreased production of protein (liver disease), or increased excretion of protein (renal disease) • Other chronic inflammatory or neoplastic disease can also produce these changes.

Table 21.3. Changes in the buffy coat.

Measurement	Possible Cause
Increased buffy coat (>1% of entire column)	• If buffy coat is increased, it can suggest infection, inflammation, or cancer (i.e., lymphoma, mast cell leukemia, etc.). • When noted, a buffy coat smear is recommended. (See blood cell differential.) • The presence of abnormal cells in the buffy coat may suggest white blood cell cancer (i.e., lymphoma, leukemia).
Decreased buffy coats (<1%)	• Decreased buffy coat layer size is associated with decreased white blood cell counts. They can be seen with severe viral infections that cause immunosuppression by decreasing the white blood cell numbers. • Decreased white blood cell counts can also be seen with neoplastic, hormonal, and severe inflammatory disease.

tion of early serious disease. In order to evaluate blood cell morphology, the team member must be able to produce a good blood film. There are many ways to produce a good blood film. Here is one method.

1. Place a single drop of blood at the end of a microscope slide.
2. Place another slide in front of the drop of blood at a 45-degree angle to the first slide.
3. Draw the angled slide back into the drop of blood and then quickly push it forward across the bottom slide, producing a feathered edge (see Figure 21.3). The feathered edge is a tapering at the end of a blood film where the cells are not touching. This is where the bulk of the blood film evaluation occurs.

Once produced, the slide should be heat fixed and stained with a differential stain such as a Wright-Giemsa stain or Diff-Quik stain. The stain is dried, and the slide is initially examined under low power. The entire slide should be scanned to appreciate the overall blood film density, qualitatively observe white blood cell number, and determine if

there are any heartworm parasites, platelet clumps, or large abnormal cells present on the blood film. The parasites, platelet clumps, and abnormal cells are often at the feathered edge (see Figure 21.4).

Once the slide is scanned at low power, the slide is then examined under higher power (high dry and oil immersion objectives) and the slide is moved to the feathered edge region where the red blood cells are touching but not overlapping each other. This area is where cell morphology is evaluated.

The Red Blood Cell

Mammalian red blood cells are non-nucleated biconcave discs without internal organelles. Each cell is bound by a bi-layered lipid membrane and contains 35% hemoglobin by volume. Hemoglobin is a large protein molecule closely associated with iron. Hemoglobin gives the cells their ability to carry oxygen and CO_2.

Function

Red blood cells function to carry oxygen to and remove CO_2 from the tissue to be expelled by the lungs. Oxygen is needed by every cell in the body to take sugar and produce CO_2, water, and energy in a process called respiration. Without this process, cells cannot produce energy and will die.

Life Cycle

Red blood cells are produced primarily in the bone marrow. A small amount of red blood cell production occurs in the liver and spleen. All blood cells, including platelets, are derived from bone marrow stem cells (see Figure 21.5). When

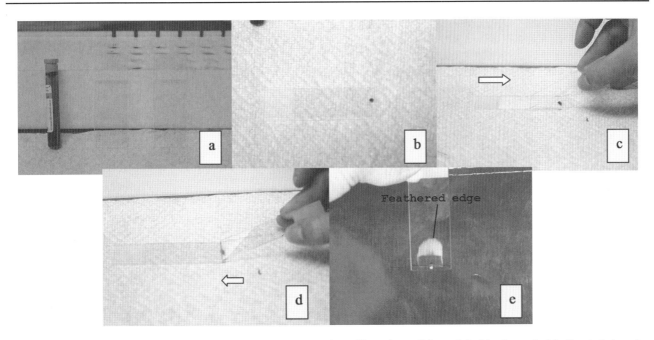

Figure 21.3. To obtain a good feathered edge smear the team member will need two slides and the blood sample (a). One technique is to place a small bleb of blood on the lower slide (b), then back the advancing slide into the drop (c). Allow the drop of blood to expand over the lower margin of the advancing slide and then push the advancing slide forward (d), producing a slide with a rounded feathered edge (e).

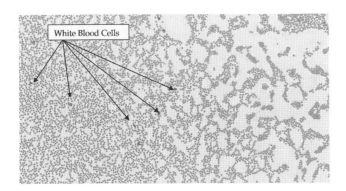

Figure 21.4. Blood smear viewed under low-power lens. This smear should be evaluated for blood parasites such as heartworms, changes in the white blood cell population, and changes in red blood cell population, suggestive of disease conditions. On this slide 8–10 white blood cells can be seen without any obvious large blood parasites seen.

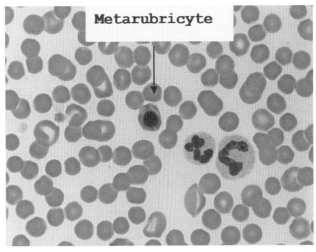

Figure 21.5. Image of normal red blood cells and a nucleated red blood cell (metarubricyte) that has been pushed out from the bone marrow. Increased numbers of nucleated red blood cells can suggest a regenerative response due to an acute or chronic blood loss (anemia).

stem cells divide, one daughter cell remains a stem cell and the other can go on to develop into any of the blood cell types, depending on the hormonal stimulus it receives. If the cell is destined to be a red blood cell, it will differentiate into a **rubriblast**, the first cell that can be recognized as being in the red blood cell series. Once the process of differentiation begins, by repeated cell division (mitosis), the immature red blood cells mature through recognizable stages. In order from least mature to most mature, the red blood cell stages are rubriblast, **rubricyte, metarubricyte, polychromato-**

philic red blood cell, and **mature red blood cell.** The metarubricyte and polychromatophilic red blood cell are often seen on the blood film, especially with a regenerative anemia. The term *nucleated red blood cell* (NRBC) is used for any red blood stage with a nucleus; the metarubricyte is the NRBC most commonly seen on the blood film.

The average life span of a mature red blood cell is

90–120 days. As the cells age, the lipid membranes become fragile after continuous daily wear and tear as the cells move through veins and arteries at high speed. As the cells filter through the spleen, damaged and weakened cells are destroyed. The leftover hemoglobin is degraded to bilirubin, sent to the liver, and excreted in the bile.

Changes in Red Blood Cell Number

With low red blood cell count (low PCV) the major concern associated with a decrease in red blood cell number is loss of red blood cells through active bleeding or decreased production of red blood cells in the marrow. A lower than normal red blood cell count or PCV is called an **anemia**.

Significant anemia can be life threatening because the patient has decreased ability to oxygenate tissues. A decrease in red cell number results in a bone marrow response to produce new red cells: this response takes 3–5 days.

As the bone marrow and other tissues respond to the increased demand, immature red blood cells can be released into the peripheral blood.

Metarubricytes (nucleated red blood cells), polychromatophilic red blood cells (see below), and Howell-Jolly bodies (see below) are commonly seen on the blood film when there is an appropriate response to a decrease in red blood cell numbers. When these cells are seen in significant number on a blood film from an anemic patient, this is termed a **regenerative anemia.**

To confirm a regenerative anemia, a special stain process is used so that the number of immature red blood cells may be counted. This stain is **new methylene blue,** and the immature red blood cells seen when this stain is used are called reticulocytes. Their number often, but not always, correlates with the number of polychromatophilic red cells seen on the routine Diff-Quik or Wright–Giemsa stain.

With increased red blood cell count, as discussed above, elevations in the red blood cell count is generally associated with dehydration. However, there are diseases that are associated with an increased red blood cell count without any evidence of dehydration.

Evaluating the Red Blood Cell Morphology on the Blood Film

Normal red blood cells should be evaluated for size, shape, and central **pallor.** Although sample handling can produce cell artifacts, any significant change to the cell morphology should be discussed with the veterinarian immediately. (Please see the Red Blood Cell flowchart and Table 21.4).

Evaluating Normal Blood Films

A systematic approach to blood film evaluation is necessary to ensure accurate identification of changes in blood cell morphology. After scanning the slide under low power, the region just inside the feathered edge (the counting region) should be scanned under the oil immersion objective. As the slide is scanned, the observations discussed next should be made.

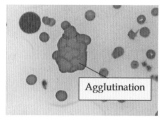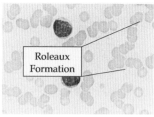

Figure 21.6. At left, agglutination caused by an immune-mediated disease. At right, roleaux formation, a nonpathologic change in the red blood cell smear.

Is There Agglutination or Roleaux Formation?

As discussed above, **agglutination** is the clumping of red blood cells associated with an immune-mediated disease. These cells precipitate out of the blood and can be seen microscopically and in the EDTA blood tube. Agglutination suggests serious life-threatening disease.

Roleaux formation is a stack of red blood cells like a stack of coins. In the horse this is a normal nonpathlogical event as blood settles. In the dog and cat it is often seen with increased total protein or changes in the type of proteins in the blood. It is often seen in inflammatory diseases (see Figure 21.6).

> **Practice Tip:** To differentiate between roleaux and agglutination, make a saline prep of a blood drop. Roleaux formation will break apart in normal saline; Agglutinated red blood cells continue to stay together.

Is There a Variance in the Central Pallor or Color of the Red Blood Cells?

The central pallor refers to the light area at the center of each cell. Dogs have a more pronounced area of central pallor compared with the cat. The central pallor is due to the concave disc shape of the dog's red blood cell. The cat's red blood cell is less concave and therefore has a much less-pronounced central pallor.

Hypochromasia refers to an increase in the size of the area of central pallor and is most often due to a decrease in the concentration of hemoglobin within the red blood cell.

- The two most common causes for increased central pallor are immature red blood cells and blood loss associated iron deficiency.
- These cells are larger than mature red blood cells and have a lower hemoglobin concentration for the larger cell volume. They therefore appear to have increased cental pallor.
- Significant chronic blood loss results in iron deficiency and, as a consequence, decreased concentration of hemoglobin within red blood cells.

- In some cases, there can be a small region of increased central color making a targetlike apperance. These cells are called **target cells** and are most often nonspecific changes seen with numerous diseases. Target cells are often polychromatophilic as well (see Plate I).
- Hypochromasia should not be confused with punched out red blood cells. Punched out red blood cells are a drying artifact in which the hemoglobin in the red blood cell moves to the perephery of the cell. Usually, this cell type has a more regular, even appearance, with the hemoglobin near the cell wall (see Plate II).

Polychromasia refers to a bluish coloration in the red blood cells due to remnants of nuclear material. This pattern is typically seen when red blood cells are released early from the bone marrow as the body responds to loss or destruction of red blood cells (**regenerative anemia**) (see Plate III).

Is There Significant Abnormality in the Red Blood Cell Shape and Internal Structure?

The slide should be evaluated for overall changes in cell shape. The most important aspect of the evaluation is to identify consistent abnormalities in the cells. Many early disease conditions can be detected by the technical team scanning the slide for changes in red cell morphology and reporting any abnormal cell shapes to the veterinarian or a clinical diagnostic lab. Some possible abnormalites of red blood cell morphology are discussed next.

Echinocytes

Echinocytes are red blood cells with clublike projections from the cell surface (see Plate IV). This cell shape change can occur in association with

- diseases affecting **fat metabolism**, which produces alterations in cell membrane formation.
- a **vascular tumor** (i.e., hemangiosarcoma) in which blood is moved through irregular vascular channels within the tumor at a high rate of speed.
- **snake bites** (i.e., rattlesnake, diamondback, sidewinder), whereby blood is exposed to specific snake venoms and the red blood cell membrane becomes altered.
- **crenation**, which is produced by the slow drying of blood films producing **artifactual** echinocytes. If crenation is noted, another blood film should be prepared and evaluated for echinocytes.

Schistocytes

Schistocytes are fragmented red blood cells that are produced by colliding with intravascular fibrin strands as the body attempts to form clots within the blood vessels (see Plate V). These cell types can be associated with the following.

- **Heartworm disease:** Generalized heartworm disease produces chronic inflammatory reactions in the lungs' vascular supply as the patient deals with the adult heart-

worms. This chronic inflammatory disease can produce strands of fibrin and clots and can shear red blood cells.
- **Splenic and hepatic disease:** With chronic inflamatory liver and splenic disease, fibrin stands can be produced, also causing red blood cell shear.
- **Neoplasia** Vascular neoplasms such as hemangiosarcoma can cause shearing of the red blood cells due to small clots within the vascular channels.

Spherocytes

Spherocytes are small, dense red blood cells without the normal central pallor. Spherocytes are difficult to identify in cat blood due to the small size and lack of central pallor in the normal cat red blood cell (see Plate VI). Although spherocytes appear smaller on the blood film, they do not have a significant decrease in cell volume. They are usually seen with immune-mediated hemolytic anemia. When serum antibodies adhere to the surface of the red blood cell, the macrophages in the spleen and liver recognize the damaged protion of the red cell membrane and pinch it off. The loss of cell membrane changes the shape of the red blood cell to a sphere. Spherocytes should be suspected when there is large variability in red blood cell size.

Intracellular Structures

Changes in intracellular structures can be subtle and hard to identify. Recognition of abnormal internal cellular structures can be the key to early detection of asymptomatic disease. A possible internal structure is intracellular parasites, which are not uncommon in the dog and cat. *Mycoplasma* (formerly *Hemobartonella*), *Babesia*, and *Cytauxoon* are parasites that can be found in red blood cells (see Plate VII). Some of these parasites can produce significant disease and others can be asymptomatic. Identification of these parasites and diagnosis at a clinical pathology lab can help prevent acute severe illness in the patient.

Other Abnormalities

- **Howell-Jowell bodies** are nuclear remnants seen within the cytoplasm as dark-staining bodies. They are typically seen with regenerative anemias as the body increases production of red blood cells (see Plate VIII).
- **Heinz bodies** are denatured hemoglobin fused to the cell membrane. Heinz bodies are associated with a specific toxic injury to red blood cells (oxidative injury). It is commonly associated with toxins such as acetaminophen and onions or garlic. Heinz bodies are often difficult to see on a routine Diff-Quik or Wright-Giemsa stain. They are more easily seen on the new methylene blood stain for reticulocytes (see Plate IX).

The Immune System and the White Blood Cell Population

The immune system is a complex cellular defense that recognizes foreign substances and infectious agents and

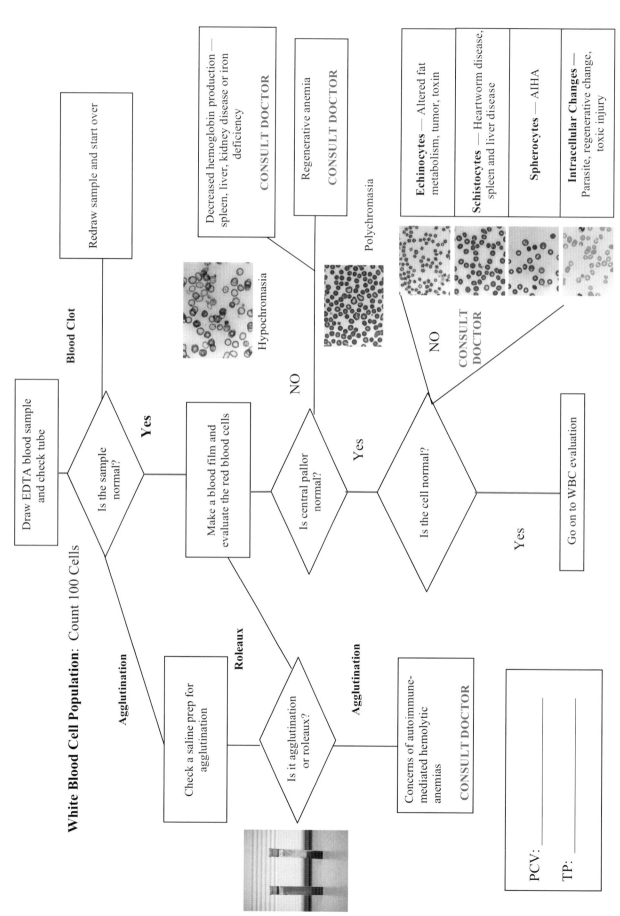

White Blood Cell Population: Count 100 Cells

Draw EDTA blood sample and check tube

Is the sample normal?

Blood Clot — Redraw sample and start over

Yes

Agglutination

Roleaux — Check a saline prep for agglutination

Is it agglutination or roleaux?

Agglutination — Concerns of autoimmune-mediated hemolytic anemias

CONSULT DOCTOR

Make a blood film and evaluate the red blood cells

Is central pallor normal?

NO — Hypochromasia — Decreased hemoglobin production — spleen, liver, kidney disease or iron deficiency

CONSULT DOCTOR

Yes

Is the cell normal?

NO — Polychromasia — Regenerative anemia

CONSULT DOCTOR

NO — **CONSULT DOCTOR**

Echinocytes — Altered fat metabolism, tumor, toxin

Schistocytes — Heartworm disease, spleen and liver disease

Spherocytes — AIHA

Intracellular Changes — Parasite, regenerative change, toxic injury

Yes — Go on to WBC evaluation

PCV: _____

TP: _____

Flowchart 21.1. Complete Blood Count Differential Flow Chart—Red Blood Cell Evaluation.

Cell type[1]	Description	Normal Values	Number Seen
Neutrophils	Neutrophils have segmented nuclei with a pink staining cytoplasm.		
Bands	Band neutrophils have unsegmented nuclei (monocyte-like) with a pink-staining cytoplasm. **Increased Bands Suggest Acute Disease**		
Eosinophils	Eosinophils have segmented nuclei with a pink cytoplasm and dark red granules in the cytoplasm. **Eosinophils respond to fungal infections or allergic reactions.**		
Monocytes	Monocytes have unsegmented nuclei with a purple staining cytoplasm. They are seen with chronic infections.		
Lymphocytes	Lymphocytes are small round cells with round nuclei and purple-staining cytoplasm. They are responsible for producing immunoglobulin.		

  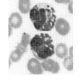 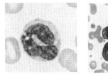 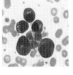

Source: Images reprinted with permission from Heska Corp., 3760 Rocky Mountain Avenue, Loveland, CO 80538.

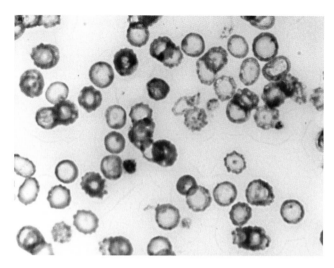

Plate I: Hypochromasia occurs secondary to iron deficiency. The lack of iron limits hemoglobin production and produces red blood cells with marked increase in central pallor and margination of normal color to the periphery of the cell.

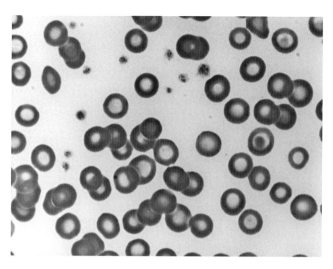

Plate II: Punched-out red blood cells are cells that have their hemoglobin pushed out to the cell margin. These are produced as a drying artifact and suggest no pathology. Punched-out red blood cells can be mistaken for hypochromasia.

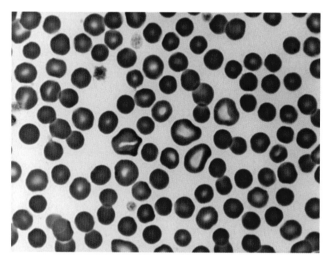

Plate III: Polychromasia refers to an increased blue tinge of the cytoplasm due to nuclear remnants still present in the immature red blood cells. Changes in these red blood cells suggest a regenerative response to anemia.

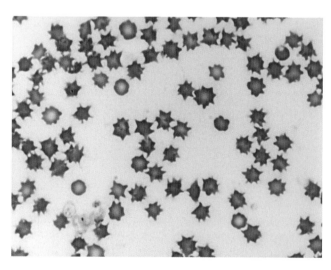

Plate IV: Echinocytes are alterations in the red blood cell membrane produced by improper drying of the slide (crenation), disease affecting fat metabolism, vascular tumor (i.e., hemangiosarcoma), or snake bite envenomation.

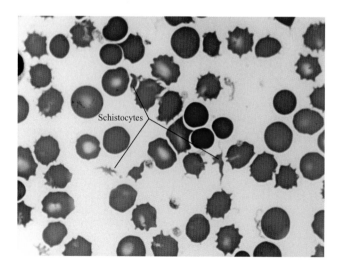

Plate V: Schistocytes are fragmented red blood cells that are produced by colliding with intravascular fibrin strands as the body attempts to form clots within the blood vessels. These cell types can be associated with heartworm disease, spleen and hepatic disease, and cancer.

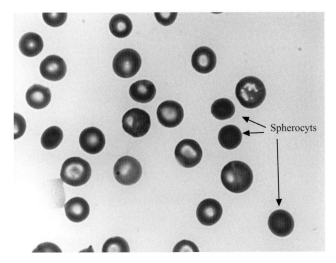

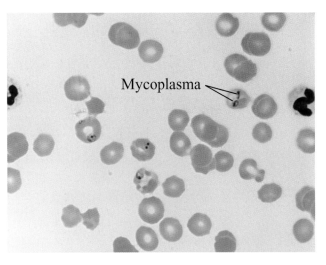

Plate VI: Spherocytes are small, dense red blood cells without the normal central pallor. Spherocytes are difficult to identify in cat blood due to the small size and lack of central pallor in the normal cat red blood cell. Although spherocytes appear smaller on the blood film, they do not have a significant decrease in cell volume. They are usually seen with immune-mediated hemolytic anemia. When serum antibodies adhere to the surface of the red blood cell, the macrophages in the spleen and liver recognize the damaged protion of the red cell membrane and pinch it off. The loss of cell membrane changes the shape of the red blood cell to a sphere. Spherocytes should be suspected when there is large variability in red blood cell size.

Plate VII: *Mycoplasma* (formerly *Hemobartonella*), *Babesia, Cytauxoan* are parasites that can be found in red blood cells. Some of these parasites can produce significant disease whereas others can be asymptomatic. Identification of these parasites and diagnosis at a clinical pathology lab can help prevent acute severe illness in the patient.

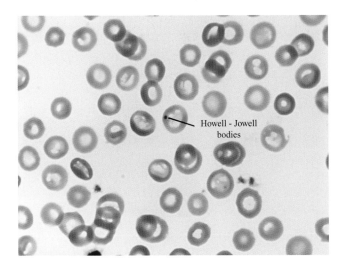

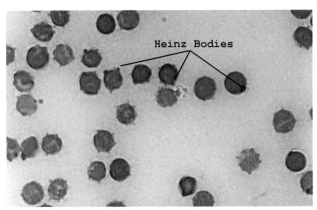

Plate IX: Heinz bodies are denatured hemoglobin fused to the cell membrane. Heinz bodies are associated with a specific toxic injury to red blood cells (oxidative injury). It is commonly associated with toxins such as acetaminophen and onions or garlic. Heinz bodies are often difficult to see on a routine Diff-Quik or Wright-Giemsa stain. They are more easily seen on the new methylene blood stain for reticulocytes.

Plate VIII: Howell-Jowell bodies are nuclear remnants seen within the cytoplasm as dark staining bodies. They are typically seen with regenerative anemias as the body increases production of red blood cells.

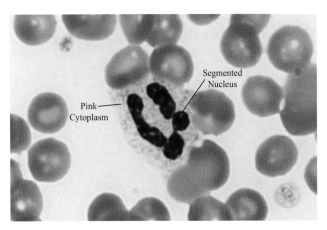

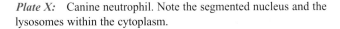

Plate X: Canine neutrophil. Note the segmented nucleus and the lysosomes within the cytoplasm.

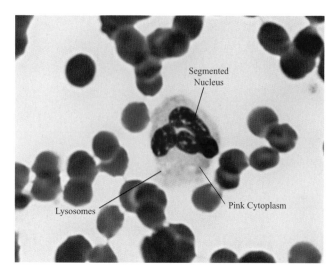

Plate XI: Feline neutrophil. Note the segmented nucleus and the lysosomes within the cytoplasm.

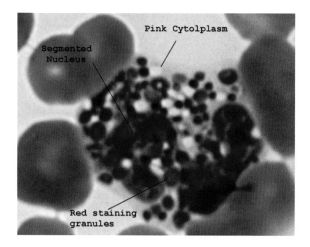

Plate XIII: Canine eosinophil. Note the pink cytoplasm, segmented nucleus, and red granules. When noted in increased numbers, fungal, parasitic, and allergic reactions (rare) are chief concerns.

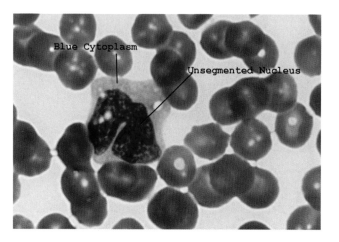

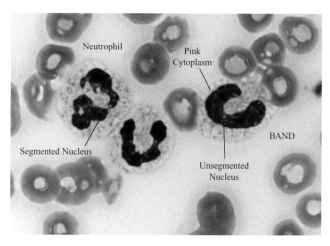

Plate XII: Canine band neutrophil. Note the unsegmented neutrophil, the pink-staining cytoplasm, and the vacuoles in the nucleus. Increased bands suggest a response to an acute inflammatory or infectious disease. If observed, increased bands should be reported to the veterinarian.

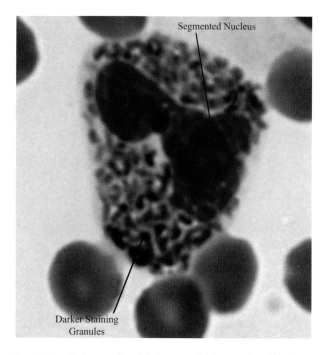

Plate XIV: Feline eosinophil. Image of feline eosinophil; these cells contain segmented nuclei, dark-staining granules, and a pink cytoplasm.

Plate XV: Canine monocyte. Note the blue-staining cytoplasm and unsegmented nucleus, It is important to differentiate these cell types from band neutrophils. Monocytes are seen with more chronic infections.

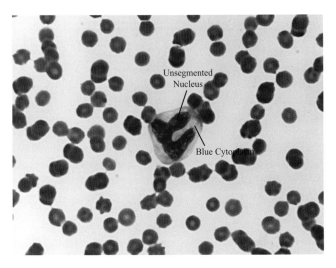

Plate XVI: Feline monocyte. Note the blue cytoplasm and unsegmented nucleus.

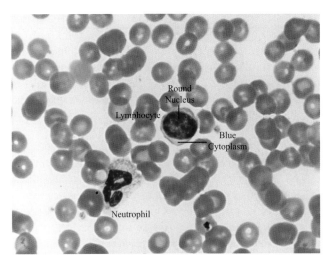

Plate XVII: Canine lymphocyte. Note the round large nucleus with dark blue cytoplasm. These cells produce immunoglobulin protein to help identify foreign invaders and mount an immune response.

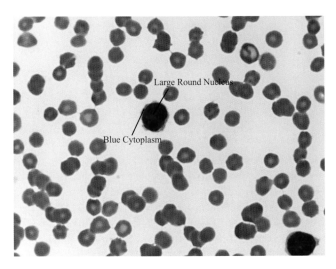

Plate XVIII: Feline Lymphocyte. Note the round large nucleus with dark blue cytoplasm. These cells produce immunoglobulin protein to help identify foreign invaders and mount an immune response.

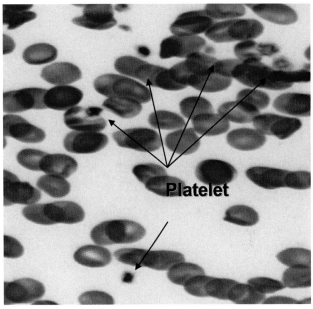

Plate XIX: Image of smaller platelet clumps evident.

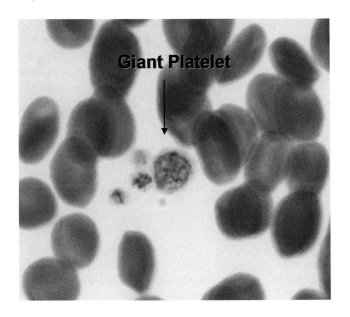

Plate XX: Image of a giant platelet that can sometimes be seen in a peripheral blood smear.

mounts a reaction to destroy the foreign agent. The system responds to infectious agents (bacterial, fungal, and viral), parasites, and foreign material. The response often results in an inflammatory or allergic reaction. The components of the immune system are listed next.

- **Lymph nodes:** Lymph nodes are small round or oval structures within the subcutaneous tissue and abdominal and thoracic cavities that function to filter extracellular fluid (lymph) for foreign material and produce white blood cells (specifically lymphocytes) that then produce antibodies in response to foreign infection.
- **White blood cells:** These are specific cell types that respond to foreign material and infectious agents (see below). The white blood cells involved in the immune system are
  — monocytes,
  — neutrophils,
  — lymphocytes,
  — basophils, and
  — eosinophils.
- **Immunoglobulin**: Proteins produced from lymphocytes that recognize specific foreign material are called *immunoglobulin*. Antibodies are part of the final stage of the immune response. They can "neutralize" infectious agents (viruses), promote the phagocytosis and killing of bacteria, and assist in recruiting white blood cells to the site of inflammation or infection.
- **Recognition of self:** In order for the immune system to work effectively, the body must be able to differentiate foreign cells and material from the patient's cells. To accomplish this, all cells of the body have proteins on their surface that are specific only to those individuals cells. This allows the immune system to differentiate between "self" and "non-self." Foreign cells do not have these specific proteins; when specific white blood cells encounter them, they stimulate an immune response.

Overall Changes in White Blood Cell Populations

Increase in white blood cells (**leukocytosis**) is generally seen when the patient has an infectious, parasitic, or inflammatory disease. It can also be seen with certain types of cancers of the white blood cells (i.e., lymphoma, leukemia, etc.).

Decrease in white blood cells (**leucopenia** is observed when the patient is infected with specific infectious diseases (i.e., parvo or distemper virus), the patient is suffering from a severe inflammatory disease process that depletes their ability to produce normal cell numbers, or the patient is undergoing chemotherapy. Animals with significantly low counts of white blood cells are susceptible to massive infections and can go into shock (septic shock; see Chapter 30).

Cells of the Immune System

Each white blood has a specific function and responds to different types of infection. There are two overall categories of white blood cells: the granulocyte and the agranulocyte.

Granulocytes
Mature Neutrophils

Neutrophils are medium-sized cells one to two times larger than red blood cells and have multiple variations in the nucleus diameter (a **segmented nucleus**). The cytoplasm is clear to light pink. There can be vacuoles in the cytoplasm, and with extensive bacterial infection, the cytoplasm can appear foamy, light blue (basophilic), and bacteria can occasionally be seen within the cytoplasm (see Plates X–XI).

Functions

Neutrophils are the first responders to the site of infection. They function to engulf bacteria and foreign debris. Once the material is phagocytized, it is exposed to membrane-bound vesicles (**lysosomes**) that contain enzymes that can destroy the foreign agent. The neutrophil will also secrete chemicals to attract and stimulate other white blood cells, inducing a more extensive inflammatory response. Neutrophils are the major cellular component of a purulent (pus) discharge as they respond to foreign material and bacterial, fungal, and viral infections.

Normal Blood Values
- Canine: 3000–11,500/μl
- Feline: 2500–12,500/μl

Changes in Neutrophil Population

An increase in the neutrophil population number is referred to as a **neutrophilia** and can be associated with acute and chronic infectious or inflammatory diseases. Sharp decreases in the neutrophil population number are referred to as a **neutropenia** and can be seen with patients undergoing chemotherapy, suffering from specific viral infections (i.e., canine parvovirus, canine distemper, or feline panleukopenia), or from overwhelming inflammatory or infectious disease that exceeds the bone marrow's ability to produce neutrophils.

Immature Neutrophil (Bands)

Immature neutrophils are medium-sized cells one to two times larger than red blood cells, which have a uniform U-shaped nucleus. Although a band can be mistaken for a monocyte, the cytoplasm stains clear or light pink (in Romanowski or Diff-Quik stain kits). As with mature neutrophils, there can be vacuoles in the cytoplasm, and with extensive bacterial infection, the cytoplasm can appear foamy and bacteria occasionally seen in the cytoplasm (see Plate XII).

Functions

The band neutrophils have the same function as the mature neutrophils. Identification of band neutrophils is very important when evaluating a blood film. Most automated hematology analyzers cannot differentiate band cells from other types of white blood cells in the blood. They are most often miscounted as monocytes. Identification of band neutrophils is most accurately done on examination of the blood film.

Band neutrophils indicate early release of immature neutrophils when the bone marrow cannot keep up with the demand for neutrophils in the face of a significant inflammatory or infectious disease process. These patients often show signs of serious illness. In some cases the white cell count is normal, and the severity of the inflammatory disease is only determined by the white blood cell differential and identification of band neutrophils. Increased bands suggest a patient has a severe infection. When identified, these patients may require more intensive care to control the infection.

Normal Blood Values
- Canine: 0–500/μl
- Feline: 0–500/μl

Changes in Band Neutrophil Numbers
Increases in the band neutrophil number are referred to as a **left shift** and can be associated with an acute massive early infectious or inflammatory disease (i.e., septic shock; see Chapter 30).

Eosinophils
Eosinophils are medium-sized cells one to two times the size of a red blood cell. They are often slightly larger than the neutrophil. Just as with mature neutrophils, they contain nuclei with variable thickness (**segmented**). The cytoplasm appears pink in Diff-Quik and Romanowski stain systems. The most noticeable difference in these cells is the red granules. Different eosinophilic species have different shapes and numbers of red granules; all eosinophils have similar architecture (see Plates XIII–XIV).

Functions
Eosinophils respond to fungal and parasitic infections and foreign bodies, and they participate in allergic reactions. Common fungal and parasitic agents associated with an eosinophilic response in the tissues include *Cryptococcus, Coccidioides, Blastomyces, Histoplasma,* heartworm, intestinal parasites, and fleas). These cells are often a significant part of allergic reactions and result in some of the adverse effects associated with allergies.

Normal Blood Values
- Canine: 100–1250/μl
- Feline: 0–500/μl

Changes in Eosinophil Numbers
An increase in eosinophil numbers is referred to as an **eosinophilia** and, as discussed previously, can be seen with systemic fungal-, parasitic-, and allergy-related disease.

Basophils
Basophils are medium-sized cells one to two times the size of a red blood cell and have a segmented nucleus. Like the eosinophil, they have distinct granules within their cytoplasm, except their granules are deep to light purple. The granules in the basophil also vary in size and number in different species. Their cytoplasm, when visible between the granules, is clear to lightly blue.

Functions
The function of basophils is not well understood. Basophils are rare in peripheral blood and thought to be related to allergic reaction. **Basophilia** often accompanies an eosinophilia.

Normal Blood Values
- Canine: 0/μl
- Feline: 0/μl

Changes in Basophil Population
An increase in basophil numbers is referred to as **basophilia** and can be seen with allergenic conditions.

Agranulocytes
Monocyte
The monocyte is the largest white blood cell, three to four times the red blood cell size. It has a round- to irregular-shaped nucleus with blue cytoplasm. Vacuoles can sometimes be seen within its cytoplasm (see Plates XV–XVI).

Function
Monocytes respond to chronic infections to help clear up debris and inflammatory products from an on-going inflammatory response. Like neutrophils, monocytes contain lysosomes that have specific enzymes and nonenzyme chemicals inside that kill and degrade bacteria.

Normal Blood Values
- Canine: 150–1350/μl
- Feline: 0-850–/μl

Changes in Monocyte Population
An increase in monocyte number is referred to as **monocytosis** and can be associated with chronic infectious or inflammatory diseases.

Small and Large Lymphocytes
Lymphocytes vary in size from a small lymphocyte, just larger than a red blood cell, to a larger lymphocyte, the same size or larger than a neutrophil. Lymphocytes are round cells with light to deep blue cytoplasm and round to slightly oval or indented nuclei. The nucleus often makes up the majority of the cell with only a small, thin rim of light blue cytoplasm surrounding it. Nuclei are rarely lobulated (see Plates XVII–XVIII).

Function
Lymphocytes produce specific blood proteins called **immunoglobulins** (antibodies). After the lymphocytes are exposed to proteins from foreign material or infectious agents by macrophages, the lymphocytes produce specific immu-

noglobulin proteins. These proteins will recognize and attach to the invading bacteria, parasite, fungus, or virus. Once attached, these proteins activate other white blood cells and blood proteins that help destroy the pathogen. When first exposed to a new foreign agent, the production of immunoglobulin takes about 14 days. The second time lymphocytes are exposed to the same foreign agent, there is a more rapid and effective immune response. This second rapid response is due to specific lymphocytes, **memory cells**, that remain after the previous infection was cleared. These cells are already primed to respond to the same agent within a few days rather than 2 weeks. Memory cells are responsible for the protection provided by vaccination for specific infectious diseases.

Normal Blood Values
- Canine: 100–1250/µl
- Feline: 1500–7000/µl

Changes in Lymphocyte Numbers
An increase in lymphocyte number is referred to as **lymphocytosis** and can be associated with chronic infection or some cancers. A decrease in lymphocyte number is a **lymphopenia** and can be associated with stress, acute viral infection, some cancers, and chemotherapy.

Platelets

Platelets are small cell components of blood that are several times smaller than normal red blood cells. They can be present in clumps. They are cytoplasmic fragments that break off large cells within the bone marrow (**megakaryocytes**) (see Plates XIX–XX).

Function
Platelets are necessary for normal blood clotting. They form the initial blood clot at the site of vessel injury. After this "platelet plug" is formed, circulating proteins (clotting factors) are deposited on the platelet plug to strengthen it and "cement" it in place.

Normal Blood Values
- Canine: 164,000–500,000/µl
- Feline: 170,000–600,000/µl

Changes in Platelet Number
An increase in platelet number is a thrombocytosis. Increased platelet numbers can be seen with certain metabolic diseases and often is seen in markedly regenerative anemia. Thrombocytosis can also be associated with cancer, including cancers arising from megakaryocytes (the cells that form platelets). A decrease in platelets is **thrombocytopenia**. There are many causes for thrombocytopenia, including infectious disease, neoplasia, bone marrow injury, and immune-mediated disease.

Evaluating Platelet Number
The platelet count can be determined by automated or manual methods. It is essential to review a blood film before any platelet count is accepted. Especially if there are clumps of platelets at the feathered edge or within the body of the blood film, the platelet count will be artifactually decreased and should not be reported. A quick method for estimation of platelet numbers can be done from a blood film. Using the following method:

Estimated platelet number = the average number of platelets $\times$ 15,000

The platelet estimate should be done on the area of the blood film where the red blood cells are overlapping, not in the counting area where the differential is performed. The number of platelets seen on a $100\times$ high-power immersion field are then averaged. Note that this is not accurate in anemic animals.

CD-ROM 2 will focus on concepts of understanding and discussing clinical diagnostics and the disease conditions represented. The exercises can be done individually or as case rounds as they explore specific topics in veterinary medicine that discuss clinical diagnostics and treatment.

Chapter 22

Organ, Hormonal, and Drug Level Clinical Pathology

Chemistry

A blood chemistry analysis (chemistry profile) and other chemical diagnostics allow the veterinarian to evaluate the patient's physical condition, metabolic function, and response to treatment. No single clinical test can evaluate an animal's overall condition; the assessment of the animal depends on the history, physical exam, clinical diagnostics, and response to treatment. The goal of this chapter is to give the team member an understanding of clinical assays, how they are performed, how changes can reflect disease processes, and how to discuss these clinical tests with the client. *The veterinarian is always responsible for interpreting the clinical diagnostics and outlining treatment option.* It is important for the team member to understand why specific diagnostics are performed to more efficiently determine the veterinarian's needs, to properly monitor the hospitalized patient, and to educate the client.

Sample Handling

When obtaining blood samples for chemistry profiles or drug levels, the medical team must be able to perform a blood draw in a clean environment with a clean venipuncture. *The way in which the sample is handled impacts the accuracy of results.* For example, **hemolysis**, red blood cell breakdown with release of hemoglobin in the serum, can occur if there is difficulty in puncturing the vein or if excess pressure is applied to the syringe during collection. Lipemia, fat accumulation in the serum, is most common and is caused by collection of blood after the patient has eaten. Both hemolysis and lipemia occur as a result of the disease process or as an artifact (see Table 22.1). These changes can also falsely increase or decrease other clinical pathology values; each in-house chemistry and lab test should list how changes in the serum will affect specific chemistries. *If there are abnormalities noted in the serum, it should be noted in the record and discussed with the veterinarian.*

For clinical chemistry profiles, most samples collected should be placed in a clot tube (red-topped tube) or a serum-separator tube (red/yellow or red/gray tube). Once the blood is in the tube, it must sit until a clot forms completely. This may take anywhere from 10 to 15 minutes. *If a clot does not form in this time, a doctor should be notified immediately because this can suggest problems with the animal's ability to clot.*

After the clot forms, the sample is placed in a centrifuge and spun for 10–15 minutes or according to the centrifuge manufacturer's instructions. Centrifugation separates the red blood cells from the serum. If a sample is spun that does not have a serum separator gel, it is necessary to immediately separate the serum from the clot once it has finished spinning. *If the serum is allowed to lie on top of the clot, the prolonged exposure of the serum to the red blood cells will decrease the level of glucose and increase the level of phosphorus, causing an inaccurate measurement.* Do not pour the serum off the clot. A pipette should be used to remove the serum to avoid any red blood cell contamination.

There are many organ systems that can be evaluated generally with clinical chemistry examination (see Table 22.2).

Individual Clinical Chemistry

Alanine Aminotransferase

Alanine aminotransferase (ALT)is an indicator of liver damage in the dog and cat. *It does not aid in evaluation of liver function.*

Function

ALT is a hepatic intracellular enzyme that is responsible for the conversion of 2-oxoglutarate to pyruvate and glutamate in the liver cells (hepatocytes).

Where It Is Produced

ALT is an enzyme produced in the liver cell (hepatocyte).

Abnormalities

Changes in ALT activities generally occur when hepatocytes are damaged, causing a leakage of cellular contents into the bloodstream.

Decreased ALT activity is not generally associated with disease conditions. In rare cases, low activity has been mildly associated with congenital porto-systemic shunts (see Chapter 14).

Increased ALT activity of the enzyme in the blood occurs when there are alterations in the lipid membrane of the hepatocytes secondary to injury, inflammations, or infection within the liver**.** Significant increases of ALT activity are associated with acute hepatic disease, which affects many hepatocytes simultaneously.

The degree of increase in activity does not indicate the

Table 22.1.   Changes in serum—artifact vs. disease.

Change in Serum	How Change Can Occur in Patients
Lipemia	**Artifactual:** Occurs if pet has eaten a fatty meal before blood draw.
WHITE SERUM	**Disease** Hyperlipidemia: Rare disease, usually in schnauzers. Hypercholesterolemia: Common secondary abnormality associated with liver, metabolic, and endocrine diseases.
Hemolysis	**Artifactual:** Occurs if the venipuncture was traumatic. A traumatic venipuncture can cause lysis of the red blood cells and release of hemoglobin.
RED SERUM	**Disease** Hemolysis: Can be noted in immune-mediated hemolytic anemia in which the red blood cells are being lysed by antibodies that have attached to their surface.
Icterus	**Artifactual:** None
YELLOW SERUM	**Disease** Can occur with liver, immune-mediated hemolytic anemia (IMHA), anemia, or gall bladder obstruction. The buildup of bilirubin can be due to inability of the liver to clear bilirubin from the body, the inability to secrete the gall bladder contents back into the intestine, or a massive destruction of red blood cells in the vessels.

Table 22.2.   Organ systems and correlating clinical diagnostic components.

Organ System	Clinical Diagnostic Examination
Kidney dysfunction	Blood urea nitrogen Creatinine Phosphorous Potassium Albumin
Liver damage	ALT (alanine aminotransferase) AST (aspartate aminotransferase) SAP (serum alkaline phosphatase) GGT (gamma-glutamyltransferase) Triglycerides Cholesterol
Liver function	Albumin Total bilirubin Blood urea nitrogen Glucose
Exocrine pancreatic function	Amylase Lipase Cholesterol
Endocrine pancreatic function	Glucose Cholesterol
Adrenal dysfunction (hypoadrenocorticism)	Sodium (Na) Potassium (K) Chlorine (Cl)
Adrenal dysfunction (hyperadrenocorticism)	Cholesterol Alkaline phosphatase Glucose
Muscle function	CK (creatinine kinase)
Gall bladder function	Alkaline phosphatase Gamma-glutamyltransferase Bilirubin

severity of the damage to the hepatocytes or degree of reversibility of the disease process.

With chronic liver disease causing only mild liver damage over a longer period of time, there may be significant disease evident, and enzyme activity may be normal or only mildly increased. Increases in ALT activity only imply liver degeneration but do not assess liver function.

ALT activity can also be increased secondary to

- trauma (i.e., hit by car),
- anticonvulsants,
- steroids,
- cardiac disease,
- hypoxia, and
- severe anemia.

Symptoms Associated with Increases in ALT Activity
The symptoms vary, depending on the severity of the disease and its underlying cause. Many signs are nonspecific and include

- anorexia,
- depression,
- weight loss,
- vomiting,

- diarrhea,
- jaundice (although not always directly associated with elevations of ALT), and
- neurologic signs.

Other Clinical Diagnostic Tests
Other clinical diagnostic tests are used to help evaluate the cause of increased ALT activity. These diagnostics suggest that hepatocyte degeneration or cholestasis (decreased bile flow) can be helpful in determining the cause of increased ALT activity.

- Aspartate aminotransferase (AST)
- Alkaline phosphatase/skeletal alkaline phosphatase (ALP/SALP)
- Gamma-glutamyltransferase (GGT)

(Please also see algorithm for liver disease on p. 332.)

Other diagnostics that suggest decreased liver function and can assist in determining the cause of increased ALT activity are for

- blood urea nitrogen (BUN),
- albumin,

- total bilirubin,
- cholesterol, and
- bile acids (paired).

> **Discussing Changes in Alanine Aminotransferase Level with the Client**
> - Alanine aminotransferase (ALT) is a hepatic intracellular enzyme necessary for metabolism of specific nutrients within the liver.
> - Decreasing ALT activity is not generally associated with disease.
> - Increasing activity can be associated with acute or ongoing damage to the liver, causing the leakage of ALT into the blood.
> - A normal ALT level does not rule out chronic liver disease or dysfunction where mild liver damage occurs over a long period of time with a cumulative effect.
> - Increases in ALT activity can be of concern, but the blood test must also be fully evaluated, along with the pet's condition, history, other diagnostics, and response to treatment, before conclusions can be reached.

Albumin

Albumin is monitored to help evaluate the patient for

- hydration status,
- blood loss,
- liver dysfunction/liver disease,
- protein-losing nephropathy/renal disease (glomerular), and
- protein-losing enteropathy/intestinal disease (i.e., inflammatory bowel disease).

Function

Albumin is a small carrier protein that binds to hormones and other components in the bloodstream to maintain and move necessary elements throughout the body. Because albumin is a protein molecule, it maintains a constant pull of fluid from the tissue into the bloodstream. This effect, called **oncotic pressure,** helps maintain blood pressure because these protein molecules help draw and hold fluid inside the vessels.

Where It Is Produced

Albumin is produced in the liver.

Abnormalities

Hypoalbuminemia

Decreases in blood albumin concentration can occur generally with a number of disease syndromes that affect production or loss of the protein molecule. Some disease concerns are as follows:

- **External or internal bleeding:** Acute blood loss (i.e., trauma) or chronic loss (i.e., gastrointestinal bleeding) can produce decreased blood and protein levels. As an animal bleeds, both red blood cells and serum (with albumin) are lost. When there are concerns for acute blood loss, both the packed cell volume (PCV) and total protein (TP) must be monitored closely (see Chapter 21).
- **Liver disease:** Any disease that significantly decreases the number of functioning hepatocytes will compromise the liver's ability to produce albumin. As a general rule, at least 75% of normal liver function must be lost before albumin concentration is decreased due to lack of production by hepatocytes. When attributable to liver disease, hypoalbuminemia is an indicator of decreased liver function (see Chapter 14; see also the liver disease diagnosis algorithm on p. 332).
- **Kidney disease:** The kidneys function to filter toxins from the body, regulate electrolytes, and concentrate urine. The fine openings within the filtration barrier of the glomeruli can be damaged secondary to diseases affecting the glomeruli. This allows larger molecules such as proteins to leak into the urine. This syndrome is called **protein-losing nephropathy** and is denoted both by hypoalbuminemia and significant **proteinuria** (see Chapter 13; see also the kidney disease diagnosis algorithm on p. 331).
- **Intestinal disease:** The intestines loose the ability to absorb necessary proteins and other food stuffs because of specific forms of intestinal disease and cancer (i.e., **inflammatory bowel disease, intestinal lymphoma**). These patients are unable to produce enough albumin in the liver to compensate for the excessive loss by the intestine. This syndrome is called **protein-losing enteropathy** and is usually seen in patients with chronic gastrointestinal signs (i.e., vomiting and diarrhea) and weight loss (see Chapter 10).
- **Hyperalbunemia:** Although not linked to a disease entity, hyperalbunemia is associated with significant dehydration because the amount of fluid decreases within blood, concentrating the albumin and PCV (see hypovolemic shock; Chapter 30).

Symptoms Associated with Changes in Albumin Level
- **Hypoalbuminemia:** With chronic low albumin concentration, patients can lose oncotic pressure, which is produced from the albumin concentration in the blood. As albumin decreases, fluid begins to pool within the tissue, causing swelling of the limbs (**peripheral edema**) and ventral neck and jaw, and buildup in the lungs (**pulmonary edema**). When this happens, patients should be monitored for
  — swelling of the digits and distal limbs,
  — swelling under the neck and jaw,
  — moist cough,
  — increased respiratory effort,
  — abdominal breathing,

— poor capillary refill time,
— cyanotic mucous membranes: purple to blue to gray, and
— decreased ability to exercise.

- **Hyperalbuminemia:** Physical signs are directly attributable to dehydration, and the proper monitoring of the patients is discussed in Chapter 28 and Chapter 30.

Other Clinical Diagnostic Tests
Bleeding
Monitoring PCV and TP can help determine if there is continued bleeding.

Liver Disease
Evaluating other chemistry tests that suggest liver damage may support decreased production by the liver as the cause of hypoalbuminemia (please see the algorithms for liver disease and kidney disease on pp. 331 and 332). These tests are for

- AST,
- ALT,
- ALP or SALP, and
- gamma-glutamyltransferase (GGT).

Evaluating chemistry tests that suggest liver function may also indicate the cause of hypoalbuminemia. These tests are for

- BUN,
- total bilirubin,
- cholesterol,
- glucose, and
- bile acids (paired).

Kidney Disease
Some clinical diagnostic tests that help determine if glomerular disease is the cause of the hypoalbuminemia are

---

Discussing Changes in Albumin Levels with the Client
- Albumin is a small protein produced by the liver to carry other nutritional and hormonal components through the blood.
- Marked elevations in albumin are associated typically with marked dehydration because albumin concentration increases with decreasing fluid levels in the blood.
- Decreasing albumin levels can be associated with acute and chronic bleeding or chronic disease of the liver, kidneys, or intestines.
- Changes in albumin concentration can be of concern, but the blood test must also be fully evaluated, along with the pet's condition, history, other diagnostics, and response to treatment, before a diagnosis can be made.

- BUN,
- creatinine,
- urinalysis, and
- urine protein/creatinine ratio.

Intestinal Disease
Clinical diagnostic tests that help determine if intestinal disease is the cause of hypoalbuminemia are

- fecal floatation/smear,
- pancreatic lipase inhibitor (PLI),
- trypsin-like immunoassay (TLI),
- endoscopy, and
- intestinal biopsy.

Alkaline Phosphatase
Alkaline phosphatase (ALP) and skeletal ALP (SALP) is monitored to help evaluate the patient for

- hormonal disease/hyperadrenocorticism,
- liver disease, and
- gall bladder disease or obstruction.

Function
ALP removes inorganic phosphate molecules from many compounds, such as glucose phosphates.

Where It Is Produced
ALP refers to a large number of intracellular enzymes that are present within the liver, intestine, bone, kidneys, and placenta. On most chemistry panels, ALP activity represents the combined activity of all ALP sources of the body. Realistically, since all non-liver ALP has very a short half-life, serum ALP activity reflects that of the liver enzyme. Exceptions to this include increased bone origin activity during active bone growth in young animals or active bone destruction in neoplasia.

Abnormalities
Increased ALP activity can come from several possible pathological and nonpathological conditions. Unlike ALT and AST, SALP activity does not increase due to "leakage" from hepatocytes; its activity increases because of increased production of the enzyme (induction) by the hepatocytes in response to disease. Some conditions that increase ALP activity are as follows.

- **Hyperadrenocorticism:** Although not a specific test for hyperadrenocorticism (Cushing's disease; see Chapter 17), chronic increases in ALP activity may suggest the effects on the liver of an overproduction of corticosteroids from the adrenal gland. In addition, the administration of corticosteroids can cause increased ALP activity.
- **Liver and gall bladder disease:** With chronic disease of the liver and/or gall bladder (infection, obstruction, cancer), increases in ALP activity can be observed.

- **Long-term medication:** Long-term administration of specific medication (i.e., phenobarbital, prednisone) can affect the liver and increase ALP activity in the serum.
- **Bone growth:** Increases in bone ALP can be seen in rapidly growing animals and can also be elevated in bone disease.

Symptoms Associated with Elevations of Alkaline Phosphatase

Symptoms associated with elevation of ALP can be seen in liver disease/gall bladder obstruction or hyperadrenocorticism. The symptoms can vary depending on the severity of disease and its cause.

Liver Disease/Gall Bladder Obstruction

Signs for these diseases include

- anorexia,
- depression,
- weight loss,
- vomiting,
- diarrhea,
- increased thirst (polydipsia),
- increased urination (polyuria),
- painful abdomen (gall bladder obstruction),
- jaundice (although not always directly associated with elevations of ALP), and
- neurologic signs.

Hyperadrenocorticism (Cushing's Disease)

Signs of this disease include

- increased thirst (polydipsia),
- increased urination (polyuria),
- lethargy,
- poor hair coat—especially bilateral over the flank, and
- pot-bellied appearance.

Other Clinical Diagnostic Tests
Liver Disease

Evaluating other liver enzymes that suggest liver damage may indicate the cause of increased ALP activity. These diagnostic tests are

- ALT,
- AST, and
- GGT.

Evaluating other diagnostic tests that suggest altered liver function may indicate the cause of increased ALP activity. These diagnostic tests are

- BUN,
- total bilirubin,
- cholesterol,
- bile acids (paired), and
- glucose.

Hyperadrenocorticism (Cushing's Disease)

Diagnostic tests for hyperadrenocorticism are

- adrenocorticotropic hormone (ACTH) stimulation test,
- low-dose dexamethasone suppression test, and
- urine cortisol/creatinine ratio.

Discussing Changes in Alkaline Phosphatase Levels with the Client

- Alkaline phosphatase (ALP) and skeletal ALP (SALP) are hepatic intracellular enzymes evident in many body tissues (i.e., gall bladder, liver, muscle, bone).
- A decrease in SALP or ALP levels is not generally associated with disease.
- Increased levels can be associated with multiple organ systems. Some examples of diseases in this case are
  —liver or gall bladder disease,
  —hormonal disease (hyperadrenocorticism), and
  —exposure to chronic medication (i.e., prednisone, phenobarbital).
- Elevations in SALP or ALP can be of concern, but the blood test must also be fully evaluated, along with the pet's condition, history, other diagnostics, and response to treatment, before conclusions can be reached.
- Often, other forms of clinical diagnostic tests are necessary to identify possible causes in elevations of SALP or ALP.

Amylase

Amylase is an indicator of pancreatitis in the canine. *It is not helpful in evaluation of feline pancreatitis.*

Function

Amylase is an enzyme that helps break down larger, more complex sugars into small 1-unit sugars for absorption.

Where It Is Produced

Amylase is produced in the pancreas and enters the duodenum through the pancreatic ducts to break down sugars for digestion.

Abnormalities

Amylase is released when there are changes within the pancreatic cells that produce a leakage of the enzyme into the bloodstream. This pancreatic damage is secondary to infection and inflammation of the pancreas (pancreatitis; see Chapter 15) or pancreatic cancer.

Symptoms Associated with Increases in Amylase Activity

Symptoms associated with increases in amylase activity are due to the infection or inflammation of the pancreas and resulting pancreatitis. Common signs of acute severe pancreatitis in the dog are

- anorexia,
- depression,
- vomiting,
- diarrhea,
- jaundice, and
- sepsis.

Other Clinical Diagnostic Tests

Tests that are used to help evaluate the cause of increased amylase activity are as follows (see the algorithm for exocrine pancreatic disease on p. 333).

- Lipase
- TLI
- Pancreatic lipase immunoreactivity (PLI)
- Complete blood count
  — Elevation of white count
  — Increased band neutrophils
  — Total bilirubin

Discussing Changes in Amylase Levels with the Client

- Amylase is an enzyme produced by the pancreas to help break down sugar for absorption in the small intestine.
- In the dog, elevations in amylase can suggest an infection or inflammation of the pancreas (i.e., pancreatitis). The disease process causes the enzyme to leak out of normal pancreatic cells and into the bloodstream.
- In the cat, elevation of pancreatic enzymes does not directly correlate with pancreatitis.
- Rarely, elevations of amylase may suggest pancreatic cancer in the dog and cat.
- It is important to note that patients, especially with chronic disease, can have severe pancreatitis without elevations of lipase.
- Elevations of amylase can be of concern, but the blood test must also be fully evaluated, along with the pet's condition, history, other diagnostic tests, and response to treatment, before conclusions can be reached.

Aspartate Aminotransferase

Aspartate aminotransferase (AST)is an indicator of acute liver damage in the dog and cat. It does not aid in evaluation of liver function.

Function

AST is an intracellular enzyme that is in all cells, but is predominant in muscle and liver cell damage. AST transfers

α-amino groups between specific amino acids as a part of normal protein metabolism.

Where It Is Produced

AST is an enzyme produced in the hepatocytes.

Abnormalities

Changes in AST activity generally occurs when hepatocytes are damaged, causing a leakage of cellular contents into the bloodstream.

Decreased AST activity is not generally associated with disease conditions. In rare cases, low activity is seen in congenital porto-systemic shunts (see Chapter 14).

AST activity is increased for many of the same reasons ALT activity is increased. Increased activity of the enzyme in the blood occurs when there are alterations in the lipid membrane of the hepatocytes secondary to injury, inflammation, or infection within the liver.

- Significant increases of AST activity are associated with acute hepatic disease that affects many hepatocytes simultaneously.
- The degree of increase in activity does not indicate the severity of the damage to the hepatocytes or the degree of reversibility of the disease process.
- With chronic liver disease causing only mild damage over a protracted period of time, there may be significant disease, and enzyme activity may be normal or only mildly increased.
- Increases in ALT activity only imply liver degeneration but does not assess liver function. AST can also be elevated with
  — muscle disease or disease that affects muscle acutely (i.e., trauma or seizure).
  — destruction of red blood cells due to disease or as an artifact.

Symptoms Associated with Elevations of AST

Symptoms of elevated AST are associated with liver disease (see Chapter 14). The signs can vary depending on the cause and severity of the disease and may include

- anorexia,
- depression,
- weight loss,
- vomiting,
- diarrhea,
- jaundice (although not always directly associated with elevations of AST), and
- neurologic signs.

Other Clinical Diagnostic Tests
Liver Disease

Evaluating other liver enzymes that suggest liver damage or cholestasis may indicate the cause of increased AST levels.

(Please see the algorithm for liver disease on p. 332.) These diagnostic tests are

- ALT,
- SALP or ALP, and
- GGT.

Evaluating other diagnostics that suggest liver function may indicate the cause of increased AST. These diagnostic tests are

- BUN,
- total bilirubin,
- cholesterol,
- bile acids (paired), and
- glucose.

Discussing Changes in Aspartate Aminotransferase Levels with the Client

- Aspartate aminotransferase (AST) is a hepatic intracellular enzyme involved in protein metabolism within the liver.
- Decreasing AST activity is not generally associated with disease.
- Increasing activity can be associated with acute damage to the liver, causing the leakage of AST into the bloodstream.
- Normal AST activity does not rule out chronic liver disease or dysfunction where only small numbers of hepatocytes are damaged per day.
- Although elevations of AST can be of concern, the blood test must also be fully evaluated, along with the pet's condition, history, other diagnostics, and response to treatment, before conclusions can be reached.

Bilirubin

Bilirubin is used to evaluate the liver's ability to detoxify and to eliminate toxins from the body. It is a liver function test. Increased levels of bilirubin can also suggest increased intravascular red blood cell destruction in immune-mediated hemolytic anemias.

Function

Bilirubin is a potentially toxic metabolite produced from the breakdown of hemoglobin and other pigments in the body.

Where It Is Produced

Heme pigments are broken down by the liver and excreted into the small intestine as a part of bile. Normally, a small amount of bilirubin is excreted by the urogenital system in dogs. Larger amounts of bilirubin can be excreted by the kidneys in both dogs and cats with **hyperbilirubinemia**.

Abnormalities

Physical signs occur as bilirubin builds up in the tissue secondary to liver disease, gall bladder obstruction, or massive destruction of red blood cells in the body, producing high levels of free hemoglobin (hemoglobin to bilirubin). *If the buildup of bilirubin is caused secondary to liver disease, the presence of increased bilirubin concentration can suggest functional liver disease.*

Symptoms Associated with Increases in Bilirubin Concentration

Physical signs can be associated with the liver disease, gall bladder obstruction, or immune-mediated hemolytic anemia, producing the increases in bilirubin in the blood and tissue (see Chapter 14 and Chapter 21). The signs can vary depending on the cause and severity of the disease.

Liver Disease

Signs of liver disease are

- anorexia,
- depression,
- weight loss,
- vomiting,
- diarrhea,
- jaundice, and
- neurologic signs.

Gall Bladder Obstruction

Signs of gall bladder obstruction are

- abdominal tenderness/pain,
- jaundice (directly linked to obstruction of the gall bladder),
- vomiting,
- anorexia,
- dehydration, and
- diarrhea.

Immune-Mediated Hemolytic Anemia

Signs of immune-mediated anemia are

- pale mucous membranes—possible jaundice,
- weakness,
- lethargy,
- jaundice (directly linked to massive red blood cell breakdown and release of hemoglobin in the vessels),
- vomiting,
- diarrhea, and
- anorexia.

Other Clinical Diagnostic Tests
Liver Disease

Evaluating other liver enzymes that suggest liver damage may indicate the cause of hyperbilirubinemia. (Please see the algorithm for liver disease on p. 332.) The diagnostic tests are

- ALT,
- SALP or ALP,
- AST, and
- GGT.

Evaluating other diagnostics for liver function may indicate the cause of hyperbilirubinemia. These diagnostic tests are

- BUN,
- cholesterol,
- bile acids (paired), and
- glucose.

Gall Bladder Obstruction

Tests for gall bladder obstruction are

- ALP,
- GGT,
- abdominal x-rays, and
- abdominal ultrasounds.

Immune-Mediated Hemolytic Anemia

Diagnostic tests for immune-mediated hemolytic anemia are

- PCV/TP,
- complete blood count, and
- blood film—agglutination, spherocytes.

Discussing Changes in Bilirubin Level with the Client

- Bilirubin is a breakdown product of hemoglobin.
- Bilirubin is delivered to the liver to be detoxified and excreted through the gall bladder and intestinal system.
- When there is a liver dysfunction, gall bladder obstruction, or massive breakdown of red blood cells in the body, bilirubin builds up in the serum and tissue.
- Although increases in bilirubin concentration can be of concern, the blood test must also be fully evaluated, along with the pet's condition, history, other diagnostics, and response to treatment, before conclusions can be reached.

Blood Urea Nitrogen

BUN concentration evaluates the patient's kidney function. With decreased production, BUN also can be an indicator of liver dysfunction.

Function

BUN is a potentially toxic metabolite produced during protein metabolism. BUN is produced in the liver as a means of eliminating ammonia from the body and is excreted by the kidneys.

Where It Is Produced

BUN is produced from ammonia in the liver and transported by the bloodstream to the kidneys, where it is largely excreted through the glomerular filters.

Abnormalities

Increases in BUN concentration can be associated with the following.

- **Decreased glomerular filtration rate:** BUN concentration is generally increased when there is a decrease in the patient's glomerular filtration rate. Causes of decreased glomerular filtration rate include
  — **Pre-renal azotemia:** When the patient is dehydrated, the body cannot maintain adequate perfusion through the kidneys at a rate adequate to produce a normal filtration rate.
  — **Renal azotemia:** When damage to the kidneys results in loss of normal renal tissue, glomerular filtration rate of the kidneys is not sufficient to clear toxins and metabolites such as BUN from the body.
  — **Postrenal azotemia:** When the lower urinary tract is obstructed (i.e., blocked tomcat), the increased pressure and lack of urine outflow inhibits normal filtration. As a result, substances normally excreted by the kidney build up in the serum.
- **Gastrointestinal bleeding:** Intestinal bleeding can produce increases in BUN. Gastrointestinal diseases that produce intestinal ulceration and bleeding (i.e., parvoviral infection) can secondarily increase BUN levels in the blood. Blood contains a large amount of protein that is digested just like a high-protein meal.
- **High-protein meal:** If a blood sample is taken following a meal high in protein, there will be a transient increase in serum BUN as the protein is metabolized.

Decreases in BUN concentration can be associated with the liver's inability to produce BUN. When attributable to liver disease, it is an indicator of severe liver dysfunction. A low BUN by itself does not always indicate liver dysfunction. Low-protein diets can also result in a low BUN.

Symptoms Associated with Changes in BUN Concentration

Increased BUN concentration is generally associated with decreases in glomerular filtration, producing increasing serum BUN concentration. As the pet becomes more toxic (**azotemic**), physical signs include the following.

With acute azotemia signs are

- vomiting,
- diarrhea,
- anorexia,

- dehydration, and
- neurologic signs—seizures.

With chronic azotemia signs are

- weight loss,
- chronic vomiting,
- chronic diarrhea,
- muscle loss,
- increased thirst (polydipsia), and
- increased urination (polyuria).

Decreased BUN concentration is generally associated with diseases that produce liver dysfunction. For a more complete discussion on these signs, please refer to Chapter 14.

Other Clinical Diagnostic Tests

Other clinical diagnostic tests are used to help evaluate changes in BUN concentration, as well. (Please see the algorithma for liver disease and kidney disease on p. 331, 332.)

Increased BUN may occur due to decreased renal glomerular filtration. Diagnostic tests are

- creatinine,
- phosphorus,
- urinalysis—urine specific gravity, and
- serum electrolytes (especially potassium).

Gastrointestinal bleeding may also result in increased BUN. Diagnostic tests are

- PCV/TP,
- parvo cite test,
- fecal examination, and
- endoscopic examination of the gastrointestinal tract.

Decreased BUN concentration may be associated with liver dysfunction. Evaluating other liver enzymes that suggest liver damage may indicate the cause of decreased BUN concentration. The diagnostic tests are

- ALT,
- SALP or ALP,
- AST, and
- GGT.

Evaluating other diagnostics that suggest liver function may indicate the cause of decreased BUN concentration. These diagnostics are

- albumin,
- bilirubin,
- cholesterol,
- bile acids (paired), and
- glucose.

Discussing Changes in Blood Urea Nitrogen Concentration with the Client

- Blood urea nitrogen (BUN) is a metabolite produced in the liver to remove ammonia from the body. Once produced, the body transports BUN to the kidneys for excretion in the urine.
- Marked increase in BUN concentration is typically associated with the body's inability to filter toxins (glomerular filtration) through the kidneys. This can be caused by marked dehydration, kidney disease, or urinary obstruction.
- Occasionally, increases in BUN concentration can be associated with diseases that can produce gastrointestinal ulceration and bleeding.
- Decreased BUN concentration levels can be associated with liver dysfunction.
- Although changes in BUN concentration can be of concern, the blood test must also be fully evaluated, along with the pet's condition, history, other diagnostics, and response to treatment, before conclusions can be reached.

Calcium

When elevated, calcium can suggest certain endocrine diseases or some forms of cancer (i.e., lymphoma, anal sac apocrine gland adenocarcinoma, osteosarcoma, fibrosarcoma). In lactating dogs, low levels of calcium can suggest **eclampsia** (see Chapter 18).

Function

Calcium is a mineral that is used by the body for production of bone, many chemical reactions (blood clotting, many enzymatic reactions), and muscular contractions. It is essential for body function, milk formation, and reproduction.

Where It Is Produced

Calcium is absorbed from the diet and stored in the bone. As it is needed, calcium is reabsorbed from the bone and carried in the bloodstream for numerous body functions.

Abnormalities

Increased blood calcium concentration (hypercalcemia) can be associated with specific types of tumors and rare hormonal disease. Hypercalcemia is a significant clinical finding associated with cancers that produce the **hypercalcemia of malignancy**. In fact, in the dog and cat, the most common cause of hypercalcemia is cancer.

Decreased blood calcium concentration (hypocalcemia) is generally associated with female dogs immediately after whelping that are producing large amounts of milk for many puppies. This syndrome is called **eclampsia** (see Chapter 18).

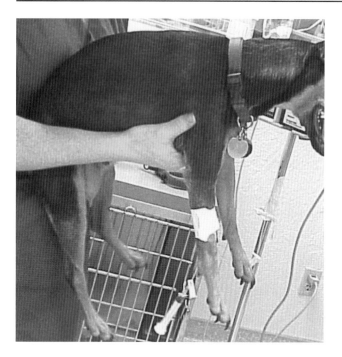

Figure 22.1.   Image of a female dog with eclampsia. Notice the rigid limbs and sawhorse position. This patient is unable to have normal muscle contraction and is rigid and stiff.

Symptoms Associated with Changes in Blood Calcium Concentration

- **Hypercalcemia:** Significantly increased blood calcium concentration can produce calcification of abdominal organs and potential organ disease (i.e., kidneys, liver, lungs). Physical signs are generally associated with the organs and the diseases produced. Hypercalcemia can cause a significant increase in urination (polyuria).
- **Hypocalcemia:** With low blood calcium concentration the pet is unable to sustain normal muscle control, heart rate, and coordination because calcium is needed for muscular contraction. Affected female pets present with
  — rigid limbs (see Figure 22.1),
  — muscular tremors,
  — hyperthermia (due to constant muscular spasms),
  — weakness, and
  — bradycardia.

Other Clinical Diagnostic Tests

Diagnostic tests that are used to help evaluate cause of increased calcium concentration include the following.

- **Hypercalcemia:** With concerns of significant hypercalcemia, a complete blood count, blood chemistry, radiographs, and ultrasound may be needed to evaluate the cause of the increased blood calcium concentration and assess organ damage.
- **Hypocalcemia:** With the history of a postwhelping dog with a large litter, physical signs and blood calcium concentration are often sufficient for the diagnosis of eclampsia.

Discussing Changes in Calcium Concentration with the Client

- Calcium is a mineral that is used for production of bone, chemical reactions in the body, and muscular contraction. Calcium is absorbed from the diet and stored in the bone.
- Abnormal increases in calcium concentration are a significant concern and can be associated with certain types of malignant cancers or hormonal diseases.
- Decreased calcium concentration is associated with serious diseases in the postwhelping dog that is producing large amounts of milk for numerous pups.
- Although changes in calcium concentration can be of concern, the blood test must also be fully evaluated, along with the pet's condition, history, other diagnostics, and response to treatment, before conclusions can be reached.

Creatinine
Tests for creatinine evaluate the patient's kidney function.

Function
Creatinine is a small amino acid that is a metabolite of muscle creatinine and is excreted by the kidneys.

Where It Is Produced
Creatinine is produced in the body during normal muscle metabolism.

Abnormalities
Increases in creatinine concentration can be associated with changes in glomerular filtration rate. Creatinine concentration is generally increased when there is a decrease in the kidney's glomerular filtration rate. Causes of decreased glomerular filtration rate include the following.

- **Prerenal azotemia:** When the body has decreased fluid (i.e., dehydration), the heart cannot pump blood through the kidneys at a rate adequate to produce a normal filtration rate. As a result, creatinine concentration is increased.
- **Renal azotemia:** When damage to the kidneys results in loss of normal renal tissue, the glomerular filtration rate of the kidneys is not sufficient to clear toxins and metabolites such as creatinine from the body.
- **Postrenal azotemia:** When the lower urinary tract is obstructed (i.e., blocked tomcat), the increased pressure and lack of urine outflow inhibit normal filtration. As a result, substances normally excreted by the kidney, such as creatinine, build up in the serum.

A decrease in creatinine is not indicative of disease.

Symptoms Associated with Changes in Creatinine Concentration

Increased creatinine concentration is generally associated with decreased glomerular filtration rate. As the pet becomes more toxic (**azotemic**), physical signs can be as follows.

With acute azotemia signs are

- vomiting,
- diarrhea,
- anorexia,
- dehydration, and
- neurologic signs: seizures.

With chronic azotemia signs are

- weight loss,
- chronic vomiting,
- chronic diarrhea,
- muscle loss,
- increased thirst (polydipsia), and
- increased urination (polyuria).

Other Clinical Diagnostic Tests

Diagnostic tests that are used to help evaluate increases in creatinine include

- phosphorus,
- urinalysis—urine specific gravity,
- BUN, and
- serum electrolytes (especially potassium).

(Please see the algorithm for kidney disease on p. 331.)

Discussing Changes in Creatinine Concentration with the Client

- Creatinine is a metabolite produced during muscle metabolism that is excreted by the kidneys.
- Marked increase in creatinine concentration is typically associated with the body's inability to filter toxins (glomerular filtration rate) through the kidneys. This can be caused by marked dehydration, kidney disease, or urinary obstruction.
- Decreasing creatinine levels can be associated with muscle wasting but are usually not significant.
- Although changes in creatinine levels can be of concern, the blood test must also be fully evaluated, along with the pet's condition, history, other diagnostics, and response to treatment, before conclusions can be reached.

Gamma-Glutamyltransferase

Gamma-glutamyltransferase (GGT) is an indicator of nonmovement of the gall bladder (**cholestasis**) in the dog and cat. It does not aid in evaluation of liver function.

Function

GGT is an intracellular enzyme responsible for cleaving C-terminal glutamyl groups from one substrate or molecule to another. It is thought to be involved in pathways used to protect cells from oxidative injury.

Where It Is Produced

All cells except muscle contain GGT; however, renal epithelial, bile duct, and hepatic cells contain the highest activity.

Abnormalities

Increased GGT activity can be seen with decreased bile flow (**cholestasis**). GGT can increase with liver damage that results in cholestasis. *Significant increases in GGT are associated with hepatic disease and bile duct obstruction.* Unlike AST and ALT, GGT does not "leak" from hepatocytes; its activity is increased due to increased production (induction) of the enzyme in response to disease. Increases in GGT activity can be the result of pathologic and nonpathologic conditions.

Symptoms Associated with Changes in GGT Activity

Changes in GGT activity can be associated with liver disease or bile duct obstruction (see Chapter 15). The symptoms can vary depending on the severity and cause of the disease.

Liver Disease

For liver disease, symptoms include

- anorexia,
- depression,
- weight loss,
- vomiting,
- diarrhea,
- jaundice (although not always directly associated with elevations of GGT), and
- neurologic signs.

Gall Bladder Obstruction

For gall bladder obstruction, symptoms include

- abdominal tenderness/pain,
- jaundice (directly linked to obstruction of the gall bladder),
- vomiting,
- anorexia,
- dehydration, and
- diarrhea.

Other Clinical Diagnostic Tests

Diagnostic tests that are used to help evaluate the cause of increased GGT activity include those for liver disease and gall bladder obstruction.

Liver Disease

Evaluating other liver enzymes that suggest liver damage may indicate the cause of increased GGT activity. These diagnostic tests are

- ALT,
- SALP or ALP, and
- AST.

Other diagnostic tests for **liver function** may indicate the cause of increased GGT activity. These diagnostic tests are

- BUN,
- total bilirubin,
- cholesterol,
- bile acids (paired),
- glucose, and
- TP.

Gall Bladder Obstruction

Some clinical diagnostic tests that help determine if gall bladder obstruction is the cause of changes in GGT activity are

- total bilirubin,
- alkaline phosphatase,
- abdominal X-ray, and
- abdominal ultrasound.

Discussing Changes in Gamma-Glutamyltransferase Activity Levels with the Client
- Gamma-Glutamyltransferase (GGT) is a hepatic intracellular enzyme that is involved in protecting cells from cellular injury.
- Decreased GGT activity is not generally associated with disease.
- Increased activity can be associated with damage to the liver, causing increased production of GGT by the hepatocytes and release into the bloodstream.
- A normal GGT activity level does not rule out liver disease or dysfunction where only small amounts of liver tissue has decreased function.
- Although elevations in GGT activity level can be of concern, the blood test must also be fully evaluated, along with the pet's condition, history, other diagnostics, and response to treatment, before conclusions can be reached.

Glucose

Glucose is the body's energy source obtained from ingestion of carbohydrates and other food stuffs.

Function

Glucose is metabolized intracellularly into adenosine triphosphate (ATP) energy through a process called **respiration**.

Where It Is Produced

Glucose is absorbed through the intestines from digestion of carbohydrates and obtained by fat and protein metabolism in the liver.

Abnormalities

Hyperglycemia

Hyperglycemia is defined by glucose levels, as follows:

- Canine: Blood glucose >300 mg/dl
- Feline: Blood glucose >200 mg/dl

Some patients become hyperglycemic due to stress and can produce blood glucose levels above 200–300 mg/dl.

Diabetes mellitus can cause pathologic increases in blood glucose (see hyperglycemia values above) due to lack of insulin production or insulin resistance in the tissue (see Chapter 15).

Hypoglycemia

Low blood sugar (hypoglycemia <60 mg/dl) is produced by insulin overdose, massive body infection, or tumor. It can also occur in young neonates that do not have enough body reserve to maintain normal blood sugar levels (i.e., juvenile hypoglycemia). *Hypoglycemia is a life-threatening concern that should be brought to the veterinarian's attention immediately.*

Practice Tip: When dealing with a potential hypoglycemia there are two factors the team member should evaluate:

1. **Has the blood sample been sitting for too long?** It is important to note that if a blood sample is left sitting for too long, the red blood cells will continue to consume the glucose in the tube, producing artifactual hypoglycemia.
2. **Is a human glucometer being used?** When using a human glucometer, blood glucose levels can be higher by 30–40 mg/dl. The manufacturers set the glucometer high to ensure that human diabetics will eat before their blood sugar level is too low, hence a blood sugar of 80 may show up as 40 on a human machine.

Symptoms Associated with Changes in Glucose Levels

Symptoms can vary depending on the severity and cause of the disease and may include the following.

Hyperglycemia associated with diabetes mellitus presents with

- increased thirst (polydipsia),
- increased urination (polyuria),
- increased appetite (polyphagia), and
- weight loss.

Hypoglycemia is a life-threatening condition affecting the central nervous system directly, producing

- weakness,
- lethargy,

- coma,
- seizure,
- death.

Other Clinical Diagnostic Tests
The following changes can be associated with diabetes mellitus (hyperglycemia).

Complete Blood Count
There is no overall change in CBC blood work.

Chemistry
Tests are as follows:

- Hyperglycemia
- Increased liver enzymes
  — ALT
  — AST
- Lipemic serum
- Increased cholesterol
- Increased fructosamine
- Urinalysis
  — Glucosuria
  — Ketonuria
  — Evidence of secondary urinary tract disease, such as proteinuria, hematuria, crystals, etc.

Hypoglycemia, which if present, needs to be brought to the attention of the medical team immediately.

Discussing Changes in Glucose with the Client
- Glucose is the energy source of the body that is converted into cellular fuel called ATP by the cells of the body.
- Low blood sugar (hypoglycemia) commonly occurs secondary to massive infection, insulin overdose, or cancer. It also occurs in small newborns that do not have the body reserves to maintain normal body blood sugar levels.
- Hypoglycemia is an emergency condition that can produce coma, seizures, and death, and it must be treated immediately.
- High blood sugar levels (hyperglycemia) occur secondary to stress or disease conditions such as diabetes mellitus.
- Persistent hyperglycemia may require the medical team to do further diagnostic testing to help differentiate if the patient has diabetes or has a stress-induced hyperglycemia.

Lipase
Lipase is an indicator of pancreatitis in the dog. It is not helpful in evaluation of feline pancreatitis.

Function
Lipase is an enzyme that helps break down larger lipid molecules for absorption.

Where It Is Produced
Lipase is produced in the pancreas and enters the duodenum through the pancreatic ducts to break down lipids for digestion.

Abnormalities
Lipase is released when there is damage to the pancreatic cells that produce leakage of the enzyme into the bloodstream. Pancreatic damage is secondary to infection and inflammation of the pancreas (pancreatitis; see Chapter 15) or pancreatic cancer.

Symptoms Associated with Increased Lipase Activity
Increased lipase activity is associated with the infection or inflammation of the pancreas and the resulting pancreatitis. Common symptoms of acute severe pancreatitis in the dog are

- anorexia,
- depression,
- vomiting,
- abdominal pain,
- diarrhea, and
- jaundice.

Other Clinical Diagnostic Tests
Diagnostic tests that are used to help evaluate the cause of increases in lipase activity include

- amylase,
- TLI,
- pancreatic lipase immunoreactivity,

Discussing Elevations of Lipase with the Client
- Lipase is an enzyme produced by the pancreas to help break down sugar for absorption in the small intestine.
- In the dog, elevations in Amylase can suggest an infection or inflammation of the pancreas (i.e. pancreatitis). The disease process causes the enzyme to leak out of normal pancreatic cells and into the blood stream.
- In the cat, increased pancreatic enzyme activity does not directly correlate with pancreatitis.
- Rarely, increased lipase activity may suggest pancreatic cancer in the dog and cat.
- It is important to note that patients, especially with chronic disease, can have severe pancreatitis without elevations of lipase.
- Although increased lipase activity can be of concern, the blood test must also be fully evaluated, along with the pet's condition, history, other diagnostics, and response to treatment, before conclusions can be reached.

- complete blood count,
  — elevation of white count
  — increased band neutrophils
- total bilirubin.

(Please see the algorithm for exocrine pancreatic disease on p. 333.)

Phosphorus

Increased phosphorus concentration is associated with decreased kidney function secondary to acute or chronic renal disease.

Function

Phosphorus is a mineral that plays an important part in many cell functions, including bone formation, energy metabolism, muscle contraction, and acid–base balance.

Where It Is Produced

Phosphorus is absorbed from the diet and stored with calcium in a complex structure in the bone. The combination of calcium and phosphorus architecture gives bone its strength. Phosphorus is also a key element needed for energy production in the cell.

Abnormalities

Increased blood phosphorus concentration (**hyperphosphotemia**) is associated with both acute and chronic renal disease. Phosphorus is eliminated by glomerular filtration. As with BUN and creatinine, kidney disease that results in decreased glomerular filtration rate can cause an increase in phosphorus concentration in the blood. Parathyroid hormones can also affect serum phosphate concentration. Serum phosphorus can also be increased by ingestion of high-phosphate substances (i.e., many antifreeze products have high phosphorus concentration).

Decreased phosphorus concentration (**hypophosphotemia**) is not generally associated with disease conditions. However, significant hypophosphatemia can result from acid–base imbalance and aggressive insulin therapy.

Symptoms Associated with Increased Phosphorus Concentration

Generally associated with kidney disease are decreased glomerular filtration rate and retention of increased amounts of phosphorus in the bloodstream. Physical symptoms can be

- weight loss,
- chronic vomiting,
- chronic diarrhea,
- muscle loss,
- increased thirst (polydipsia), and
- increased urination (polyuria).

Other Clinical Diagnostic Tests

Diagnostic tests that are used to help evaluate the cause of increases in phosphorus concentration associated with renal disease include

- BUN,
- creatinine,
- urinalysis—urine specific gravity, and
- serum electrolytes (especially potassium).

(Please see algorithm for kidney disease, p. 331.)

Discussing Increases in Phosphorus Concentration with the Client

- Phosphorus is a mineral that is used for stability of bone and is a key element in the production of cellular energy. Phosphorus is absorbed from the diet and stored in the bone.
- Abnormal increases in phosphorus concentration are generally associated with renal disease because the kidneys lose their ability to filter out phosphorus in the urine.
- Although changes in phosphorus can be of concern, the blood test must also be fully evaluated, along with the pet's condition, history, other diagnostics, and response to treatment, before conclusions can be reached.

Potassium

Significant changes in potassium can produce severe whole body disease. Changes in potassium concentration can suggest

- hormonal disease—hypoadrenocorticism (Addison's disease),
- feline lower urinary tract disease (FLUTD),
- renal disease, and
- gastrointestinal disease.

Function

Potassium is an intracellular electrolyte necessary for producing skeletal and cardiac contraction muscle, depolarization of nerves, and other metabolic functions.

Where It Is Produced

Potassium is an electrolyte that is absorbed through the digestive system through dietary elements, stored intracellularly, and excreted through the kidneys.

Abnormalities

Increased blood potassium concentration (**hyperkalemia**) is a life-threatening derangement of the body's electrolyte balance. It is generally associated with hormonal dysfunction, kidney disease, and urinary obstruction.

- **FLUTD:** Animals with obstruction of their lower urinary tract are unable to eliminate potassium from the body. Over 8–12 hours, the hyperkalemia can be so severe that it produces weakness, muscle fasciculations, and cardiac arrhythmias.
- **Hypoadrenocorticism:** Hypoadrenocorticism (Addison's disease; see Chapter 16) is a lack of the hormone

aldosterone from the adrenal gland. This hormone stimulates the release of potassium in the kidneys while reabsorbing sodium. Addisonian animals can have significant alterations in normal sodium and potassium concentration, causing generalized weakness, bradycardia, muscle fasciculations, and collapse.

Decreases of body potassium (**hypokalemia**) are associated with disease entities that cause increased loss of fluids from the body (i.e., vomiting or diarrhea, polyuric renal disease) or increased fluid excretion through the kidneys (i.e., diuresis). Common diseases that can produce profound hypokalemia are listed below.

- **Gastrointestinal disease:** Severe hypokalemia (<2.5 mEq/dl) can be associated with diseases that cause significant fluid losses from vomiting and diarrhea. Diseases such as colitis, parvoviral infection, panleukopenia, gastric foreign body, and others can produce severe low body potassium levels.
- **Kidney disease:** Animals with kidney disease lose the ability to concentrate their urine (see Chapter 13). To compensate, these patients must drink large amounts of water and excrete large amounts of urine. This mechanical diuresis increases the amount of potassium excreted.
- **Hospitalized animals on IV fluids:** When anorexic animals are on intravenous fluid support in the hospital setting, they may demonstrate diuresis-associated hypokalemia.

Symptoms Associated with Increased Potassium Concentration

Physical signs of hyperkalemia can be life threatening because the body's normal balances of sodium and potassium are affected, decreasing the body's ability to produce electrical impulses required for normal cell function. The cells most severely affected are nerves, skeletal muscle, and cardiac muscle. Symptoms of hyperkalemia are

- anorexia,
- weakness,
- muscle fasciculations,
- abnormal heart rhythms—ventricular premature contractions,
- pulse deficits,
- collapse, and
- bradycardia.

Although less severe, hypokalemia also affects the body's ability to produce normal electrical impulses. Common symptoms of hypokalemia are

- weakness,
- ventroflexion of the neck (see Figure 22.2),
- anorexia,
- depression, and
- cardiac arrhythmia.

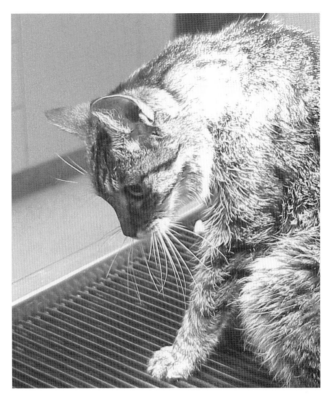

Figure 22.2. Image of a cat with severe ventroflexion of the neck secondary to profound hypokalemia.

Discussing Changes in Potassium Concentration with the Client

- Potassium is an electrolyte that is responsible for normal contractions of the heart and skeletal muscle and nerve impulses as well any many other intracellular metabolic functions.
- Abnormal increases in potassium concentration are serious, life-threatening conditions generally associated with urinary obstruction or hormonal dysfunction.
- Abnormal decreases in potassium are associated with gastrointestinal losses (vomiting and diarrhea) or increased fluid loss through the kidneys (i.e., kidney disease).
- Although changes in potassium concentration can be of concern, the blood test must also be fully evaluated, along with the pet's condition, history, other diagnostics, and response to treatment, before conclusions can be reached.

Other Clinical Diagnostic Tests

Diagnostic tests that are used to help evaluate the changes in potassium concentration include the following.

For hyperkalemia tests are:

- BUN,
- creatinine,

- phosphorus,
- sodium and chloride,
- ACTH stimulation test (see below),
- abdominal radiographs, and
- electrocardiogram.

For hypokalemia tests are:

- BUN,
- creatinine, and
- urinalysis—urine specific gravity.

Total Protein

Total protein (TP) is monitored to help evaluate the patient for hydration status and blood loss.

Function

TP is the sum of albumin and globulin in the bloodstream. Albumin has already been discussed earlier in this section. Globulin is a protein produced from the lymphocytes of the body (white blood cell) to fight off infection, for example, immunoglobulin.

Where It Is Produced

Albumin is produced from the liver. Immunoglobulin is produced by lymphocytes in the bloodstream in response to infectious organisms or other foreign substances (see Chapter 21).

How Level Is Evaluated

TP can be evaluated two ways: using a refractometer and through clinical blood chemistry tests.

An estimate of TP concentration can be determined using the spun PCV microcapillary (hematocrit) tube.

- After the sample is spun down and the PCV recorded, the hematocrit tube is broken in the serum region above the red blood cell column and buffy coat.
- The serum is then placed on a refractometer and read on a scale from 1 to 12 mg/dl.
- The value is recorded along with the PCV.

TP can also be obtained through a clinical chemistry or an individual in-house chemistry unit. Blood should be obtained through a red-topped tube or serum separator.

Abnormalities

Changes in TP depend on overall changes in albumin and immunoglobulin.

As discussed earlier (see albumin), decreased albumin concentration can suggest liver, renal, and intestinal disease, as well as acute or chronic blood loss. Increased albumin concentration is generally associated with dehydration.

Immunoglobulin concentration is generally increased in the body with chronic infectious disease and specific types of cancer (i.e., lymphoma, myeloma). Decreased immunoglobulin concentration can suggest an inability of the white blood cells to produce immunity because of immunosuppression or chemotherapy.

Symptoms Associated with Changes in Total Protein Concentration

Increased TP concentration can be associated with dehydration, similar to the increase in albumin concentration. It can also be associated with chronic infection, inflammation, or cancer.

Decreased TP concentration can be associated with conditions that produce decreased albumin concentration (see above). Further decreases can be seen with diseases that lower the body's response to infection (**immunosuppression**).

Other Clinical Diagnostic Tests

Diagnostic tests are used to help evaluate changes in TP concentration. For increased TP, associated with increased albumin concentration, the tests are

- PCV,
- albumin, and
- urine specific gravity.

For increased TP associated with increased globulins, secondary to chronic infection, inflammation, or cancer, the tests are

- complete blood counts—white blood cell count,
- globulin blood level, and
- infectious disease titers, including
  — fungal screens,
  — rickettsial screens, and
  — feline infectious peritonitis (feline corona virus).

Discussing Changes in Total Protein Levels with the Client

- Total protein (TP) is a combination of blood albumin and globulin proteins in the blood.
- Albumin is produced by the liver as a carrier protein to carry nutrients and hormones through the bloodstream.
- Globulins are proteins produced from a type of white blood cell (lymphocytes) to help fight off infection.
- Elevations in TP can suggest increases in albumin, secondary to dehydration, or elevations in globulin, secondary to chronic infection.
- Decreases in TP can be associated with chronically low albumin due to external bleeding or chronic kidney, liver, or intestinal disease. Rarely, decreased production by lymphocytes (immunosuppression) can be associated with a low globulin.
- Although elevations in TP can be of concern, the blood test must also be fully evaluated, along with the pet's condition, history, other diagnostics, and response to treatment, before conclusions can be reached.

For decreased TP due to decreased albumin tests are

- PCV/TP (blood loss),
- liver enzymes (liver disease),
- BUN/creatinine (protein-losing enteropathy), and
- TLI/PLI (inflammatory bowel disease).

For decreased TP due to decreased globulins, secondary to immunosuppression, the diagnostic test used is a complete blood count.

Advanced Diagnostics for Adrenal Gland Function

Advanced blood clinical pathology diagnostics are tests that are run in-hospital or through reference laboratories to detect specific infectious, metabolic, or organ-associated diseases. The diagnostic tests are used to help differentiate specific diseases that cannot be evaluated through normal blood chemistries. Each section below outlines the clinical protocols used to perform each test; however, every reference laboratory is different in their approach. It is important to discuss the testing protocols with the each lab prior to performing the clinical diagnostic test.

The veterinarian is always responsible for interpreting the clinical diagnostic tests and outlining treatment options. It is important for the team member to understand why specific diagnostic tests are performed to better anticipate the veterinarian's needs, to properly monitor the hospitalized patient, and to educate the client.

Diagnostic tests for adrenal gland function help to evaluate overproduction of cortisol from the adrenal gland (**hyperadrenocorticism**) or decreased adrenal production of aldosterone (**hypoadrenocorticism**) (see Chapter 17).

How the ACTH Stimulation Test is Performed
The patient is fasted for 12 hours. The patient cannot be on any topical, injectable, or oral prednisone medication.

1. A baseline (pre-ACTH) blood sample is drawn in a red-topped or serum separator tube.
2. ACTH can be given as a liquid suspension or as a corticotrophin gel. It is given as follows:
   —ACTH dose: 2.2 IU/kg IM
   —Corticotrophin gel: ACTH can be given as a liquid suspension or as a corticotrophin gel.
3. A post-ACTH blood draw is performed as follows:
   - If ACTH is given, draw the cortisol baseline 1 hour after injection in a red-topped or serum-separator tube.
   - If Corticotrophin is given, draw cortisol baseline 2 hours after injection in a red-topped or serum-separator tube.

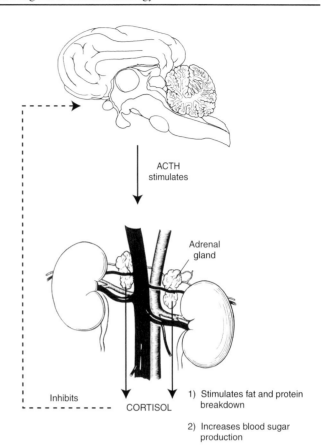

Figure 22.3. Illustration of normal release of ACTH to stimulate the release of cortisol. Cortisol then stimulates production of glucose from fat and protein, while also decreasing the production of ACTH. This type of model is called a negative feedback loop.

ACTH Stimulation Test

The ACTH stimulation test helps evaluate overproduction of cortisol produced by hyperadrenocorticism (Cushing's disease). It does not differentiate between a pituitary- or adrenal-dependent form. Furthermore, the ACTH stimulation test helps assess for decreased production of cortisol produced by hypoadrenocorticism (Addison's disease).

Function
ACTH is the hormone produced by the pituitary gland to stimulate production of cortisol by the adrenal gland. Cortisol is used in times of stress and emergency to provide glucose to the cell by metabolism of fat and proteins (see Figure 22.3).

Where It Is Produced
ACTH is produced in the pituitary gland.

Evaluation of the Test
The test evaluates both overproduction of cortisol in hyperadrenocorticism (Cushing's disease) and decreased cortisol production due to decreased response to ACTH associated with hypoadrenocorticism (Addison's disease).

Abnormalities

Alterations in the ACTH response test suggest abnormalities in adrenal gland function.

Increased response suggests hyperadrenocorticism (Cushing's disease). It does not differentiate whether the disease is occurring within the pituitary (with increased release of ACTH) or within the adrenal gland (overproduction of cortisol by an adrenal tumor).

Decreased response can suggest hypoadrenocorticism due to decreased production of cortisol and/or aldosterone from the adrenal gland.

Other Clinical Diagnostic Tests

Diagnostic tests are used to help evaluate changes in ACTH stimulation.

For increased response, further clinical diagnostic tests are used to help differentiate the type of Cushing's disease present (i.e., adrenal versus pituitary disease). Some of these diagnostic tests listed next.

- **Low-dose dexamethasone suppression test:** (See below for more detail.) If the ACTH stimulation test is inconclusive, a low-dose dexamethasone test may be performed because it may be a more sensitive indicator of adrenal function.

Discussing Changes in the Adrenocorticotropic Hormone Response Test with the Client

- The adrenocorticotropic hormone (ACTH) response test is used to help detect abnormal increases or decreases in the body's cortisol level in response to stimulation.
- ACTH is a hormone that is produced from the pituitary gland in the brain to help stimulate cortisol production in the adrenal gland.
- To evaluate the pet for changes in normal cortisol production, a blood sample for determination of baseline cortisol concentration is drawn from your fasted pet.
- The patient is then given ACTH and a second blood sample for determination of cortisol concentration is drawn 1–2 hours later.
- Increased response to the ACTH stimulation test suggests that the pet is suffering from hyperadrenocorticism. However, it does not differentiate between pituitary and adrenal causes of Cushing's disease.
- Decreased response of ACTH stimulation is suggestive of hypoadrenocorticism.
- Although derangements in cortisol production in the ACTH response test can be of concern, the blood test must also be fully evaluated, along with the pet's condition, history, other diagnostics, and response to treatment, before conclusions can be reached.

- **High-dose dexamethasone suppression test:** (See next page for more detail.) If the ACTH stimulation test identifies hyperadrenocorticism, the high-dose dexamethasone suppression test helps determine if the cause of the increased cortisol is pituitary or adrenal in origin.
- **Abdominal radiography:** Radiography can be used to help examine the mid-dorsal abdomen for suspicious masses that may be suggestive of an adrenal tumor.
- **Abdominal ultrasound:** Ultrasound allows the patient's adrenal glands to be visualized and examined for changes that could indicate pituitary-dependent disease or adrenal tumor.

Low-Dose Dexamethasone Suppression Test

Similar to the ACTH stimulation test, the low-dose dexamethasone suppression test screens for hyperadrenocorticism. The test evaluates the normal suppression of cortisol that should occur as increased amounts of dexamethasone (a cortisol-like steroid) are administered to the body. It is important to note that different labs require different protocols for the diagnostic test; the lab should be consulted prior to the test to ensure that their protocol is followed.

The low-dose dexamethasone suppression test helps evaluate overproduction of cortisol produced by hyperadrenocorticism (Cushing's disease). *It does not differentiate between a pituitary- or adrenal-dependent form.*

Function

In a normal patient, by giving a small amount of exogenous steroid to the body, the pituitary will decrease ACTH production and normal cortisol levels will decrease. This is called a negative feedback loop. In animals with Cushing's disease, the production of cortisol does not depend on normal ACTH secretion, and the cortisol levels continue to be secreted at increased rates (see Figure 22.3).

How the Low-Dose Dexamethasone Suppression Test Is Performed

The patient is fasted for 12 hours. The patient cannot be on any topical, injectable, or oral prednisone medication.

1. A (pre-LDD suppression) blood sample for determination of the baseline cortisol concentration is drawn in a red-topped or serum-separator tube.
2. A low dose of dexamethasone is given intravenously (0.01 mg/kg).
3. A blood sample for determination of post-LDD suppression of cortisol concentration is drawn as follows:
   - A sample is drawn at 6 hours in a red-topped or serum-separator tube.
   - Another sample is drawn at 8 hours in a red-topped or serum-separator tube.

Evaluation of the Test

The test evaluates the patient's ability to suppress cortisol production when exogenous steroids are injected. Normal patients will show a 50% suppression (reduction) in cortisol levels within 6–8 hours.

Abnormalities

If there is no obvious suppression within 6–8 hours, it suggests hyperadrenocorticism. The test usually does not differentiate whether the disease is occurring within the pituitary (with increased release of ACTH) or within the adrenal gland (overproduction of cortisol).

Other Clinical Diagnostic Tests

Further clinical diagnostic tests are used to help differentiate the type of Cushing's disease present (i.e., adrenal versus pituitary disease). Some of these diagnostic tests are

- high-dose dexamethasone suppression test (discussed below);
- abdominal radiography, which can be used to help examine the mid-dorsal abdomen for suspicious masses that may be suggestive of an adrenal tumor; and
- abdominal ultrasound, which allows the patient's adrenal glands to be visualized and examined for changes that could indicate pituitary-dependent disease or adrenal tumor.

High-Dose Dexamethasone (HDD) Suppression Test

The high-dose dexamethasone suppression test is performed after hyperadrenocorticism has been diagnosed with a screening test (i.e., ACTH stimulation or low-dose dexamethasone suppression test). The test uses a dose of dexamethasone 10 times higher than that used in the low-dose dexamethasone suppression test to help differentiate pituitary-dependent adrenal disease from adrenal-dependent forms.

The high-dose dexamethasone suppression test helps to determine if the diagnosed hyperadrenocorticism patient is suffering from a pituitary- or adrenal-dependent form of the disease.

Function

In pituitary-dependent adrenal disease (see Chapter 17), higher doses of dexamethasone usually produce suppression of cortisol levels in 6–8 hours. With adrenal-dependent disease, the cortisol concentration in the serum of three out of four patients with adrenal tumors will not be suppressed when the patient is given higher levels of dexamethasone.

Discussing Results of the Low-Dose Dexamethasone Suppression Test with the Client

- A low-dose dexamethasone suppression test is used to help detect abnormal increases in the body's cortisol level caused by increased production of a releasing hormone within the pituitary or overproduction of cortisol from an adrenal tumor.
- To evaluate the pet for changes in normal cortisol production, a baseline blood cortisol concentration is drawn from your fasted pet.
- The patient is then given a low dose of dexamethasone (a cortisol-like drug) intravenously and two more blood cortisol concentrations are drawn 6 and 8 hours later.
- In normal patients, the blood cortisol concentration decreases by 50% as the body detects increasing levels of steroid and decreases production.
- Hyperadrenocorticism patients do not normally suppress after 6–8 hours.
- The test helps to diagnose Cushing's disease but does not differentiate between the diseases caused by pituitary or adrenal glands. Although derangements in cortisol production in the low-dose dexamethasone suppression test can be of concern, the blood test must also be fully evaluated, along with the pet's condition, history, other diagnostics, and response to treatment before conclusions can be reached.

How the HDD Suppression Test Is Performed

The patient is fasted for 12 hours. The patient cannot be on any injectable or oral prednisone medication.

1. A blood sample for determination of baseline (pre-HDD suppression) cortisol concentration is drawn in a red-topped or serum-separator tube.
2. A high dose of dexamethasone is given intravenously (0.1 mg/kg).
3. A blood sample for determination of post-HDD suppression of cortisol concentration is drawn as follows:
- A sample is drawn at 6 hours in a red-topped or serum-separator tube.
- Another sample is drawn at 8 hours in a red-topped or serum-separator tube.

Evaluation of the Test

The test determines the patient's ability to suppress cortisol production when exogenous steroids are injected. Most patients with pituitary-dependent Cushing's disease will show 50% suppression of serum cortisol concentration within 6–8 hours. Most patients with adrenal-dependent disease will not show suppression of serum cortisol concentration at any time during the test.

Abnormalities

If there is suppression within 6–8 hours, it suggests pituitary-dependent hyperadrenocorticism. If there is no suppression, adrenal disease is suspected.

Other Clinical Diagnostic Tests

Further clinical diagnostic tests are used to help differentiate the type of Cushing's disease present (i.e., adrenal versus pituitary disease). Some of these diagnostics are as follows.

- **Abdominal radiography:** This can be used to help examine the mid-dorsal abdomen for suspicious masses that may be suggestive of an adrenal tumor.
- **Abdominal ultrasound:** This allows the patient's adrenal glands to be visualized and examined for changes that could indicate pituitary-dependent disease or adrenal tumor.

Discussing Results of the High-Dose Dexamethasone Suppression Test with the Client

- A high-dose dexamethasone suppression test is used to help differentiate if the patient is suffering from an adrenal or pituitary form of hyperadrenocorticism.
- A baseline blood sample for determination of cortisol concentration is drawn from your fasted pet.
- The patient is then given a high dose of dexamethasone (a cortisol-like drug) intravenously, and two more blood samples for determination of cortisol concentration are drawn 6 and 8 hours later.
- In animals affected by pituitary-dependent hyperadrenocorticism, the blood cortisol concentration decreases by 50% as the body detects increasing levels of steroid and decreases production.
- In animals affected by adrenal-dependent hyperadrenocorticism, there is generally no suppression noted in blood cortisol concentration.
- Although derangements in cortisol production as seen in the high-dose dexamethasone suppression test can be of concern, the blood test must also be fully evaluated, along with the pet's condition, history, other diagnostics, and response to treatment, before conclusions can be reached.

Advanced Blood Diagnostics and Drug Assays

Monitoring Therapeutic Drug Levels

These diagnostic tests help evaluate if a prescription medication is reaching effective levels within the bloodstream without crossing over into a toxic range. The most common drug levels evaluated are phenobarbital and potassium bromine (KBr), which are used for long-term control of seizures. Although these drugs are the only two discussed in this text, therapeutic drug levels are also available for other long-term medications (i.e., thyroxine, fluconazole, ketoconazole).

Function

Phenobarbital and KBr are given continually to help decrease the severity, occurrence, and length of seizures in the patient.

How the Phenobarbital/Potassium Bromide Level Test Is Performed

The patient has a blood sample for determination of the drug concentration drawn 4–6 hours after the last dose of the medication is given.

The blood sample is drawn into a red-topped tube or a specialized serum-separator tube that does not interfere with evaluation of blood drug levels.

Evaluation of the Test

The test measures the concentration of KBr or phenobarbital in the body to determine if the level is below, within, or above therapeutic ranges.

Abnormalities

Alterations in drug levels can suggest overall response to treatment. With each specific drug, the following is noted.

- **Phenobarbital:** Low therapeutic levels suggest there is not enough drug present in the blood to help control seizures. Elevated concentration may suggest that the patient is receiving too much medication, which can produce hepatic toxicity.
- **KBr:** Low therapeutic levels suggest there is not enough drug present in the blood to help control seizures. Increased levels of KBr are rarely associated with organ toxicity.

Other Clinical Diagnostic Tests

There are diagnostic tests that are used to help evaluate the changes in phenobarbital. For KBR no other tests are indicated.

It is important to note that for phenobarbital an elevated level does not indicate liver damage or dysfunction. *Furthermore, phenobarbital within the normal drug ranges can still produce liver damage dysfunction.* To better evaluate liver damage and disease, the following tests may be indicated.

Evaluating other liver enzymes that suggest liver damage may indicate the phenobarbital liver toxicity. These diagnostic tests are

- ALT,
- SALP or ALP, and
- AST.

Evaluating other diagnostics that suggest liver function may indicate phenobarbitol liver toxicity. These diagnostic tests are

- BUN,
- total bilirubin,
- cholesterol,
- bile acids (paired),

> **Discussing Changes with Phenobarbital/**
> **Potassium Bromide Drug Levels with the Client**
> - Phenobarbital or potassium bromide (KBr) levels are being tested to help evaluate if the concentration of drugs in the blood is within therapeutic range needed to help control seizure episodes.
> - The blood samples for determination of drug concentration are drawn 4–6 hours after a dose of the medication.
> - Decreased concentration may suggest that there is not enough drug within the system to help control seizures effectively.
> - Increased concentration of phenobarbital could be associated with toxicity and must be monitored closely.
> - There are limited toxicity concerns with elevated concentration of KBr.
> - Although changes within the phenobarbital or KBr levels are of concern, the overall change in blood work must be further evaluated, along with how the pet is responding to medication and other blood work diagnostics.

- albumin, and
- glucose.

Liver Function (Bile Acids Assay)

A test for bile acids is a true liver function test. With chronic liver disease there can be extensive liver damage with normal liver enzymes (i.e., ALT, AST) and bilirubin. A bile acids assay evaluates normal liver function.

Function

Bile acids are secreted by the liver into the small intestine when an animal eats to help emulsify and increase the digestibility of fat.

> **How the Bile Acids Assay Test Is Performed**
> The patient is fasted for 12 hours.
>
> 1. A sample of blood is drawn to detect preprandial (before eating) bile acid concentration.
> 2. The animal is then fed a small amount of high-energy food.
> 3. Two hours after eating, a blood sample is drawn to determine the postprandial bile acids concentration.
>
> The blood samples are drawn into a red-topped tube or a specialized serum-separator tube that does not interfere with evaluation of blood drug levels.

Where It Is Produced

Bile acids are produced by the liver for secretion into the small intestine.

Evaluation of the Test

The test determines the patient's ability to excrete bile acids in response to eating and then normally reabsorb the acids in a 2-hour time frame. Patients with decreased liver function have decreased ability to reabsorb bile acids postprandially. The greater the postprandial bile acids, the greater the liver dysfunction.

Abnormalities

Alterations can suggest functional liver disease. *The test does not help in diagnosing the cause of the liver disease but does indicate that the liver is not functioning normally.* It is usually of no further diagnostic use to measure bile acids if the bilirubin concentration is already increased.

Other Clinical Diagnostic Tests

Diagnostic tests that are used to help diagnose the cause of liver dysfunction are

- abdominal ultrasound and ultrasound-guided liver biopsy,
- laparoscopic surgery and biopsy, and
- exploratory surgery.

> **Discussing Changes in Bile Acids Assay with the Client**
> - Bile acids are salts that are excreted into the small intestine to help emulsify fats for digestion.
> - When there are concerns of liver dysfunction, assessing bile acids helps determine if the liver is able to excrete and reabsorb bile acid normally.
> - In a fasted patient, a blood sample to determine prefeeding bile acids concentration is drawn. The patient is then fed, and 2 hours later another blood sample is taken to determine postfeeding bile acids concentration.
> - Animals with liver dysfunction may have normal or significantly increased bile acids concentration prior to eating and significantly increased bile acids concentration after eating.
> - Although this test is a valuable indicator of liver function, it does not help determine the cause of the liver damage. When abnormal, it indicates that further diagnostic tests and biopsies are necessary to help diagnose the liver disease.
> - Although changes within the bile acids are of concern, the overall change in blood work must be further evaluated, along with how the pet is responding to medication and other blood work diagnostics.

Pancreatic Function

The trypsin-like immunoreactivity (TLI) test measures the activity of specific digestive enzymes (trypsinogen) in the blood. The test helps detect if there is decreased production of these enzymes suggesting pancreatic enzyme insufficiency (PEI; see Chapter 15).

Function

Trypsinogen is a digestive enzyme produced in the pancreas and secreted into the duodenum to cleave proteins into smaller amino acids for digestion.

Where It Is Produced

Trypsinogen is produced in the **acinar cells** of the pancreas.

> **How the Trypsin-Like Immunoassay Test is Performed**
> The patient is fasted for at least 12 hours prior to the test. Eating will artifactually bump up the trypsin-like immunoassay (TLI) to the low-normal range in some animals with early exocrine pancreatic insufficiency.
>
> The blood sample is drawn into a red-topped tube or a specialized serum-separator tube that does not interfere with evaluation of blood drug levels.

Evaluation of the Test

The test determines the serum concentration of trypsinogen.

Abnormalities

Decreased production of trypsinogen is suggestive of pancreatic exocrine insufficiency, a condition in which the pancreas loses its ability to produce normal digestive enzymes.

Other Clinical Diagnostic Tests

Diagnostic tests are used to help evaluate pancreatic dysfunction or disease.

- **Fecal parasites screens:** floatation, smears, ELISA (see Chapter 23).
- **Fecal fat evaluation:** Increased amounts of fat in the feces can suggest abnormal digestion or absorption of fat due to pancreatic or intestinal disease.
- **Blood folate levels:** Changes in blood folate concentration can suggest chronic inflammatory changes in the bowel and pancreatic exocrine insufficiency.

Thyroid Function—Total T_4 and Free T_4 Levels

Total T_4 and free T_4 levels help evaluate the patient for diseases causing overproduction (hyperthyroidism) and underproduction (hypothyroidism) of the primary hormone produced by the thyroid gland.

Function

Thyroid hormone is produced to help cells set the **basal metabolic rate** of the body, the rate at which cells burn energy.

> **How the Thyroid Level Test Is Performed**
> In initial evaluation of the thyroid function, the patient can have a thyroid hormone concentration determined from a general blood sample without fasting or preparation. However, if the patient is on a thyroid medication and hormone concentrations are being rechecked, it is recommended that the level be evaluated 4–6 hours after the medication is given.
>
> The blood sample is drawn into a red-topped tube or a specialized serum-separator tube that does not interfere with evaluation of blood drug levels.

Where It Is Produced

The thyroid produces thyroid hormone, which is released in the blood to set the basal metabolic rate of cells. The primary circulating thyroid hormone is the transport form, and it is present in the bloodstream as active free T_4 and T_4 bound to albumin. The metabolically active form of the hormone is T_3.

Evaluation of the Test

The test determines the patient's serum concentration of total T_4 and free T_4.

Abnormalities

Decreased levels of T_4 production can be associated with a lack of production at the pituitary or thyroid level (**hypothyroidism**). An increase in T_4 is associated with an overproduction of thyroid hormone due to benign (most common in cats) or malignant (most common in dogs) tumors of the thyroid gland (**hyperthyroidism**). Free T_4 levels are used to evaluate animals with borderline increases and decreases in total T_4. Free T_4 levels can change more dramatically in early disease than total T_4 levels and hence may be a good indicator of early thyroid disease. *It is important to remember that many dogs and cats with low total and free T_4 have decreased concentration of thyroid hormone because of nonthyroid disease (euthyroid sick syndrome).*

Other Clinical Diagnostic Tests

There are clinical tests that are used to help evaluate potential diseases of the thyroid gland.

For decreased thyroid function the tests are as follows:

- **Cholesterol/triglyceride levels:** With low thyroid function, serum fat and triglyceride concentration can be increased.
- **Complete blood count:** Some hypothyroid animals will have a mild nonregenerative anemia.

For increased thyroid function the tests are as follows:

- **Liver enzymes:** Prolonged hyperthyroidism can increase ALT, AST, and ALP levels.

Algorithm for Kidney Disease[i]

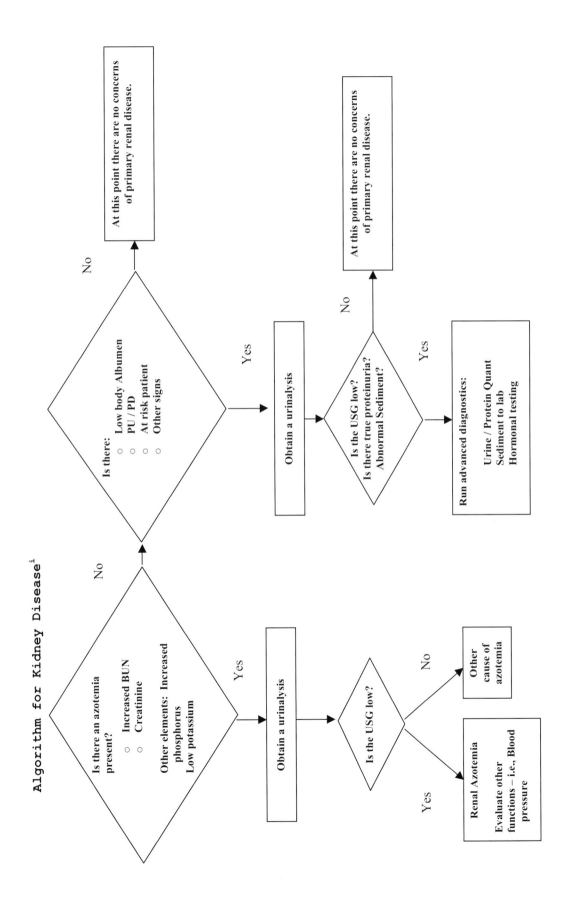

[i]Images reprinted with permission from Heska Corp., 3760 Rocky Mountain Avenue, Loveland, CO 80538.

Algorithm for Liver Disease[ii]

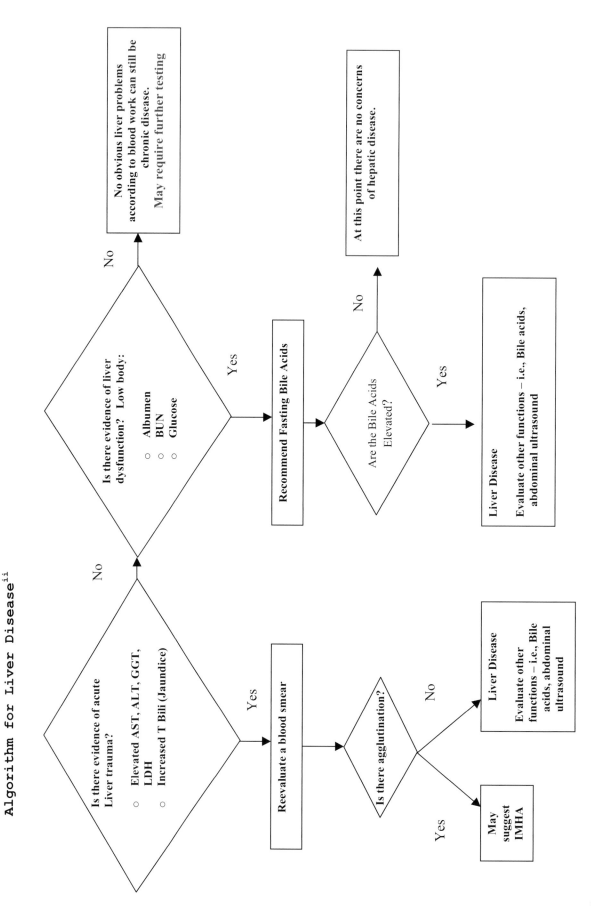

[ii]Images reprinted with permission from Heska Corp., 3760 Rocky Mountain Avenue, Loveland, CO 80538.

Algorithm for Exocrine Pancreatic Disease (i.e., Pancreatitis) [iii]

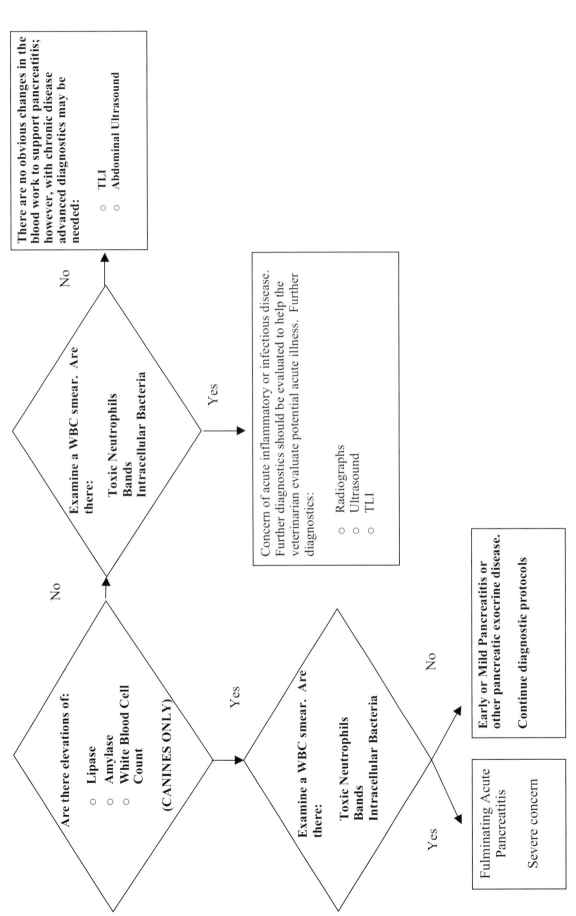

[iii]images reprinted with permission from Heska Corp., 3760 Rocky Mountain Avenue, Loveland, CO 80538.

Algorithm for Endocrine Pancreatic Disease (Diabetes) [iv]

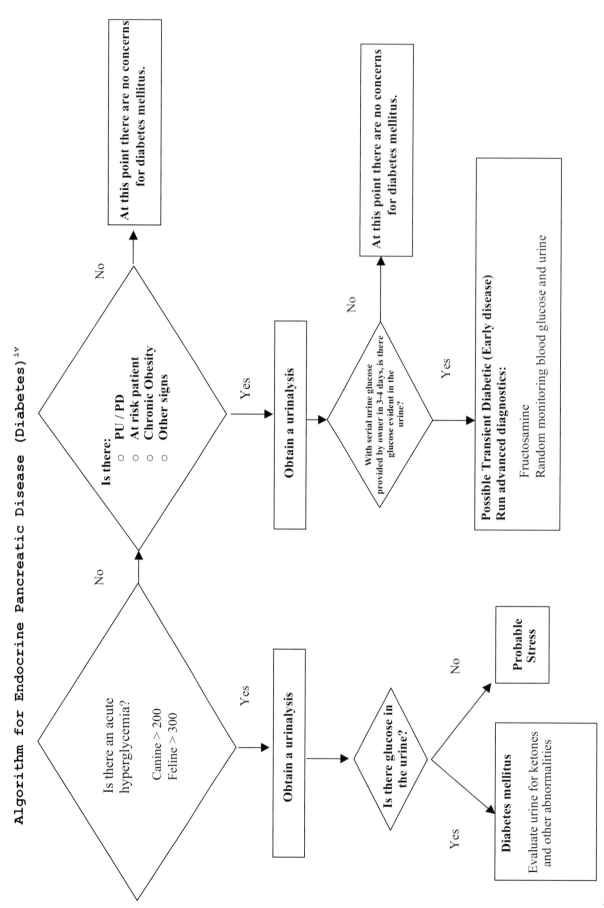

Is there an acute hyperglycemia?

Canine > 200
Feline > 300

No → **Is there:**
○ **PU / PD**
○ At risk patient
○ **Chronic Obesity**
○ Other signs

No → **At this point there are no concerns for diabetes mellitus.**

Yes → **Obtain a urinalysis**

Yes → **Obtain a urinalysis** → **Is there glucose in the urine?**

With serial urine glucose provided by owner in 3-4 days, is there glucose evident in the urine?

No → **At this point there are no concerns for diabetes mellitus.**

Yes → **Possible Transient Diabetic (Early disease)**
Run advanced diagnostics:
Fructosamine
Random monitoring blood glucose and urine

No → **Probable Stress**

Yes → **Diabetes mellitus**
Evaluate urine for ketones and other abnormalities

[iv]Images reprinted with permission from Heska Corp., 3760 Rocky Mountain Avenue, Loveland, CO 80538.

- **Hypertension:** High blood pressure is a common secondary disease of the hyperthyroid animal.

Discussing Changes in Thyroid Level with the Client

- A thyroid hormone concentration determines the amount of active hormone being produced from the thyroid gland.
- A decrease in thyroid hormone concentration can suggest a lack of hormone production within the thyroid gland (hypothyroidism).
- An increase in thyroid hormone concentration can suggest an overproduction of thyroid hormone due to benign or malignant tumors within the thyroid gland (hyperthyroidism).
- Although derangements in thyroid production can be of concern, the blood test must also be fully evaluated, along with the pet's condition, history, other diagnostics, and response to treatment, before conclusions can be reached.

Table 22.3. Normal values for canine/feline chemistry.

Test	Canine Normal Range	Feline Normal Range
ALP	10–150 U/l	0–62 U/l
ALT (SGPT)	5–60 U/l	27–76 U/l
AST (SGOT)	5–55 U/l	5–55 U/l
GGT	0–14 U/l	0–6 U/l
Albumin	2.5–3.6 g/dl	2.3–3.3 g/l
TP	5.1–7.8 g/dl	5.9–8.5 g/l
Globulin	2.8–4.5 g/dl	3.6–5.6 g/l
Total bilirubin	0–0.4 mg/dl	0–0.4 mg/dl
BUN	7–27 mg/dl	15–34 mg/dl
Creatinine	0.4–1.8 mg/dl	0.8–2.3 mg/dl
Glucose	60–125 mg/dl	70–150 mg/dl
Calcium	8.2–12.4 mg/dl	8.2–11.8 mg/dl
Phosphorus	2.1–6.3 mg/dl	3.0–7.0 mg/dl
Chloride (Cl)	105–115 mEq/l	111–125 mEq/l
Sodium (Na)	141–156 mEq/l	147–156 mEq/l
Potassium (K)	4.0–5.6 mEq/l	3.9–5.3 mEq/l

CD-ROM 2 will focus on concepts of understanding and discussing clinical diagnostics and the disease conditions represented. The exercises can be done individually or as case rounds as they explore specific topics in veterinary medicine that discuss clinical diagnostics and treatment.

Chapter 23

Urinalysis and Fecal Clinical Diagnostics

Both fecal and urine clinical diagnostic tests are commonly performed within the hospital for a thorough evaluation of the patient's medical condition. As with the blood film in evaluation of the complete blood count, microscopic evaluation of fecal and urine samples must be practiced to identify abnormalities and suggest disease conditions. Sample handling and preparation are key in obtaining reliable consistent results. To achieve this goal, the client must be educated in how to properly obtain and store the fecal and urine samples before bringing them into the hospital. Improper sample storage, old samples, and poor sample handling can produce artifacts in the sample that can mimic serious disease. The goal of this chapter is to give the team member the tools to discuss the importance of each diagnostic test, to obtain and handle the sample, to perform the diagnostic test, and to discuss the test and its outcome with the client.

Urinary Clinical Diagnostic

Urinalysis
The urinalysis is one of the most important clinical diagnostics used to help evaluate the patient for renal disease, diabetes mellitus, hyperadrenocorticism, hypoadrenocorticism, urinary tract infection, and cancer. Used in conjunction with routine blood work, this diagnostic test provides a baseline for evaluation of the patient's overall metabolic function.

Sample Collection
Urine collection is achieved in a variety of ways, depending on what type of clinical diagnostic tests are to be performed.

Free Catch
In this protocol, the urine is collected while the animal is voiding its sample or collected fresh from a litter box. In canine collection, a midstream sample is collected using a specimen cup or other sampling device. A few milliliters (1–2 teaspoons) are sufficient to perform the necessary tests. With cats, the litter box is cleaned thoroughly and lined with strips of plastic, glass beads, or specially produced crystals that do not absorb the moisture. The sample should be collected as soon as possible after it has been voided and without fecal contamination. *Free-catch or voided samples cannot be used for culture or sensitivity of potential bacterial pathogens.*

Cystocentesis
This procedure is generally done by the veterinarian. In this protocol, the patient is placed on its side or back and restrained while the bladder is palpated. A small-gauge needle (i.e., 20–22 gauge) on a 15-ml syringe is then introduced into the bladder through the abdominal wall and urine is collected. This sterile sample can be used for culture and sensitivity of potential bacterial pathogens. *This collection method can produce a small amount of blood in the urine that is not related to bladder disease.*

Catheterization
In this protocol, a urinary catheter is placed through the penis or vulva to obtain a sterile urine sample. This sample can be used for culture and generally does not produce artifactual blood in the urine. Furthermore, this diagnostic helps the veterinarian assess possible lower urinary tract obstruction secondary to a stone, mass, or prostatic disease.

Sample Handling
Urine samples should be evaluated as soon as possible to avoid changes in the urine that could mimic actual disease-induced abnormalities. If samples must be stored before they can be evaluated, they can be refrigerated up to 12 hours. Once the urine is ready for evaluation, it must be allowed to warm up to room temperature. Many components of urine will not be accurately measured if the urine does not reach room temperature. Conversely, if the urine is allowed to sit at room temperature too long, urinary crystals (i.e., struvite, calcium oxalate, and other types) may form as the urinary components precipitate over time. This may erroneously suggest the patient has been forming urinary crystals.

Performing a Urinalysis
The urinalysis is composed of three diagnostic steps, which are presented next.

Urinary Chemical Strip
This strip is dipped into the room-temperature urine to determine the chemical composition of the urine. Each strip has small chemical reagent squares that are sensitive to one specific component of the urine (see below). Each reagent square reacts and changes color within 30–120 seconds and is read at the appropriate time by comparing the color change to the guide on the container's label.

Refractometer

The refractometer evaluates the concentration of the urine, the **urine specific gravity (USG)**. A few drops are placed on the refractometer's reading surface and the refractometer is held up to the light. USG is read from 1.001 to 1.045 (or >1.045). The USG is a very important diagnostic test to evaluate kidney function. *Although some urine chemical strips do have a reagent square for USG, a refractometer reading should always be completed to get an accurate evaluation of concentration of urine.*

Urine Sediment

Lastly, the urine is placed in a test tube and spun for 6 minutes at low speeds in a centrifuge. This separates the cellular components from the urine. Once spun down, the liquid portion (**supernatant**) is poured off and the sediment is mixed with a small amount of saline or stain and evaluated under the microscope. Changes in cellularity can suggest infection, inflammation, formation of dietary crystals, or cancer of the kidneys or bladder.

Evaluating the Urinalysis

Urine Color

Urine color can suggest disease conditions of the kidneys and lower urinary tract. Any abnormal colors should be reported to the veterinarian. Possible color changes are red, orange, and yellow.

Red

A red color change could indicate increased red blood cells (**hematuria**) in the urine from infection, cancer, or spontaneous bleeding in the kidneys or urinary tract. Red coloration can also be due to increased red blood cell destruction and release of hemoglobin (**hemoglobinuria**) or muscle cell destruction and release of myoglobin (**myoglobinuria**) in the urine. Hemoglobinuria can be associated with diseases in which red blood cells are destroyed at increasing levels in the body from immune-mediated disease (immune-mediated hemolytic anemia).

Myoglobinuria is associated with significant muscle damage. To differentiate hemoglobinuria and myoglobinuria from hematuria, the urine sample should be spun down. Red blood cells will be concentrated in the pellet, and the urine will lose its red color. Hemoglobin and myoglobin will remain in the supernatant.

It is more difficult to differentiate hemoglobinuria from myoglobinuria. Because myoglobin is more rapidly cleared from the serum by the kidneys than hemoglobin, the serum in myoglobinuria will be clear and in hemoglobinuria will be red.

Orange or Yellow

An orange or yellow color change can suggest increased bilirubin and liver disease or increased breakdown of red blood cells from immune-mediated hemolytic anemia.

Urine Appearance

Urine samples can be turbid (cloudy) or clear. The turbidity of urine samples is related to the concentration of cell, crystals, or mucin in the sample.

Urine Specific Gravity

USG is the measure of urine concentration compared with distilled water (USG 1.000).

USG is a major indicator of primary renal function. As discussed in Chapter 13, the kidneys serve two major functions: to filter out toxins and concentrate urine. The kidneys also function to control blood pressure and acid/base and electrolyte balance. With serious renal disease, the kidney loses its ability to filter toxins and concentrate urine. Since there are major diseases and syndromes that can decrease glomerular filtration and azotemia (i.e., blood urea nitrogen, or BUN, and creatinine), the USG can help distinguish between primary kidney disease or other causes of azotemia, such as prerenal azotemia due to dehydration.

Increases in USG are normal, and increased concentration (USG >1.045) does not suggest disease, just normal ability of the kidneys to concentrate urine. Increased USG is seen in dehydration.

Decreased USG (USG <1.015) can suggest the patient has adequate to increased hydration and does not need to concentrate urine at this time. However, if the patient is dehydrated, azotemic (increased BUN/creatinine), or generally ill, a low USG can suggest renal or other systemic disease that is inhibiting normal concentrating ability of the kidneys.

How Is It Evaluated

USG is evaluated by placing a drop of urine on a refractometer and reading where the urine line forms on the USG line.

Normal values of USG.

Species	Range
Canine	USG >1.015: 1.025–1.040
Feline	USG >1.022: 1.025–1.045 (or greater)

Terminology

- **Isosthenuria** refers to urine that has the same specific gravity as plasma or serum: USG 1.010–1.015.
- **Hyposthenuria** refers to urine that has more dilute specific gravity than plasma or serum: USG <1.008.

Physical Symptoms Associated with Changes in USG

Generally patients with chronic low USG are drinking more water (**polydipsia**) and producing more urine (**polyuria**) than normal patients. Because patients cannot concentrate their urine, they must drink larger amounts of water to keep up with their increased urine production.

Other Clinical Diagnostic Tests

The other clinical diagnostic tests that will help evaluate kidney function are

- BUN,
- creatinine,
- phosphorus,
- urine protein/creatinine ratio, and
- electrolytes.

Urine Chemistries
Bilirubin

Bilirubin is a hemoglobin breakdown product produced as red blood cells are lysed and hemoglobin is released in the body. The bilirubin is then absorbed by the liver, detoxified, and passed into the intestine for excretion. Increased levels of bilirubin in the blood can suggest underlying liver disease in which the liver cannot take up bilirubin and excrete it, causing large amounts of bilirubin to be excreted in the urine. Increased urine bilirubin concentration can also be associated with **immune-mediated hemolytic anemia,** where red blood cells are being lysed. In the dog, **bilirubinuria** can be normal, especially in concentrated urine. However, in the cat, *any evidence of bilirubinuria is abnormal and should be reported to the veterinarian immediately.*

How It Is Evaluated
Bilirubin is evaluated by dipping a urine stick into urine and allowing a specific time interval to pass and then examining the chemical square for color change.

Normal values of bilirubin.

Species	Range
Canine	Negative to weakly positive
Feline	Negative

Terminology
Bilirubinuria refers to the presence of bilirubin in the urine.

Physical Signs Associated with Changes in Bilirubin
Animals with increased bilirubinuria will present with jaundice, vomiting, diarrhea, and anorexia secondary to the presence of diseases associated with decreased liver function or hemolytic anemia.

Other Clinical Diagnostic Tests
To help evaluate liver disease clinical tests include

- aspartate aminotransferase,
- alanine aminotransferase,
- gamma-glutamyltransferase,
- alkaline phosphatase,
- bilirubin,
- bile acids,
- BUN, and
- glucose.

Tests to help evaluate for immune-mediated hemolytic anemia tests include

- packed cell volume,
- bilirubin, and
- blood film—agglutination/spherocytes.

Blood
Blood in the urine consists of red blood cells, hemoglobin, or myoglobin.

Blood in the urine can be suggestive of active inflammation of the bladder, the kidney, the reproductive organs, or a tumor within the urinary tract. Blood in the urine occurs most commonly secondary to urinary tract disease, **urolithiasis** (bladder stones), or prostate disease. Blood occurs as the bladder wall becomes thickened and inflamed and the irritated tissue bleeds into the urine. Occasionally, blood in the urine can also be secondary to kidney disease, problems clotting blood, and tumors of the bladder and kidneys. *Evidence of blood in the urine is a concern and should be reported to the veterinarian.* The blood reagent pad measures intact red blood cells, hemoglobin, and myoglobin. Determination of which condition is present is done by evaluation of the urine color and the sediment evaluation.

How It Is Evaluated
Blood in the urine is evaluated by dipping the urine stick into urine, allowing a specific time interval to pass, and then examining the chemical square for color change.

Normal values red blood cells, hemoglobin, or myoglobin.

Species	Range
Canine	Negative
Feline	Negative

Terminology
Hematuria refers to blood in the urine.

Physical Signs Associated with the Presence of Blood in Urine
Physical signs of blood in the urine are generally associated with blood spotting or the passing of blood clots in the urine. If it is secondary to lower urinary tract disease (i.e., urinary tract infection, urolithiasis, mass), other associated signs can be

- straining to urinate,
- polyuria/polydipsia,
- urinating small amounts, and
- urgency while urinating.

Other Clinical Diagnostic Tests
To help evaluate urinary tract infection/urolithiasis these tests include

- urine protein,
- urine sediment,
- urine leukocytes, and
- urine culture.

To help evaluate for other possible diseases, tests include

- BUN,
- creatinine,
- abdominal radiographs,
- abdominal ultrasound, and
- clotting times.

Glucose

Glucose in the urine can be suggestive of diabetes mellitus, other systemic diseases (rare), or stress. In the dog, glucose in the urine occurs generally when the patient is diabetic and cannot use blood glucose. Serum glucose concentration increases and passes into the urine. **Glucosuria** is also evident when patients become stressed in a hospital setting and produce enough blood glucose to spill into the urine. Glucosuria due to stress is most common in the cat. *Evidence of glucose in the urine is a concern and should be reported to the veterinarian.*

How It Is Evaluated

Glucose in the urine can be evaluated by dipping urine stick into urine, allowing a specific time interval to pass, and then examining the chemical square for color change.

Normal values of glucose concentration.

Species	Range
Canine	Negative
Feline	Negative

Terminology

Glucosuria refers to glucose in the urine.

Physical Signs Associated with Changes in Glucose in Urine

Increased thirst and urination are associated with chronic glucosuria in diabetic animals. The patient must drink more water to replace fluid lost due to the diuretic effect of glucosuria. The increased urination causes increased thirst and polydipsia.

Other Clinical Diagnostic Tests

To help evaluate for diabetes mellitus, the following clinical diagnostics are helpful.

- **Blood glucose:** Blood glucose (see Chapter 22) between 200 and 300 mg/dl can be related to stress and result in glucosuria. Blood glucose concentration above 300 is more suggestive of diabetes.
- **Fructosamine:** Measuring another form of glucose that increases when there is persistent hyperglycemia is helpful. Serum fructosamine measurement allows the veterinarian to evaluate how the patient is controlling glucose metabolism over the past several days.

Ketones

Ketones are a metabolite of fat metabolism associated with unregulated diabetes mellitus.

Ketones in the urine can be suggestive of a severe life-threatening syndrome, diabetic **ketoacidosis,** caused by excessive uncontrolled diabetes mellitus. As the patient continues with uncontrolled diabetes, the body cannot use glucose and must turn to fat metabolism. The end products of fat metabolism are ketoacids, including acetone. *Evidence of ketones in the urine is a concern and should be reported immediately to the veterinarian (see Chapter 15).*

How Is It Evaluated

Ketones are measured by dipping the urine reagent stick into the urine, allowing the specific time interval to pass, and then examining the chemical square for color change.

Normal values of ketones.

Species	Range
Canine	Negative
Feline	Negative

Terminology

Ketonuria refers to ketones in the urine.

Physical Signs Associated with Changes in Urine Ketone Concentration

Ketoacidotic diabetics are generally significantly ill due to the buildup of ketones in the blood, which produces a life-threatening acidosis. Common signs are

- vomiting,
- diarrhea,
- anorexia,
- weakness,
- dehydration, and
- depression.

Other Clinical Diagnostic Tests

To help evaluate for diabetes mellitus the following clinical diagnostics can be performed.

- **Complete blood count and chemistry** evaluate the patient for primary diabetes or other systemic disease that could make the patient diabetic secondarily (i.e., **hyperadrenocorticism**).
- Testing **blood gases** help evaluate blood pH and determine the degree of acidosis in the patient.

Protein

Urinary protein levels reflect the amount of protein from the blood that enters the urine secondary to kidney, bladder, and other systematic disease.

Protein in the urine can be an indicator of renal, bladder, or other systematic diseases. The presence of increased urine protein concentration can suggest the following:

- **Kidney disease:** Proteins are large molecules that normally do not cross through the glomerular filters into the urine. With kidney disease, damage to the glomerular filters can allow protein to leak into the urine. The presence of protein without other signs of urinary tract infection (i.e., hematuria, leukocytes, active sediment) can be an indicator of glomerular disease.
- **Urinary tract disease:** Protein can also increase in the urine due to infection and inflammation in the bladder. When the bladder wall becomes inflamed and irritated, protein and blood can leak into the urine.
- **Other systemic diseases**: Other chronic inflammatory and neoplastic disease may increase protein concentration in the urine.

How It Is Evaluated

Urine protein is measured by dipping the urine reagent stick into urine, allowing the specific time interval to pass, and then examining the chemical square for color change. There are some key points to monitor when evaluating protein concentration in the urine.

- **Urinary pH:** Alkaline pH (>7.5) will produce an *artifactual proteinuria*. Animals being evaluated for signs of early kidney disease with proteinuria in the presence of alkaline urine must be resampled at another time or begin medications to acidify their urine to more adequately evaluate renal protein loss.
- **Bladder infection:** There is no test available to differentiate between protein produced from a bladder infection and protein that is leaked by damaged kidneys. *If a bladder infection is prevalent, the resulting infection must be cleared before protein can be evaluated as an early indicator of renal disease.*

Normal values of protein.

Species	Range
Canine	Negative to trace
Feline	Negative

Terminology

Proteinuria refers to the presence of high protein levels in the urine.

Physical Signs Associated with Changes in Urine Protein Concentration

Physical signs associated with proteinuria are generally associated with urinary tract disease (i.e., urinary tract infection, urolithiasis, acute renal disease).

For urinary tract disease the signs are as follows:

- Straining to urinate
- Polyuria/polydipsia
- Urinating small amounts
- Urgency while urinating

For renal disease, the symptoms are as follows. (Note that in early stages of disease, the patient may be asymptomatic.)

- Polyuria/polydipsia
- Anorexia
- Weight loss
- Chronic vomiting
- Diarrhea

To help evaluate for renal or bladder infection, inflammation, or cancer the following clinical diagnostics can be performed.

- **Complete blood count** and **chemistry** tests evaluate the patient for increases in renal enzymes, other organ enzymes, and changes in the complete blood count that could suggest a kidney or other systemic disease.
- **Urine sediment** evaluates changes in the cellularity of urine for red blood cells, white blood cells, casts, and cells that can suggest infection, inflammation, or cancer of the kidney or bladder (see below).
- **Urine culture and sensitivity** isolates possible bacterial pathogens and determines their sensitivity to specific antibiotics secondary to urinary or renal disease.
- **Urine protein/creatinine ratio** determines a quantitation of the amount of protein to the amount of creatinine excreted for comparison. It is used when there is concern about protein loss in the kidneys (glomerular disease). In healthy kidneys, there is very little protein excreted compared with creatinine (urine protein/creatinine ratio <1). The more leakage from the glomeruli, the higher the urine protein/creatinine ratio and the worse the kidney glomerular disease (see Chapter 13).

pH

Although not directly associated with disease, abnormalities in urinary pH can precipitate crystals in the urine as well as produce artifacts in the urinalysis.

Urinary pH is an extremely important indicator when evaluating a patient for urolithiasis. Urinary crystals and stones form from dietary elements in the presence of urinary tract infection and proper pH of the urine (see Table 23.1). Many treatment options are focused on correcting pH of the urine to help control the formation of future stones or crystals. Furthermore, alkaline urinary pH can produce an artifactual proteinuria (see proteinuria).

Table 23.1. Changes in urine depending on pH.

Acidic Urine (pH <6.5)	Alkaline Urine (pH >7.5)
Calcium oxalate urolithiasis	Struvite (triple phosphate) urolithiasis Artifactual proteinuria

How It Is evaluated

Urine pH is determined by dipping the urine reagent stick into urine, allowing the specific time interval to pass, and then examining the chemical square for color change.

Normal values of urinary pH.

Species	Range
Canine	6.5–7.5
Feline	6.5–7.5

Terminology

- pH <7: Acidic
- pH >7: Alkaline

Other Clinical Diagnostics

To help evaluate for bladder urolithiasis and bladder infection, the following clinical diagnostics can be performed.

- **Urine sediment** evaluates changes in the cellularity of urine for red blood cells, white blood cells, casts, and cells that can suggest infection, inflammation, or cancer of the kidney or bladder (see below).
- **Urine culture and sensitivity** isolates possible bacterial pathogens and determines their sensitivity to specific antibiotics secondary to urinary or renal disease.

Urine Sediment Evaluation

The examination of urine sediment is a very important part of urinalysis. The identification and quantification of formed elements (cells, casts, crystals, infectious agents) in the urine are necessary for a full evaluation for urinary tract disease.

Urine sediment examination assists in identification of infectious and inflammatory disease in the urinary tract. Occasionally, urine sediment can also assist in the diagnosis of urinary tract cancer and certain toxicities, such as ethylene glycol (antifreeze) poisoning.

How It Is Evaluated

Urine sediment is examined microscopically. Specific formed elements are identified and quantified at low and high power. The quantification of formed elements is an estimate (semiquantitative) due to the large number of factors that need to be standardized. The sediment can be stained prior to viewing it under the microscope or it may be examined without stain.

To perform the test a clean urine sample is obtained, preferably by cystocentesis or catheterization. A sample obtained first thing in the morning provides the most information.

1. Pour 10 ml of urine into a conical centrifuge tube and process in the centrifuge at a low setting (1500 rpm) for 5 minutes.
2. Pour off the supernatant, leaving about 0.5 ml of fluid in the centrifuge tube to resuspend the sediment.
3. After thoroughly mixing the sediment, place a drop on a clean glass slide and cover with a large coverslip.
4. Examine the slide by lowering the microscope condenser or closing the iris diaphragm to increase the contrast.
5. On low (10×) power, scan the slide to get an overall view of the cellularity and number of other formed elements such as casts and crystals. Large epithelial cells (squamous epithelial cells and transitional epithelial cells) can be quantitated at this power and noted as number of cells per low-power field (lpf).
6. On high (40×) power, all formed elements can be quantified as number per high-power field (hpf). Bacteria are usually noted as few, moderate, or many, rather than counted.

Normal values of urine sedimentation.

Formed Element	Number/hpf in normal urine
Epithelial cells	Few to many
Red blood cells	0–5/hpf
White blood cells	0–8/hpf
Casts	Rare hyaline and granular casts (<2/lpf)
Crystals	Few dihydrate calcium oxalate or phosphate crystals
Bacteria	None

Terminology

- **Hematuria** refers to increased numbers of red blood cells in the urine.
- **Pyuria** refers to increased numbers of white blood cells in the urine.
- **Cylinduria** refers to increased numbers of casts in the urine.
- **Crystalluria** refers to increased numbers of crystals in the urine.
- **Bacteriuria** refers to the presence of bacteria in the urine.

Cellular Elements

The cellular elements that are identified within the urine sediment include squamous epithelial cells, transitional epithelial cells, red blood cells, and white blood cells.

- **Squamous epithelial cells:** Squamous cells are seen in free-catch and catheter samples. These cells are from the urethra and are considered insignificant findings. They are the largest cells and often have angular sides. They may or may not have a nucleus.
- **Transitional epithelial cells:** Transitional cells are usually smaller than squamous cells. They can vary considerably in size and are round with round nuclei. They are commonly shed into the urine as a normal process of bladder mucosal epithelial cell turnover. Increased numbers are often shed when there is inflammation in the bladder.
- **Red blood cells:** Red blood cells should not be present in normal urine. They are slightly refractile and may have a slight red coloration. They can vary from their normal bi-

concave discs to crenated cells, depending on the specific gravity of the urine.

High specific gravity causes crenation.

Low specific gravity (less than 1.005) can cause lysis of the red blood cells. When the cells lyse, they may appear as "ghost" cells with little hemoglobin left inside. Unlike epithelial cells, they are small and do not have internal structures. They can be confused with lipid droplets. They will be in focus with the rest of the formed elements that have settled to the surface of the glass slide, whereas lipid droplets will be in a focus plane above the rest of the cellular elements. If red blood cells are seen upon sediment examination, there should be a positive blood reaction of the chemical urine strip.

- **White blood cells:** Urine sediment can contain white blood cells as a result of inflammation or hemorrhage. When present as a result of hemorrhage, white blood cells will be in much smaller numbers compared with red blood cells. With inflammation, white blood cells may outnumber red blood cells. In most cases, inflammation of the bladder or kidney will be associated with some degree of hemorrhage. White blood cells are slightly larger than red blood cells and smaller than most epithelial cells. They have internal structure and often "glitter" when viewed with increased contrast. A sediment stain can be used to confirm the presence of white blood cells if they cannot be definitively identified on the unstained preparation. In most cases, the most numerous white blood cells seen in urine sediment are the neutrophils. However, eosinophils, lymphocytes, and monocytes or macrophages can be present.

Importance of Identification of Elements in Urine

- **Squamous and transitional cells:** These cells are usually common and have no significance. Increased numbers of transitional cells without any evidence of inflammation are sometimes seen with bladder cancer.
- **Red blood cells:** Red blood cells indicate hemorrhage in the urinary tract. If the sample was obtained by cystocentesis, blood may be present due to hemorrhage at the time the sample was taken (iatrogenic hemorrhage). The hemorrhage may be occurring in the bladder or the kidney.
- **White blood cells:** In urine samples obtained by cystocentesis or catheterization increased numbers of white blood cells indicate inflammation in the bladder or kidney. In free-catch samples, the inflammation may also be present in the urethra, vagina, or prepuce.
- **Casts:** Casts are aggregates of protein or cells that form inside the kidney tubules. They are "casts" of the tubular lumen. There are cellular casts (red cell, white cell, epithelial cell, and granular casts), protein casts (hyaline), and waxy casts. Casts have linear sides and rounded ends.

Types of casts are as listed next.

- **Epithelial casts:** Epithelial casts are composed of sloughed epithelial cells that have not degenerated. The epithelial cells can still be discerned within the cast and are held together by a protein matrix.
- **Granular casts:** Granular casts form within the renal tubules and are composed of sloughed renal epithelial cells. The casts can be coarsely or finely granular depending on how long the cast stayed in the tubules before being flushed out. The longer the cast is retained in the tubule, the finer the granularity will be when viewed in the sediment examination. When viewed with increased contrast, granular casts often have ill-defined internal structure that gives them their granular appearance. Their width is often approximately three times the diameter of a white blood cell.
- **Waxy casts:** Waxy casts are granular casts that have remained in the renal tubule until all the cellular components have degenerated completely. They have straight ends and cracks along the sides. They are often larger than most granular casts and may form in the larger collecting ducts of the kidney rather than the proximal or distal tubules or loops of Henle.
- **White blood cell casts:** White blood cell casts are formed when white blood cells migrate into the renal tubule as a result of inflammation within the nephron. They can be difficult to differentiate from epithelial cell casts. The cells within a white blood cell cast are usually smaller than those seen in an epithelial cast. White blood cells tend to have the same tendency to "glitter" in the cast as they do when present free in the urine sediment.
- **Hyaline casts:** Hyaline casts are composed of a protein matrix and can be found in low numbers in normal urine. They are similar to the waxy cast in that they do not contain internal structure. In contrast to waxy casts, they have rounded ends and no cracks on their sides. They are usually smaller than waxy casts.
- **Miscellaneous casts:** Bilirubin casts (bilirubin-stained granular casts and protein casts), lipid casts, hemoglobin casts, and myoglobin casts can also be seen in urine sediment. They are relatively uncommon.

Importance of Cast Identification in Urine

The presence of epithelial cell and granular casts indicate sloughing of renal epithelial cells. These casts can be seen as a result of acute or chronic renal disease. They are often increased as a result of hypoxia. Increased numbers of granular casts can be seen following prolonged dehydration or kidney disease that results from renal epithelial cell necrosis or degeneration.

Waxy casts are strongly suggestive of chronic renal disease.

Red blood cell casts form in the tubules as a result of hemorrhage into the nephron. They are composed of red blood cells, fibrin, and may contain a few other cell types. They will have red-orange coloration and will have distinct cellular outlines in fresh urine. They can degenerate over time if the sample is not evaluated promptly. As they degenerate, the red blood cells may lyse and the color may take on a more yellow-red hue. Red blood cell casts indicate hemorrhage within the renal tubule.

The presence of white blood cell casts indicates inflammation within the kidney tubule.

When present in significant numbers, hyaline casts indicate increased protein loss into the renal tubule. Increased numbers can be seen following strenuous exercise.

Crystals

Crystals are formed by precipitation of minerals and salts. Their presence can be normal or indicate underlying disease processes. The most common crystals seen in dog and cat urine include triple phosphate, dihydrate calcium oxalate, monohydrate calcium oxalate, bilirubin, and ammonium biurate. There are a few crystals, such as cysteine, associated with inherited metabolic diseases. In addition, medications such as antibiotics can be associated with crystals that may precipitate out in the urine as the drug is excreted. The most common drugs associated with crystalluria are antibiotics such as sulfadiacine and ampicillin and contrast agents used in radiography.

Types of crystals include the following.

- **Triple phosphate:** Triple phosphate crystals (struvite, magnesium ammonium phosphate) are common findings in dog and cat urine. They are usually present in alkaline urine and are colorless, prismlike crystals that often resemble a coffin lid.
- **Calcium oxalate:** Two types of calcium oxalate crystals can be found in urine sediment. Both crystals are colorless. Monohydrate calcium oxalate crystals are most often elongate crystals with pointed ends (resembling the slats of a picket fence). However, they can be spindle, oval, or dumbbell shaped. Dihydrate calcium oxalate crystals are usually square with intersecting diagonal lines that form an "envelope" appearance.
- **Bilirubin:** Bilirubin crystals are light to darkly yellow or yellow-brown in color. They form structures resembling bundles of wheat sheaths or needlelike structures. They are common in concentrated urine (especially in the male dog).
- **Ammonium biurate:** Ammonium biurate crystals are often light to dark brown in color. They have a distinct round shape with irregular spikes extending out from the body of the crystal (thorny apple form). This appearance is striking, making this crystal difficult to confuse with others.
- **Miscellaneous crystals:** Additional crystals that are rarely seen in urine sediment examination are uric acid, cysteine, leucine, and tyrosine. Leucine, cysteine, and tyrosine crystals are associated with loss of these amino acids into the urine and usually are the result of inherited metabolic diseases.

Importance of Identification of Crystals in Urine
- **Triple phosphate crystals** may be found in normal animals, animals with septic or nonseptic urinary tract disease, or associated with struvite uroliths. They are a nonspecific finding.

- **Dihydrate calcium oxalate crystals** are found in normal dog and cat urine. They can be seen in association with oxalate uroliths. Monohydrate calcium oxalate crystals are not found in normal urine. When present in large numbers, ethylene glycol (antifreeze) poisoning should be the first consideration. In small numbers, they may indicate hypercalciuria (increased loss of calcium in the urine).
- **Bilirubin crystals** are relatively normal in the dog, but when present in large numbers, especially in dilute urine, they may indicate increased serum bilirubin. In the cat, their presence may be more significant because bilirubinuria usually indicates hyperbilirubinemia in this species.
- **Ammonium biurate crystals** are associated with hyperammonemia (increased serum ammonia) and usually seen in animals with altered liver function. Classically, these crystals are associated with portal vascular shunts, developmental anomalies that allow blood from the intestinal tract to bypass the liver. They can be seen as the result of metabolic abnormalities in the Dalmatians and English bulldogs. They are rare in normal dogs and cats.

Pathogenic Organisms

Bacteria

Bacteria are the most difficult elements to accurately identify. It is not uncommon for inexperienced team members to misidentify amorphous granular material in the urine as bacteria.

- **Rod-shaped bacteria** are often motile and will be seen moving in a progressive manner across the field of view.
- **Coccoid bacteria** are rarely motile and are most often confused with amorphous granular material. Coccoid bacteria should be seen in chains or in clusters. Staining the urine sediment may assist in confirming the presence of bacteria. However, care should be taken to ensure stain precipitate is not confused with bacteria.

Fungal Elements

The presence of fungal mycelia or yeast bodies is not uncommon in urine. If seen, they should be confirmed by examination of a stained preparation and submission of the sample to a diagnostic laboratory for assistance in identifying the type of fungal organism.

Both bacteria and fungi in urine sediment indicates an infectious process that should be confirmed by culture of the urine.

There are several elements that are commonly found in free-catch urine samples that can be confused with other formed elements, especially microorganisms such as fungal elements and parasite eggs. Plant pollen can be a contaminent, especially in a free-catch urine sample from a male dog, and may be confused with a pathogenic organism.

Overview of Urinalysis Evaluation

The following flowcharts are meant to help the team member understand the urinalysis evaluation and what the abnormalities can suggest. Pathologic changes in urine can suggest disease and further suggest other clinical diagnostics that may need to be evaluated. The flowcharts are not meant to be used by the team members to diagnose a disease condition, but rather to make them aware of concerns so they can inform the doctor of serious pathology, be more prepared to run other diagnostics, and help educate the client.

Discussing Urinalysis with the Client
- A urinalysis is an important part of the evaluation of an animal's metabolic baseline because it allows the veterinarian to evaluate kidney function, urinary tract disease, systemic disease, and neoplasia that can occur in the patient.
- A component of the urinalysis is the evaluation of chemical reagents that allow the veterinarian to evaluate abnormal components (i.e., blood sugar, blood, protein, or toxins) in the urine that can suggest disease.
- Furthermore, the urinalysis evaluates concentrating ability of urine, which can serve as a direct evaluation of kidney function.
- Finally, the urine sediment is appreciated to evaluate cellular components of the urine that could suggest infection, inflammation, or cancer.
- With many patients in early disease such as kidney disease, diabetes mellitus, and other systemic diseases, early changes may be seen in urine and blood work before physical signs are noted in the patient.

Advanced Urinary Diagnostics
Urine Culture and Sensitivity
Urine culture and sensitivity tests are used to identify urine pathogenic bacteria stemming from a kidney or bladder infection and identify nonresistant antibiotics.

The patient can have a urine culture and sensitivity test completed without fasting or special preparation. A large sample of urine is collected from the patient (>6 ml) by catheter or cystocentesis. A sterile sample must be taken for the test to be accurate. It can take 48–72 or more hours for test results to be available.

How It Is Evaluated
Growth of pathogenic bacteria suggests infection of the kidneys or bladder. The antibiotics that stop the growth of the bacteria are indicated.

Normal values of bacteria

Test	Normal Canine Results	Normal Feline Results
Urine culture and sensitivity	No growth	No growth

Other Clinical Diagnostic Tests
Other diagnostic tests are helpful in diagnosing the cause of urinary disease problems.

- Complete blood count—increased white blood cell population, changes in white blood cell on blood film
- Chemistry (renal enzymes)
- Abdominal ultrasound

Discussing Changes in Urine Culture and Sensitivity with the Client
- A urine culture and sensitivity test has been recommended by the veterinarian to evaluate the urine for possible pathogenic bacteria in the urine.
- The presence of the bacteria suggests infection within the kidney or bladder.
- Once the bacteria are isolated, further tests help evaluate which antibiotics are the best choice to treat the infection.

Urine Protein/Creatinine Ratio
To evaluate protein loss in the urine caused by early kidney disease, a urine protein/creatinine ratio is determined. Protein loss suggests damage to the glomerular filters, which allow larger protein molecules to pass into the urine.

Function
As discussed in Chapter 13, proteins are large blood molecules that cannot pass through the glomerular filters into the urine. When these filters are damaged, protein can leak into the urine at increased amounts. This test evaluates the amount of normal protein in the urine in comparison to creatinine, a small amino acid normally secreted in the urine.

How Test Is Performed
For the urine protein/creatinine ratio, the patient does not need fasting or special preparation. A large sample of urine is collected from the patient (>6 ml) by catheter or cystocentesis. Depending on the type of container used, a free-catch sample may add external protein from the sample container. The sample should be immediately submitted to the lab or run in-hospital.

Evaluation of Test
In healthy patients, the amount of protein lost in the urine is generally much less than the amount of creatinine in the urine. Increasing amounts of protein suggest glomerular disease and may be an indicator of renal disease.

- It is important to understand that this test will produce an increased ratio if the patient is suffering from a urinary tract infection due to increased protein loss from an inflamed bladder wall.

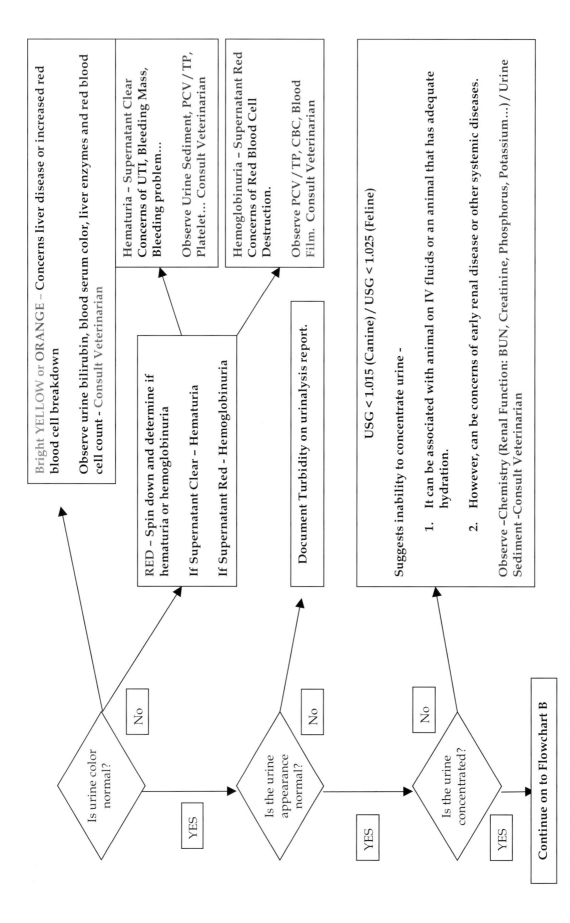

Is urine color normal?

- **No** → Bright YELLOW or ORANGE – Concerns liver disease or increased red blood cell breakdown

  Observe urine bilirubin, blood serum color, liver enzymes and red blood cell count - Consult Veterinarian

  RED – Spin down and determine if hematuria or hemoglobinuria

  If Supernatant Clear – Hematuria → Hematuria – Supernatant Clear Concerns of UTI, Bleeding Mass, Bleeding problem...

  Observe Urine Sediment, PCV / TP, Platelet... Consult Veterinarian

  If Supernatant Red - Hemoglobinuria → Hemoglobinuria – Supernatant Red Concerns of Red Blood Cell Destruction.

  Observe PCV / TP, CBC, Blood Film. Consult Veterinarian

- **YES** ↓

Is the urine appearance normal?

- **No** → Document Turbidity on urinalysis report.

- **YES** ↓

Is the urine concentrated?

- **No** → USG < 1.015 (Canine) / USG < 1.025 (Feline)

  Suggests inability to concentrate urine -

  1. It can be associated with animal on IV fluids or an animal that has adequate hydration.
  2. However, can be concerns of early renal disease or other systemic diseases.

  Observe –Chemistry (Renal Function: BUN, Creatinine, Phosphorus, Potassium...) / Urine Sediment -Consult Veterinarian

- **YES** ↓

Continue on to Flowchart B

Flowchart A. Evaluating Urine Color, Turbidity, and Specific Gravity

346

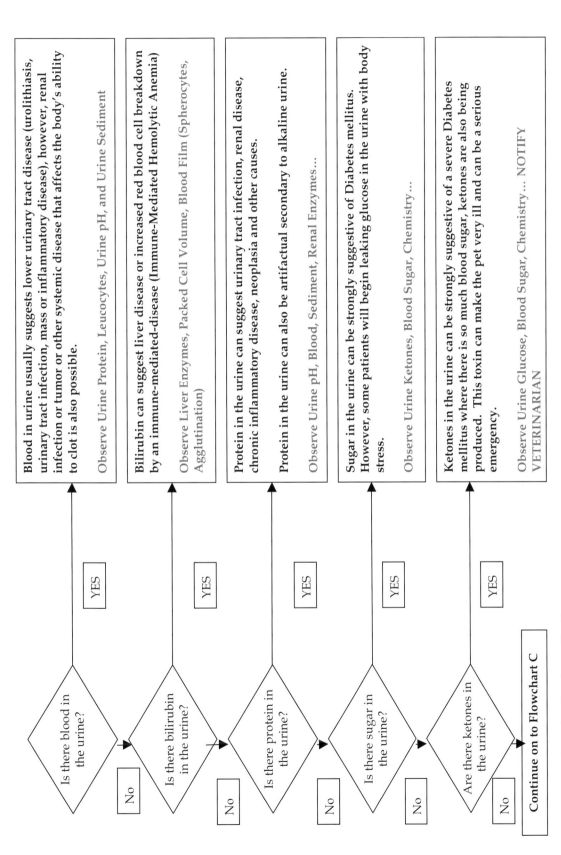

Flowchart B. Evaluating Urine Chemistry—Key Factors

Is there blood in the urine? — YES →

Blood in urine usually suggests lower urinary tract disease (urolithiasis, urinary tract infection, mass or inflammatory disease), however, renal infection or tumor or other systemic disease that affects the body's ability to clot is also possible.

Observe Urine Protein, Leucocytes, Urine pH, and Urine Sediment

No ↓

Is there bilirubin in the urine? — YES →

Bilirubin can suggest liver disease or increased red blood cell breakdown by an immune-mediated-disease (Immune-Mediated Hemolytic Anemia)

Observe Liver Enzymes, Packed Cell Volume, Blood Film (Spherocytes, Agglutination)

No ↓

Is there protein in the urine? — YES →

Protein in the urine can suggest urinary tract infection, renal disease, chronic inflammatory disease, neoplasia and other causes.

Protein in the urine can also be artifactual secondary to alkaline urine.

Observe Urine pH, Blood, Sediment, Renal Enzymes…

No ↓

Is there sugar in the urine? — YES →

Sugar in the urine can be strongly suggestive of Diabetes mellitus. However, some patients will begin leaking glucose in the urine with body stress.

Observe Urine Ketones, Blood Sugar, Chemistry…

No ↓

Are there ketones in the urine? — YES →

Ketones in the urine can be strongly suggestive of a severe Diabetes mellitus where there is so much blood sugar, ketones are also being produced. This toxin can make the pet very ill and can be a serious emergency.

Observe Urine Glucose, Blood Sugar, Chemistry… NOTIFY VETERINARIAN

No ↓

Continue on to Flowchart C

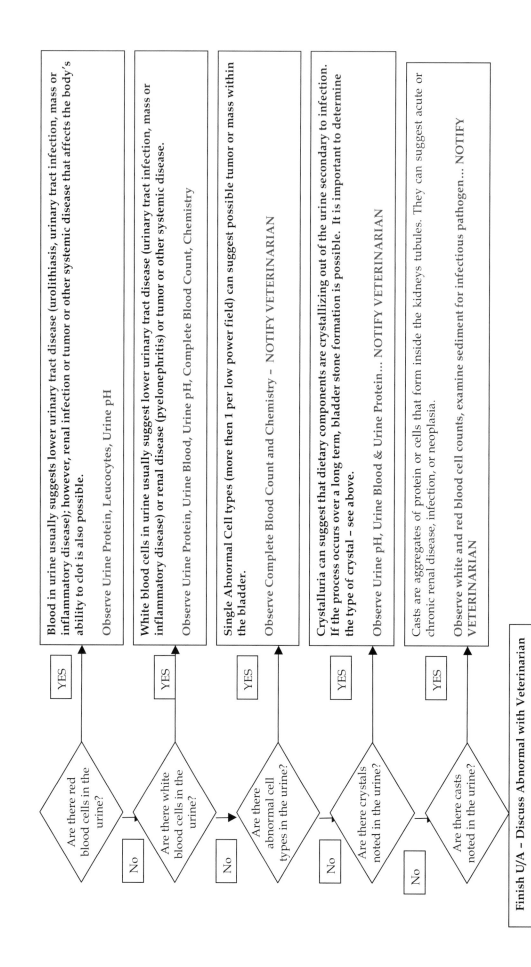

Are there red blood cells in the urine?

YES → **Blood in urine usually suggests lower urinary tract disease (urolithiasis, urinary tract infection, mass or inflammatory disease); however, renal infection or tumor or other systemic disease that affects the body's ability to clot is also possible.**

Observe Urine Protein, Leucocytes, Urine pH

No →

Are there white blood cells in the urine?

YES → **White blood cells in urine usually suggest lower urinary tract disease (urinary tract infection, mass or inflammatory disease) or renal disease (pyelonephritis) or tumor or other systemic disease.**

Observe Urine Protein, Urine Blood, Urine pH, Complete Blood Count, Chemistry

No →

Are there abnormal cell types in the urine?

YES → **Single Abnormal Cell types (more then 1 per low power field) can suggest possible tumor or mass within the bladder.**

Observe Complete Blood Count and Chemistry – NOTIFY VETERINARIAN

No →

Are there crystals noted in the urine?

YES → **Crystalluria can suggest that dietary components are crystallizing out of the urine secondary to infection. If the process occurs over a long term, bladder stone formation is possible. It is important to determine the type of crystal – see above.**

Observe Urine pH, Urine Blood & Urine Protein... NOTIFY VETERINARIAN

No →

Are there casts noted in the urine?

YES → **Casts are aggregates of protein or cells that form inside the kidneys tubules. They can suggest acute or chronic renal disease, infection, or neoplasia.**

Observe white and red blood cell counts, examine sediment for infectious pathogen.... NOTIFY VETERINARIAN

Finish U/A – Discuss Abnormal with Veterinarian

Flowchart C. Evaluating Urine Sediment

- Patients with an alkaline pH (pH >7.5) will have artifactual proteinuria that could also increase this ratio.

Normal protein–creatinine ratios.

Cortisol Level	Normal Canine Ranges	Normal Feline Ranges
Urine protein/creatinine ratio	<1	<1

Reference values can vary from lab to lab. It is important to refer to normal reference values for the lab that performs the diagnostic trial.

Other Clinical Diagnostic Tests

Diagnostic tests that are helpful in diagnosing the cause of kidney function are

- complete blood count/chemistry (renal enzymes), and
- abdominal ultrasound and ultrasound guided renal biopsy.

Discussing Changes in Urinary Protein/Creatinine Ratio with the Client
- The urine protein/creatinine ratio is an important diagnostic test in evaluating early protein loss that could suggest early kidney disease.
- The kidneys' filters (glomeruli) are microscopic filters that filter the blood, removing toxins and small particles.
- When the filters are damaged, the larger protein molecules work their way through the damaged filters and enter the urine.
- Increased urine protein loss can suggest early renal disease before physical signs may be evident.

Fecal Diagnostics

The intestinal parasites and their life cycles are outlined in Chapter 10. Clinical diagnostics of feces allow the medical team to evaluate the patient for intestinal parasites, pathogenic bacteria, white blood cells, and skin parasites (occasionally). Samples should be as fresh as possible (ideally less than 4 hours old) to prevent degradation of fecal ova and bacteria. If samples are obtained the night before, they should be refrigerated. Samples should be free of debris, gravel, or kitty litter. When brought in to the hospital for evaluation, a direct visual examination should occur prior to clinical diagnostics. The sample should be opened and evaluated for

- blood,
- mucus,
- parasites,
  — roundworms,
  — tapeworms, and
  — maggots (nonintestinal parasites).
- foreign debris (plant material, foreign bodies).

Any abnormalities should be recorded and pointed out to the veterinarian. Furthermore, the presence of maggots that were deposited by flies after the feces were excreted should be pointed out to the owner, since these are not an intestinal parasite but an environmental contamination.

Routine Fecal Diagnostics
Fecal Floatation
Fecal floatation is the standard fecal clinical diagnostic test to evaluate the patient for intestinal ova.

Importance
The fecal floatation test is an important diagnostic evaluation to find intestinal parasites in patients. Many young and adult animals may be carrying asymptomatic infections that can produce a more severe gastrointestinal infection secondary to an initial gastrointestinal disease. Furthermore, these patients continue to increase the parasite load to the environment, acting as a reservoir for the parasites.

Discussing Fecal Floatation with the Client
- A fecal floatation allows the medical team to evaluate the feces for the presence of microscopic parasites and eggs that can suggest a parasitic infection.
- Many intestinal parasites are microscopic as adults and will not appear grossly in the feces.
- Furthermore, many adult pets will shed parasites into the environment without showing physical signs.
- Fecal examination allows the veterinarian to determine if the patient has a parasitic infection that can be treated and thus reduce the parasite load within the environment.

How It Is Evaluated
A fresh fecal sample (<4 hours old) is placed into a container and mixed with a dense fluid medium (i.e., zinc sulfate, dextrose). The container is covered with a coverslip or slide and allowed to sit for a minimum of 15 minutes. After the allotted time, the slip is placed on the microscope slide and examined at 10× and 40× objective. Intestinal ova vary depending on the geographic location, but typical intestinal parasites are seen in Figure 23.1.

Fecal Smear
A fecal smear is the standard fecal clinical diagnostic test used to evaluate the feces for obvious protozoa (i.e., giardia), increased bacteria, abnormal cell types, and possibly ova.

Importance
The fecal smear is an important diagnostic to evaluate the feces for motile protozoa. Mobile forms of many protozoa can be appreciated under high dry power as they move through the microscope field. In some instances, placing a

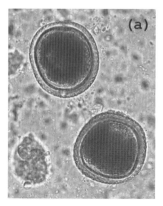
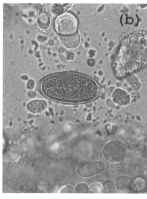
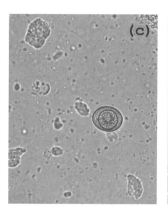
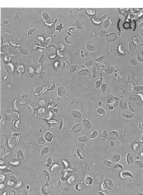

Figure 23.1. Common parasites seen on 40× objective. Parasite ova present are *Toxocara* (hookworms) (a), *Trichuris* (whipworms) (b), *Isospora* (Coccidia)(c), and *Giardia* oocysts (d).

small amount of dilute betadine can make the small single-celled organisms easier to evaluate.

How It Is Evaluated

A small fresh fecal sample (<4 hours old) is placed on a slide with physiological saline, and then a coverslip is placed on top. The slide is immediately evaluated on high dry power for giardia (see Figure 23.2) and other coccidia evident. Normal values may be seen in Figure 23.1.

> **Discussing Fecal Smears with the Client**
> - A fecal smear allows the medical team to evaluate the feces for the presence of protozoal parasites and eggs that can suggest a parasitic infection.
> - Many intestinal parasites are microscopic as adults and will not appear grossly in the feces.
> - Furthermore, many adult pets will shed parasites into the environment without showing physical signs.
> - Fecal examination allows the veterinarian to determine if the patient has a parasitic infection that can be treated and thus reduce the parasite load within the environment.

Fecal Cytology

Fecal cytology is a useful diagnostic used to evaluate patients with significant diarrhea for bacterial pathogens and abnormal cell types (i.e., white blood cells).

Importance

The fecal cytology evaluates the feces for abnormal levels of bacterial pathogens (i.e., *Clostridium* spp.) and white blood cells to help evaluate the patient for a primary or secondary bacterial gastroenteritis. Although not always the primary cause of a patient's symptoms, observation and treatment of the infection may help decrease or resolve gastrointestinal signs.

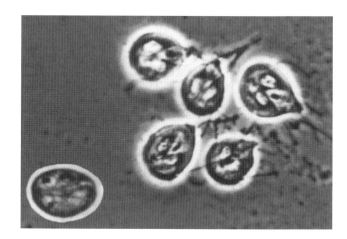

Figure 23.2. Image of the motile form of giardia on 40× magnification (high dry).

How It Is Evaluated

A small, fresh fecal sample is smeared on a slide and heat fixed. The cytology sample is then stained with a Gram stain or Diff-Quik protocol. The slide is dried and then evaluated under high-power oil immersion. The slide is evaluated for pathogenic bacteria and white blood cell or abnormal cell types that may suggest disease. *There is always a bacterial component evident in feces; the presence of increased bacterial pathogens and white blood cells are abnormal.*

Normal values for levels of bacterial pathogens.

Fecal Flora and Cells	Normal Canine Ranges	Normal Feline Ranges
Fecal white blood cells	Negative	Negative
Clostridium spp.	<1/hpf	<1/hpf

Discussing Fecal Cytology with the Client

- A fecal cytology allows the medical team to assess the feces for the presence of pathogenic bacteria and white blood cells that can suggest a primary or secondary bacterial infection of the intestines (**bacterial gastroenteritis**).
- Although not always the primary cause of intestinal disease, proper diagnosis and treatment of the bacterial infection can decrease physical signs and treatment time for the patient.

Fecal Enzyme-Linked Immunoassay Tests

Fecal enzyme-linked immunoassay (ELISA) tests help detect surface proteins (antigens) of specific viral, bacterial, and parasitic pathogens in the feces.

Importance

Many of these infectious diseases can be insidious and hard to diagnose based on blood work and fecal examination. ELISAs examine the feces for antigens of specific pathogens. These tests can be run in-hospital or sent out to a medical laboratory. Each clinical diagnostic evaluates the following pathogens.

- **Parvo ELISA:** Detects for antigens against **canine parvovirus** infection. It can also aid in the diagnosis of **feline panleukopenia** (see Chapter 10). The test can produce a false negative if the patient is not shedding large amounts of the virus. Furthermore, the test may show a weak positive if the patient has been vaccinated for parvovirus within 10 days of the test. The test is available in-hospital and at a veterinary laboratory.
- **Giardia ELISA:** Detects for antigens against the intestinal parasite, giardia. It is an excellent screening test for chronic diarrhea patients in which the animal has no visible giardia evident and does not respond to medication. The test is available in-hospital and at a veterinary laboratory.
- **Cryptococcus:** Detects for antibodies against the intestinal parasite, cryptococcus, a very small intestinal parasite (smaller than toxoplasma). It is an excellent screening test for chronic diarrhea patients in which the animal has no visible parasites evident and does not respond to medication. The test is available at a veterinary laboratory.
- **Clostridium toxin:** A screening test for animals exposed to the clostridium toxin. These patients may have severe gastrointestinal signs without obvious clostridium overload in the feces. The test is available at a veterinary laboratory.

How It Is Evaluated

Fecal samples are collected and checked for the presence of surface proteins (antigens) for specific infections. In these ELISA tests, positive results indicate an active infection.

Normal values for pathogen antigens.

Fecal Flora and Cells	Normal Canine Ranges	Normal Feline Ranges
Parvo cite	Negative	Negative
Clostridium toxin	Negative	Negative
Cryptococcus spp.	Negative	Negative
Giardia	Negative	Negative

Discussing Fecal ELISA with the Client

- A fecal ELISA test allows the medical team to evaluate the feces for proteins on the cell wall (antigens) of specific infectious and parasitic disease organisms of the intestine.
- In specific intestinal disease (i.e., parvo, clostridium, giardia, cryptococcus), where normal fecal and blood work clinical diagnostics cannot identify the pathogen, these tests can help isolate the specific pathogen.
- The test does require that the pet has a sufficient population of the infectious agent to produce a positive response. Therefore, in some cases, the patient may have a negative ELISA test and still have the infection.
- A positive test is strongly suggestive of an active infection from the specific pathogen.

Cytology Samples—Ears

Diseases of the ear are discussed in Chapter 20. Clinical diagnostics of the ears allow the medical team to evaluate the patient for bacterial, fungal, or parasitic infections. Samples should be taken in-hospital and evaluated microscopically for

- bacteria,
- fungi (malasezzia and cocci),
- ear mites (*Otodectes*), and
- white blood cells.

Any abnormalities should be recorded and pointed out to the veterinarian. The procedures for the clinical diagnostics are discussed next.

Ear Cytology

A diagnostic test is performed to detect pathogenic bacteria, parasites, and fungal pathogens within the ear canal.

Importance

This diagnostic test allows the medical team to determine the type of infectious agent producing the ear infection.

How It Is Evaluated

Similar to the fecal cytology, a sample of ear debris is collected with a nonsterile swab and placed on a microscope slide. The cytology sample is then stained with a Gram or Diff-Quik stain. The slide is dried and then evaluated under high power–oil immersion. The slide is evaluated for bacteria, fungi, and white blood cells. The following should be noted on each smear.

- **Bacteria:** The type of bacteria should be noted (i.e., rod, cocci) and as well as if bacteria are also evident within the white blood cell. The amount of bacteria is qualitatively gauged from mild to severe.
- **Fungi:** The presence of the peanut-shaped dimorphic malasezzia and the single cocci fungi can suggest a fungal infection. The amount of fungi is qualitatively gauged from mild to severe.
- **White blood cell:** The presence of white blood cells can suggest a more severe chronic infection in which the body is now trying to mount an immune response to fight off the ear infection. The evidence of white blood cells should be pointed out to the veterinarian because the pet may require systemic medications to help resolve the infection.
- **Ear mite swab:** In this diagnostic test, the ear debris is collected with a nonsterile swab and mixed with mineral oil on a microscope slide. The slide is then covered, and the debris is examined for ear mites or mite eggs.

Discussing Ear Cytology with the Client
- Ear cytology has been recommended by the veterinarian to help distinguish the type of organism producing the ear infection.
- Common infectious agents are bacteria, fungus, and ear mites.
- The course of treatment depends on the type of pathogen found.
- In some chronic severe cases, further diagnostics (i.e., culture and sensitivity) may be needed to evaluate if there is a specific bacterial pathogen evident and what antibiotics would be successful in treating the infection.

Normal values of bacteria, fungi, and white blood cells.

Fecal Flora and Cells	Normal Canine Ranges	Normal Feline Ranges
Bacteria	Negative	Negative
Fungi	Negative	Negative
Mites	Negative	Negative
White blood cells	Negative	Negative

Ear Culture and Sensitivity

The culture and sensitivity test is performed to identify pathogenic bacteria from a chronic ear infection and identify nonresistant antibiotics.

How Test Is Performed

The patient can have an ear culture and sensitivity completed without fasting or special preparation. A sample of ear debris is collected from the patient on a sterile culturette. The sample is then plated and incubated or sent to the lab for identification. It can take 48–72 or more hours for test results to be available.

How It Is Evaluated

Growth of pathogenic bacteria suggests infection of the ear canal. The antibiotics that stop the growth of the bacteria are indicated.

Normal values of pathogenic bacteria.

Test	Normal Canine Results	Normal Feline Results
Ear culture and sensitivity	No growth	No growth

Discussing Changes in Ear Culture and Sensitivity with the Client
- Ear culture and sensitivity has been recommended by the veterinarian to evaluate the ear for possible pathogenic bacteria.
- The presence of the bacteria suggests infection within the ear canal.
- Once the bacteria are isolated, further tests help evaluate which antibiotics are the best choice to treat the infection.

CD-ROM 2 will focus on concepts of understanding and discussing clinical diagnostics and the disease conditions represented. The exercises can be done individually or as case rounds as they explore specific topics in veterinary medicine that discuss clinical diagnostics and treatment.

Chapter 24

Electrocardiogram

To understand the basic concepts of the electrocardiogram (EKG), the team member must have a working knowledge of the flow of blood through the heart in diasystole and systole (see Chapter 12). The heart is an electrical pump that produces normal electrical rhythms that then stimulate muscular contractions. These electrical impulses are stimulated within the heart muscle itself; the heart initiates its own electrical rhythm without any outside stimulation. The ability to produce this rhythm is called **automaticity**. The central nervous system does increase and decrease the heart rate in response to the body's needs, but the heart initiates its signal, carries the electrical depolarization throughout its muscle cells, and contracts as one unit.

The EKG is a modified oscilloscope that graphs electrical changes within the heart. As the electrical wave moves toward the EKG sensor, the graphed wave goes upward. As the electrical wave moves away from the sensor, the graphed wave moves downward (see Figure 24.1). By understanding normal electrical patterns, cardiac arrhythmias can be diagnosed.

Performing the EKG

To perform an EKG the team member places three to five metal clips on the patient on regions of the forelimb and hind limb, and possibly the chest. These clips are the sensors that evaluate the electrical rhythm of the heart. The location of the observation point of the electrical signal can be switched from one clip to the next. In doing this, the EKG can evaluate the heart from **six different leads.** These leads are I, II, III, AVL, AVR, and AVS.

Although EKG machinery can vary from company to company, a basic protocol for performing an EKG is as follows.

1. The animal should be placed on a nonconductive surface. If a metal table or grate is being used, a towel should be placed over the work surface (see Figure 24.2). If the metal clip comes in contact with a metal table, artifactual images could be produced that could be misread as cardiac arrhythmias.
2. The patient should be placed in **right lateral recumbency** or, if the animal isn't nervous, the test can be done with the animal standing (see Figure 24.3). If at all possible, minimal to no chemical restraint should be used because these drugs can affect heart rate.

3. The electrode clips are placed.
   - The right and left forelimb clips are placed at the level of the elbow on the caudal surface.
   - The right and left hind limb clips are placed at the medial aspect of the knees.
   - A cardiac electrode (the fifth lead "C") is found on some machines and is placed on the ventral aspect of the thorax (see Figure 24.4).
4. Alcohol is placed on the lead to increase conductivity of the signal.
5. The EKG is started on lead II at either the 25 mm or 50 mm/second rate. Some machines cannot set the rate of speed at which the EKG reads the patterns.
6. The sensitivity should be adjusted until a large enough complex is printed within the margins of the paper or screen. On some machines sensitivity cannot be set.

Conduction Anatomy

Although evaluation of the EKG is the responsibility of the veterinarian, the team members should be able to perform and evaluate the EKG rhythm for changes in rate or rhythm, since EKG monitoring is often incorporated in anesthesia monitoring and evaluation. To evaluate the electrocardiogram, the team member must understand the conduction anatomy of the heart.

The initiator of the conduction signal is high in the right atrium in a region called the **sino-atrial node (S-A node)**. Because the S-A node has the highest automaticity of the heart fibers, it can stimulate a wave of depolarization on its own without outside stimulation. Because the S-A node produces the initial rhythm that starts the heartbeat, it is called *the pacemaker of the heart*. The S-A node is closely integrated with the parasympathetic and sympathetic nervous systems (part of the autonomic nervous system) to control heart rate, depending on the body's need for oxygenated blood and maintenance of blood pressure. However, the heart stimulates its own contraction.

Once the S-A node fires, it begins waves of depolarization over the atrium to produce an atrial contraction. As the current runs from the S-A node toward the EKG monitor it produces a positive deviation. The electrical wave then spreads over the atrium away from the EKG sensor, and the wave returns to baseline. This is called the **P wave.** After the P wave is produced, both atria contract, producing diasystole (see Figure 24.5).

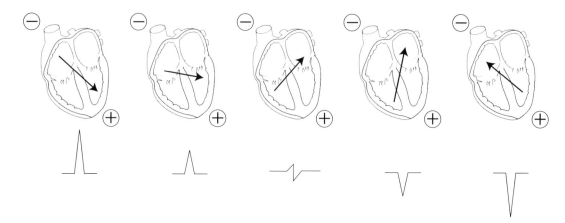

Figure 24.1.   Image of how the electric current through the heart is read and displayed by the EKG. An electrical wave toward the sensor displays as a positive deviation, an impulse across the heart reads as a small positive deviation, and a wave away from the sensor is shown as a negative deviation

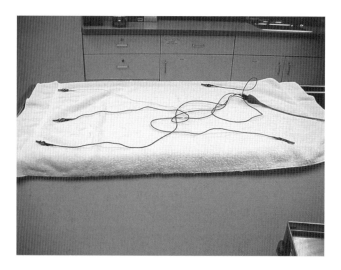

Figure 24.2.   Image of an EKG setup in a hospital.

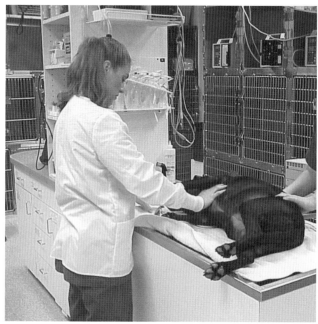

Figure 24.3.   The patient is placed on right lateral recumbency.

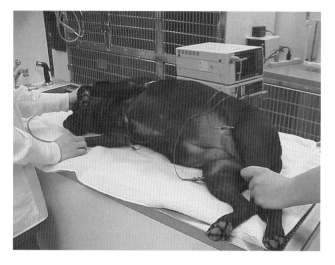

Figure 24.4.   The clips are placed on the forelimbs, hind limbs, and on the chest. Some machines will have only have three or four leads.

As the P wave occurs, the current from the S-A node travels toward the top of the interseptal wall where a collection of fibers, called the **atrial-ventricular node (A-V node),** focuses the signal down the septal wall. After the P wave is completed, the current travels down toward the ventricles via a number of specific conductive fibers called the **Purkinje fibers (bundle of His).** As the current spreads through the septal wall, it produces a slight negative deviation away from the EKG, producing a downward deviation; this is the **Q wave.** The current then moves directly toward the sensor as it approaches the base of the heart, producing the **R wave.** Once the electrical wave reaches the heart base, it begins to

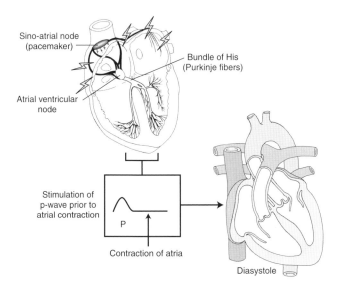

Figure 24.5. The illustration shows the production of the P wave (a small positive deviation wave that washes over the atrium) that stimulates atrial contraction.

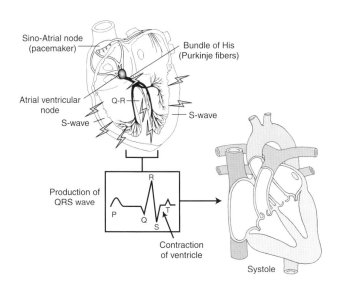

Figure 24.6. Image of the A-V node focusing energy down the septal walls via the Purkinje fibers and up and around the ventricular wall, producing the QRS patter and stimulating ventricular contraction.

move up the outside ventricle wall; this produces the **S wave.** Shortly after the QRS complex is produced, the ventricles contract (see Figure 24.6).

After the full heartbeat occurs, the muscle goes through a wave of repolarization in which the electrolytes of the body are rebalanced to make the heart ready for the next beat. This is called the **T wave.** This wave of repolarization can be directed toward, away from, or parallel to the EKG. Thus the T wave can be positive, negative, or have no deviation after the QRS complexes

Evaluating the Electrocardiogram

The EKG is typically read in lead II; however, if the electrical wave is small or hard to evaluate, it can be read in other leads that may have more identifiable P-QRS complexes. For nonanesthetized patients, EKG evaluation should be run for at least 30–60 seconds.

Arrhythmias occur due to

- disease, infection, or trauma in the S-A node,
- an obstruction in the A-V node or in the bundle of His,
- a region of muscle that becomes irritated and begins transmitting its own depolarization wave, and
- an electrolyte abnormality that decreases the electrical potential of the heart.

Although a full evaluation of the EKG can be an in-depth process, the technical team should be able to perform a basic evaluation using these steps (see Algorithm: Evaluating the EKG).

Step I: Calculate the Heart Rate

Although many EKG machines will calculate the heart rate, abnormal complexes and artifactual rhythms could alter the underlying heart rate. The team member should evaluate the heart rate on the printed report using the following.

- **25 mm/second speed:** Count 75 mm (75 boxes; 3 seconds). Count the number of **normal rhythms** and multiply by 20 to get beats per minute (see Figure 24.7).
- **50 mm/second count:** Count 150 mm (150 boxes; 3 seconds). Count the number of beats within the 150 mm and multiply by 20 to get beats per minute. (See Figure 24.7; see also Table 24.1 for normal heart rates.)

Step II: Identify Changes in the Pattern

Tachycardia refers to rapid heart rates above normal limits. In the example below, the calculated heart rate shows a persistent tachycardia (see Figure 24.8). *Tachycardia should be reported to the veterinarian immediately.*

Bradycardia refers to slow heart rates below normal limits. In the example below, the calculated heart rate shows a persistent bradycardia (see Figure 24.9). *Bradycardia should be reported to the veterinarian immediately.*

Table 24.1. Normal heart rates.

Species	Normal Heart Rates	When To Be Concerned
Canine	80–120 bpm	Heart rate <60 bpm Heart rate >200 bpm
Feline	120–180 bpm	Heart rate <80 bpm Heart rate >220 bpm

Algorithm: Evaluating the EKG

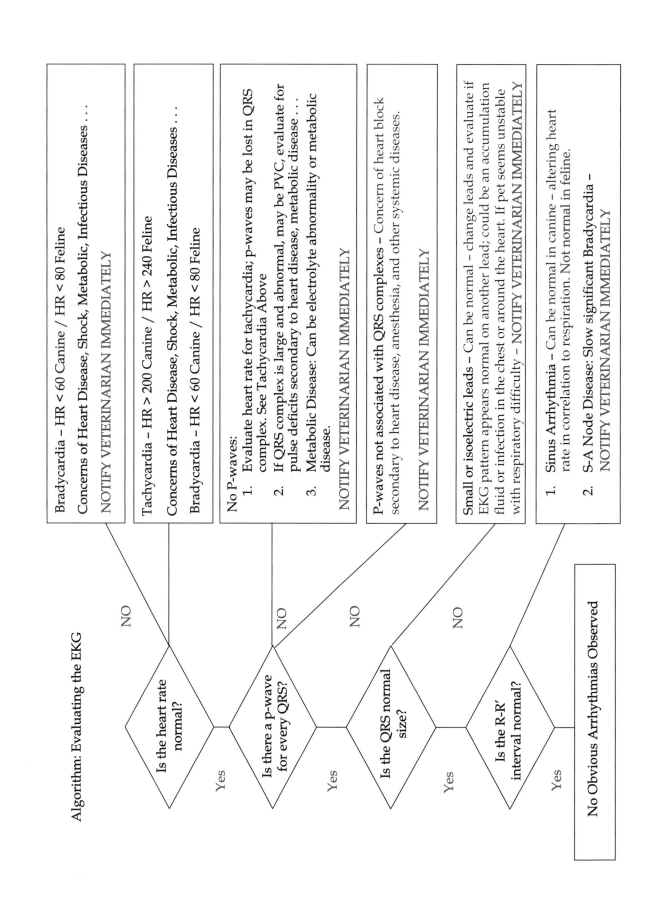

Is the heart rate normal?

NO → Bradycardia – HR < 60 Canine / HR < 80 Feline

Concerns of Heart Disease, Shock, Metabolic, Infectious Diseases . . .

NOTIFY VETERINARIAN IMMEDIATELY

Tachycardia – HR > 200 Canine / HR > 240 Feline

Concerns of Heart Disease, Shock, Metabolic, Infectious Diseases . . .

Bradycardia – HR < 60 Canine / HR < 80 Feline

Yes ↓

Is there a p-wave for every QRS?

NO → No P-waves:
1. Evaluate heart rate for tachycardia; p-waves may be lost in QRS complex. See Tachycardia Above
2. If QRS complex is large and abnormal, may be PVC, evaluate for pulse deficits secondary to heart disease, metabolic disease . . .
3. Metabolic Disease: Can be electrolyte abnormality or metabolic disease.

NOTIFY VETERINARIAN IMMEDIATELY

Yes ↓

Is the QRS normal size?

NO → P-waves not associated with QRS complexes – Concern of heart block secondary to heart disease, anesthesia, and other systemic diseases.

NOTIFY VETERINARIAN IMMEDIATELY

Yes ↓

Is the R-R' interval normal?

NO → Small or isoelectric leads – Can be normal – change leads and evaluate if EKG pattern appears normal on another lead; could be an accumulation fluid or infection in the chest or around the heart. If pet seems unstable with respiratory difficulty – NOTIFY VETERINARIAN IMMEDIATELY

Yes ↓

1. Sinus Arrhythmia – Can be normal in canine – altering heart rate in correlation to respiration. Not normal in feline.
2. S-A Node Disease: Slow significant Bradycardia – NOTIFY VETERINARIAN IMMEDIATELY

No Obvious Arrhythmias Observed

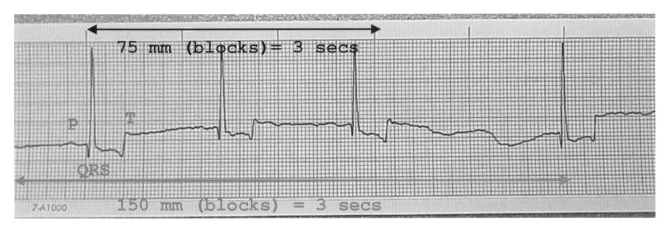

Figure 24.7.   EKG strip. The black arrow (top) is 75 blocks (75 mm). The gray arrow (bottom) is 150 blocks or 150. Depending on the rate of speed the EKG was reading, the heart rate could be calculated as

25 mm/sec: Heart rate = 3 normal beats in 3 seconds × 20 seconds = 60 bpm
50 mm/sec: Heart rate = 4 normal beats in 3 seconds × 20 seconds = 80 bpm

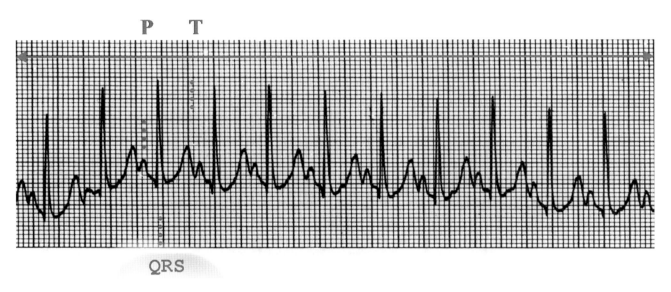

Figure 24.8.   At a 50-mm/second reading speed, if the above strip represents a 3-second strip, the heart rate is

50 mm/second speed for 3 seconds = 11 beats × 20 seconds = 220 bpm

It is important to note that with this tachycardia, the P-waves are beginning to be obscured by the last QRS-T complex

Step III: Identify Each P-Wave and Ensure a QRS Complex Is Associated With It

Each normal heart contraction should have a P-wave with an associated QRS complex. If there are no P-waves or if the P-waves are not associated with a QRS pattern, it can suggest an arrhythmia. P-waves can be absent or not associated with a QRS complex when there are no obvious P-waves.

No Obvious P-waves
Tachycardia
In times of extreme tachycardia, the heart rate can be so fast that the P-wave can become obscured in the QRS complex,

typically seen when heart rates are greater than 220 (see Figure 24.8). This can sometimes be seen secondary to excitement or stress but can also be seen with serious disease conditions. *Tachycardia should be reported to the veterinarian immediately.*

Premature Ventricular Contraction
One of the most important arrhythmias to detect is the premature ventricular contraction (PVC). In this situation a region of ventricular muscle becomes irritated by trauma, disease, or infection. This region is so irritated that it produces a depolarization wave that stimulates a ventricular contrac-

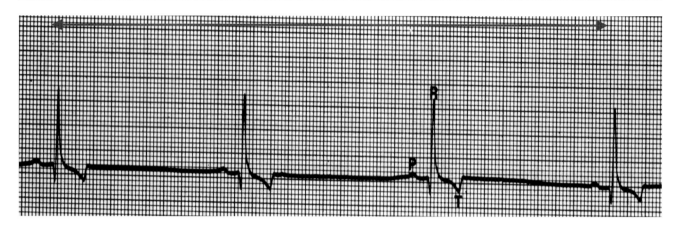

Figure 24.9. At a 50-mm/second reading speed, if the above strip represents a 3-second strip, the heart rate is

50 mm/second speed for 3 seconds = 3 beats × 20 seconds = 60 bpm

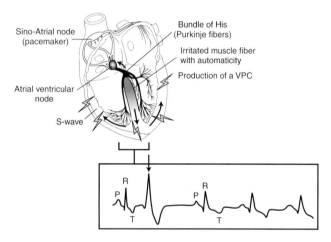

Figure 24.10. Illustration of a PVC in which irritated muscle fiber with greater automaticity than the S-A produces an abnormal ventricular contraction. The resulting arrhythmia produces a large, wide abnormal rhythm with no associated P-wave. This animal could present with an abnormal heart rhythm and pulse deficits.

tion independent of the S-A node. The PVC occurs because the affected muscle fiber has greater automaticity than the S-A node (see Figure 21.10). PVCs can occur when there is no blood within the ventricle. This produces an abnormal or skipped beat that produces no perceivable pulse (**pulse deficit**). *Persistent PVC can be life threatening and should be reported to the veterinarian immediately.*

Metabolic Disease

Sodium, potassium, and other electrolytes are necessary to produce the electrical current that produces the heart rhythm. When there are metabolic diseases that affect the normal electrolyte population, abnormal EKG rhythms can be observed (see Figure 24.11). Specific diseases that affect the P-waves are

- Addison's disease (hypoadrenocorticism; see Chapter 27),
- renal disease (see Chapter 13),
- urinary obstruction (FLUTD; see Chapter 13),
- ketoacidotic diabetes (DKA; see Chapter 15), and
- shock (see Chapter 30).

P-Waves Not Associated with QRS Complexes

If there is infectious, traumatic, neoplastic, or inflammatory disease of the A-V node or Purkinje fibers (bundle of HIs), normal electrical impulses cannot be passed from the atrium to the ventricle (see Figure 24.10). This condition is called **heart block** and can vary from mild signal interruption (**primary heart block**), to moderate interruption (**secondary heart block**), to complete interruption (**complete heart block**). Affected patients will show P-waves that are not directly associated with QRS complexes. There can be normal P-QRS complexes as well when the depolarization wave does enter the ventricle. With complete heart block, there is no communication between atria and ventricle, and the ventricle produces an escape beat to move blood throughout the body (see Figure 24.12).

Step IV: Small (Isoelectric) QRS Complexes

Small or isoelectric patterns can suggest a number of disease conditions that interfere with evaluation of the EKG or decrease normal electrical output.

Normal Rhythm

Some machines have decreased ability to evaluate felines or specific patients, depending on their body conformation and position of the heart in the chest. If the EKG pattern is small, changing to other leads may differentiate a true pathologic condition from an isoelectric lead.

Disease Conditions

There are disease conditions in which an accumulation of fluid, air, or infection within the chest (see Figure 24.13), around the heart or within the lungs, can decrease the signal. Some of these disease entities are

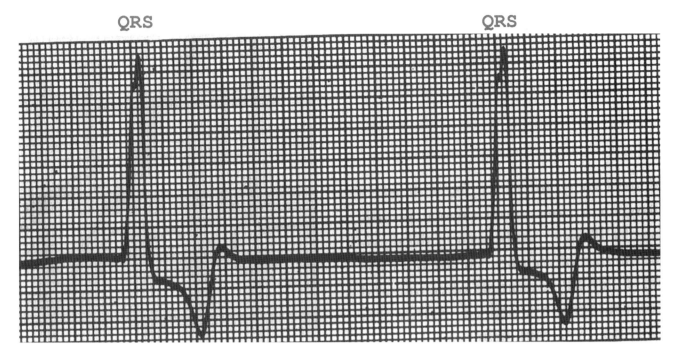

Figure 24.11. Image of QRS complexes without obvious P-waves.

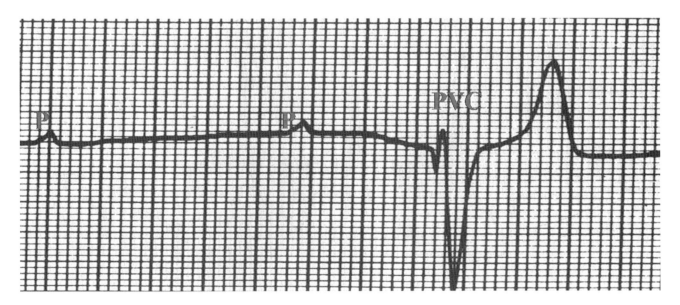

Figure 24.12. Image of complete heart block. Here there are P-waves with no associated QRS. The ventricle stimulates its own escape beat to help pump blood into the body.

- pericardial effusion,
- pneumothorax,
- pleural effusion, and
- pulmonary disease.

Step V: Evaluate the Distance between Complexes
The distance between complexes (from one positive R spike to the next; R-R′ interval) can suggest a disease process in the A-V node. Disease, inflammation, or trauma of the node can slow normal signals, producing severe bradycardia (see

Figure 24.14) or bursts of normal heart rhythms with a sudden sino-atrial pause. Changes in the R-R′ interval can occur due to sinus arrhythmia and sick sinus syndrome.

Sinus Arrhythmia
Sinus arrhythmia is an alternating rhythm of rapid heart rate with a slowing rhythm that corresponds to the patient's respiratory rate. *This is a normal rhythm in canines and does not suggest pathology.* In other breeds, this suggests a potential arrhythmia.

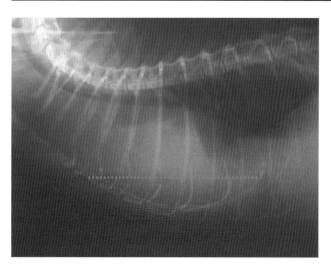

Figure 24.13.   X-ray of a chest with a pleural effusion evident. The fluid (evident by a lack of detail below the dotted line) around the heart and lungs is decreasing the ability of normal electrical signals to be evaluated by the sensor.

Sick Sinus Syndrome

Sick sinus syndrome is a disease of the S-A node in which the disease process slows the normal waves of depolarization that produces the heartbeat (see Figure 21.14).

When To Perform an Electrocardiogram

Although the veterinarian is responsible for indicating the need for an electrocardiogram, the medical team should be ready to perform an EKG in any situation. Some indications are as follows.

Trauma

Any patient that suffers from a significant trauma (i.e., fall, hit by car, shake injury) should have an EKG to monitor the heart for arrhythmia. The most common arrhythmia is PVC caused by irritated muscle fibers secondary to trauma (see below).

Cardiac Disease

As discussed in Chapter 12, any form of cardiac disease (i.e., cardiomyopathy, valvular disease, cardiac tumor, cardiovascular shock) can have an arrhythmia component. An EKG should be performed as long as the patient is stable and not stressed.

Anoxia/Surgical Monitoring

Decreasing oxygen concentration to the heart muscle can commonly produce abnormal rhythms (i.e., PVC). While under anesthesia the patient can have decreasing amounts of oxygen concentration, producing arrhythmias. These events can be small and isolated and are simply treated by increasing oxygen concentration in the bloodstream.

Metabolic Disease

Patients with severe metabolic or emergency disease can irritate cardiac muscle fibers producing life-threatening arrhythmias. Some diseases are as follows:

*   Gastrodilatation volvulus (GDV; Chapter 10)
*   Tumors/masses of the spleen (hemangiosarcoma)
*   FLUTD/obstruction (Chapter 13)
*   Ketoacidotic diabetes (Chapter 15)
*   Shock (Chapter 30)

R-R′ interval

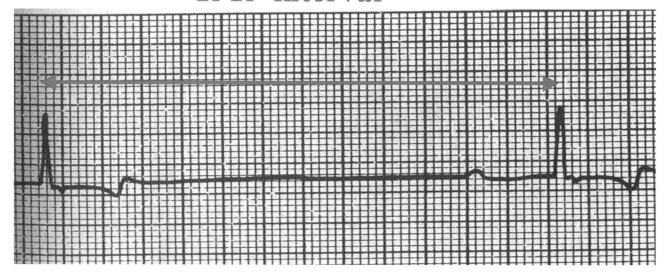

Figure 24.14.   The line denoting the R-R′ interval is prolonged, suggesting disease of the S-A node or other heart or systemic disease process.

Preanesthetic Evaluation

In the geriatric animal (patients older than 7–8 years of age) and in specific breeds that are prone to heart disease (i.e., boxer, Doberman pinscher, cocker spaniel, Maine coon cat), EKGs may be indicated to help screen for patients with any early or silent arrhythmias who could be poor candidates for anesthesia.

Wellness Examination

As discussed with preanesthetic evaluation, performing a routine EKG on breeds predisposed to heart disease may aid in early diagnosis and treatment of a silent cardiac disease.

Key Points in Discussing the Electrocardiogram with the Client

- An electrocardiogram (EKG) evaluates the electrical current through the heart.
- The heart is a specialized muscle that initiates its own electrical heart rhythm to stimulate heart contraction.
- Specific diseases can alter and affect the heart's electrical rhythm and ultimately affect its ability to beat correctly. This is called a cardiac arrhythmia.
- In many cases, the arrhythmias do not produce obvious symptoms until the patient is in an emergency life-threatening situation.
- Diseases that can produce an EKG are heart disease, trauma, metabolic disease, infectious disease, cancer, shock, and many others.
- If not detected and treated, arrhythmia can be life threatening.
- Many types of arrhythmias can be controlled with medication.

Diseases of the Cardiac System

Although not all diseases are mentioned below, the common arrhythmias are discussed, with the main goal being to identify the arrhythmia and to understand and be able to explain to the client what the abnormalities are, how they can present themselves, and what can be the overall short- and long-term concerns of each disease. Any discussion of overall diagnostic and treatment protocols should be discussed based on the recommendations of the doctor and the medical team. Please use the following information as a basis to discuss and educate the client, *but never to diagnose a patient.*

Premature Ventricular Contraction

PVC is a rhythm initiated within irritated ventricular muscle fibers instead of the S-A node. This rhythm produces an abnormal contraction when there may be limited blood in the ventricles, producing a heart sound without a corresponding pulse (**pulse deficit**).

Etiology

A PVC is caused by disease that irritates ventricular muscle fibers, increasing automaticity and initiating an abnormal cardiac rhythm. Disease processes that can affect the ventricular muscle fibers are

- trauma,
- cardiac disease,
- anoxia/anesthesia,
- metabolic disease, and
- shock.

Signalment

PVC is commonly seen in large breed dogs with **cardiomyopathy**, especially boxers and Dobermans, but can also be seen in felines with a history of cardiomyopathy or hyperthyroidism.

Complications

If gone untreated, PVCs can develop into runs called **ventricular tachycardia** that can produce severe weakness and anoxia. If not treated, it can develop into ventricular fibrillation and cardiac failure.

Common Points in Medical History

PVC can be asymptomatic in the affected patients until severe cardiac disease is evident. Clients may note the following changes:

- Weakness
- Inability to exercise
- Collapse
- Coughing

Common Points on Initial Assessment

Severely affected animals may be life threatened and may require immediate attention. These patients must be handled with minimal stress because they can collapse and die with any excitement. Common physical changes can be

- pulse deficits,
- escape beats/third beat of the heart,
- cyanotic mucous membrane color/capillary refill time (CRT),
- cough,
- dyspnea,
- collapse/syncope, and
- sudden death.

Diagnostics
EKG Pattern

PVC is represented as wide, irregular QRS waves without the presence of P-waves (see Figure 24.15). These rhythms do not tend to have a pulse associated with the contraction because of decreased cardiac output. Multiple complexes of PVC are called ventricular tachycardia.

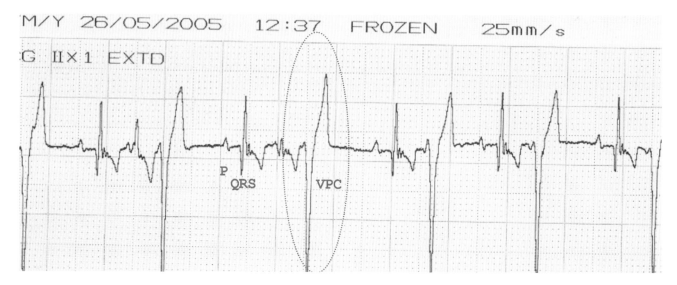

Figure 24.15. EKG strip of VPC and regular rhythms, not the normal P-QRS complex with the alternating wide VPC (dotted circle) without obvious P-wave.

Complete Blood Count/Chemistry

Changes in electrolytes, especially in potassium and sodium, can precipitate PVC.

Thyroid Profile

In cats, checking thyroid levels is very important to help distinguish if the causes of PVC are from hyperthyroidism (see Chapter 16).

Radiology/Ultrasound

A full radiographic evaluation of the heart and lung fields can help determine if there are changes in the cardiac silhouette and lung fields suggestive of heart, infectious, or cancerous disease that may be predisposing the patient to arrhythmias. Further internal ultrasound examination of the heart can help evaluate cardiac muscle thickness, valvular disease, or cardiac cancer.

Treatment

Treatment options depend on physical symptoms of the patient and the extent of the arrhythmias. Some treatment options are listed here.

- **Oxygen therapy:** By increasing oxygen concentration in the body, the heart does not have to work as hard. By increasing oxygen concentration in a low-stress environment, it may decrease heart rate, oxygen need, and arrhythmias.
- **Monitoring:** The animal should be treated as an inpatient with cage rest activity restrictions. Frequent ECG and blood pressure monitoring may be recommended if the they can be completed without stressing the patient.
- **Medications:** Anti-arrhythmatic medications help to improve conduction through the ventricle and help convert

the PVC to normal rhythms. Examples of these medications are lidocaine, procainimide, and quinidine.

Prevention

There is no way to prevent PVCs. However, through routine clinical diagnostics in older animals and breeds that are more sensitive to heart disease, early diagnosis and treatment can help increase quality of life and life span of the pet.

Discussing Premature Ventricular Contractions with the Client

- Premature ventricular contraction (PVC) occurs when an area of ventricular muscle becomes diseased, inflamed, infected, or traumatized.
- The affected muscle releases a depolarization wave that produces a premature contraction of the ventricles.
- The contraction can occur when little to no blood is evident in the ventricles, producing a heart rhythm without a pulse.
- Continued contractions can produce weakness, collapse, and even cardiovascular shock if the arrhythmia is not controlled and normal circulation restored.
- The diagnosis is based on history, physical exam, and EKG studies to evaluate the heart's electrical rhythm.
- Most forms of PVC can be controlled with medication, monitoring, and hospitalization.
- If not corrected, PVC can produce life-threatening cardiac shock

Atrioventricular Block (Heart Block)

This arrhythmia is produced by a blockage of the conduction of the electrical signal through the A-V node and the bundle of His. The obstruction prevents the normal transmission of the signal from the S-A node to the ventricle.

Etiology

Heart block produces atrial contraction independent of ventricular contractions. If there is a long enough pause between ventricular stimulation, the ventricle will produce an escape rhythm. The escape rhythm produces a VPC wave. *The key to diagnosis is the observation of multiple P-waves without a normal QRS pattern.* There are different degrees of heart block, from partial to complete.

- **First-degree heart block:** This is usually an asymptomatic form where an occasional P-wave will fire with no resulting QRS complex. This can be associated with anesthetic procedures.
- **Second-degree heart block:** This block is a more significant obstruction of the A-V node and bundle of His. There are still some normal P-QRS complexes; the disease process can still be asymptomatic. If this is caused from a heart disease, it can develop into complete heart block.
- **Complete heart block:** These patients have a complete blockage through the A-V node and bundle of His. P waves are not associated with wide PVC escape beats. The patient can be severely affected.

Signalment

Heart block is commonly seen in older dogs and cats with thickening and fibrosis of the conduction pathways. Common breeds affected are

- Doberman pinschers,
- pugs,
- dachshunds,
- cocker spaniels, and
- cats with **hypertrophic cardiomyopathy.**

Furthermore, underlying diseases that can produce heart block are

- congenital cardiac disease,
- cardiomyopathy,
- toxicity to cardiac medication (i.e., digitalis),
- infection or inflammation of the heart muscle (**myocarditis**), and
- electrolyte disorder.

Complications

With mild forms of heart block, there may be no physical symptoms or deterioration of the heart. If more serious forms go untreated, complete heart block can develop into weakness, collapse. and sudden death.

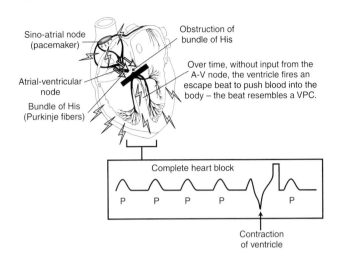

Figure 24.16. Illustration of a complete heart block. Here the normal depolarization waves cannot transmit through the bundle of His. P-waves are produced normally; however, they are not associated with the QRS complex. The ventricle produces an escape beat (PVC) to push blood out of the ventricles and into the body.

Common Points in Medical History

With mild heart block, the patient may be asymptomatic. With more severe heart blocks, clients may observe

- weakness,
- inability to exercise, and
- collapse.

Common Points on Initial Assessment

Severely affected animals may be life threatened and may require immediate attention. *These patients must be handled with minimal stress because many patients can collapse and die with any excitement.* Common physical changes can be

- bradycardia,
- abnormal heart sounds,
- cyanotic mucous membranes,
- poor capillary refill time, and
- cardiovascular shock.

Diagnostically

- **EKG pattern:** The P-waves look normal but are often without normal QRS complexes. The QRS complexes can be wide, bizarre, and PVC-like, depending on the location of where the escape beat is produced. The ventricular rate QRS pattern (usually less than 40–60 bpm) is slower than the atrial rate P-wave (see Figure 24.16).
- **Complete blood count/chemistry:** Changes in electrolytes, especially in the potassium and sodium, can precipitate heart block.
- **Thyroid profile:** There are possible arrhythmias that can be produced from changes in normal thyroid production.
- **Radiology/ultrasound:** A full radiographic evaluation of the heart and lung fields can help determine if there are

changes in the cardiac silhouette and lung fields suggestive of heart, infectious, or cancerous disease that may be predisposing the patient to arrhythmias. Further internal ultrasound examination of the heart can help evaluate cardiac muscle thickness, valvular disease, or cardiac cancer that can also produce heart block.

Treatment

In milder cases, treatment is not necessary unless there is an underlying cause of the heart block. In more advanced cases, treatment may be focused on the following.

- **Treatment of the underlying disease causing the heart block.**
- **Oxygen therapy:** By increasing oxygen concentration in the body, the heart does not have to work as hard. By increasing oxygen concentration in a low-stress environment, heart rate, oxygen need, and arrhythmias may be decreased.
- **Monitoring:** The animal should be treated as an inpatient with cage rest activity restrictions. Frequent ECG and blood pressure monitoring may be recommended.
- **Medications:** Parasympatholytic drugs (e.g., atropine, glycopyrrolate) that block the normal neurologic input from the parasympathetic nervous system, which slows the heart rate, can be used to increase the normal heart rhythm.
- **Surgery:** With severe heart block, an electronic pacemaker may need to be implanted under the skin with leads that attach to the heart. This electronic device can then produce an initial depolarization signal that can aid in complete atrial and ventricular contraction.

Prevention

There is no way to prevent heart block. However, through routine clinical diagnostics in older animals and breeds that are more sensitive to heart disease, early diagnosis and treatment can help increase quality of life and the life span of the pet.

Discussing Heart Block with the Client

- Heart block is an arrhythmia of the heart that blocks normal conduction of electrical signals from the atrium into the ventricles, blocking the normal wave of energy that stimulates ventricular contraction.
- There are many mild forms of the disease that occur without symptoms or need for treatment.
- With severe obstruction, the patient can become weak, cannot exercise, and can collapse due to the decreased blood flow out of the ventricles.
- These patients can develop cardiac collapse and life-threatening disease.
- Severe heart block is controlled with medication and possibly implantation of a pacemaker.

CD-ROM 2 will focus on concepts of understanding and discussing clinical diagnostics and the disease conditions represented. The exercises can be done individually or as case rounds as they explore specific topics in veterinary medicine that discuss clinical diagnostics and treatment.

Chapter 25

Radiology, Ultrasound, and Endoscopy Techniques

The goal of this chapter is to focus on discussion of the technology of each diagnostic test, safety measures needed while performing these evaluations, indications of when the diagnostics are recommended, and how to communicate the importance of the evaluation to the client.

Radiology

Radiographs are one of the most commonly used diagnostic tools within veterinary medicine. The radiograph allows the doctor to noninvasively (i.e., no surgery is needed) view internal structures within the pet. Radiographs can be evaluated almost immediately by the veterinarian. Animals often require no anesthesia to minimal sedation for radiographic tests; therefore, they are able to go home the day of the study.

Technology

X-ray radiation is focused, nonluminous electromagnetic radiation with a very short wavelength. The short wavelength allows x-rays to penetrate solid objects. X-rays are produced when the electrons emitted from a tungsten filament within the x-ray machine are stopped by a solid structure (i.e., an animal's body).

The amount of electrons released is based upon the amount of energy applied to the filaments; this measure of the energy applied is called **kilovoltage (kV).** The greater the kilovoltage, the more electrons are produced and the deeper the electrons can penetrate into tissue. Therefore, the larger or broader the animal the more kilovoltage is used.

The length of time the electrons are exposed to the tissue is called the **milliamperage seconds (MaS).** The combination of kilovoltage and milliamperage seconds defines the depth and contrast needed to produce a diagnostic image (see Figure 25.1).

The collision of the electrons into tissue produces 99% heat energy, with 1% x-ray energy. The more energy fired off, the more x-rays are produced. The x-rays that come in contact with the x-ray film help to expose it, producing an image.

Safety

X-ray radiation, in enough quantity, can destroy healthy living tissue. *The x-ray radiation that is produced from the x-ray tube does not all stream through the patient and onto the cassette.* Some x-rays are transferred directly to the film, and some scatter off in all directions (**scatter radiation**). The scatter radiation is of concern to the hospital staff. Absorbed radiation builds up over time and never dissipates once absorbed into the body. To prevent excessive damage from compounding exposure to radiation, safety standards and recommendations should be set up by the hospital team. Although radiation safety varies slightly from hospital to hospital, some basic safety guidelines are as follows.

- **All nonessential personnel should stay away from the x-ray area while films are being taken.** Employees that are not assisting and not wearing protective gear should be away from the machine. Clients should never be allowed in the area while their pet is being x-rayed. Furthermore, clients should not be allowed to help restrain the pet even with protective gear. They have no formal training in restraint and x-ray safety. *Pregnant women or young children should never be allowed in the area while x-rays are being taken; there are too many health risks.*
- **Protective clothing should always be worn at all times when x-rays are being taken.** Leaded aprons with thyroid shields, leaded goggles, and leaded gloves should always be used to help minimize exposure to the hands while restraining the pet. X-ray gloves should never be included in the x-ray film. Even these leaded gloves are not enough to protect the holder's hands from x-rays in the primary field. They are meant to protect the holder only from scatter radiation.
- **All protective clothing should be x-rayed regularly.** This is to make sure that the lead is still thick enough to prevent x-ray penetration. With time, large holes can develop in the aprons and gloves and produce areas where scatter radiation can easily pass through.
- **X-ray monitoring badges should always be worn by the medical team taking the film.** These badges monitor the exposure to scatter radiation. They are generally changed every month, and a radiation report is sent to the hospital. The radiation report should be either posted or available to all employees. Significant changes or elevations in radiation exposures warrant a review of radiation safety and a recheck of the x-ray unit.
- **Technique charts should be developed and used to maximize the efficiency of the films.** Technique charts are a recording of exposure times and power settings

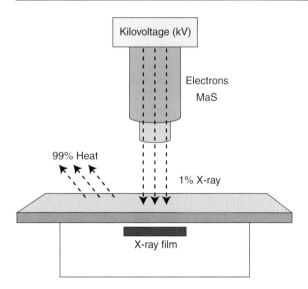

Figure 25.1. Illustration of x-ray radiation being produced. The tungsten filaments within the x-ray unit produce electrons. The greater the amount of energy (kV), the more x-rays are released and the deeper the penetration of the beam into the tissue. The duration of exposure (MaS) dictates the level of clarity and contrast the image produces.

based on the thickness of the body region x-rayed. They allow the best technique to be used for each body part and its thickness measurement. If done correctly, it minimizes the amount of x-rays needed and prevents more exposure to scatter radiation.

- **X-ray equipment should be regularly checked and monitored.**

Radiographs as Part of the Medical Record

Radiographs are part of the medical record and the property of the veterinary hospital. Although state laws vary, radiographs are generally required to be maintained on site for 3 years. In some states, radiographs may need to be available to the hospital for 7 years.[1] Radiographs should be available for loan to the client or referring veterinarian. The client should fill out a form that gives the following information.

- Where the x-rays are going
- For what purpose they are being lent out
- When they are to be returned to the hospital

This form should stay with the medical record until the films are returned. The radiograph folder itself should state that the x-rays are the property of your hospital and they need to be returned to your hospital when the referring veterinarian is done with them. If the owner needs a copy or is permanently changing hospitals and wants all files trans-

---

[1]Required radiographic log information varies from state to state. The veterinary hospital should consult with state legal statutes to ascertain what types of information should be available within the radiographic log.

ferred, radiographs can be copied through a human radiology service.

All radiographs should be permanently labeled with the following information:

- Name of animal
- Patient identification number
- Date of exam
- Name of hospital
- Section of body being x-rayed

Labeling of the x-rays can be done by leaded letters and numbers, label tape, light-flasher system, or a film label camera. Furthermore, all radiographs should also be filed in an x-ray log. These logs should contain the following information.

- Log number identifying the radiographic study
- Date the x-ray was taken
- Patient name
- Machine settings
- Number of films taken

Types of Studies
The following section outlines types of radiographic studies and gives examples of normal and abnormal structures. The goal of this section is to understand the important structures and pathology observable in each radiographic study.

Orthopedic Films
As discussed in Chapter 8, an orthopedic study refers to an evaluation of bone and bony detail. These studies allow the veterinarian to assess bone health.

The Density of Bone Tissue
Changes in bone density can suggest bone cancer (i.e., osteosarcoma and other neoplasia), inflammation (panosteitis), and bony infection (osteomyelitis). The veterinarian can determine loss and increased or abnormal calcification. Significant changes in bone density may suggest the need for further diagnostics (i.e., complete blood count and chemistry, infectious titers, bone biopsy; see Figure 25.2).

Bone Fractures
If there is an obvious fracture or break in the bone, radiographs help the doctor evaluate the location, the extent of damage, and type of repair needed for the fracture (see Figure 25.3). As discussed in Chapter 8, common types of fractures are

- greenstick,
- transverse, and
- comminuted.

Evaluation of the Joint
The soft tissue structures of the joint (i.e., ligament, menisci, joint cartilage) do not show up on radiographs; however, x-rays allow the veterinarian to evaluate the joint for

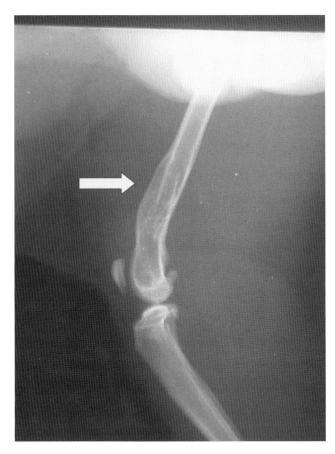

Figure 25.2. Changes in bone density seen in this femur can be an old fracture that has healed irregularly or it can suggest cancer or bony infection.

- arthritis (see Figure 25.4),
- dislocation (**subluxation**) of the bones,
- Orthopedic Foundation of America (OFA)'s Penn hip, screenings of hip dysplasia, and
- joint infection.

Soft Tissue Studies

Soft tissue studies allow the veterinarian and the veterinary team to evaluate the soft tissue structure within the chest and abdomen for changes in organ size, masses, foreign material, fluid, or infection. Although radiographs are not able to visualize internal changes within organs, changes in organ size, position, and external silhouette can indicate serious disease. Examples of soft tissue studies are discussed next.

Thoracic (Chest) Studies

Thoracic studies allow visualization of the normal anatomy while identifying changes that suggest trauma, infection, cardiac disease, or cancer (see Figure 25.5).

Abdominal Studies

Abdominal studies allow visualization of the normal anatomy while identifying changes that suggest trauma, infection, disease, or cancer.

Normal architectures (see Figure 25.6) that can be appreciated are

- liver,
- stomach,
- small and large intestines,
- spleen,
- kidney,
- bladder,
- abdominal lymph nodes, and
- uterus/prostate.

Examples of diseases (see Figure 25.7) that can be appreciated with normal abdominal radiographs are

- masses/tumors,
- kidney/bladder stones,
- torsed or rotated stomach (gastrodilatation volvulus),
- fluid in the abdomen, and
- changes in abdominal organ size.

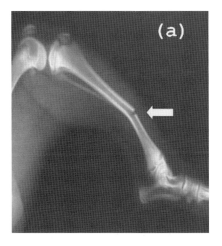
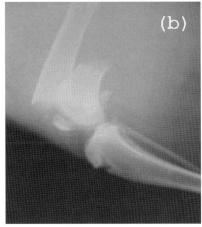
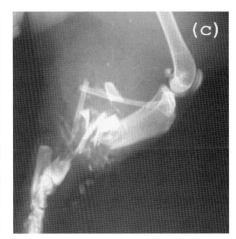

Figure 25.3. Radiographs of different types of fractures: greenstick fracture (a); transverse fracture (b); comminuted fracture (c). The x-ray allows the veterinarian to assess the potential damage and what type of repair is recommended.

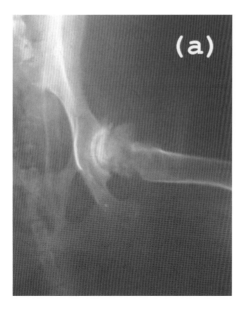
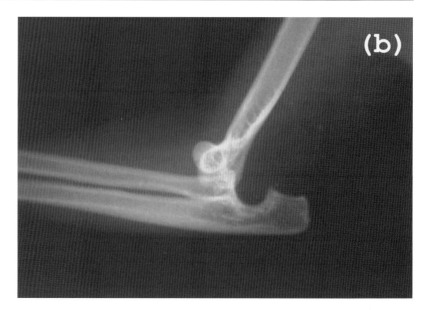

Figure 25.4.   Radiographs of joint evaluations. The x-ray shows significant arthritis within the hip (a). The humerus is subluxated out of the elbow joint (b).

Contrast Studies

Contrast studies are x-rays taken with the aid of some chemical or material that allows a change in the contrast of the surrounding tissue. This change of contrast allows the veterinarian to image structures, obstructions, or masses that may not show up on a regular film. Types of contrast material can be air (carbon dioxide), barium, iohexal (Omnipaque), or renograffin.

Specific materials (i.e., bone, metal, stone) are radio dense and will show up on a radiograph. Other material (i.e., plastic, paper, and fabric) are not dense enough to observe on a normal x-ray. To increase contrast, these materials (i.e., air, barium, etc.) are administered orally or injected. The veterinarian then takes a series of x-rays to monitor the normal flow of the material through the specific organ or cavity to assess if there is an obstruction or obstructive density.

- **Upper GI:** An upper GI is a radiographic study in which the patient ingests barium and x-rays are taken at set intervals to evaluate possible obstruction, mass, or ulceration of the esophagus, stomach, and intestine. Radiographs are generally taken until the barium flows into the large colon (see Figure 25.8). If the barium stops at a given point or is retained within a section of intestine; it can suggest an intestinal obstruction (see Chapter 10).

   Although there are many possible protocols for performing an upper GI barium series, one suggested protocol is as follows.

   1. **After plain films are taken:** Administer 3–5 cc/lb barium orally. Care should be taken to slowly administer the barium through a feeding syringe to prevent barium aspiration.

   2. **Change of radiograph settings:** From the plain film settings increase the kilovoltage by 2–3 kV to produce a sharper image because of the increased contrast material in the intestine. The time of the study (i.e., 30, 60, 120 minutes) should be written or encoded on each film.

   3. **Schedule of x-rays:** Radiographs are taken over 4 hours (it can be longer) or until the barium has moved entirely into the large colon. Radiographs should be taken on the following schedule:

      —Time 0—lateral and ventrodorsal (V/d)
      —Time 15—lateral and V/d
      —Time 30—lateral and V/d
      —Time 60—lateral and V/d
      —Time 120—lateral and V/d
      —Time 240—lateral and V/d

- **Myelogram:** This dye study of the spinal cord uses a water-soluble iodine-based solution, called iohexital, to check for strictures and pressures in the spinal cord caused by intervertebral disc extrusion or spinal masses.

   This procedure is usually performed by specialty hospitals and requires general anesthesia and careful monitoring of the patient. The dye is injected into the space around spinal cord. Lateral and V/d x-rays are taken. Normally, the upper and lower dye lines should flow down the spinal column without obstruction (see Figure 25.9).

Limitations of Radiology

Although an extremely useful diagnostic tool, radiographs have specific limitations that should be discussed with the client when applicable.

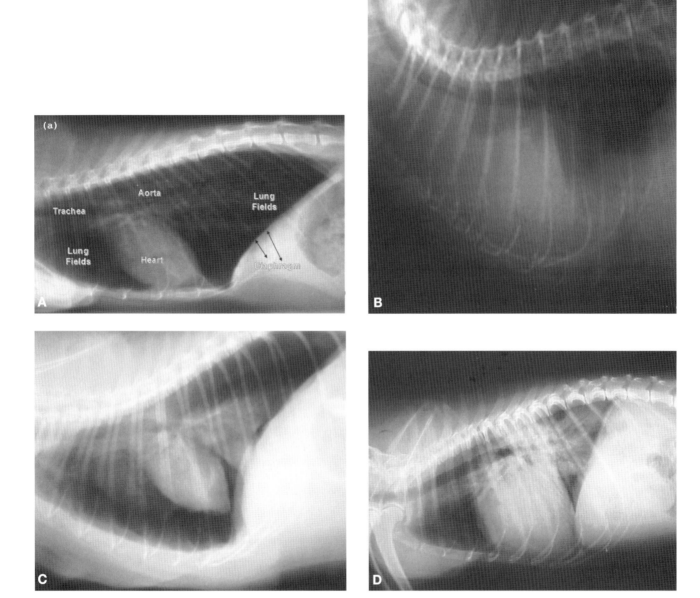

Figure 25.5. Thoracic radiographs allow the veterinarian to assess normal chest anatomy (a) and disease pathology. Examples of disease process that can be appreciated on an x-ray are seen in (b–d). Pleural effusion (b). In this film, normal anatomical definition is being obscured by a fluid line secondary to infection, cardiac disease, trauma, or other diseases of the chest. Pneumothorax (c). In this study, the heart is floating on a cushion of air as it rushes into the chest after a trauma, destroying the vacuum, and collapsing the lungs. Enlarged heart (d). This image shows a very large globelike heart suggestive of heart disease.

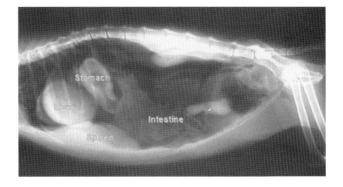

Figure 25.6. X-ray image of an feline abdomen. In this study, increased gas helps highlight each organ to increase abdominal contrast.

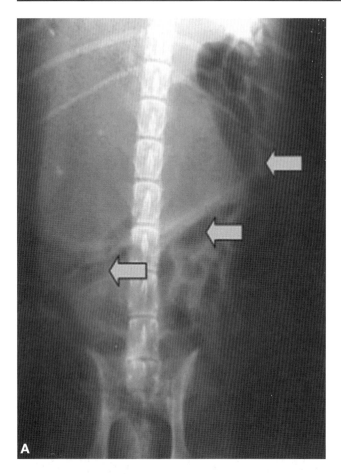

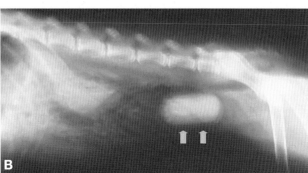

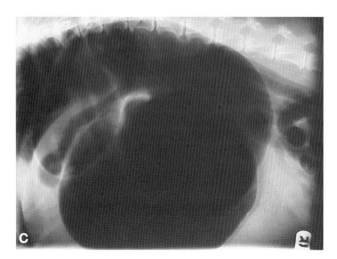

Key Points in Discussing the Importance of a Radiographic Evaluation with the Client

- Radiographs allow the doctor to assess the normal structures of the body and determine if there are any abnormalities that could suggest disease.
- There can be changes to the organs and bone (i.e., stones, areas of enlargement, masses, fluid, changes in bone density) that cannot be seen without an x-ray image.
- In some cases, repeat films (upper GI, animal with heart disease with fluid on the lungs, drowning animals) may need to be taken to assess the animal's status, its response to treatment, and the need for further diagnostics.
- With the concerns of abdominal foreign bodies, there are certain materials and items that will not show up on a plain film x-ray.
- Items such as cloth, plastic, wood, and other non-dense items may not be seen. However, the veterinarian is also examining changes in the intestinal pattern that may suggest a soft tissue obstruction.
- If your pet still is vomiting and a plain film x-ray is not enough to detect an obstruction, a barium series (an upper GI) may be needed.
- An upper GI is done when barium is given to the pet. Barium will light up and allow the veterinarian to see the liquid flow through the intestines.
- If the barium fails to move through the intestines in a set amount of time or there are areas that continue to retain barium, this could be suggestive of a mass, ulceration, or obstruction.
- X-rays are a very helpful diagnostic tool; however, they have limitations, and even the best x-ray studies or contrast studies may not be completely inclusive. Other diagnostics may be suggested.

- **Radiographs do not visualize non-radio dense material or soft tissue structures.** X-rays do not allow the appreciation of non-radio dense foreign material (i.e., cloth, plastic, paper, string) that could cause severe gastrointestinal obstruction. Furthermore, orthopedic radiographs cannot visualize soft tissue structures associated with joints, the spinal column, and limbs. Therefore, an injured ligament, an extruded intervertebral disc, or a torn tendon will not show up on an x-ray.
- **Radiographs cannot distinguish pathology in internal organ disease:** X-rays can suggest changes in organ size

Figure 25.7. Examples of diseases that can be detected with abdominal radiography. Abdominal masses (a). A large mass (arrows) is pushing the intestines to the right and taking up a large portion of the middle abdomen. Stones (b). A large calcified bladder stone is evident. Stomach torsion (c). The stomach is twisted around its own axis (gastrodilatation volvulus).

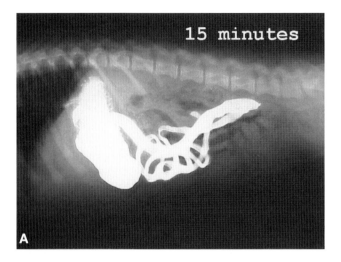

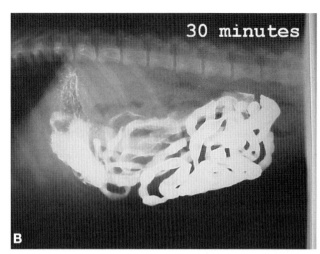

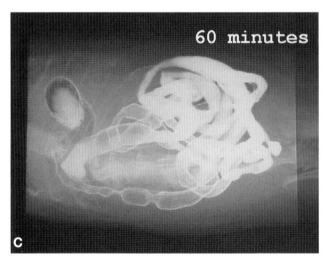

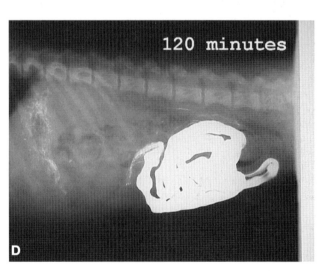

Figure 25.8. Radiographic images of an barium series. Although both lateral and V/d radiographs were taken at each time interval, the lateral x-rays show a progression of dye through the stomach and small intestine and into the lower small intestine.

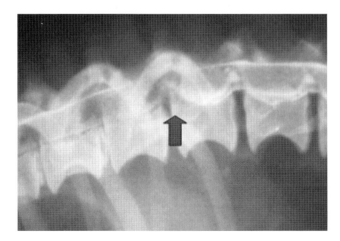

Figure 25.9. Radiograph of a myelogram series. Note the dye lines on the dorsal and ventral aspect of the spinal cord. The arrow delineates an area where the ventral line is pushed dorsally and the dye line thins. This could be suggestive of a mass or disc pushing upward on the spinal column.

suggesting disease pathology. However, merely seeing abnormally enlarged organs (i.e., kidney, liver, spleen) cannot distinguish the cause of the organ enlargement.

- **Radiographs are a health hazard to the medical team:** As stated previously, radiograph radiation can be a health hazard to the medical team. Standardized protocols in performing and restraining animals must be in place to minimize radiation exposure and risk to the team and the patient.

Ultrasound

Ultrasound examination allows imaging of internal thoracic and abdominal organs without the need for surgery. Most units are portable and pose no radiation risk. Ultrasound exams allow a visualization of internal structures and architecture that can suggest disease, infection, inflammation, or pathology.

Technology

Sound is defined as a mechanical pressure wave made up of a series of compressions and rarefactions transmitted through a specific medium. Ultrasound uses focused sound waves that are emitted at a specific frequency (speed) that then encounter a tissue density. Some of these waves are reflected back to the ultrasound emitter. Different densities of tissues reflect the sound waves at different speeds and amounts. These waves are visualized as images of gray; the stronger the echoed wave, the brighter the image. Thus increased density means increased echo and a brighter image.

Ultrasounds use piezo crystals. The electrical energy in the crystal produces mechanical sound waves that echo back after hitting dense structures. The piezo crystals then reabsorb the sound waves and turn their amplitude into a physical image that is transmitted on a monitor. These crystals listen for rebounding waves 99.9% of the time and emit sound waves .1% of the time, so there is very little sound energy released while performing an ultrasound. Ultrasounds are able to produce and rebound their sound waves through solid and liquid interfaces but are unable to visualize through an air interface (i.e., the lungs).

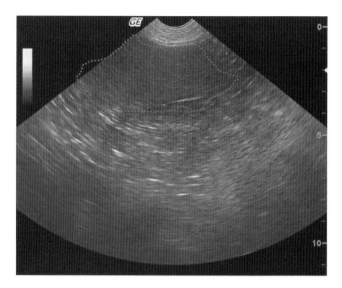

Figure 25.10. Image of a spleen surrounded by abdominal fat. Both the spleen (surrounded by dots) and surrounding fat are echoic structures, but the fat is hyperechoic (brighter) in comparison with the spleen.

Safety

Because ultrasounds emit only a small amount of sound waves, there are no health concerns to patients or the medical team secondary to ultrasound exposure.

Preparation of Animal

- Hair contains air pockets and hence ultrasound waves cannot go through the hair coat.
- The animal must be shaved and a conduction gel must be applied to allow the passage of sound waves.
- Most healthy animals will tolerate an ultrasound exam without any form of sedation or anesthesia, just proper restraint.

Terminology

Ultrasound studies produce grayscale images of internal structures. Veterinary evaluation of the images compares the brightness and density of one organ to another tissue. These grayscale comparisons have specific terminology.

- **Echogenicity:** The strength or amplitude of the returning echo is referred to as echogenicity. **Echogenic** structures produce echoes, and **anechogenic** structures are unable to produce echoes (i.e., lung tissue).
- **Density:** Images are discussed in terms of density (see Figure 25.10) as
  - **Hyperechoic:** Structures that are brighter than the surrounding tissue.
  - **Isoechoic:** Structures that have the same brightness as surrounding tissue.
  - **Hypoechoic:** Structures that have decreased brightness as surrounding tissue.

Ultrasound Exam

Types of ultrasound studies used can vary from species to species.

For large animals, ultrasound studies can be used for the following purposes.

- **Pregnancy diagnosis:** Ultrasound studies are used for intrarectal examination in the horse and large ruminant (i.e., cow) or abdominal detection in the small ruminant; it is an excellent tool to use to diagnose and follow pregnancy. Furthermore, the ovaries can be imaged to aid in estimation of the heat cycle and breeding times.
- **Tendon examination:** Ultrasonic exam of the limb allows the imaging and evaluation of deep tendons and muscles for damage, infection, or masses. Furthermore, the ultrasound can help obtain a cellular aspirate of a mass or drain fluid-filled regions in damaged tissue.
- **Abdominal disease:** As with the small animal examination, ultrasound examination of internal organs can be performed to detect infection, inflammation, or masses in abdominal structures.

For small animals ultrasound studies can be used for the following purposes.

- **Abdominal:** Abdominal studies allow the veterinarian to assess if there are changes in normal tissue pattern or changes in tissue brightness, internal masses, or fluid-filled structures that can suggest disease (see Figure 25.11). Furthermore, the abdomen can be evaluated for evidence of free fluid, suggesting liver disease, bleeding,

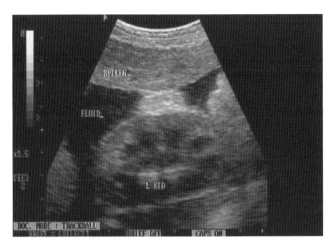

Figure 25.11. Ultrasound image of a spleen and left kidney. The ultrasound allows an evaluation of internal structure as well as a comparison of echogenicity to other tissues, which could suggest organ disease.

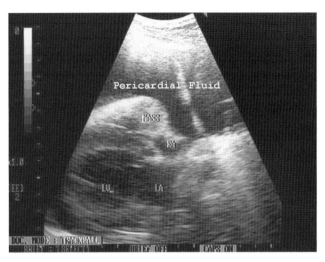

Figure 25.12. An ultrasound of the long axis of the heart. This heart is surrounded by fluid due to a mass on the right atrium (RA).

cancer, and other potential causes. Lastly, the ultrasound can aid in guiding biopsy instruments so tissue and fluid samples can be obtained.

- **Chest:** Cardiac ultrasound is an extremely important diagnostic tool to evaluate changes in the cardiac wall, changes of the valves within the heart, evaluation of contractility of the heart, evidence of masses or tumors, and appreciation of fluid around the heart, or pericardial effusion (see Figure 25.12). Furthermore, the region between the heart and lungs, the **mediastinum,** can be evaluated for masses or fluid from infection or cancer.

Limitations of Ultrasound Diagnostics
Thoracic Studies
Ultrasound waves cannot be carried through an air medium. Therefore, lung tissue cannot be evaluated with an ultrasound exam. Masses within the lungs must be in direct contact within the chest wall in order to be visualized. Furthermore, the lung fields can obscure and limit the exposure of the heart or mediastinal region.

Abdominal Studies
Ultrasound is very good at detecting changes within tissue that can suggest organ disease or cancer. However, without a biopsy, ultrasound cannot identify the type of disease affecting an organ system. Multiple diseases (i.e., infection, cancer, inflammation, metabolic disease) can all appear as similar diffuse organ disease on ultrasound diagnostics. In many cases, (i.e., liver, kidney, spleen, and other organ diseases), owners must understand that although the ultrasound can help distinguish if an organ seems affected, it cannot help diagnose the cause of the process without a tissue biopsy.

Discussing Ultrasound with the Client
- Ultrasound is a noninvasive diagnostic test that allows the veterinarian to image the internal architecture of the abdominal organs and the heart.
- Ultrasound cannot image the lung fields because the sound waves cannot reflect back through air.
- There are many times when the ultrasound will reveal a mass or fluid-filled area that can directly relate to a disease problem.
- However, there are times when the ultrasound will only suggest changes in organs based on the brightness or change in tissue density.
- Ultrasounds are not a replacement for x-rays, because radiographs allow the veterinarian to get specific information about sizes of organs, changes in the chest cavity, and changes in the bone that ultrasounds cannot always pick up.
- A cardiac ultrasound can help the veterinarian understand the inner anatomical changes and function of the heart so that the best medical recommendations are available to treat the underlying disease.
- Ultrasound can be a very powerful diagnostic test, but there are times when further diagnostics may need to be recommended to more fully understand the disease process.

Endoscopy

Endoscopy is the use of a fiber-optic camera that can be passed into the upper gastrointestinal system, the lower intestinal system, and the respiratory system to help image and diagnose disease. The procedures are done under general anesthesia, but are not invasive because there is no surgical incision. The endoscope allows access to regions that normally would be unreachable without major surgery. Some of these regions are

- esophagus,
- trachea,
- bronchi,
- nasal sinus, and
- the vulva.

There are both rigid and flexible endoscopes of different sizes and for different purposes. One endoscope does not have the ability to handle all sizes of animals and all needs.

Technology
The fiber-optic endoscope allows for intestinal exploration of the upper gastrointestinal system (the esophagus, stomach, and possibly early small intestines). The lower colon can also be imaged by introducing the endoscope through the rectum. Finally, the trachea and bronchi can be examined through a special connecter in the anesthesia machine that allows the scope to enter through the endotracheal tube (see Figure 25.13).

Safety
Because endoscopy requires general anesthesia, there is a mild anesthetic risk to the patient (see Chapter 29).

Types of Studies
Removal of Foreign Bodies/Foreign Material
In some cases certain foreign material can be removed with the endoscope from the early intestinal system without the need for surgery. These items are usually small enough to grasp with the endoscope's basket or graspers and removed through the esophagus. Items that can sometimes be removed with this procedure include

- hooks and needles,
- bone spurs, and
- other small foreign debris.

Examination of Intestinal or Bronchial Lining (Mucosa) and Biopsy
The endoscope can image the intestinal lining and take tissue for biopsy. The biopsy tissue is a very small, partial-thickness section of the region that will be examined to aid in the overall diagnosis of the disease.

Culture and Sensitivity/Brushings of the Respiratory Tract
When there are concerns of chronic infection or potential cancer in the trachea and lungs, the endoscope can be passed through the trachea into the deeper bronchi. Once there, samples of debris and purulent material can be collected to

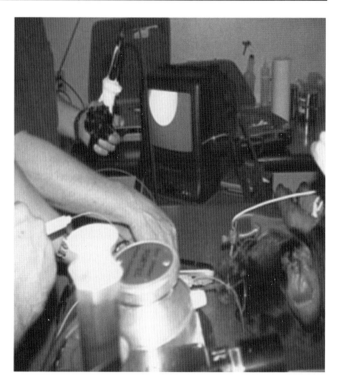

Figure 25.13. Endoscopy allows access to many regions of the body without surgery. It can further aid in the removal of certain foreign material, biopsy of sites, or even perform culture and sensitivity tests for potential infections.

help diagnose the bacterial infection or to obtain cell samples that may suggest the infectious cause or evidence of cancer.

Preparation
Animals need to fast for at least 12–18 hours prior to the endoscopy to ensure that the stomach is empty. The endoscopy does not work well navigating through intestinal contents. For a lower endoscopy (colonoscopy), multiple enemas are generally given the day before with a solution called **Golytely** to aid in cleansing the colon prior to the test. All animals undergoing an endoscopy should be good anesthetic candidates for the procedure.

Limitations to Endoscopy
Depending on the size of the endoscope, the pet, and its anatomy, the endoscope cannot always get into the regions that need to be examined, especially going into the small intestine or smaller bronchi. Not all foreign bodies can be removed due to their size, thickness, and location. If they cannot be removed with the endoscope, the foreign bodies will need to be removed surgically.

Obtaining Biopsy Tissue
The tissue for biopsy obtained are small samples of the intestine. The samples are surface layers and do not go to full

thickness. The endoscope can only take tissue from the upper gastrointestinal tract or lower colon. If the tissues are not inclusive enough, the animal may need to have exploratory surgery so that full thickness of the entire intestinal system and other organs can be taken to biopsy.

Endoscopy of the Trachea and Bronchi

The endoscope can penetrate to the level of the deeper bronchi but not to the level of the bronchioles or alveoli. Some diseases will not be evident at the bronchi level, and some tumors will not shed enough cells to suggest disease at this level either. In some cases when an endoscopy is not helpful, other procedures such as an MRI or CAT scan may be needed to help visualize the entire lung field. In other cases a surgical approach to the chest (**thoracotomy**) may be needed to examine the chest and possibly remove a mass or severely infected lung lobe.

CD-ROM 2 will focus on concepts of understanding and discussing clinical diagnostics and the disease conditions represented. The exercises can be done individually or as case rounds as they explore specific topics in veterinary medicine that discuss clinical diagnostics and treatment.

Discussing the Endoscopy with Clients

- An endoscopy is an exploration of the stomach and early small intestines, the colon, or trachea and bronchi with a fiber-optic or rigid camera.
- An endoscopy requires anesthetic, and the animal must be a good candidate for anesthesia.
- An intravenous catheter, with or without fluids, presurgical blood work, and full anesthetic monitoring may be needed to fully evaluate and maintain the patient while under anesthesia.
- An endoscopy is limited to the ability of the scope to access the sites in question. Depending on the animal's anatomy and the size and length of the scope, some areas cannot be reached. The endoscope cannot reach all areas of the intestines or lungs.
- If there is a foreign body evident, it may not be possible to retrieve it with an endoscope, and the pet may still require surgery. Furthermore, if the animal has eaten prior to ingesting the foreign body, it may be impossible to navigate around the intestinal contents to retrieve the material with an endoscope.
- With respect to a biopsy, the endoscope can take small, partial (not full thickness) samples of the areas that are within reach. The partial-thickness tissue biopsy can help in the diagnosis, but at times full-thickness samples of the entire intestine may be needed. In order to do this, an exploratory surgery may be needed.
- The endoscope can go only into a certain depth of the trachea and bronchi (bronchoscopy). Culture and sensitivity and brush samples may be very helpful in diagnosis of the disease; however, other procedures may need to be done to more fully explore the chest cavity, such as a CAT scan, MRI, or a surgical exploration into the chest (a thoracotomy).

Section 4

Understanding the Concepts of Disease and Treatment

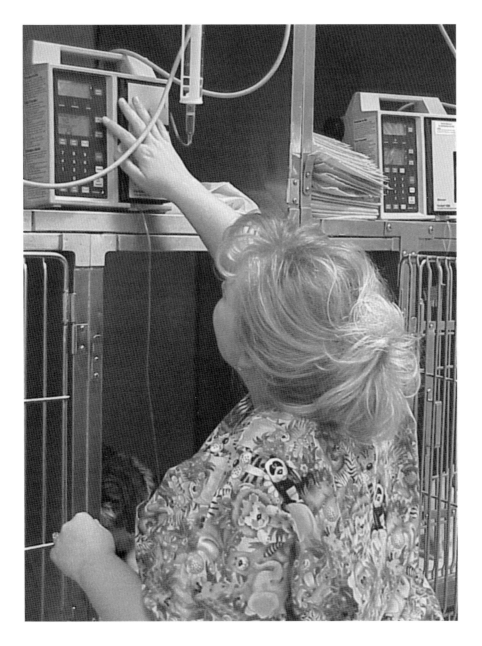

The goal of this section is to understand the concepts of treatment so the team member can monitor the patient, identify symptoms of shock, and help the veterinarian treat the hospitalized animals.

Chapter 26

Pharmacology

Introducion

A drug is defined as a substance used therapeutically in the treatment of a disease or illness. In veterinary medicine drugs fall into many categories, such as treatment of disease, anesthesia, behavioral modification, treatment of pain, and other needs. For the purpose of this book, the drugs will be limited to prescription medications, wormers and antiparasitics, and emergency injectable medication. A list of commonly used drug categories is as follows:

- Antibiotics
- Fluids
- Antifungals
- Antiparasitics
- Antivirals
- Chemotherapeutics
- Anesthesias
- Sedatives
- Behavioral modifiers
- Non-steroidal anti-inflammatory medications
- Steroids
- Vaccines

Drug Delivery Systems

Drugs can be given by various routes depending on the disease process, the drug, and the needs of the patient. It is important for the medical team member to understand the goals and risks of medicating the patient using each route of administration.

Intravenous Route

Intravenous (IV) drugs are sterile drugs that are safe to give through an intravenous catheter or syringe. Only drugs marked safe for IV use can be given intravenously. If a drug not labeled for this use is given intravenously, an animal could die instantly of anaphylactic shock. In general, IV drugs should be given slowly and the patient monitored for reactions. If there is any concern regarding giving a drug intravenously, a veterinarian should be consulted prior to administration of the drug. IV drugs tend to have an instantaneous or quick-acting effect on the animal.

Intramuscular Route

Intramuscular (IM) drugs are meant to go into a large muscle mass for slightly slower absorption than those given by IV administration. Drugs that are delivered intramuscularly should be labeled for IM use. Some drugs can be very irritating if not given intravenously and may cause severe reactions if not given by their normal route. Commonly, IM injections are given in the large muscle mass of the hind limbs or in the muscle of the lumber spine (canine). Caution should be used when giving IM injections into the large hind limb muscle mass; improperly injected, it can accidentally enter into the sciatic nerve, a long nerve of the hind limb. This can produce long-standing paralysis and inability to use the leg properly.

Subcutaneous Route

Subcutaneous (Sq) drug administration is the safest and easiest route of drug delivery. However, it is also the slowest route for the drug to take effect for the animal. Some drugs (i.e., dextrose or fluids with dextrose) can be irritating and should not be given subcutaneously because severe skin reaction or skin sloughing can occur. If there are any questions consult your veterinarian.

Dosing Terminology

As with most fields of veterinary medicine, drug dosing and anatomical charting has its own nomenclature for prescription documentation. The basic abbreviations are as follows.

For dosing, the nomenclature is

- SID: 1×/day
- BID: 2×/day
- TID: 3×/day
- QID: 4×/day
- EOD: Every other day
- ETD: Every third day
- PRN: As needed.

For anatomical nomenclature, the terms are as follows.

- Eyes
  — OU: Both eyes
  — OD: Right eye
  — OS: Left Eye

- Ears
  — AU: Both ears
  — AD: Right ear
  — AS: Left ear
- By Mouth: Per OS (PO)

- **Example A:** Give 100 mg amoxicillin BID PO × 14 days: translates into 1 tablet twice a day by mouth for 14 days.
- **Example B:** Give 1/8-inch strip of Triple Antibiotic ophthalmic medication TID OU × 14 days: translates into give 1/8 inch in both eyes three times per day for 14 days.
- **Example C:** Give 300 mg cefazolin TID IV × 3 days: translates into give 300 mg intravenously every 8 hours for the next 3 days. (This would be an in-hospital treatment).

Drug Dosing

To properly medicate a patient, all team members should be able to calculate the proper drug dose. Although it is the veterinarian's responsibility to make sure the proper dose and route is used, the team members should be able to calculate the proper dose and administer the medication when requested. The following protocol is meant to help make sure the proper dose is always calculated and administered safely.

Step 1: **Never give any medication by any route of which you are unsure.** If a team member is faced with giving a new medication or giving a known medication by an unusual route (i.e., giving a subcutaneous medication intravenously), the medication should not be given without first discussing it with the veterinarian.

Step 2: Convert the pet's weight into the proper units (i.e., kilograms to pounds or pounds to kilograms). Many doses of medication can be milligrams per kilogram or milligrams per pound. It is very important that the medical team dose for the correct weight measurement. A miscalculation can overdose or severely underdose a patient. The conversions from pounds to kilograms or kilograms to pounds are as follows.

---

1 kg = 2.2 lb or 11 lb = 5 kg

- **Example A:** Convert 33-pound dog to its weight in kilograms:

    33 = 3 × 11 lb = 3 × 5kg = 15 kg or
    33 lb/2.2 = 15 kg

- **Example B:** Convert a 20-kilogram dog to its weight in pounds:

    20 kg × 2.2 lb/kg = 44 lb

Step 3: Calculate the patient's dose requirement. Often this step is calculated by the veterinarian; however, there are doses that may be common knowledge to the team members (i.e., dose of amoxicillin: 10 mg/lb). To calculate the patient's dose:

Patient's dose = Dose in mg/kg or mg/lbs × weight (kg or pounds

- **Example A:** 40 pound dog requires 10 mg/pound dose of Amoxicillin Sq:

    Dose = 10 mg/pound × 40 pounds = 400 mg IM

- **Example B:** 30 kg dose requires a dose of 1.5 mg/kg of a drug IM

    Dose = 1.5 mg/kg × 30 kg = 45 mg

Step 4: Calculate milliliters needed for the dose. Once the patient's dose has been calculated, the amount of milliliters needed is the final step. To accomplish this, the team member multiplies the number of milligrams needed divided by concentration of the drug (mg/ml).

Milliliters needed for dose = dose ÷ concentration of drug

- **Example A:** 400 mg of ampicillin/100 mg/ml ampicillin = 4 ml or cc.
- **Example B:** 45 mg of drug/20 mg/ml of drug = 2.25 ml or cc.

When dealing with solutions with a percentage of concentration (i.e., 2% lidocaine, 50% dextrose, etc.), the percent solution refers to the fact that 100% solution = 1000 mg/mg or 1000 g/l. To calculate how many milligrams per milliliter are in a percent solution, perform the following:

Mg/ml = % solution × 10, then as above.
Milliliters needed for dose = dose ÷ concentration of drug.

- **Example A:** 2% lidocaine solution contains = 2 × 10 = 20 mg/ml. Dose needed is 200 mg. Milliliters needed = 200 mg/20 mg/ml = 10 ml.
- **Example B:** 50% dextrose contains = 50 × 10 = 500 mg/ml. Dose needed is 25 mg. Milliliters needed = 25 mg/500 mg/ml = 0.05 ml.

Responsibilities of the Medical Team

Although the liability of prescription medication is ultimately the responsibility of the veterinarian, all team members are responsible for filling prescriptions and medicating patients. Each team member must be responsible for understanding the following information about each drug before administering or filling any medication.

Type of Drug Administered
Each team member should have an understanding of the drug given, its function, and why it is being administered. *If team members do not have a basic understanding of why the medication is being given, they cannot monitor if the patient is responding properly to medication.* Furthermore, certain drugs (i.e., chemotherapy drugs) must be handled and disposed of carefully because they can pose a danger to the medical team or the client.

Route of Administration
As discussed previously, all medications have safe routes of administration. Specific drugs cannot be given intravenously without concern of massive anaphylactic reaction and death, whereas other drugs should not be given subcutaneously due to irritation or skin sloughing.

Date of Expiration
It is always important to evaluate the expiration date to make sure the drug is still effective. Furthermore, specific medications that may need to be reconstituted with sterile saline may have only a limited date of effectiveness. For example, certain intravenous antibiotics once reconstituted may be usable for only 72–96 hours with refrigeration.

Contraindications
Specific drugs may be contraindicated for a specific age group, sex, or species. It is extremely important that the medical team be aware of the most common drugs' contraindications to make sure that certain drugs are not administered or prescribed. For example, acepromazine (tranquillizer) should not be administered to pets prone to seizures (see below).

Side Effects
As with contraindications, some drugs produce moderate to serious side effects. The medical team should be aware of these concerns to monitor the patient for any significant changes and to forewarn the client of potential changes in their pet. For example, oral and injectable steroidal medications can increase thirst, urination, and appetite in canines.

Drug Interactions
Many drugs can have serious to life-threatening side effects if given in combination with other medication. The medical team should be aware of the more common drug interactions and make sure the patient is not on medications that interfere with others. For example, steroidal medication and other types of nonsteroidal anti-inflammatory medication (i.e., aspirin) should never be given together unless the veterinarian and client are both aware of the potential concern of gastric ulceration and/or perforation.

Drug Classes

Antibiotics
Antibiotics are drugs that stop the growth of or kill infectious bacterial pathogens. Antibiotics have different modes of function to stop or destroy bacterial cell growth. There are two overall groups:

- **Bacteriostatic antibiotics:** These antibiotics stop the growth of foreign bacteria, but do not kill them. The patient must have an active immune system to destroy the inactivated bacteria.
- **Bactericidal antibiotics:** These antibiotics destroy bacteria populations and wipe out the possible infections. Bactericidal antibiotics are generally not used with other bacteriostatic antibiotics because bactericidal medications rely on large populations of rapidly dividing normal bacteria to stop bacterial action. If the bacterium is being wiped out from another bacterial agent, bacteriostatic bacteria are less effective.

Penicillin Family
Antibacterial activity is accomplished by inhibition of bacterial wall synthesis. It has broad bacterial activity against gram-negative and gram-positive bacteria. Access to mammalian tissue is generally adequate to combat bacterial infections with exception of intraocular and intracerebral sites. Inflammation to these sites may enhance penetrability to the site of the infection. Penicillins are very safe because they target a process in bacterial cell walls that are not present in mammalian cells.

Forms of Drug
- Penicillin (Procaine Pen-G)
- Amoxicillin trihydrate/clavulanate potassium (Clavamox/Unasyn)
- Ampicillin (Polyflex, Ampicillin IV)
- Amoxicillin (Amoxi-Tabs)

Route of Administration
The route of drug administration depends on the preparation of the penicillin. There are penicillins that are only to be given subcutaneously or intramuscularly (i.e., Polyflex, Amoxi-Inject, Procaine Pen-G). There are other groups that are safe for intravenous administration (i.e., Unasyn, ampicillin IV injectable). Care should be taken to make sure medication is safe for administering intravenous penicillin. Almost all forms of penicillin have an oral form.

Contraindications
The penicillin family is generally safe for use in mammals. However, these drugs should not be used with animals that are allergic to the penicillins. Furthermore, for animals with impaired renal function, the dosage of the drug should be decreased with the extent to which renal function is impaired. (i.e., creatinine clearance).

Side Effects

Side effects are rare but can include the following.

- Gastrointestinal upsets: Vomiting and diarrhea
- Allergic reaction: Animals sensitive to penicillins can have
    — mild allergic reactions: Rashes, erythema, pruritus, and hives.
    — anaphylaxis (rare): Collapse, weakness, bronchoconstriction, respiratory wheezes, and death.

Drug Interactions

It is generally recommended that penicillins not be used with bacteriostatic (i.e., tetracycline) antibiotics because these drugs impair bacterial wall synthesis.

Cephalosporin Family

Antibacterial activity is accomplished by inhibition of bacterial wall synthesis. The antibiotics generally have broad bacterial activity against gram-negative and poor response to gram-positive bacteria. Access to mammalian tissue is generally adequate to combat bacterial infections, with exception of intraocular, prostatic, and intracerebral sites. Inflammation of these sites may enhance penetrability to the site of the infection. Cephalosporins are very safe because they target a process in bacterial cell walls that is not present in mammalian cells.

Forms of Drug
- Cephalexin
- Cefazolin sodium (cefazolin)
- Cefadroxil (Cefa-Tabs)
- Cefoxitin (Mefoxitin)
- Simplecef

Route of Administration

The route of drug administration depends on the preparation of the cephalosporin. Care should be taken to make sure medication is safe for intravenous administration.

Contraindications

The cephalosporin family of antibiotics is generally safe in mammals. However, these drugs should not be used for animals that are allergic to the cephalosporins. Furthermore, the dosage of the drug should be decreased in animals with impaired renal function, depending on the severity of renal dysfunction (i.e., creatinine clearance).

Side Effects

Side effects are rare, but can include

- gastrointestinal upsets (i.e., vomiting/diarrhea),
- allergic reaction (animals sensitive to cephalosporin), producing
    — mild allergic reactions: rashes, erythema, pruritus, and hives

    — anaphylaxis (rare): collapse, weakness, bronchoconstriction, respiratory wheezes, and death.

Drug Interactions

It is generally recommended that cephalosporins not be used with bacteriostatic (i.e., tetracycline) antibiotics because these drugs impair bacterial wall synthesis.

Cephalosporins may enhance nephrotoxicity (kidney damage) of aminoglycoside (i.e. Gentacin, amikacin).

Fluoroquinolone Family

A fluoroquinolone antimicrobial drug is a bactericidal antibiotic that affects a wide spectrum of gram-negative and gram-positive aerobic bacterial pathogens. It is ineffective against anaerobic bacteria and has variable effectiveness against streptococci. The fluoroquinolone's mechanism of antimicrobial action is an inhibition of enzymes necessary for bacterial DNA replication and is unique among antibiotics. The drug's ability to penetrate tissue, including difficult to access regions such bone, prostate, and cerebrospinal sites, supersedes that of most antimicrobial agents. Penetration into mammalian cells makes it effective for infections at intracellular sites (chlamydia, mycoplasma, mycobacterium). Since high concentrations of active fluoroquinolones and metabolites are eliminated in the urine, the drug is valuable in the treatment of genitourinary tract infections.

Forms of Drug
- Enrofloxacin (Baytril)
- Marbofloxacin (Zeniquin)
- Ciprofloxacin (Cipro)

Route of Administration

The route of drug administration depends on the preparation of the fluoroquinolone. Care should be taken to make sure medication is safe to administer intravenously. Most of this family comes in oral medication; however, enrofloxacin is also available in injectable and otic preparations.

Contraindications

The drug should be used cautiously in skeletally immature animals (including pregnant females) because the drug may cause microscopic cartilage lesions leading to lameness in weight-bearing joints of the body. Age restriction should be longer (up to 18 months) in larger breed dogs. Also reported to cause retinal lesions in cats.

Higher doses of fluoroquinolones may promote seizure activity. This tendency may be enhanced in epileptics and in animals with structural central nervous system (CNS) disease.

Side Effects

Side effects are rare but can include

- gastrointestinal upsets (i.e., vomiting/diarrhea), and
- retinal lesions in felines when doses exceed 2.5–5 mg/ kg/day.

Drug Interactions
Caution should be exercised when fluoroquinolones are used with the following drugs.

- **GI protectants:** Drugs such as sulcrafate, magnesium- and aluminum-containing antacids, and calcium- and iron-containing dietary supplements decrease oral absorption of enrofloxacin.
- **Chloramphenicol:** The antibiotic chloramphenicol may decrease enrofloxacin efficacy.
- **Theophylline:** The bronchodilator's metabolism may be slowed by fluoroquinolones leading to accumulation of toxic (CNS stimulatory) levels of the latter drug.

Tetracycline Family
Tetracyclines act by inhibition of microbial protein synthesis. It is a bacteriostatic and affects a broad spectrum of aerobic and anaerobic bacterial and nonbacterial pathogens, including *Mycoplasma, Chlamydia,* and *Rickettsia* species. As a group, tetracyclines affect spirochetes, including Lyme disease-causing organisms.

Forms of Drug
- Doxycycline
- Tetracycline
- Oxytetracycline

Route of Administration
Most of this family comes in oral medication; however, some forms of the drug are available in injectable preparations. Care should be taken to make sure medication is safe for administration intravenously.

Contraindications
The drug should be used cautiously in skeletally and dentally immature patients (i.e., no permanent teeth descended) because tetracyclines can damage developing bone and teeth, leading to permanent lesions. These drugs should be avoided throughout pregnancy because they readily cross the placenta and also should be avoided in neonatal life (until bone/teeth development is completed) if possible.

Side Effects
Side effects are rare but can include

- gastrointestinal upsets (i.e., vomiting/diarrhea),
- fevers (hyperthermias) in cats, which are more sensitive to tetracyclines and may have aberrant increases in body temperature (rare), and
- rashes or irritations of mucous membranes (photosensitization), causing lesions on the skin and mucocutaneous tissue when exposed to ultraviolet light (rare).

Drug Interactions
Caution should be exercised when tetracyclines are used with the following drugs:

- **GI protectants and supplements:** Drugs such as nutritional supplements and drugs (antacids, antiemetics, and antidiarrheal preparations) containing calcium, magnesium, aluminum, zinc, iron, and bismuth can bind tetracyclines and lower their overall activity.
- **Bactericidal antibiotics:** In general, it is recommended that bacteriostatic antibiotics such as tetracycline not be administered simultaneously with bactericidal drugs (i.e., penicillins, cephalosporins) that affect bacterial cell wall formation.

Trimethoprim—Sulfa Family
The trimethoprim family disrupts folic acid metabolism and nucleic synthesis. Against bacteria it generally exerts a bactericidal action. The drug has a relatively broad spectrum of antibacterial activity against gram-negative and gram-positive bacteria and generally has a greater effect against aerobic than against anaerobic organisms. A specific drug in this family (i.e., Tribrissen) also inhibits the growth of protozoa (i.e., coccidia, toxoplasma).

Form of the Drug
- Trimethoprim-Sulfa (Tribrissen)
- Trimethoprim/sulfamethoxazole (Bactrim)
- Ormetoprim/sulfadimethoxine (Primor)

Route of Administration
Most drugs in this family come in oral medication; however, some forms of the drug are available in injectable preparations. Care should be taken to make sure medication is safe to administer intravenously.

Precautions/Contraindications
- **Organ disease:** Caution should be used in animals with extensive liver or kidney disease.
- **Breed sensitivity:** The drug should be avoided in animals with breed susceptibilities (see below) and in animals with ocular disorders.
- **Pregnancy:** Caution should be used with pregnant animals, since birth defects have been reported with certain sulfa drugs.

Side Effects
- **Gastrointestinal system:** Upsets (anorexia, vomiting, and diarrhea) may result from flora alterations.
- **Urinary tract:** Trimethoprim sulfa can precipitate in the urine to cause crystalluria (especially if urine is acidic).
- **Anaphylaxis:** Too rapid intravenous administration may lead to a shocklike state with weakness, tremors, and collapse.
- **Blood populations:** Particularly with prolonged therapy, blood population abnormalities, such as anemia, thrombocytopenia, and granulocytopenia have been noted; this may be prevented/treated with folic acid therapy.
- **Dry eye:** Keratoconjunctivitis sicca is a side effect of sulfonamide therapy in dogs.

- **Autoimmune conditions:** Large breed dogs (e.g., Dobermans, rotteweilers) have demonstrated a higher incidence of hypersensitivity reactions (polyarthritis, hemolytic anemia, hepatic disorders).
- **Hypothyroidism:** Long-term therapy in dogs may lead to thyroid dysfunction.

Drug Interactions

Because trimethoprim sulfa drugs are extensively bound to plasma proteins, concurrent use with other plasma protein-bound drugs (e.g., aspirin) may affect the bioavailability by displacement from binding sites.

Metronidazole

Metronidazole is a synthetic antimicrobial agent. Following intracellular conversion to metabolic products, it interacts with microbial nucleic acids, leading to a lethal effect on the organism. It has a limited spectrum of antibacterial activity, affecting primarily anaerobic organisms. It also has widespread antiprotozoal activity and is used to treat Giardia and Trichomonas infections. In mixed aerobic and anaerobic bacterial infections, additional antibiotics are required to eliminate the aerobic organisms.

Form of Drug

Metronidazole (Flagyl) is available in tablets, liquid suspension, and injectable form.

Route of Administration

Metronidazole is available in an oral and injectable form.

Contraindications

- **Hepatic disease:** Dosage should be decreased for animals with hepatic disease.
- **Pregnancy:** Because of its teratogenic effects, the drug should not be administered to animals that are in their first trimester of pregnancy unless there is no other drug alternative.
- **Neurologic disease:** Animals with neurologic dysfunction may be more susceptible to the concentration-dependent neurotoxicity of metronidazole.

Side Effects

- **Gastrointestinal upsets:** Vomiting and diarrhea may occur if medication is not given with food.
- **CNS toxicity:** Metronidazole causes concentration-dependent CNS dysfunction producing signs of
  — ataxia,
  — lethargy,
  — tremors, and
  — seizure.
- **Birth defects:** Flagyl can produce birth defects in pregnant animals due to metronidazole's ability to affect cellular DNA.

Drug Interactions

Due to metronidazole's reliance on hepatic biotransformation for elimination, drugs that induce drug metabolism may lead to a diminished effect of metronidazole or drugs that affect biotransformation may increase its activity. The following drugs should be used with caution with concurrent administration of metronidazole.

Drugs that promote hepatic metabolism and decrease Metronidazole activity are

- phenobarbital, and
- primidone.

Drugs that reduce hepatic metabolism and increase metronidazole activity are

- cimetidine, and
- chloramphenicol.

Antihistamine Medication

Antihistamines prevent and reverse the pathological effects of endogenously released histamine (e.g., in allergic disorders, by concurrent drug administration, with histamine-producing tumors such as mast cell tumors). These medications also exert an antiemetic action, especially in cases of motion sickness. The sedative effect may be of value in animals with severe pruritus, with the tendency to cause self-mutilation.

Form of the Drug

There are many different types of antihistamine medications. Most medications come in oral tablets, syrups, and suspensions. A few types (i.e., diphenhydramine) come in injectable medication. Antihistamine effects can be extremely variable from animal to animal. Common types of antihistamines are

- diphenhydramine (Benadryl),
- hydroxyzine (Atarax),
- clemastine (Tavist), and
- chloraphenaramine maleate (Chlor-Trimeton).

Route of Administration

Most of this family comes in oral form; however, some forms of the drug are available in injectable preparations, which can be given subcutaneously, intramuscularly, or intravenously. Care should be taken to make sure specific medication is safe to administer intravenously.

Precautions

- **Anticholinergic side effects:** Antihistamines can block aspects of the parasympathetic nervous system, which is responsible for maintaining normal body function (i.e., intestinal motility, slowing heart rate, constriction of the eye, production of salivary glands). Antihistamines can aggravate conditions such as glaucoma, urinary obstruction, and gut hypomotility disorders.
- **Effects in cardiac patients:** Animals with cardiovascular disease may be more susceptible to toxic effects.

- **Effects in pregnant patients:** Some antihistamines (i.e., hydroxyzine [Atarax]) in high doses have produced teratogenic effects in laboratory animals; use caution in pregnant or potentially pregnant animals.

Side Effects
- **Depression:** Antihistamines can cause significant CNS depression (sedation, ataxia).
- **CNS excitement:** Large doses may cause CNS stimulation with tremors, aggressive behavior, and possibly convulsions.
- **Anticholinergic side effects:** As stated previously, antihistamines can block the parasympathetic nervous system, producing side effects of dry mouth, tachycardia, and possibly constipation.

Drug Interactions
- **CNS depressants:** The CNS depressant effects of antihistamines may add to that of any other class of CNS depressants (e.g., anesthetics, tranquilizers, narcotic analgesics, sedatives).
- **Atropine/glycopyrrolate:** Anticholinergic side effects (ileus, tachycardia, pupil dilation) of antihistamines could add to those produced by atropine and glycopyrrolate (see Chapter 29).

Anti-Inflammatory Medications
This classification of drugs belongs to steroidal and nonsteroidal medication (NSAID) that is used to decrease whole-body inflammation, pain, and swelling. These medications can be used for short-term injury or for chronic long-term disease (i.e., arthritis).

Nonsteroidal Anti-Inflammatory Medications (NSAIDs)
Function
This group of drugs reduces pain and inflammation in the body caused by trauma, fever, wear and tear, and athletic injury. By decreasing inflammation, the body reduces its response to white blood cells and the animal has less pain.

Form of Drug
Prescription drugs include

- carprofen (Rimadyl),
- meloxicam (Metacam),
- deracoxib (Deramaxx),
- etodolac (Etogesic), and
- phenylbutazone (Bute).

Over-the-counter drugs are very potent and are generally not recommended in dogs, and NEVER in cats. These drugs should only be prescribed by the veterinarian.

Over-the-counter drugs occasionally prescribed by veterinarians for canines include

- aspirin,
- ibuprofen, and
- acetaminophen.

Naproxen (Aleve) should never be prescribed for any animal.

Route of Administration
All NSAIDs are available in oral tablet form. Some newer medication is also available in injectable form.

Side Effects
- **Gastric ulceration:** All NSAIDs can cause gastric ulceration, producing vomiting and diarrhea. Often it is recommended that the medication be given with food to help decrease the chance of ulceration.
- **Kidney toxicity (nephrotoxicity):** At higher doses (toxic levels), NSAIDs can produce kidney damage. This concern is much more common if a patient has had an overdose of medication, is given a potent over-the-counter drug (i.e., Naprosyn), or has a significant underlying kidney disease.
- **Liver disease:** Rarely, in some cases some prescription NSAIDs can affect liver function.

Contraindications
The following animals should not take a NSAID.

- Animals with gastrointestinal ulcers.
- Animals with kidney and/or liver disease.
- Animals on steroids, because this greatly increases the chance of gastrointestinal ulceration (see Figure 26.1).
- Cats, because they are extremely sensitive to most of these drugs. Their livers are unable to break down the drug, and the drug can cause severe side effects. Some NSAIDS are now used with caution by veterinarians.

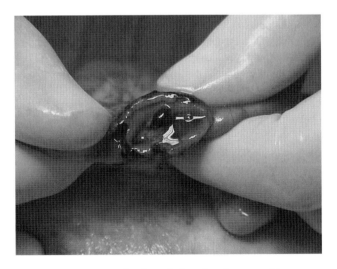

Figure 26.1. Image of an intestinal perforation caused by concurrent use of steroid and NSAID medication.

Drug Interactions

Use of these drugs with other NSAIDs or steroidal anti-inflammatory agents may lead to additive toxic effects in the gastrointestinal system.

Other drugs that are avidly bound to plasma proteins (e.g., sulfonamides, digoxin) may be displaced if used simultaneously with a NSAID.

The diuretic effects of furosemide (Lasix) may depend, in part, on the generation of vasodilatory prostaglandins. NSAIDs decrease prostaglandin production and may diminish the diuretic action of Lasix. Furthermore, concurrent diuretic therapy may lead to volume depletion and enhancement of the nephrotoxicity of carprofen.

Steroidal Medication

This family of drugs is used for its anti-inflammatory effects, immunosuppression, shock, and emergency. Each effect is dose dependent, requiring increasing dosage as the medication's effect goes from anti-inflammatory to immunosuppression to emergency stabilization. The goal of each dose level is as follows.

- **Anti-inflammatory doses:** At lower doses these drugs decrease white blood cell activity that responds to infection and inflammation. These steroids reduce the body's response to inflammation, hence reducing pain (i.e., arthritis, back pain).
- **Immunosuppression:** At higher doses these drugs serve to slow or completely suppress the white blood cell response to the body, causing an immunosuppression. Animals are more likely to become secondarily infected because the white blood cells and the immune system have decreased function. This dose level is used for lymphoma (certain forms), immune-mediated hemolytic anemia, or in conjunction with specific treatment protocols in certain types of cancer.
- **Shock doses:** Although potentially controversial, in case of severe shock (anaphylactic and other forms), a short-term steroid at an extremely high dose can be given. It is thought to help stabilize the body from shock by increasing blood sugar supplies, stabilizing and protecting the cell membrane, and maintaining blood pressure.

Form of Drugs
- Prednisone (Solu-Delta-Cortef)
- Dexamethasone (dexamethasone SP)
- Triamcinolone (Vetalog)
- Methyl prednisone (Depo-Medrol)

Routes of Administration
- Most steroidal medications come in injectable, oral, and topical forms. Care should be taken to ensure medication is safe to administer intravenously.
- The use of oral corticosteroids must be slowly tapered, not stopped quickly.

- An example of normal dosing regimes is 1 tab 2×/day for *x* days, then 1 tab 1×/day for *x* days, then 1 tab EOD.
- Once steroids are given, the animal's body begins to slow normal production of its steroid, cortisol.
- Cortisol is used to help produce sugar from the breakdown of fats and proteins.
- Similar to an Addisonian reaction (see Chapter 17), if oral corticosteroids are withdrawn too abruptly, the animal's body does not have time to adjust and the animal can become weak, lethargic, collapse, have poor pulse, and have vomiting and diarrhea.

Side Effects

Steroidal medication has both short- and long-term side effects.

Short-term side effects occur as the pet is exposed to increased amounts of the medication. These conditions usually subside as the patient is withdrawn from medication. These side effects are

- polyuria/polydipsia (increased thirst/urination),
- increased appetite,
- changes in behavior,
- panting, and
- vomiting/diarrhea (gastric ulceration).

Long-term side effects are systemic conditions that occur as the pet is exposed to corticosteroids over long periods of time (i.e., months to years). These conditions can produce long-term disease that may require hospitalization and long-term care.

- Muscle breakdown (long term)
- Secondary infection
- Liver disease
- Hyperadrenocorticism (see Chapter 17)

Contraindications

Corticosteroids can produce serious and life-threatening side effects if given to patients with underlying conditions or disease. Some concerns are listed here:

- **Pregnant animals:** In most species, systemic corticosteroids can induce labor and produce abortion. Care should be taken, even with topical steroidal medications, because some of these medications can have enough systemic absorption to induce premature labor.
- **Congestive heart failure:** Corticosteroids initiates a medullary wash out within the kidneys, reducing their ability to reabsorb water from the urine (see Chapter 13). These effects increase water consumption and urine output. Secondary to polydipsia, patients with congestive heart disease and failure can begin to build up fluid within the lung field, producing pulmonary edema.
- **Hepatic disease:** Care should be taken when using corticosteroids in patients with certain forms of liver disease.

Over the long term, steroidal medication can produce chronic damage to hepatocytes.

- **Animals with existing infection:** As stated previously, increasing doses of corticosteroids can produce an immunosuppression, which can worsen a preexisting infection.
- **Animals on concurrent NSAIDs:** As discussed previously, concurrent use of corticosteroids and steroidal medication can produce additive effects of gastrointestinal ulceration and possible perforation.

Drug Interactions

- Phenobarbital induces the rate of hepatic metabolism, which can increase the rate of corticosteroid elimination.
- Concurrent administration with NSAIDs (aspirin, carprofen, deracoxib) may increase the likelihood of developing gastrointestinal ulceration.
- Corticosteroids increase blood sugar, increasing requirements for insulin in the diabetic animals.
- Corticosteroids can attenuate the immunologic response to vaccines.
- Cyclosporine, cyclophosphamide, estrogens, mitotane, or erythromycin can increase corticosteroids' effect if given concurrently.

Miscellaneous Anti-Inflammatory Agents

This group of medications is commonly used with NSAIDs and corticosteroids to decrease inflammatory response, disable chronic pain pathways in the spinal cord, and help increase joint movement and protect hyaline cartilage.

Dimethyl Sulfoxide

Dimethyl sulfoxide (DMSO) is an organic solvent with numerous pharmacological actions. It is used primarily as an anti-inflammatory agent, particularly to reduce acute soft tissue swelling associated with trauma. Among other effects, DMSO is a free radical scavenger, which accounts for its potent anti-inflammatory action. Anti-inflammatory effects have been reported in musculoskeletal injuries, CNS inflammatory processes, and CNS trauma.

Form of the Drug

The drug comes in a liquid solvent, an otic preparation (synoptic), and an oral powder, methylsulfonylmethane (MSM).

Routes of Administration

DMSO is meant for topical, otic, and oral administration. Care should be taken to wear gloves when administering this drug topically. This drug is absorbed readily and can produce similar side effects in the administrator.

Side Effects

There are some common observable side effects.

- **Localized dermatological reactions:** Reddening, itching, blister formation, and dry skin may occur with

chronic topical application. This may disappear with continued use and is readily reversed by discontinuing DMSO application.

- **Halitosis:** The oysterlike odor on the breath may be noted.

Contraindications

Caution must be exercised to prevent inadvertent contamination of DMSO with other drugs or toxins whose absorption into the systemic circulation may be facilitated by DMSO.

Use in pregnant animals is questionable because DMSO exerts teratogenic effects in laboratory animals.

Drug Interactions

DMSO is a cholinesterase inhibitor. It can potentiate the effects of other drugs (organophosphate and carbamate insecticides, neuromuscular blocking agents such as succinylcholine), which also inhibit cholinesterase.

Glucosamine

For the management of severe osteoarthritic disease (traumatic or degenerative in origin) in dogs, these drugs can be used in conjunction with NSAIDs or corticosteroids. Glucosamine is a complex molecule of high molecular weight. Chemically, it is a sulfated polysaccharide similar to that found endogenously in cartilaginous tissues. Used for the management of osteoarthritic disease, these drugs are believed to have a number of effects that may lead to a restoration of damaged cartilage. They inhibit the synthesis of inflammatory prostaglandins and counteract the adverse effects of catabolic enzymes released in the arthritic joint. It may stimulate the production of endogenous hyaluronic acid, which leads to an increased viscosity and cushioning of the joint fluid. Glycosaminoglycans are components of proteoglycans, which provide structural integrity to cartilage.

Form of the Drug

Glucosamine is available in an injectable liquid (Adequan) or in an oral tablet combined with chondroitin (i.e., Cosequin).

Route of Administration

The injectable form is meant to be given intramuscularly; the tablets are given orally.

Side Effects

The following side effects can be observed.

- **Pain at injection site:** There may be transient pain at the intramuscular injection site.
- **Hypersensitivity:** Repeated administrations may provoke hypersensitivity reactions.
- **Gastrointestinal upset:** Occasionally vomiting and diarrhea can be observed with administration of glucosamine.

Precautions
Glucosamine is not for use in animals that have exhibited hypersensitivity to it.

Drug Interactions
No interactions have been reported.

Tramadol
Tramadol is an opiate agonist for the treatment of pain or cough in the dog.

Form of the Drug
Tramadol is available in tablet form.

Route of Administration
Tramadol is administered orally.

Side Effects
Tramadol appears to be well tolerated by dogs. However, it can produce the following side effects:

- **CNS excitement:** Agitation, anxiety, tremor, and dizziness.
- **Gastrointestinal upset:** Anorexia, vomiting, constipation or diarrhea.
- **Chemical dependence (low risk):** Pets have been taking tramadol long term should be withdrawn slowly from the drug.

Precautions
- **Opioid sensitivity:** Tramadol should not be used in patients that have shown allergic or hypersensitive reaction to other opioid drugs.
- **CNS disease:** Tramadol should be used with caution in patients with underlying CNS disease.
- **Geriatric/debilitated patients:** Due to its potential for CNS depression, tramadol should be used with caution in debilitated or older animals.
- **Hepatic/renal disease:** Due to how it is metabolized, tramadol should be used with caution in patients with underlying liver or kidney disease.

Drug Interactions
Due to its affects on the CNS, tramadol should be used with caution with other drugs that affect neurochemical levels (i.e., serotonin) within the CNS. Examples of these drugs are

- SAM-E and
- selegine (Anipryl).

Antiparasitic Agents
Although types of antiparasitic medications can vary from hospital to hospital, the main prescription drugs will be covered here.

Ivermectin/Avermectin
Ivermectin is approved for use in dogs and cats as a heartworm (*Dirofilaria immitis*) preventive; it is administered once per month. It is active against the third- and fourth-stage larvae.

Form of Drug
Ivermectin and similar drugs come in oral tablets and chews for monthly administration. An injectable and oral solution is also available. Common forms of ivermectin are

- Heartgard,
- Interceptor, and
- Ivomec.

Route of Administration
Ivermectin/avermectin are administered orally or are injected subcutaneously.

Side Effects
Ivermectin is an extremely safe drug under most circumstances due to its restriction from the CNS in mammalian species.

- **CNS depressant effect:** Lethargy, ataxia, tremors progressing and prolonged (days to weeks), and coma may occur with extremely high dosages or if given to breeds (e.g., collies and shelties) that apparently accumulate more of the drug in the CNS.
- **Anaphylaxis:** When used as a microfilaricide to kill larval heartworms in the treatment of heartworm disease, an anaphylactic shocklike effect may occur due to the massive death of the parasite. It is recommended that animals be observed for adverse effects for 12–24 hours after the drug is used in this manner.

Precautions/Contraindications
- **Breed specificity:** Dosages in excess of those used for heartworm prevention should not be used in collies and collie-type dogs.
- **Neonates:** The drug is not recommended for dogs and cats less than 6 weeks of age.
- **Patients with heartworm disease:** Animals should be checked for an existing heartworm infection prior to initiating ivermectin preventive therapy.

Drug Interactions
Although no interactions are commonly reported, the possible additive CNS depressant effect of ivermectin and other drugs that affect mammalian CNS should be noted. Drugs that would fall into this class are as follows:

- Barbiturates: morphine, oxymorphone
- Benzodiazepine: Valium, Telazol
- Tranquilizers: acepromazine

Pyrantel Pamoate
Pyrantel pamoate is used for the removal of ascarids (*Toxocara canis, Toxascaris leonina*) and hookworms (*Ancylo-*

stoma caninum, Uncinaria stenocephala) in dogs and puppies. Although not approved for use in cats, it has effectiveness against similar parasites in this species.

Form of Drug
Pyrantel comes in a liquid suspension and a tablet form (Nemex).

Route of Administration
Pyrantel is administered orally.

Side Effects
Although pyrantel is extremely safe, occasionally animals may experience vomiting following pyrantel administration.

Complications
Caution must be employed if using pyrantel in sick or debilitated animals.

Drug Interactions
Pyrantel should not be administered simultaneously with other antiparasitic drugs that also affect the acetylcholine-type receptors in the parasite, and, potentially, in the host; for example,

- levamisole,
- piperazine,
- organophosphates, and
- diethylcarbamazine.

Fendbendazole
Fenbendazole is approved for the control and removal of ascarids (*Toxocara canis, Toxascaris leonina*), hookworms (*Ancylostoma caninum, Uncinaria stenocephala*), whipworms (*Trichuris vulpis*), and tapeworms (*Taenia pisiformis*) in dogs. Extra-label use includes the removal of *Capillaria, Filaroides, Paragonimus,* and *Giardia* in dogs and for the treatment of gastrointestinal and lungworm (*Aelurostrongylus, Capillaria*) infections in cats.

Form of Drug
The drug is available in granules or in powder form as Panacur.

Route of Administration
The drug is administered orally.

Precautions
There are no known contraindications, although animals with extensive hepatic disease may be in greater jeopardy of adverse effects.

Side Effects
Minor gastrointestinal upsets (vomiting) may occur infrequently.

Drug Interactions
No drug interactions are reported in small animals.

Praziquantel
Praziquantel is approved for the removal and control of the following tapeworms in dogs:

- *Diplydium caninum*
- *Teania pisiformis*
- *Echinococcus granulosus*
- *Echinococcus multiocularis*

In cats, praziquantel is recommended for the removal and control of

- *Taenia taeniaeformis,* and
- *Diplydium caninum.*

Because the worms are likely to be digested in the gastrointestinal tract of the host, there may be no evidence of drug efficacy by seeing worms in the feces.

Form of Drug
The drug is available in tablet or injectable form as Droncit.

Route of Administration
The drug is administered in the oral or injectable form. The injectable form is typically given by subcutaneous or intramuscular route.

Precautions
There are no known contraindications for the use of praziquantel in dogs and cats, including breeding or pregnant animals. The drug is not intended for puppies less than 4 weeks of age or kittens less than 6 weeks of age.

Side Effects
- **Pain:** Pain at the site of injection is a common side effect.
- **Gastrointestinal side effects:** Vomiting, anorexia, diarrhea, excessive salivation may occur.
- **Mild CNS signs:** Drowsiness, lethargy, mild ataxia may occur with the oral or parenteral preparation.

Drug Interactions
No drug interactions have been reported.

Sulfadimethoxine
Sulfadimethoxine is used for the treatment of coccidiosis where it exerts a coccidiostatic action.

Form of Drug
Sulfadimethoxine (ALBON) comes in a tablet and liquid suspension.

Route of Administration
The drug is administered orally.

Contraindications

- **Renal/hepatic disease:** Administration of sulfadimethoxine to animals with extensive liver or kidney disease should be done carefully.
- **Large breed dogs:** Large breed dogs (Dobermans, rottweilers) have demonstrated a high incidence of hypersensitivity reactions with the sulfonamides. Some conditions noted are
  — polyarthritis,
  — hemolytic anemia, and
  — hepatic disorders.
- **Ocular disorders:** Animals with ocular disorders should also be treated with caution.
- **Pregnant animals:** Teratogenesis is noted with animals in early pregnancy treated with sulfa drugs.

Side Effects

- **Urinary tract:** Sulfonamides and its metabolites tend to precipitate in the urine, causing crystalluria (especially if the urine is acidic), although this is generally less prominent with sulfadimethoxine.
- **Ocular:** Sulfa drugs have been shown to cause keratoconjunctivitis sicca (dry eye).

Drug Interactions

Because sulfadimethoxine and other sulfa drugs are extensively bound to plasma proteins, concurrent use with other plasma protein-bound drugs (e.g., NSAIDs) may affect the bioavailability by displacement from the binding sites.

Tylosin Tartrate

Tylosin is used for the elimination of cryptosporidium, a microscopic parasite producing profuse diarrhea. Furthermore, tylosin can be used for the management of chronic large bowel diarrhea/colitis. Modulation of intestinal flora in the large bowel (e.g., anaerobes) by tylosin contributes to this effect.

Form of the Drug

Tylosin comes in a powder form as Tylan powder.

Route of Administration

Tylosin is administered orally.

Precautions

Because tylosin is eliminated in the bile, decreasing the dosage in animals with extensive hepatic disease is recommended.

Side Effects

Gastrointestinal side effects (vomiting, anorexia, and diarrhea) may accompany oral administration of tylosin. This may be attributable to alterations in bowel flora or to direct irritation of the gut mucosa.

Drug Interactions

Lincosamide antibiotics (clindamycin, lincomycin) and tylosin may produce mutually antagonistic effects on these drugs' antimicrobial action due to competition at a similar site of action in microbial protein synthesis.

Gastrointestinal Drugs

These categories of drugs focus on reducing stomach acidity, which decreases nausea, blocking vomiting and lining and protecting the intestinal mucosa in case of gastrointestinal ulceration.

Decreased Acid Producers

These drugs are used for the prevention and management of vomiting and other clinical signs associated with gastroduodenal hyperacidity states. These may be related to infectious, drug (corticosteroids, NSAIDs), stress, or concurrent disease (e.g., uremia, mast cell tumors) phenomena. It exerts a prophylactic and curative effect in gastric and duodenal ulcers.

Form of the Drug

In general, all medications are available as over-the-counter tablet medication. There is also an injectable form. Examples of these drugs are

- cimetidine (Tagamet),
- famotidine (Pepcid), and
- ranitidine (Xantac).

Route of Administration

Tablet form is given orally. The injectable form can be given subcutaneously, intramuscularly, or intravenously.

Precautions

- **Renal disease:** Since most acid blockers are eliminated by direct renal excretion, dosage adjustments may be needed with patients suffering from renal disease.
- **Hepatic disease:** Hepatic disease may also impair elimination, especially with orally administered cimetidine.

Side Effects

- Gastrointestinal signs (anorexia, vomiting, and diarrhea) may be observed during drug therapy, but these may be related to the gastrointestinal diseases being treated.
- Massive overdoses (especially with IV administration) may lead to cardiovascular toxicity with hypotension, tachycardia, and syncope.

Drug Interactions

- **Carafate:** Although controversial, some clinicians believe that concurrent use with acid blockers may impair the ability of Carafate to disperse and protect the gastric mucosa. It is recommended that administration of Carafate and acid blockers be staggered, with a 2-hour separation.
- **Medication requiring acidic conditions for absorption:** Concurrent administration with drugs that require acidic conditions in the gut for optimum absorption (e.g., ketoconazole) may diminish the efficacy of the latter unless they are staggered as above.

- **Medication detoxified by the liver:** Some acid blockers, such as cimetidine, have been documented to inhibit the biotransformation and elimination of drugs from the liver or alter hepatic blood flow, potentially increasing the toxicity of these agents. Examples of these drugs are
  — theophylline,
  — metronidazole,
  — propranolol, and
  — lidocaine.

Gastrointestinal Protectants
Sucrafate
Sucrafate has a nonspecific beneficial effect in the management of gastrointestinal ulcers, ulcers related to infections, drugs (e.g., corticosteroids, NSAIDs), stress or concurrent disease (uremia, mast cell tumor). It is particularly useful in counteracting the gastric ulceration associated with NSAID therapy. It exerts a prophylactic effect in gastric and duodenal ulcers and may possibly help esophageal ulceration.

Form of Drug
Sucrafate (Carafate) comes in an oral tablet form or liquid suspension.

Route of Administration
Sucrafate is administered orally.

Precautions
Dehydrated animals or animals with a history of constipation may be more vulnerable to the constipating side effects of sucrafate.

Side Effects
Because sucrafate is not absorbed systemically, it generally is an innocuous substance. Excessive amounts of sucrafate may produce constipation.

Drug Interactions
Sucrafate may bind to simultaneously administered oral drugs and prevent their systemic bioavailability. To help prevent this occurrence, administration of Carafate should be given 2 hours before the administration of any other medication. Examples of these medications are as follows.

- **Tetracyclines:** Tetracycline, oxytetracycline, doxycycline
- **Fluoroquinolones:** Enrofloxacin (Baytril), ciprofloxacin (Cipro), marbofloxacin (Zeniquin)
- **Decreased acid producers:** Cimetidine (Tagamet), ranitidine (Xantac), famotidine (Pepcid)
- **Cardiac drugs:** Digoxin (Lanoxin)

Antiemetic Medication
Chlorpromazine
Chlorpromazine is used for the management of vomiting in dogs and cats. The antiemetic action in cats may be less pro-

found than in dogs. The drug is especially valuable in cases where there is a centrally mediated component to the vomiting due to circulating endogenous or exogenous toxins. Furthermore, chlorpromazine may be used prophylactically to inhibit vomiting induction by drugs (i.e., chemotherapeutic agents).

Form of the Drug
Chlorpromazine is available as an oral suspension, tablet, and timed-released capsule. It is also available as an injectable solution.

Route of Administration
Chlorpromazine is generally used as an injectable drug for subcutaneous, intramuscular, and intravenous administration. The oral forms are given by mouth.

Side Effects
- **Sedation:** Excessive amounts of chlorpromazine may cause profound CNS depression and hypotension, especially in debilitated or dehydrated animals that have suffered prolonged emesis.
- **Parasympathetic nervous system effects:** These include xerostomia (dry mouth), pupillary dilation, gut hypomotility (ileus), and tachycardia.
- **CNS effects:** Phenothiazine tranquilizers can produce tremors, muscle rigidity, and spasms.

Drug Interactions
- **Other sedatives or analgesics:** Chlorpromazine may accentuate the CNS depression produced by virtually any other type of drug that is capable of producing this action (injectable and inhalation anesthetics, butyrophenone and benzodiazepine tranquilizers, sedatives, narcotic analgesics, etc.).
- **Atropine/glycopyrrolate:** The activity of chlorpromazine could add to that of the antiparasympathetic effects of these drugs, producing more significant tachycardia, ileus, and pupil dilation.
- **Antihistamines:** Chlorpromazine can enhance the sedative effects of antihistamines, such as diphenhydramine (Benadryl) and hydroxyzine (Atarax).
- **Chloramphenical/fluoroquinolone:** These drugs slow hepatic biotransformation, which is instrumental in chlorpromazine elimination and can therefore enhance the duration/effect of chlorpromazine.

Precautions
- **Cardiac:** Chlorpromazine can lead to profound hypotension; caution should be used in animals with cardiovascular disease.
- **Seizure patients:** Animals with a history of seizures may have this condition worsened by chlorpromazine.
- **Hepatic disease:** Animals with hepatic disease have decreased ability to eliminate this drug, causing potential toxicity.

Metoclopramide

Metoclopramide is used for the management of severe emesis (e.g., that is associated with cancer chemotherapy or other circulating toxins) or nausea and vomiting associated with gastroesophageal reflux, gastric ulceration, or delayed gastric emptying. Furthermore, the drug can be used as a motility modifier, which may have value in preventing gastroesophageal reflux (increased tone of the lower esophageal sphincter) and management of ileus, especially that involving the upper small intestine.

Form of the Drug

Metoclopramide (Reglan) is available in tablet, liquid suspension, and injectable form.

Route of Administration

The tablet and suspension are for oral administration. The injectable medication can be given subcutaneously, intramuscularly, intravenously, or in fluids in a constant rate infusion medication.

Precautions

- **Seizure disorders:** Metoclopramide is not to be used in patients with seizure disorders. Metoclopramide may aggravate seizure activity.
- **Gastrointestinal obstruction:** Reglan is contraindicated in obstructive disease of the gastrointestinal tract.

Side Effects

- **Neurologic:** Metoclopramide may produce dose-dependent CNS side effects (nervousness, restlessness, and tremors).
- **Gastrointestinal:** Excessive drug doses may cause colic, diarrhea, or constipation.

Drug Interactions

Specific drugs can block the gastrointestinal stimulatory effect of metoclopramide. These drugs are as follows.

- **Anticholinergic drugs:** Atropine, glycopyrrolate
- **Opioid narcotic analgesics:** Morphine, oxymorphine
- **Antihistamines:** Diphenhydramine (Benadryl)
- **Tranquilizers:** Certain tranquilizers may potentiate the adverse CNS effects of metoclopramide. Examples of these drugs are
  — phenothiazine tranquilizers*:* Acepromazine
  — butyrophenone tranquilizers: butorphanol (Torbutrol), and
  — bupronorphine (Buprenex).

Emergency Drugs

This category of drugs is used in emergency situations to stabilize patients in critical condition. Although not all medications are listed, the basic emergency drugs are discussed.

Furosemide

Furosemide is used for the treatment of ascites, hydrothorax, pulmonary edema, or any pathological accumulation of non-inflammatory fluid. In emergency settings, this drug is used to help reduce fluid accumulation within the lung fields (pulmonary edema) associated with congestive heart failure, drowning, and electrical injury.

Form of the Drug

Furosemide (Lasix) is available in tablet and syrup form, as well as in an injectable solution.

Route of Administration

Furosemide (Lasix) can be given orally or by subcutaneous, intramuscular, or intravenous injection.

Precautions

- **Severe renal disease:** Therapy with Lasix should be discontinued in cases of progressive renal disease with increasing azotemia and lack of urine production (anuria).
- **Hepatic disease:** Animals with hepatic disease may have the condition exacerbated by the fluid/electrolyte shifts caused by the diuretic and must be closely monitored.
- **Diabetes:** Diabetic patients should be monitored closely because furosemide has a mild tendency to cause hyperglycemia.
- **Sulfa antibiotic sensitivity:** Individuals sensitized to sulfonamides may respond adversely to furosemide due to its sulfalike chemical structure.

Side Effects

Excessive increased urinary output (diuresis) produced by Lasix may lead to electrolyte wasting and deficiency (e.g., hyponatremia, hypokalemia, hypochloremia, etc.) and dehydration, producing signs of

- lethargy,
- gastrointestinal disturbances,
- tachycardia, and
- anorexia.

Drug Interactions

- **Drugs eliminated by renal excretion:** Concurrent administration with drugs eliminated largely by the kidneys (e.g., digoxin, potassium bromide) could lead to more rapid elimination of these drugs and diminished pharmacological effect.
- **Aspirin:** Because aspirin and Lasix are excreted by similar mechanisms, aspirin levels may be increased when used in conjunction with furosemide.
- **Digoxin:** Furosemide induces potassium loss, which may increase the toxicity of concurrently administered digitalis (digoxin) cardiac medication.
- **Corticosteroids:** Both steroidal medication (i.e., prednisone) and Lasix produce profound potassium loss. Concurrent use of both medications can produce an additive effect, which could produce a serious hypokalemia.

Atropine

Atropine blocks a section of the CNS (i.e., parasympathetic nervous system) that regulates normal body function to slow heart rate, produce intestinal peristalsis, produce bronchial secretion, and constrict the iris and other body functions. The principal use of atropine is as a preanesthetic agent to decrease salivary and bronchial secretions and prevent potential bradycardia associated with anesthesia. It is an antidote in cases of overdosage with drugs or pesticides that cause excessive CNS stimulation. It is also used in the management of specific cardiac arrhythmias (i.e., heart block) and is used as an ophthalmologic agent for dilation of the iris in ocular disease.

Form of the Drug

Atropine is available in an injectable solution and ophthalmic eye drop and solution.

Route of Administration

Injectable atropine can be administered subcutaneously, intramuscularly, intravenously, and intratracheally. The ophthalmic preparation is only for topical application into the eye.

Precautions

- **Glaucoma:** Both injectable and ophthalmic forms of atropine produce iris dilation that can decrease the excretion of aqueous humor from the eye. In patients with glaucoma, this can elevate ocular pressure (see Chapter 20).
- **Tachycardia:** Patients with underlying cardiac arrhythmias can produce more abnormal heart rhythms due to the secondary tachycardia produced by atropine administration.
- **Ileus:** Patients suffering from gastrointestinal hypomotility disorders may be worsened by atropine.
- **Renal/hepatic disease:** Animals with kidney or liver disease may show signs of atropine accumulation and toxicity.

Side Effects

- Atropine can produce gastrointestinal hypomotility (ileus), causing constipation or colic.
- Atropine can produce iris dilation, which can make the patient sensitive to light (photophobic).
- With excessive amounts, atropine can cause CNS stimulation that could cause seizures.
- Due to atropine's affects on the heart, excessive use may provoke cardiac arrhythmias and decrease cardiac output.

Drug Interactions

Due to the tachycardial effects of atropine on the heart, specific cardiac medications can be affected.

- Antiarrhythmic medication such as quinidine or procainamide can have additive effects on the tachycardia produced by atropine.

- Digoxin's (digitoxin) effect of slowing the heart rate and decreasing arrhythmia can be compromised by concurrent atropine administration.

Atropine can slow the effects of medications (motility modifiers) that stimulate peristalsis (contraction of the intestine) and urinary bladder contraction. Examples of these drugs are

- cisapride (Propulsid),
- metoclopramide (Reglan), and
- bethanechol (Urecholine).

Epinephrine

Epinephrine is indicated in the following situations.

- **Cardiac resuscitation:** Epinephrine is used in conjunction with other measures such as external massage or electrical stimulation in cardiac arrest or asystole. Intravenous, intratracheal, or direct intracardiac administration or epinephrine may be used to stimulate cardiac contraction and maintain heart rate and cardiac output.
- **Anaphylactic shock:** Epinephrine is extremely effective and often lifesaving in treatment of acute anaphylactic shock due to the reversal of hypotension and bronchoconstriction. Epinephrine provides immediate relief from bronchial asthma through the potent bronchodilatory action.
- **Hemostasis:** Local application (1:100,000 to 1:20,000 solution) with moistened gauze sponges or aerosol sprayed directly onto the region may be used for hemostasis from small vessels.

Form of the Drug

Epinephrine is available in an injectable solution.

Route of Administration

Injectable epinephrine can be administered subcutaneously, intramuscularly, intravenously, intracardially, and intratracheally.

Precautions

- **Cardiac arrhythmias:** Since epinephrine may promote the development of cardiac arrhythmias, extreme caution must be employed in patients with hypoxia-induced or other cardiac arrhythmias.
- **Hyperthyroidism:** Concurrent treatment with hyperthyroid also increases the likelihood of arrhythmia induction.

Side Effects

- **Cardiac arrhythmia:** Epinephrine may promote the development of tachycardia and fatal ventricular arrhythmias.
- **Hypertension:** Hypertensive crises occur from epinephrine overdosage.

Drug Interactions

Certain drugs and hormone therapies can make patients more prone to epinephrine's effects to produce cardiac arrhythmias. Some of these drugs are

- thyroid hormone,
- digitoxin (digoxin), and
- Halothane anesthetics.

Dextrose 50% Solution

Dextrose 50% solution is used to correct states of carbohydrate and energy insufficiency associated with hypoglycemia in various disease states.

Form of the Drug

The drug is available commonly.

Route of Administration

The drug can be given orally or diluted with sterile water to be given intravenously (25% solution) or in fluids as a continuous rate infusion drug (see Chapters 27 and 30).

Precautions/Contraindications

Dextrose should never be administered subcutaneously or intramuscularly because it can be very irritating and can cause tissue damage and necrosis.

Side Effects

Excessive amounts may lead to fluid overload with resultant clinical signs such as dyspnea and cardiovascular dysfunction.

Drug Interactions

No drug interactions have been reported.

Miscellaneous Drugs

This category of drugs outlines commonly used medications that are prescribed in general practice every day.

Levothyroxine Sodium/L-Thyroxine Sodium

Levothyroxine sodium/L-thyroxine sodium is used for the treatment of hypothyroidism, where life-long therapy with the hormone is required. Reversal of clinical signs of hypothyroidism may take weeks (lethargy, bradycardia, and other cardiovascular signs) to months (e.g., skin and hair coat changes).

Form of the Drug

Thyroxine comes in tablet form as Soloxine, L-thyroxine, Thyrotabs, and many other names.

Route of Administration

Thyroxine is administered orally.

Precautions/Contraindications

- **Heart disease/hypertension:** Thyroxine should be used with caution in patients with hypertension and cardiac disease.

- **Hyperthyroid/Addisonian patients:** It should not be used in patients with untreated Addison's disease and hyperthyroidism.

Form of Drug

Try to avoid switching brands of thyroxine once animals are established on a dosage regime. Commonly, there are differences in potency and bioavailability between different sources.

Side Effects

Excessive dosages may cause signs of hyperthyroidism, which can produce

- CNS stimulation/hyperactivity,
- tachycardia,
- hyperthermia,
- polyuria,
- polydipsia,
- increased appetite (polyphagia), and
- alopecia.

Drug Interactions

- **Epinephrine:** Thyroxine potentiates the effects of epinephrine.
- **Digitoxin:** Thyroxine inhibits the cardiovascular potency of digoxin.
- **Insulin:** Thyroxine exerts anti-insulin effects and may increase the dosage of insulin required by diabetics.
- **Ketamine:** Cardiovascular effects of ketamine are increased in the presence of thyroxine.
- **Anticonvulsants:** Drugs, such as phenobarbital, decrease thyroxine levels, possibly by increasing the rate of hepatic metabolism and clearance.

Phenobarbital

Phenobarbital is used orally for the long-term control of epilepsy and seizures in dogs and cats. Combination therapy with phenobarbital and other antiseizure medications (e.g., potassium bromide) is commonly employed for long-term seizure control. Administered intravenously, it may be used to abolish acute seizures (e.g., cluster seizures).

Form of the Drug

Phenobarbital is available in pill form, as an oral elixir, or as an injectable solution.

Route of Administration

Phenobarbital can be given orally or intravenously.

Precautions/Contraindications

- **Cardiovascular disease:** Animals with preexisting compromise of respiratory or cardiovascular function should be considered more vulnerable to the depressant effects of barbiturates on these systems.

- **Liver/kidney disease:** Animals with hepatic or renal disease may have altered elimination of phenobarbital, increasing the potential for phenobarbital side effects.
- **Pregnancy:** Phenobarbital crosses the placental barrier and may lead to excessive CNS depression in the fetus.
- **Injection site reaction:** Administration of phenobarbital extravascularly can lead to severe tissue damage.
- **Chemical dependence:** A form of addiction may occur with chronic use, leading to an increased likelihood of severe seizures if the drug is abruptly stopped.

Side Effects

Side effects are dose dependent and can be as follows.

- **Behavior changes:** Animals may show behavioral changes (anxiety, agitation) at the start of therapy.
- **Systemic side effects:** There may be polyuria, polydipsia, and polyphagia.
- **CNS depressants:** Sedation and ataxia occur with excessive amounts.
- **Cardiovascular side effects:** Hypotension and decreased cardiac output are potential complications.
- **Hepatotoxicity:** Long-term therapy may lead to liver damage; serial monitoring of hepatic function is recommended.

- **Blood abnormalities:** Anemia has been reported and hematological parameters should be determined serially.

Drug Interactions

- As with all barbiturates, other drugs that have CNS depressant properties, such as anesthetics will add to the extent of CNS depression produced by phenobarbital.
- Drugs that inhibit hepatic metabolism (e.g., chloramphenicol) may significantly augment phenobarbital-induced CNS depression.
- Drugs that are eliminated primarily by hepatic metabolism (e.g., theophylline, metronidazole) could be eliminated more rapidly in animals on chronic phenobarbital therapy.

CD-ROM 2 will focus on concepts of Understanding the Concepts of Disease and Treatment. The exercises can be done individually or as case rounds as they explore specific topics in veterinary medicine that discuss clinical diagnostics and treatment.

Chapter 27

Toxins and Poisons

Introduction

This chapter will examine and discuss common toxic and poisonous substances that can affect most small animal patients. The goal of this chapter is to understand how toxins can affect the animal, how to approach a history and initial assessment on potential poisonings, and understand treatment options.

In approaching a potential intoxication, the patient should first be triaged (see Chapter 6), because many patients are in shock. Once the patient is stable, a complete history should be obtained (see Chapter 5). With concerns of intoxications, the following specific questions should be asked (see also Flowchart of Treating Toxicity at the end of this chapter).

Could the Patient Have Ingested Poison or Toxin?
The hospital team member must be specific when asking this question and give examples of types of common drugs or poisons. Many clients will not consider that specific agents (i.e., antifreeze, cleaning supplies, fertilizer, plant food, and other chemicals) may be a toxin or that their pet would even ingest the chemical.

Is Your Pet on any Medications?
Some patients have been on medications for years (i.e., phenobarbital, digitoxin, thyroxine, insulin, etc.) that may now be causing toxicity. Furthermore, owners may be altering the schedule of drug administration or increasing the dose of medication without discussing these changes with the veterinarian.

Could the Pet Have Ingested Human Medications?
Often clients will not consider that the pet may have gotten into a family member's medication. Some clients feel that the medication may be too bitter for the animal to ingest or did not even consider the possibility of exposure. *If there is any concern for ingestion of prescription medication, the client should obtain the exact name of the medication, the dosage, and the number of tablets the patient could have ingested.*

Is Your Pet on any Homeopathic Medications?
Some pet owners may administer homeopathic medications to the patient without consulting a veterinarian. Because many homeopathic drugs are considered neutroceuticals, many clients administer these medications as if the patient is being placed on a vitamin supplement. However, many homeopathic herbs (i.e., nightshade, St. John's wort, etc.) can produce serious to toxic side effects.

Is the Pet on Any Over-the-Counter Medication?
As with homeopathic medications, many owners will give their pets over-the-counter medications without consulting the veterinarian. In discussing these types of medications with the client, the team member should be specific when listing the types of drugs of concern. These drugs may include

- aspirin,
- ibuprofen,
- acetaminophen (i.e., Tylenol or aspirin-free medication),
- naproxen (Aleve),
- antihistamines, and
- cough medications.

Has There Been Green Vomitus or Blue-Colored Stool?
Blue- or green-colored vomit or stool can be suggestive of specific toxins.

Patients with blue fecal contents may have ingested a third-generation rodenticide. Many of these rat poisons have a distinctive blue dye evident. However, since the poison does take 2–3 days to have effect, the feces may have been noticed 1–2 days earlier, before physical symptoms have occurred.

Often patients suffering from strychnine toxicity (i.e., gopher bait) will produce a dark green-tinged vomit. This emesis should be obtained and held for the veterinarian because strychnine levels can be detected in this fluid.

Seeking Help for the Poisoned Pet

Although some poisoning can occur as a chronic condition (i.e., heavy metal toxicity), most intoxications produce acute severe syndromes with potential life-threatening physical symptoms. Often the patient presents acutely ill without any chronic history of disease. Since toxins can affect multiple body systems producing a variety of physical signs, initial assessment should be done to evaluate the patient for instability or shock (see Chapter 6). Any patient that presents in a life-threatened status should be immediately brought to the veterinarian's attention and stabilization begun (see Chapter 30).

If a drug or poison is suspected by the owner, all infor-

mation on the type of drug or active agent, the amount ingested, and the time it was ingested should be documented. If a toxin or poison (i.e., rose food, rat bait, etc.) is suspected, the client should be instructed to bring in the packaging of the product as well. These potential toxins will have a listing of their active ingredients and often a contact phone number from the corporate producer.

There are tens of thousands of potential toxins that can affect a patient. When researching if a chemical or medication is toxic to a patient, the following resources are available to most hospital teams:

- **Corporate contact information:** On most household products there is a contact phone number for consumer information and emergencies. Most companies will have emergency information in case of ingestion or topical contact with their product. Some companies' information will be limited to human intoxication and may not have specific information for animal consumption.
- **Local poison control:** Although an excellent and free service on most toxins and poisons, local poison control numbers do not typically carry information on the effect of toxins on the animal population. Although symptoms and treatments in humans can sometimes correlate to the veterinary patient, often intoxications in animals can have varying symptoms and treatment protocols.
- **ASPCA—University of Illinois Poison Control:** This service is a database of thousands of toxins and medications that can affect the veterinary patient. The service offers the client or veterinarian direct access to a veterinary toxicologist who can aid the medical team in identifying the toxin of most concern, discuss physical signs and duration of drug effects, and outline treatment protocols and prognosis. There is a fee for the initial consultation. (Phone number: 800-548-2423.)

Just as physical symptoms can change dramatically depending on the type of poison, clinical chemistry and blood populations can vary dramatically. If the toxin has been identified, specific blood work may be recommended to evaluate the poison's effect on the body. If intoxication is suspected in a patient but the poison is unknown, complete blood work and urinalysis is generally recommended.

Common Toxins and Poisons

Although not all intoxications are mentioned below, the common poisonings are discussed with the main goal being to understand and be able to explain to the client what the intoxications and poisonings are, how they can present themselves, and what can be the overall short- and long-term concerns of each disease. Any discussion of overall diagnostic and treatment protocols should be discussed based on the recommendations for the doctor. Please use the following information as a basis for discussion and to educate the client, *but never to diagnose a patient.*

Acetaminophen Toxicosis

Acetaminophen (Tylenol) is a non-narcotic analgesic drug with a very small margin of safety in animals, causing severe effects on the liver and blood.

Etiology

In dogs, acetaminophen can affect the liver, causing an acute necrotic liver disease.

Cats are much more susceptible to acetaminophen intoxication. Acetaminophen changes **hemoglobin**, a chemical within the red blood cell that is responsible for carrying oxygen to the tissue, to **methoxyhemoglobin.** This compound is unable to carry oxygen into the body, and the animal slowly begins to suffocate.

Signalment

Acetaminophen toxicosis can affect dogs and cats of any age. There is no breed or sex predisposition.

Toxic Dose Levels

Acetaminophen is the chemical toxin found in many human headache and pain-relieving medications. Although Tylenol is the brand name for acetaminophen, there are numerous products that contain acetaminophen, so please check labels carefully, especially on products labeled, *aspirin free.* It is also important to note that some animals can show symptoms at much lower doses (see Table 27.1).

- Children's Tylenol contains 80 mg of acetaminophen.
- Regular-strength Tylenol contains 325 mg of acetaminophen.
- Extra-strength Tylenol contains 500 mg of acetaminophen.

Onset of Physical Signs

Physical signs occur shortly after ingestion.

Key Points in Medical History/Initial Assessment

Acetaminophen toxicity can produce severe organ and respiratory disease. In some cases, despite all treatment options, the patient will succumb. Physical symptoms of acetaminophen toxicosis are as follows.

In dogs, symptoms are

- vomiting,
- depression (progressive),
- abdominal pain, and
- dark-colored urine.

In cats, onset of toxicosis is acute (1–2 hours). Symptoms are

- salivation,
- not eating,
- vomiting,
- brown tinge of gums/ears/white of eyes,
- dark chocolate-colored blood and urine, and
- swelling of the face, paws, and forelimbs.

Death can occur in 18–36 hours.

Table 27.1. Toxic dose of acetaminophen.

	Cats	Dogs
Toxic dose	50 mg/kg	150 mg/kg

Table 27.2. Dose of theobromine in chocolate.

Type of Chocolate	Level of Theobromine/Oz
Milk Chocolate	45 mg/oz
Unsweetened Chocolate	400 mg/oz

Table 27.3. Theobromine toxicity per weight of animal.

Weight (kg)	Milk Chocolate	Unsweetened Baker's Chocolate
5	11 ounces	1.25 ounces
10	22 ounces	2.5 ounces
20	44 ounces	5 ounces
30	66 ounces	7.5 ounces
40	88 ounces	10 ounces
50	110 ounces	12.5 ounces

Diagnosis

Diagnosis of acetaminophen is largely based on history and evidence of physical symptoms. However, in felines, a significant symptom is brown coloration of the serum and urine as hemoglobin is transformed into methoxyhemoglobin. There can also be Heinz bodies noted in the red blood cells.

Treatment

The goal of treatment depends on physical symptoms of the patient. Overall guidelines for acetaminophen toxicity are as follows.

- **Induction of vomiting:** If the animal has recently ingested the acetaminophen, inducing vomiting may bring up any undigested medication. *However, due to the concerns of a patient accidentally pushing emesis into the lung field (aspiration), inducing vomiting should never be attempted if the patient is having seizures or cannot swallow properly.*
- **Activated charcoal:** Charcoal is an inert substance that helps absorb toxins left in the intestinal system. Activated charcoal can also be combined with Sorbitol (cathartic) to help move any remaining residues out into the feces.
- **Fluid therapy:** For more seriously affected animals (i.e., dehydration, tachycardia, shock, etc.), hospitalization and intravenous fluids are recommended to help maintain hydration and flush toxins from the body (diuresis).
- **Oxygen therapy:** In felines that are having problems oxygenating their tissue, oxygen therapy may be recommended to increase oxygen saturation in blood.
- **Medications:** Multiple administrations (5–7 doses) of acetylcysteine (Mucomyst) over 20–28 hours (every 4 hours) can help counteract the formation of methoxyhemoglobin.

Chocolate Toxicosis

Chocolate toxicosis is a possible life-threatening disease caused by the ingestion of too much chocolate, which contains theobromine and caffeine.

Etiology

The chocolate can cause severe gastrointestinal upset whereas the theobromine and caffeine affects the amounts of calcium in the cells, causing muscular tremors and increased heart activity.

Signalment

Chocolate toxicosis can affect dogs and cats of any age. There is no breed or sex predisposition.

Toxic Dose Levels

Theobromine

Symptoms occur when 100 mg/kg of theobromine is ingested. The type of chocolate contains different levels of theobromine (see Table 27.2).

It is important to note that toxic ingestion depends on how much total chocolate the patient has ingested (see Table 27.3). Many candies and sweets can be a mix of chocolate and other products (i.e., caramel, cake, nuts, etc.). Therefore, an 8-ounce candy bar may only contain only 3–4 ounces of milk chocolate.

Furthermore, some animals may have symptoms that indicate much lower doses of chocolate.

Caffeine

The toxic dose level for caffeine is 140 mg/kg.

Onset of Physical Signs

Signs occur shortly after ingestion.

Key Points in Medical History/Initial Assessment

Often patients will show signs of gastrointestinal disease prior to other symptoms due to the primary gastric upset caused by the change of diet. More severe signs can occur as larger quantities of chocolate are ingested. Common symptoms can be

- vomiting,
- diarrhea,

- hyperactivity,
- restlessness,
- increased urination,
- muscle tremors,
- increased heart rate,
- sometimes decreased heart rate,
- increased body temperature,
- seizures,
- coma, and
- death.

Treatment

The goal of treatment depends on physical symptoms of the patient. Overall guidelines for chocolate toxicity are as follows:

- **Induction of vomiting:** If the animal has recently in-gested the chocolate, inducing vomiting may be at-tempted. *However, due to the concerns of aspiration, in-ducing vomiting should never be attempted if the patient is having seizures or cannot swallow properly.*
- **Activated charcoal:** Charcoal is an inert substance that helps absorb toxins left in the intestinal system. Activated charcoal can also be combined with Sorbitol (cathartic) to help move any remaining residues out into the feces.
- **Fluid therapy:** For more seriously affected animals (i.e., with dehydration, tachycardia, shock, etc.), hospitali-zation and intravenous fluids are recommended to help maintain hydration and flush toxins from the body (diuresis).
- **Sedation:** In more hyperactive and excitable animals, the patient may need sedation to reduce muscle spasms and hyperactivity.
- **Monitor cardiovascular function:** With animals that are severely affected and that may have severe changes in heart rhythm, the heart rate and electrocardiogram may need to be monitored for severe tachycardia or arrhyth-mias that may require medications.

Ethylene Glycol Toxicity (Antifreeze Poisoning)

Antifreeze is sweet tasting and will be ingested by dogs and cats when available. Most antifreeze contains a toxin called **ethylene glycol;** this toxin begins to crystallize in the blood-stream, especially within the kidneys. As the chemical con-tinues to crystallize within the kidney tissue, the kidneys are selectively destroyed, causing acute and potential irre-versible kidney disease. The longer the toxin is in the body, the more damage is done. *If the animal is seen more than a few hours after ingestion takes place, there may be irre-versible kidney disease and a life-threatening condition.*

Etiology

Antifreeze is absorbed into the body rapidly, causing severe metabolic upset and crystallization in the kidney tissue. Over a short period of time, there is significant kidney tis-sue destruction.

Table 27.4. Minimum lethal dose of antifreeze.

Canine	2–3 ml/kg
Feline	1.4 ml (1/5 of a teaspoon)/kg

Signalment

The disease can affect any dog or cat; this problem is seen generally in the colder months of the year when radiators are winterized.

Toxic Dose Levels

Toxic dose levels for animals are very small, especially in the feline where less than 1 teaspoon can produce irre-versible kidney damage (see Table 27.4).

Onset of Physical Signs

Signs occur within hours after ingestion.

Common Points in Medical History

Unless the client witnessed the ingestion, patients come in acutely affected and may be profoundly ill. Chief complaints commonly can be

- mild to severe depression,
- nausea,
- vomiting,
- inability to balance properly,
- tripping easily,
- altered vocalization, and
- acting strangely.

Common Points on Physical Examination

Physical signs depend on the amount of toxin ingested and the elapsed time since ingestion occurred. In early disease, signs can be

- severe muscular tremors,
- tremor movements in the eyes (**nystagmus**),
- head tremors,
- increased thirst and urination,
- low body temperature, and
- acting abnormally,
  — change in vocalization,
  — acting blind, and
  — sudden aggression.

In late disease signs can be

- severe kidney disease,
- decreased to no production of urine,
- coma,
- seizure, and
- death.

Complications

If not diagnosed and treated immediately, ethylene glycol intoxication produces acute renal disease/failure and death.

Diagnostics

Clinical diagnostics for suspected antifreeze intoxication can be

- **Complete blood count:** Changes observed in the complete blood count are elevations in red blood cell count and total protein secondary to severe dehydration.
- **Chemistry:** With ethylene glycol poisoning there can be significant elevations in the renal enzymes (blood urea nitrogen, or BUN, creatinine, and phosphorus), as well as elevations in potassium and blood sugar.
- **Urinalysis:** Urinalysis can show a dilute urine, urine specific gravity (USG) of <1.015, suggesting a renal azotemia. Further evidence of antifreeze intoxication is the presence of *calcium oxalate crystals in the urine within 8 hours after intoxication.*
- **Ethylene glycol test:** A positive ethylene glycol test within 6 hours after ingestion suggests the presence of the toxin in the bloodstream. After 6 hours postingestion, the test can be falsely negative.

Treatment

Treatment depends on the animal's history, diagnostic tests, and physical exam findings upon presentation of the pet. However, it is important to note, especially in the feline, the longer the pet goes without treatment after ingestion, the worse the prognosis. Some treatment options are discussed next.

Hospitalization and Fluid Therapy

It is extremely important to make sure the pet is on intravenous fluids to continue perfusion of the kidneys and stimulate urine formation.

Vomiting and Gastric Lavage

If ingestion just occurred, the goal is inducing emesis (vomiting), removing any remaining antifreeze in the intestinal system, and administering activated charcoal to deactivate any remaining toxin. *However, inducing vomiting should never be attempted if the patient is having seizures or cannot swallow properly due to the concerns of aspiration.*

Medication

- **4-methylpyrazole:** This drug inhibits the crystallization of ethylene glycol from the bloodstream. It must be administered over 48 hours with the pet in the hospital. This drug is only indicated for the canine.
- **Ethanol:** The use of 95% grain alcohol also inhibits the formation of the crystals from the blood. It is the only available treatment in cats and must be given intravenously over 2 days.

Monitoring

The pet must be monitored very carefully in the hospital for urine formation and changes in the kidney enzymes to help

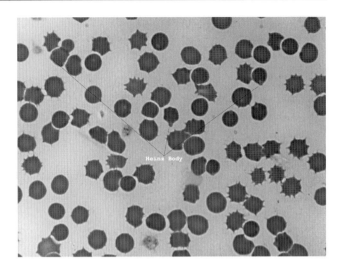

Figure 27.1. Image of red blood cells with Heinz bodies (denatured hemoglobin). Usually appear as small nodules fused to the red blood cell membrane.

the veterinarian determine the overall prognosis. *If kidney enzymes begin to climb and urine production is not present in the first 24–48 hours, the prognosis is usually grave.*

Heinz Body Anemia—Onion (and Garlic) Toxicosis

Exposure to large amounts of onions in canines and onions and garlic in felines can produce **oxidative injury** to the red blood cells, producing a life-threatening anemia.

Etiology

Exposure to onions and garlic (wild onions and store purchased) produce an oxidative injury to red blood cells, denaturing the hemoglobin in the red blood cell and forming Heinz bodies (see Figure 27.1). Other causative agents that can produce similar anemias are

- acetaminophen,
- mothballs,
- onions,
- garlic (felines), and
- zinc toxicity.

Signalment

Heinz body anemia is more common in cats, but it can affect dogs and cats without any sex, age, or breed predisposition.

Toxic Dose Levels

Toxicity depends on the type, concentration, and exposure to toxic agents that produce oxidative injury to red blood cells.

Onset of Physical Signs

Depending on how much toxin is ingested, symptoms can occur acutely to chronically.

Key Points in Medical History/Initial Assessment
This type of toxicity can produce a history of acute weakness, depression, and collapse. Physical symptoms can be

- pale mucous membranes,
- fever,
- anorexia,
- collapse, and
- reddish brown urine (**hemoglobinuria**).

Diagnosis
Diagnosis of Heinz body anemia is based on history and evidence of physical symptoms. Observed changes in the blood work can be as follows.
   In complete blood counts, changes can be

- decreased packed cell volume,
- increased reticulocytes (regenerative response),
- Heinz body formation,
- fragments of red blood cells (eccentrocytes),
- hyperbilirubinemia seen in blood chemistry, and
- bilirubinuria seen in urinalysis.

Treatment
The goal of treatment depends on physical symptoms of the patient. Overall guidelines for Heinz body toxicity are as follows.

- **Identify and remove causative agent:** Exposure to any of the above agents or addition of onion or garlic forms (raw, sliced, powder, etc.) should be removed from the pet's diet.
- **Fluid therapy:** For more seriously affected animals (i.e., with dehydration, tachycardia, shock, etc.), hospitalization and intravenous fluids are recommended to help maintain hydration and flush toxins from the body (diuresis).
- **Oxygen therapy:** In patients that are having problems oxygenating their tissue, oxygen therapy may be recommended to increase oxygen saturation in blood.
- **Blood transfusion:** In patients with severe anemia, blood transfusion may be needed to stabilize the patient.

Ibuprofen Toxicosis
Ibuprofen is a nonsteroidal anti-inflammatory drug (NSAID) with a very small margin of safety in animals, causing severe effects on the kidneys and intestinal tract.

Etiology
Ibuprofen is a potent NSAID. All drugs within this class can have ulcerative effects in the gastrointestinal tract and can be potentially toxic to the kidneys. *Each tablet of adult regular-strength ibuprofen contains 200 mg/tablet.*

Signalment
Ibuprofen toxicosis can affect dogs and cats of any age. There is no breed or sex predisposition.

Toxic Dose Levels
As with most NSAIDs, ibuprofen can produce toxic effects on the gastrointestinal system and the kidneys. Although some animals can show symptoms at much lower doses, overall symptoms can be observed at the following dose levels.

- **Gastrointestinal symptoms** occur when 150 mg/kg of ibuprofen are ingested.
- **Renal disease/failure** occur when ibuprofen levels reach 300 mg/kg.

Onset of Physical Signs
Signs occur shortly after ingestion.

Key Points in Medical History/Initial Assessment
Often patients will show signs of gastrointestinal symptoms initially, with renal disease issues occurring with higher doses. Common symptoms can be

- vomiting, possibly with blood;
- diarrhea, possibly with digested blood (melena) or frank blood;
- increased thirst;
- increased urination;
- dehydration;
- pale gums if intestinal bleeding is severe enough;
- weakness; and
- seizures with severely affected kidneys.

Diagnosis
Because ibuprofen toxicity can cause gastrointestinal bleeding and kidney disease, the following blood work profiles are recommended to monitor gastrointestinal bleeding and renal concerns.

- **A complete blood count and chemistry:** These tests will help determine if there is evidence of severe gastrointestinal bleeding, renal disease, or changes in the electrolytes that may need to be treated.
- **Urinalysis:** A urinalysis will assess the kidneys' ability to concentrate urine and expel toxins.

Treatment
The goal of treatment depends on how badly the pet is affected.

- **Induction of vomiting:** If the animal has recently ingested the ibuprofen, inducing vomiting may be recommended to bring up any undigested medication in the stomach. *However, inducing vomiting should never be attempted if the patient is having seizures or cannot swallow properly due to the concerns of aspiration.*
- **Activated charcoal:** Once the animal has vomited, the use of activated charcoal may be suggested to help absorb any drug residues left in the intestinal system. Charcoal is an inert substance that helps absorb toxins left in the intestinal system.

- **Fluid therapy:** For animals with more serious vomiting and diarrhea (with or without blood), hospitalization and intravenous fluids can help maintain hydration while giving the intestinal system time to rest. Fluids also allow toxins to be flushed from the body (diuresis).
- **Blood products:** If there is severe bleeding within the intestinal tract, the use of red blood cells and plasma may be recommended.
- **Medication:** The goal of medications would be to decrease inflammation and bleeding and protect the lining of the intestinal system. Also, if there are concerns for secondary infection, antibiotics may also be suggested.

Lead Toxicity

Lead poisoning occurs with chronic or acute ingestion of lead, producing gastrointestinal and neurologic symptoms. Exposure to lead can come from

- old paint,
- linoleum,
- car battery,
- sodder,
- golf balls, and
- lead objects (e.g., sinkers).

Etiology

Lead toxicity interferes with multiple enzyme pathways within the body, which affects production of red blood cells. Furthermore, lead may affect capillaries within the central nervous system, increasing the risk of damage to the brain and spinal cord.

Signalment

Lead intoxication can affect dogs and cats of any age. There is no breed or sex predisposition.

Toxic Dose Levels

Physical symptoms occur when lead levels >0.4 ppm in the blood.

Onset of Physical Signs

Physical symptoms depend on how much lead is ingested. Signs can occur chronically over time.

Key Points in Medical History/Initial Assessment

Initial symptoms start with gastrointestinal signs followed by central nervous system symptoms. Common symptoms can be

- vomiting,
- diarrhea,
- anorexia,
- abdominal pain,
- blindness,
- seizures, and
- death.

Diagnosis

Diagnosis is made based on medical history and physical symptoms. However, complete blood count can show increased nucleated red blood cells without obvious anemia. Anisocytosis, polychromasia, target cells, and hypochromasia may be also noted. Red blood cells may also show basophilic stippling of the red blood cell cytoplasm due to lead toxicity damage of the red blood cells (see Figure 27.2).

Treatment

The goal of treatment depends on how badly the pet is affected. Treatment may consist of the following.

- **Induction of vomiting:** If the animal has recently ingested the poison, inducing vomiting may be recommended to bring up any undigested medication in the stomach. *However, inducing vomiting should never be attempted if the patient is having seizures or cannot swallow properly due to the concerns of aspiration.*
- **Activated charcoal:** Once the animal has vomited, the use of activated charcoal may be suggested to help absorb

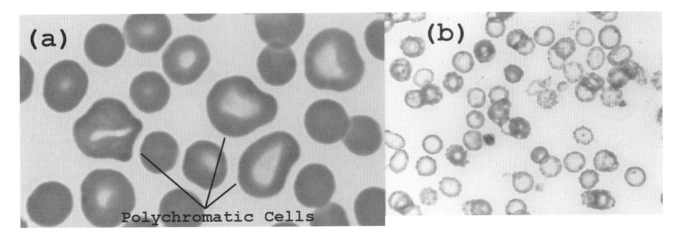

Figure 27.2. Images of polychromasia (a) and hypochromasia (b), which can be noted with lead poisoning. There may not be a true anemia present, but due to lead's effects on the red blood cell synthesis, red blood cell and hemoglobin maturation can be affected.

any drug residues left in the intestinal system. Charcoal is an inert substance that helps absorb toxins left in the intestinal system.

- **Fluid therapy:** Hospitalization and intravenous fluids can help maintain hydration while giving the intestinal system time to rest. Fluids also allow toxins to be flushed from the body (diuresis).

Medication
The goal of medications are to control seizures, excitement, and muscle spasms. Other medications are used to help inactivate lead levels in the bloodstream.

Metaldehyde Toxicity (Snail & Slug Bait)
Metaldehyde is a key poison in slug and snail bait as well as a fuel used in camp stoves. When ingested it produces a severe excitatory effect on the central nervous system.

Etiology
The cause of the toxicity is unknown. However, it is thought to affect the neurotransmitter levels within the central nervous system.

Signalment
Metaldehyde toxicosis can affect dogs and cats of any age. There is no breed or sex predisposition.

Toxic Dose Levels
Toxic dose levels depend on how methaldehyde is ingested and its concentration in the poison.

Onset of Physical Signs
Signs occur shortly after ingestion, but can take up to 3 hours to have an effect.

Key Points in Medical History/Initial Assessment
The chief complaints are changes in behavior and seizures. Common symptoms can be

- convulsions,
- muscular tremors,
- increased sensitivity to touch or pain (hyperesthesia),
- hyperthermia (>108° Fahrenheit),
- tachycardia,
- hypersalivation,
- vomiting,
- coma,
- hepatic disease (1–3 days after ingestion if the patient survives the initial episode), and
- death.

Diagnosis
Diagnosis is made based on medical history and physical symptoms. Stomach contents can be sent to the lab for evaluation of methaldehyde levels.

Treatment
The goal of treatment depends on how badly the pet is affected. Treatment may consist of the following.

- **Induction of vomiting:** If the animal has recently ingested the poison, inducing vomiting may be recommended to bring up any undigested medication in the stomach. *However, inducing vomiting should never be attempted if the patient is having seizures or cannot swallow properly due to the concerns of aspiration.*
- **Activated charcoal:** Once the animal has vomited, the use of activated charcoal may be suggested to help absorb any drug residues left in the intestinal system. Charcoal is an inert substance that helps absorb toxins left in the intestinal system.
- **Cool water bath:** For patients that present with body temperatures greater than 106° Fahrenheit, a cool water bath may be needed to reduce body temperature and control secondary side affects from heat stroke (see Chapter 30).
- **Fluid therapy:** Hospitalization and intravenous fluids can help maintain hydration while giving the intestinal system time to rest. Fluids also allow toxins to be flushed from the body (diuresis).
- **Medication:** The goal of medications is to control seizures, excitement, and muscle spasms.

Organophosphate/Carbamate Toxicosis
Organophosphates/carbamates are common ingredients in pet flea and tick control products, household insecticides, and agriculture products. When the pet is exposed to high levels of these drugs, it interferes with the normal muscle and nervous function.

Etiology
In normal muscle activation, an activated neuron releases a chemical called acetylcholine. This chemical diffuses away from the nerve toward the muscle in a space called the neuromuscular junction. The contact of acetylcholine with specific proteins (acetylcholine receptors) on the muscle stimulates muscular contraction. Shortly after activation, a chemical enzyme, called **cholinesterase**, inactivates the acetylcholine, giving the muscle time to reset and be stimulated again. With organophosphate toxicity, the toxin inhibits cholinesterase, which stops the inactivation process of acetylcholine, producing continued muscle and nervous stimulation. *Depending on the form of organophosphate, the discontinuation of the inactivation enzyme could last over days to weeks.*

Signalment
Cats are more adversely affected and more sensitive to organophosphate toxicity. The drug can be stored in fat tissue, so lean cats and thin breed dogs (e.g., sight hounds and racing breeds) also can be more susceptible to toxicosis.

Toxic Dose Levels

Toxic dose levels may vary depending on the type of organophosphate used, the concentration of the poison per milligram, and how it is absorbed or administrated. Any patient that has come in contact with an organophosphate toxin should be evaluated immediately.

Onset of Physical Signs

Physical signs can occur within minutes to hours of physical contact or ingestion of organophosphate toxins, producing a rapid and life-threatening condition. Clinical signs of organophosphate and carbamate toxicity are

- vomiting,
- diarrhea,
- increased salivation,
- small fixed pupils,
- depression (progressive),
- muscular tremors,
- high body temperature secondary to muscular contractions/ seizures,
- seizures,
- slow heart rate, and
- death.

Diagnosis

Diagnosis of organophosphate exposure is largely based on history and evidence of physical symptoms. However, there is a clinical diagnostic blood test to check for **cholinesterase activity** (the enzyme that breaks up the acetylcholine) that can be performed by sending blood to an outside lab. Animals affected by this toxin often only have 25% of normal cholinesterase levels.

Treatment

The goal of treatment depends on how badly the pet is affected. Treatment may consist of the following.

- **Induction of vomiting:** If your animal has recently ingested the organophosphate poisons, inducing vomiting may be suggested to bring up any undigested medication in the stomach. *However, inducing vomiting should never be attempted if the patient is having seizures or cannot swallow properly due to the concerns of aspiration.*
- **Cool water bath:** With patients that have high body temperatures (>106° Fahrenheit) secondary to persistent muscular tremors or seizures, a cool-down bath may need to be performed to bring down the body temperature.
- **Activated charcoal:** Once the animal has vomited, administration of activated charcoal may be recommended to help absorb any drug residues left in the intestinal system.
- **Fluid therapy:** For animals with more serious muscular tremors, weakness, seizures, high body temperatures, or gastrointestinal signs, hospitalization and intravenous fluids may be needed to help maintain hydration while giving the intestinal system time to rest. Fluids also allow toxins to be flushed from the body (diuresis).
- **Medication:** The goal of medication is to try to minimize the nervous effects, control seizures, and decrease muscular contractions.
- **Oxygen therapy:** Depending on how severe the breathing difficulty is, your veterinarian may suggest placing the pet on oxygen to help increase oxygenation of the blood.

Rodenticide (Rat Poison) Intoxication—Warfarin or Coumadin Poisons

Although there are three different types of rat poison, the most common is warfarin and anticoagulant poisons. These compounds interfere with the normal clotting agents that clot blood and stop bleeding. Animals spontaneously bleed millions of times a day, and without the necessary chemicals to stop the bleeding process, patients can quickly become life threatened.

Etiology

The anticoagulants found in rat poison interfere with the normal activation of vitamin K, a fat soluble vitamin associated with clotting of blood. Vitamin K works with several of the clotting factors to aid in the formation of a clot to prevent severe hemorrhage.

Signalment

Rat poison can affect dogs and cats of any age. There is no breed or sex predisposition.

Toxic Dose Levels

Toxic dose levels can vary depending on the generation of rodenticide used, concentration of the poison per milligram, and the amount ingested. Any patient that has ingested rodenticide should be evaluated immediately.

Onset of Physical Signs

Signs appear 2–3 days after ingestion of the toxin.

Key Points in Medical History/Initial Assessment

Patients can show the following physical symptoms associated with rat poison ingestion:

- Nose bleeds
- Spontaneous bruising
- Weakness
- Collapse
- Pale mucous membranes
- vomiting blood or dark bloody stool
- Shortness of breath
- Bloated, fluid-filled abdomen

Diagnosis

Because this disease produces clinical signs of weakness, poor color, increased chance of bleeding, and other signs that could be seen in other diseases (e.g., idiopathic thrombocytopenia; von Willebrand's disease; chronic liver disease; infectious diseases such as tick fever, Rocky Mountain spotted fever, etc.; and splenic tumor), the following diagnostic tests may be indicated.

Diagnostic Blood Work

- **Complete blood count and chemistry:** These diagnostic tests will help determine how low the red blood cell count is, the level of platelets in the blood, if the white blood cell count is elevated (suggesting a severe inflammatory response or infection), or if there are other suggestions of diseases in the kidneys, liver, or other organs.
- **Clotting times:** With concerns of bleeding, clotting times may be needed to help assess what type of bleeding problems may be occurring.
- **Infectious disease titer screens:** The veterinarian may suggest testing for specific disease in the geographical area that could be linked to bleeding problems (i.e., tick fever [ehrlichiosis], Rocky Mountain spotted fever, etc.).
- **Proteins induced by vitamin K antagonism (PIVKA):** This blood test is a highly suggestive clinical diagnostic test that detects proteins that are produced when drugs that interfere with vitamin K are present in the body.
- **Radiographs:** X-rays of the abdomen will aid in diagnosing disease in the spleen or other organs or a tumor mass that could be producing spontaneous bleeding (e.g., splenic hemangiosarcoma, tumors of the liver, etc.). Further thoracic x-rays may be suggested to evaluate the chest and lung fields for evidence of frank bleeding.
- **Ultrasound:** An ultrasound will allow the visualization of the abdomen to help assess the presence of free fluid suggestive of internal bleeding. Furthermore, the veterinarian can evaluate the abdominal organs and intestines for other causes of bleeding, weakness, and general disease.

Treatment

Treatment is based on the presentation of the animal and the severity of the disease noted and may consist of the following.

- **Induction of vomiting:** If the animal has recently ingested the poison, inducing vomiting may be recommended to bring up any undigested medication in the stomach. *However, inducing vomiting should never be attempted if the patient is having seizures or cannot swallow properly due to the concerns of aspiration.*
- **Activated charcoal:** Once the animal has vomited, the use of activated charcoal may be suggested to help absorb any drug residues left in the intestinal system. Charcoal is an inert substance that will help absorb toxins left in the intestinal system.
- **Medications:** Medications are focused on replacing vitamin K with oral or injectable medications or preventing secondary infections.

- **Hospitalization and fluids:** In animals with severe bleeding problems that may have massive blood loss, the pet may need to be hospitalized and placed on fluids to monitor and control potential life-threatening bleeding.
- **Blood products:** If the pet has severely elevated clotting times or a very low red blood cell count, red blood cells or plasma may need to be administered to help replace blood loss and clotting factors.

Strychnine Poisoning

Strychnine is a potent poison affecting the central nervous system. It is commonly found in gopher, rat, mouse, and other pest baits.

Etiology

Strychnine interferes with normal neurotransmitter levels in the central nervous and muscular systems producing profound reflex hyperactivity. If enough poison is ingested, the muscles of breathing can be affected, producing respiratory arrest (**apnea**) and death.

Signalment

Strychnine poison can affect dogs and cats of any age. There is no breed or sex predisposition.

Toxic Dose Levels

Lethal doses of strychnine are as follows:

- Canine: 0.2 mg/kg
- Feline: 0.5 mg/kg

Onset of Physical Signs

Physical signs can occur within 2 hours of ingestion.

Key Points in Medical History/Initial Assessment

Animals generally present with violent seizure activity that is made worse with loud noises. The seizures generally end with the patient in a lateral recumbency with increased rigor of all muscle groups. The limbs are locked out in space with the patient's head perpendicular to its spine (**opisthotonus**; see Figure 27.3). Other symptoms are

- muscle stiffness,
- tachycardia,
- decreased respiratory rate, and
- death.

Diagnosis

Diagnosis is made based on the pet's medical history and physical symptoms. However, urine, stomach contents, and abdominal organs can be evaluated for strychnine levels.

Treatment

The goal of treatment depends on how badly the pet is affected. Treatment may consist of the following.

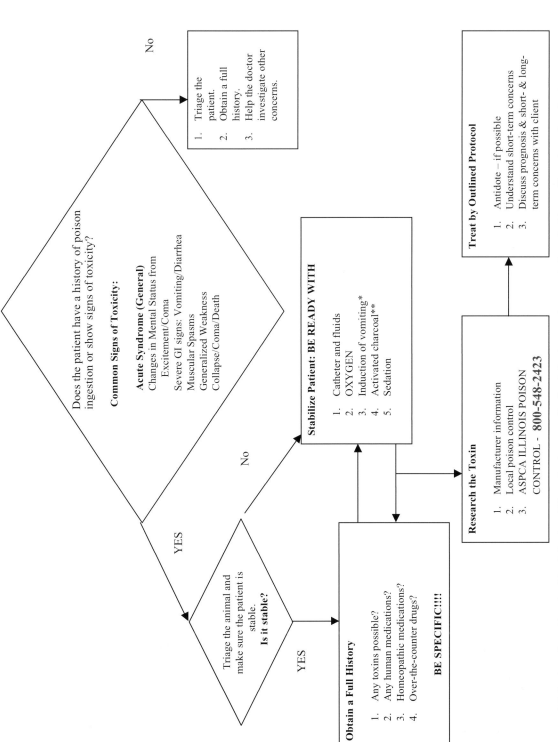

Does the patient have a history of poison ingestion or show signs of toxicity?

Common Signs of Toxicity:

Acute Syndrome (General)
Changes in Mental Status from
Excitement/Coma
Severe GI signs: Vomiting/Diarrhea
Muscular Spasms
Generalized Weakness
Collapse/Coma/Death

No

1. Triage the patient.
2. Obtain a full history.
3. Help the doctor investigate other concerns.

YES

No

Triage the animal and make sure the patient is stable.
Is it stable?

YES

Obtain a Full History

1. Any toxins possible?
2. Any human medications?
3. Homeopathic medications?
4. Over-the-counter drugs?

BE SPECIFIC!!!!

Stabilize Patient: BE READY WITH

1. Catheter and fluids
2. OXYGEN
3. Induction of vomiting*
4. Activated charcoal**
5. Sedation

Research the Toxin

1. Manufacturer information
2. Local poison control
3. ASPCA ILLINOIS POISON
   CONTROL - **800-548-2423**

Treat by Outlined Protocol

1. Antidote – if possible
2. Understand short-term concerns
3. Discuss prognosis & short- & long-term concerns with client

* Induction of vomiting should only be done if ingestion is recent. Further induction may be contraindicated with specific toxins and medications. **However, inducing vomiting should never be attempted if the patient is seizing or unable to swallow properly due to the concerns of aspiration.**
** Activated charcoal should never be attempted in comatose or seizuring patients or patients that are unable to swallow.

Flowchart 27.1. General flowchart for treating toxicity.

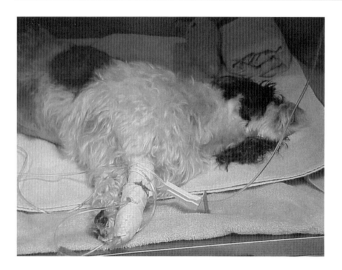

Figure 27.3. Opisthotonus. The rigidity of the forelimbs with the hyperextension of the neck and head.

- **Induction of vomiting:** If the animal has recently ingested the poison, inducing vomiting may be recommended to bring up any undigested medication in the stomach. *However, inducing vomiting should never be attempted if the patient is having seizures or is unable to swallow properly due to the concerns of aspiration.*

- **Activated charcoal:** Once the animal has vomited, the use of activated charcoal may be suggested to help absorb any drug residues left in the intestinal system. Charcoal is an inert substance that will help absorb toxins left in the intestinal system.

- **Fluid therapy:** Hospitalization and intravenous fluids can help maintain hydration while giving the intestinal system time to rest. Fluids also allow toxins to be flushed from the body (diuresis).

- **Medications:** The goal of medications is to control seizure activity and relax muscular spasms.

- **Anesthesia:** With severe cases, patients may need to be anesthetized and ventilated for 1–3 days if the patient enters respiratory arrest. These patients must continue to be supported and diuresed until the strychnine has been removed from their bodies.

CD-ROM 2 will focus on concepts of Understanding the Concepts of Disease and Treatment. The exercises can be done individually or as case rounds as they explore specific topics in veterinary medicine that discuss clinical diagnostics and treatment.

Chapter 28

Fluid Therapy

The goal of this chapter is to provide the team member with a basic understanding of the goals of intravenous therapy, including how to calculate a fluid rate for the pet, how to monitor intravenous fluids, and how to discuss treatment concerns with the client. *Administration or changes to fluid therapy should never be done without proper instruction and consent from the veterinarian.*

It is essential to have a well-educated hospital team that can monitor a patient on intravenous fluids for dehydration, fluid overload, and fluid ins/outs. In specific cases where there are increased toxins in the bloodstream secondary to renal disease, liver disease, certain forms of diabetes, or other toxic or systemic diseases, increased amounts of fluids (1.5–2 × maintenance) can aid in removing toxins from the body (**diuresis**). *The goal of fluid maintenance is to provide support to aid in rehydration, maintenance, and possibly diuresis for the pet. Fluid support is the key hallmark for stabilization in a majority of emergency care.* Necessary supplements and drugs can be added to the fluid regime to aid in the pet's recovery. Nutrients such as dextrose and potassium, and medications such as metoclopramide, lidocaine, and dopamine, can be added to intravenous fluids to provide a **continuous rate of infusion** (**CRI**) of the needed drug.

Types of Fluid Support

Fluid support can be given in two forms: subcutaneous fluids and intravenous fluids. Each type of delivery has its own strengths and weaknesses.

Subcutaneous Fluids

Subcutaneous fluids are a moderate to large bolus of fluids given under the skin to create a fluid repository that can be slowly absorbed by the pet over a 3- to 6-hour period of time.

Indications
Subcutaneous fluids are meant for slow replenishment of the mild to moderately dehydrated patient. Administration of fluids can be indicated for several reasons.

Acute Disease
Acute disease producing mild dehydration may require fluids. Disease states that may require fluids are, for example,

- mild gastrointestinal disease (see Chapter 10), and
- mild upper respiratory infections (see Chapter 11).

Chronic Disease
Subcutaneous fluids are used at regular intervals in pets with chronic disease to help maintain their hydration. These patients' diseases are usually under control, and the pets are eating, drinking, and feeling good. Examples of a chronic disease where subcutaneous fluids can be given are

- chronic renal disease (see Chapter 13), and
- chronic liver disease (see Chapter 14).

These fluids can be administered in the hospital setting, or the owner can be taught to administer subcutaneous fluids at home.

> **Practice Tip:** It is recommended that the client administering subcutaneous fluids at home be educated about and comfortable with this type of fluid administration. One suggestion is to have the client observe how to administer subcutaneous fluids and practice administration in a hospital setting with the medical team member during the first few times of administration.

Emergency Conditions
Although not as valuable as intravenous fluids in emergency situations, subcutaneous fluids can help to mildly rehydrate a patient that has severe perfusion problems. Once subcutaneous fluids are administered and absorbed, a vein may be more easily catheterized.

Contraindications
With proper administration of subcutaneous fluids, there are few contraindications. However some concerns are as follows.

- **Intravenous fluid additives:** Some caution must be exercised that certain fluid additives (i.e., dextrose), which are normally given intravenously, are not given subcutaneously. These types of fluid additives can cause irritation and damage to the overlying skin.
- **Underlying disease conditions:** Caution should be exercised with patients that have underlying disease condi-

Table 28.1.   Guidelines for subcutaneous fluid therapy.

Animal's Weight	Approximate Subcutaneous Fluid Amount*
<10 pounds	50–200 ml
11–40 pounds	200–500 ml
41–70 pounds	500–700 ml
>70 pounds +	>700–1000 ml +

*These fluids are suggested fluid ranges based on pet weights. These ranges are meant for animals without primary disease that could produce pulmonary edema and congestion (i.e., congestive heart failure, electric cord injury, etc.).

tions that have the propensity for **pulmonary edema.** Although of much less concern than when using intravenous fluids, repeated subcutaneous fluids may increase the likelihood of build up of fluid within the lung fields. Some of these conditions are

— congestive heart failure,
— severe renal disease (end stage),
— drowning, and
— electric cord injury.

Calculation of Fluid Need

The veterinarian will make recommendations for subcutaneous fluid boluses for the pet. However, the veterinary team should have an understanding of approximate fluid parameters to prevent miscommunication or overadministration of fluids (see Table 28.1).

Discussing Subcutaneous Fluid Administration (In-Patient) with the Client

- Subcutaneous fluids are the placement of sterile fluids under the skin of your pet to help rehydrate or maintain hydration during mild to moderate illness.
- The procedure is completed over 5–10 minutes as a large amount of fluid is placed in a pocket under the skin.
- Initially, the pet will have a large pocket of fluids evident in the shoulder region.
- Once the fluid is absorbed, it can migrate under the skin downward between the forearms, making them appear slightly swollen, until it is completely absorbed over the next 4–6 hours.
- The process is painless and can be done with minimal restraint.
- Subcutaneous fluids help maintain hydration of the mildly ill pet, but are more limited when dealing with patients with significant dehydration, fluid losses through vomiting and diarrhea, or acute disease producing a buildup of toxins (i.e., kidney/liver disease).

Administration

Subcutaneous fluid administration is generally given in unsedated animals over the short term to create a fluid reservoir. In most pets, administration can be done with minimal restraint (see Figure 28.1). The process is as follows:

1. With the animal restrained, a sterile needle is placed under the skin over the interscapular area (shoulder) with the needle parallel to the spine.
2. The sterile fluids are placed subcutaneously while monitoring the fluid pocket for tension and tightness.
3. If the pocket becomes tight and firm, another location is chosen until the total amount of fluid is given.
4. Once administered, there should be pressure applied to the skin where the needle was placed to prevent leakage of fluid from the repository site.

Intravenous Fluids

Intravenous fluids are one of the hallmark treatments for the hospitalized and emergency care patients in practice. Team members must be able to

- master evaluating dehydration,
- understand the benefits and concerns with different fluid types (i.e., crystalloids vs. colloids),
- understand how to calculate fluid need,
- monitor a patient on intravenous fluids, and
- properly document the fluid administration.

There are two larger groups of intravenous fluid choices, which are discussed next.

Crystalloids

The crystalloid category is made up of types of fluid that have a concentration (**isotonic**) density similar to blood. The goal of these fluids is for long-term intravenous administration for patients needing rehydration, diuresis, and emergency care. Examples of commonly used crystalloids are 0.9% NaCl, lactated Ringer's solution, and Normosol.

Colloids

The colloid category is made up of fluid types that have an increased density (**hypertonic**) as compared with blood. These fluids are separated into two further categories.

- **Natural colloids:** blood, packed red blood cells, and plasma that are meant for blood replacement products in anemic or bleeding animals (see Chapter 30).
- **Synthetic colloids:** hypertonic solutions that are used for shock and emergency patients to help increase systemic blood pressure or serve as a blood replacement product (see below).

Applications and Administration of Intravenous Fluids—Crystalloids

Crystalloids are fluids containing electrolyte and nonelectrolyte solutes capable of entering all body fluid compart-

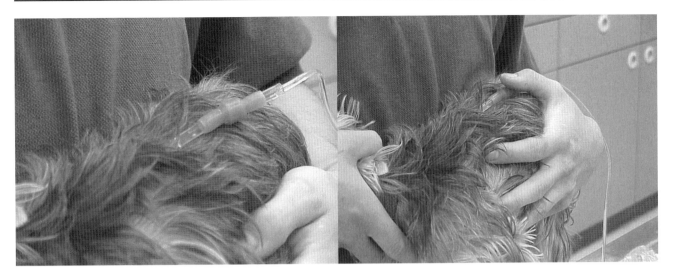

Figure 28.1.   Image of subcutaneous fluids administered to a small dog. Note the needle is entered under the skin parallel to the spine, and the pet is maintained with minimal restraint.

ments. They are the most common form of **parenteral** (nonoral) fluid therapy and are classified as replacement solutions (composition resembling extracellular fluid) or maintenance solutions (see Figure 28.2). The choice of fluid depends upon the disease process. The most useful crystalloid solutions for routine use are balanced replacement solutions such as Ringer's or lactated Ringer's solution, Normosol-R, 0.9% saline and 5% dextrose in water.

Indications
Crystalloid fluids are indicated for the treatment of ill patients that need rehydration, diuresis, or emergency care. Intravenous support can be given safely over hours to days. Nutrients such as dextrose and potassium chloride can be added to fluids to help provide minimal nutritional support as well as to balance electrolytes. Furthermore, drugs (such as metoclopramide and lidocaine) can be given for CRI of the sick patient.

Contraindications
Because intravenous fluids provide a constant flow of liquid directly into the vein, caution must be exercised with patients with specific diseases. Careful monitoring is necessary for patients with underlying disease conditions that may produce **pulmonary edema.** Because these pets cannot control the rate at which fluids enter their body, the patients can become overhydrated and begin building up fluid within the lung tissue (**pulmonary congestion**). Some diseases that require caution are

- congestive heart failure (see Chapter 12),
- severe renal disease (end stage; see Chapter 13), and
- drowning or electric cord injury.

Furthermore, animals that have diseases producing profound anemia or blood loss can be made worse with high volumes of intravenous fluids. These patients do not have enough red blood cells to carry oxygen to the body. If too much intravenous fluid is administered, the blood can become more dilute, decreasing its oxygen-carrying capacity. Some potential diseases producing a serious acute or chronic anemia include

- chronic renal disease (see Chapter 13),
- chronic liver disease (see Chapter 14),
- blood loss/trauma (see Chapter 3), and
- immune-mediated hemolytic anemia.

Calculation of Fluid Need
Calculation of fluid need depends on

- the pet,
- the disease,
- fluid losses (i.e., diarrhea and vomiting),
- the pet's level of dehydration, and
- if the pet is in shock.

The amount of fluid administered is determined by the veterinarian. However, the team member must have a concept of the types of fluids, the daily fluid needs, and rates of fluids given to ensure the pet is getting an adequate amount of fluids to rehydrate while not overloading the pet (see fluid administration algorithm on p. 417). The categories for rehydration are discussed next.

Maintenance
Maintenance fluids are the minimum amount of fluids needed for a pet that is not having significant fluid losses (i.e., vomiting or diarrhea) to maintain normal hydration. All animals require 66 ml/kg/day fluids for the body to function normally.

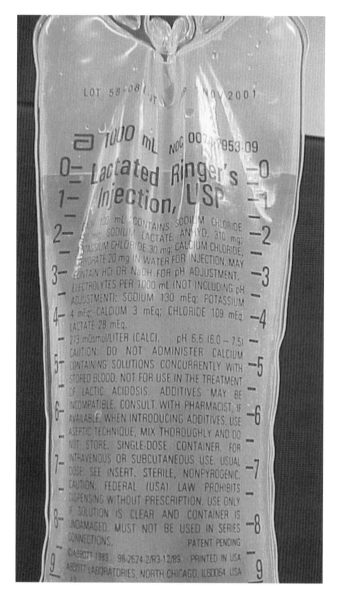

Figure 28.2. Image of crystalloids—lactated Ringer's solution fluids.

Maintenance = Body Weight (kg) × 66 ml/kg/day

In other words a 10-kg dog requires 66 ml/kg/day * 10 kg = 660 ml/day to maintain normal hydration.

This amount does not include what that animal needs for maintenance if there is any fluid losses (blood loss, vomiting/diarrhea). These pets may require larger amounts of fluids per day. Generally, with significant vomiting and diarrhea, the pet may require 1.5–2 times the maintenance dose. These maintenance rates would be:

- 1.5 × maintenance: 99 ml/kg/day
- 2 × maintenance: 132 ml/kg/day

Dehydration

Dehydration is a qualitative measurement of hydration level of the patient based on skin turgor, gums, eye appearance, and/or packed cell volume. As discussed in Chapter 6, dehydration is based on the following scale.

- **0–3%:** Undetectable dehydration secondary to an animal that has been vomiting or having mild diarrhea
- **5–7%:** Beginning of detectable dehydration with slight decrease in skin turgor and beginning of dry gums
- **7–9%:** More perceivable dehydration with much more decreased elasticity of skin, dry gums, and sunken eyes
- **9–12%:** Life-threatening dehydration with no elasticity of skin, sunken eyes, dry gums, depression, and weakness

Calculation of dehydration uses the following formula:

Dehydration = % Dehydrated in Decimal Form × wt (kg) × 1000 ml/l

For example, a 10-kg dog is 10% dehydrated.

Dehydration = (0.1) × (10 kg) × 1000 mls/l
Dehydration = 1000 mls

This animal then needs 1 l (1000 ml) of fluids just to rehydrate.

It is important to note that if the pet has reached normal hydration in the first day, there are no fluids needed for dehydration in the second 24 hours.

Total fluid need is the amount of fluid the animal needs in the first 24 hours and is the sum of maintenance plus dehydration fluids.

Total Fluid Need = Maintenance + Dehydration

Example I: A 10-kg dog with no significant fluid losses is 10% dehydrated.

Maintenance = 10 kg × 66 ml/kg/day = 660 ml/day
Dehydration = (0.1) × 10 × 1000 = 1000 ml
Total Fluid Need = 1660 ml

Thus this pet needs 1660 ml in the first day and if rehydrated will only need 660 ml each following day.

Example II: A 12-kg parvo dog with significant vomiting and diarrhea is 5% dehydrated. Here the veterinarian has recommended placing the pet on 2× maintenance.

2× Maintenance = 12 kg × 132 ml/kg/day = 1584 ml/day
Dehydration = 12 kg × (0.05) × 1000 = 600 ml
Total fluid need = 2184 ml

Thus this pet needs 2184 ml in the first day, and if rehydrated may need 1584 ml the following day (if vomiting and diarrhea continue).

Administering Intravenous Fluids
Once the total fluid need is determined by the veterinarian, fluids are administered. There usually are two administration protocols followed.

Hourly Fluid Rate
Hourly fluid rate is calculated by taking total fluid need and dividing by 24 hours per day.

> Hourly Fluid Rate = (Total Fluid Need/day)/(24 h/day)

Example III: A 10-kg dog with no significant fluid losses is 10% dehydrated.

Maintenance = 10 kg × 66 ml/kg/day = 660 ml/day
Dehydration = (0.1) × 10 × 1000 = 1000 ml
Total Fluid Need = 1660 ml
Hourly Fluid Rate = 1660 ml/24 hours = 69 ml/hr

Bolusing Fluids
In times of severe dehydration, prior to a surgery or treatment, the doctor may want to give an intravenous bolus to help replace the fluid loss more quickly. There is no specific amount of fluid administered; however, a general guide for bolusing patients can be 10–20% of total fluid for that day. The overall bolus is subtracted from total fluid need and hourly fluid rate is calculated. *When bolusing fluids, the patient must be monitored for fluid overload (see below).*

Example IV: A 12-kg parvo dog with significant vomiting and diarrhea is 5% dehydrated. Here the veterinarian has recommended placing the pet on 2× maintenance.

2× Maintenance = 12 kg × 132 ml/kg/day = 1584 ml/day
Dehydration = 12 kg × (0.05) × 1000 = 600 ml
Total Fluid Need = 2184 ml

The doctor suggests a bolus of 400 ml initially (20% of total fluid need). After the bolus, the pet requires an additional 1784 ml in the next 24 hours: 2184 ml − 400 ml (bolus).

> Hourly Fluid Rate = 1784 ml/24 h = 74 ml/h

Once the hourly rate is calculated, it can be entered into a fluid pump. The team member should still monitor hourly the fluid intake because fluid pumps can be inaccurate. If a fluid pump is not available, the team member will need to estimate hourly flow by calculating drops per second in the IV system. To do this, milliliters per second must be calculated first.

> Milliliters/sec = (hourly fluid rate)/(3600 sec/h)

Example V: A 10-kg dog with no significant fluid losses is 10% dehydrated.

Maintenance = 10 kg × 66 ml/kg/day = 660 ml/day
Dehydration = (0.1) × 10 × 1000 = 1000 ml
Total fluid need = 1660 ml

Hourly fluid rate = 1660 ml/24 h = 69 ml/h
Milliliter per second = (69 ml/h)/(3600 sec/h) = 0.02 ml/sec

To calculate drops per second, the team member must know what IV line system is being used. There are generally two systems.

- **Macro drip system:** 10 or 15 drops/ml
- **Micro drip system:** 60 drops/ml

> To calculate drops per second:
>
> Drops/sec = ml/sec × drops/ml (drip system)

Example VI: A 10-kg dog with no significant fluid losses is 10% dehydrated.

Maintenance = 10 kg × 66 ml/kg/day = 660 ml/day
Dehydration = 0.1 × 10 × 1000 = 1000 ml
Total fluid need = 1660 ml
Hourly fluid rate = 1660 ml/24 h = 69 ml/h
Milliliter per second = (69 ml/h)/(3600 sec/h) = 0.02 ml/sec

Using a 10 drop per milliliter system minus drops per second:

Drops/sec = 0.02 ml/sec × 10 drops/ml =
0.2 drops/sec or 1 drop/5 sec

Once drops per second are calculated, a *chronicity strip* can be used to make sure the animal's hourly needs are being calculated (see Figure 28.3). This type of strip, usually made of 1-inch white tape, is placed on a bag of fluids, and the times are correlated with what the estimated fluid levels should be at that given time. This allows the technician the ability to adjust the fluid rate as it is checked every 1–2 hours.

Fluid Therapy for Shock
There are times when an animal is in a life-threatening condition, such as shock or cardiovascular shutdown, and an

Fluid for
Jasper
2/12/99
69 cc/hr

1 drop / 5 sec

3 pm

5 pm

7 pm

9 pm

11 pm

1 am

3 am

5 am

7 am

9 am

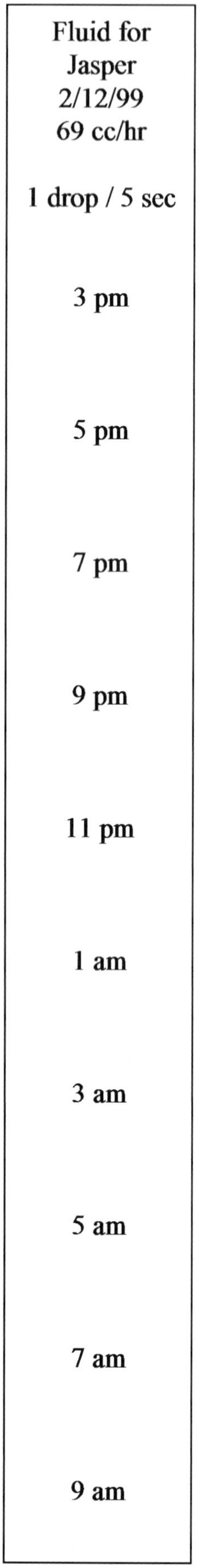

Figure 28.3. Example of a chronicity strip used to help monitor fluid rate of a patient over time.

emergency fluid dose may need to be given. At this time, this patient needs high fluid volumes to maintain their blood pressure and cardiac output. *Emergency doses of fluids are not associated or subtracted from daily need. They are given until normal perfusion and cardiac output are returned and the patient is no longer in shock.* General guidelines for emergency boluses are as follows:

- **Dogs:** 90 ml/kg /h × wt (kg)
- **Cats:** 45 ml/kg/h × wt (kg)

Example VII: A 40-kg dog is hit by a car. He has poor pulse, gum color, and is nonresponsive. He is determined to be in shock by the veterinarian, this patient can receive;

Shock Dose = weight (kg) × 90 ml/kg/h
Emergency Dose = 40 kg × 90 ml/kg/h = 3600 ml/h

Due to the life-threatening emergency, these fluids are given as quickly as possible, often with a high-pressure bag to maximize fluid administration (see Figure 28.4).

It is important to understand that these shock doses represent the maximum amount of fluids a "healthy" pet can receive in 1 hour before fluid begins to build up within the tissue. There are many patients that cannot tolerate these large doses, and the animal must be closely monitored for fluid overload while shock doses are being administered.

Once the pet is stabilized, it is re-evaluated by the veterinarian and hourly fluid rate is reassigned, depending on dehydration, medical disease, and current physical condition. Please refer to Table 28.2 for a *rough* overview of fluid need based on the patient's physical condition.

Complications—Fluid Overload
Fluid overload refers to the situation in which an animal is receiving too many intravenous fluids or receiving fluids too quickly. If too much fluid is given, the excess fluid can begin to pool outside the vessels and produce fluid buildup in the tissue. If enough fluid accumulates in the lungs, the pet can drown. Signs of fluid overload are

- clear nasal discharge as fluids are being given,
- licking lips,
- acting nauseous,
- fluid buildup in feet, under neck (edema), and
- increased respiratory effort and respiratory crackles evident.

Practice Tip: If signs of fluid overload occur, fluids should be temporarily stopped and the doctor contacted immediately.

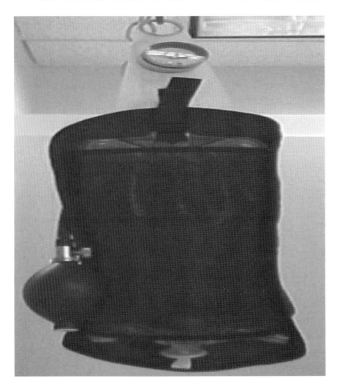

Figure 28.4. An image of a modified human blood pressure cuff. Fluid bags are slid into the pocket and the cuff inflated to 200–300 psi. This allows large amounts of fluids to be given intravenously in a matter of minutes. The patient must be carefully monitored for fluid overload while the emergency bolus is being administrated.

Administration

Intravenous fluids are administered through an indwelling peripheral vein, central line, or an intraosseous (in the bone) catheter. The fluids are administered through a sterile fluid line, extension set, and possibly a t-connector into the catheter. Each hospital has its own protocols for IV catheterization and fluid administration; the goal of the procedure is to place a sterile system in place and bandage it to support the catheter for long-term hospitalization.

Discussing Intravenous Fluid Administration (In-Patient) with the Client
- Intravenous fluids are sterile fluids delivered directly into a vein for rehydration, flushing of toxins, and fluid support of sick hospitalized patients.
- Animals on intravenous fluids must be maintained in a hospitalized setting to monitor the pet for hydration or changes in the stability of the pet.
- Animals on intravenous fluids may be supported for days in the hospital environment, depending on their disease conditions.
- Intravenous fluids are meant to maintain fluid hydration while also being able to supply the body with needed electrolytes, sugars, and medications necessary for the ill patient.

Applications and Administration of Intravenous Fluids—Colloids

Colloids are large macromolecular synthetic solutions (i.e., hetastarch, pentastarch) or natural solutions (i.e., blood, plasma, packed red blood cells) used in the treatment of shock and the maintenance of intravascular fluid balance. These large, dense molecules enter the blood vessels and increase the amount of fluid drawn into the vessels, resulting in increased blood pressure. There are two categories of colloids: natural and synthetic.

- Natural colloids include whole blood, plasma products, and albumin.
- Synthetic colloids are formulated from various sources, such as gelatins, polysaccharides (dextrans), or amylopectins (hetastarch).

Pharmacologic classification is based upon molecular weight, plasma half-life, and colloid oncotic pressure. Each colloid solution within these groups has specific characteristics, qualities, and side effects that must be considered in the selection of the appropriate therapy for each patient.

Table 28.2. Estimate of fluid need based on hydration and fluid loss status.*

Species	Condition	Significant V/D	Suggested Fluid Administration Level
Feline & canine	0–5% dehydrated/stable	N	Maintenance→ 1.5 × maintenance
Feline & canine	0–5% dehydrated/stable	Y	Bolus + 1.5–2×/maintenance
Feline & canine	7–9% dehydrated/stable	N	Bolus + maintenance→ 1.5× maintenance
Feline & canine	7–9 % dehydrated/stable	Y	Bolus + 2× maintenance
Feline & canine	9–12 % dehydrated/stable	N	Bolus + 2× maintenance
Feline & canine	9–12% dehydrated/stable	Y	Bolus + 2×/maintenance
Feline	Unstable	Y or N	Shock fluid doses (45 ml/kg/h)
Canine	Unstable	Y or N	Shock fluid doses (90 ml/kg/h)

*This table is a rough estimate of fluid need and should be used only as a reference for the medical team member to ascertain the relative fluid level needed for a sick patient. *All fluid administration rates are based solely on the veterinarian recommendations.*

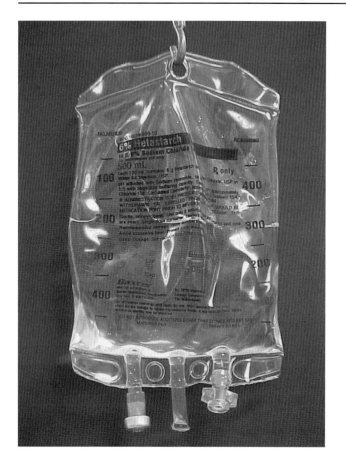

Figure 28.5.   An image of the synthetic colloid hetastarch.

Indications

Colloids can serve two overall functions. They can increase fluid uptake into the vessels from the tissue increasing blood pressure. The colloids generally used for this function are hetastarch (see Figure 28.5) and pentastarch.

Colloids can replace necessary blood factors needed for oxygenation of tissue, clotting of blood, and wound healing. The colloids used for this function are as follows.

- **Packed red blood cells:** Packed red blood cells serve as a source of red blood cells to help the patient increase its packed cell volume and increase the oxygen-carrying capacity of the blood.
- **Plasma:** Plasma is the fluid portion of blood that carries the proteins necessary for clotting blood. Furthermore, plasma is rich in a protein called albumin, which maintains blood pressure by drawing water into the blood vessels. Without proper levels of albumin in the blood, fluid can pool in the tissue, causing edema and decreasing blood pressure. Furthermore, albumin is a key protein in tissue healing.

Contraindications

Each of these colloids has its own limitations, depending on the patient's condition. The main contraindications are listed next.

- **Allergic reaction:** These chemicals can produce moderate to severe allergic reaction in the pet and should always be administered slowly in a hospital situation.
- **Dehydration:** Furthermore, because these drugs also function to pull fluid into the vascular supply, *the pet must be reasonably hydrated before administration.* Giving colloids to a dehydrated animal can lead to further dehydration and poor circulation because the body is unable to move these larger molecules to the bloodstream.

Calculation of Fluid Need

The only colloid that will be discussed for calculation information is hetastarch. Hetastarch is given in emergency cases when normal intravenous fluids are not returning normal perfusion and strong pulses to the shocky patient. As with all other fluid calculations, recommendations for fluid administration are made by the veterinarian. However, in an emergency situation, the medical staff should have an understanding of the needs of the patient and anticipate the veterinarian in order to be ready to begin treatment of a life-threatened pet.

A dose of hetastarch is based on the following.

- **Cat:** 11–15 ml/kg/day
- **Dog:** 11–22 ml/kg/day

Example VIII: A 5-kg feline with poor pulses and in shock has already been given a large bolus of intravenous fluids. The veterinarian is now recommending the use of hetastarch in conjunction with the IV fluids. Dose range would be:

5 kg × 11–15 ml/kg/day = 55–75 ml/day

Complications

Colloids can produce mild to severe allergic/anaphylactic reactions to administration (see Chapter 30). Patients should be always maintained in a hospital setting under direct supervision. Fluids should be given slowly, initially, to make sure the pet is not having any severe reaction, especially in felines. Although this is an uncommon complication, the pet must be closely monitored for

- increasing dehydration,
- increased respiratory effort,
- increasing heart/pulse rate,
- paling of the mucous membranes,
- respiratory wheezing,
- decreased mentation/responsivity,
- lateral or sternal recumbence,
- collapse, and
- cardiopulmonary arrest (severe cases).

Administration

Hetastarch can be administrated by a number of procedures. Two possible procedures follow.

IV Fluid Administration Algorithm

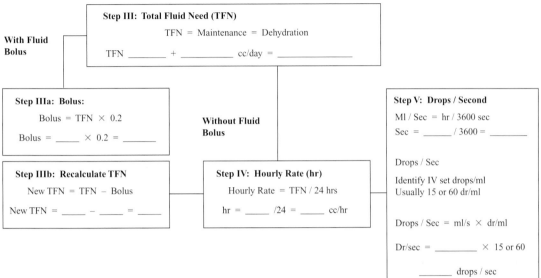

Step I: Maintenance Fluids:

_____Wt (kg) × 66 cc/kg/day = _____ cc/day

Note: Maintenance fluid may be $1\frac{1}{2}$ - 2 × maintenance (99 - 132 cc/kg/day) due to fluid losses or diuresis.

Step II: Dehydration:

_____Wt (kg) × _____ % Dehyd × 1000 ml/l = _____ cc/day

Dehydration is expressed in decimal form: (i.e., 5% dehydrated = 0.05, or 10% dehydrated = 0.1)

With Fluid Bolus

Step III: Total Fluid Need (TFN)

TFN = Maintenance = Dehydration

TFN _____ + _____ cc/day = _____

Step IIIa: Bolus:

Bolus = TFN × 0.2

Bolus = _____ × 0.2 = _____

Without Fluid Bolus

Step IIIb: Recalculate TFN

New TFN = TFN – Bolus

New TFN = _____ – _____ = _____

Step IV: Hourly Rate (hr)

Hourly Rate = TFN / 24 hrs

hr = _____ /24 = _____ cc/hr

Step V: Drops / Second

Ml / Sec = hr / 3600 sec

Sec = _____ / 3600 = _____

Drops / Sec

Identify IV set drops/ml
Usually 15 or 60 dr/ml

Drops / Sec = ml/s × dr/ml

Dr/sec = _____ × 15 or 60

_____ drops / sec

- **Small patient** (<10 pounds; requirements of <75 ml): The hetastarch can be mixed with an even volume of intravenous fluids in an IV burette system and given over 30–120 minutes.
- **Larger patient** (>15 pounds; 100–500 ml): The medication can be given directly into a catheter over 30–90 minutes. Furthermore, the drug could be drawn up into a number of syringes and injected into the IV line over the same period of time.

CD-ROM 2 will focus on concepts of Understanding the Concepts of Disease and Treatment. The exercises can be done individually or as case rounds as they explore specific topics in veterinary medicine that discuss clinical diagnostics and treatment.

Discussing Colloid Therapy (In-Patient) with the Client
- Colloids are a special class of fluid used to help increase blood pressure or return necessary blood products to the life-threatened patient.
- These liquids are slowly given intravenously in a hospitalized setting to help stabilize the patient.
- Although rare, these fluids can produce an allergic reaction, so the patient must be closely monitored for any changes in its stability.
- These fluids can greatly help in the stabilization of the patient.

Chapter 29

Anesthesia

Introduction

Anesthesia is defined as a loss of sensation in a body part (local) or the entire body (general). The anesthetic drugs depress part of the central or peripheral nervous system activity. Some goals of anesthesia are amnesia of the surgery, muscle relaxation, lack of movement, and freedom from pain. There are four stages of anesthesia.

- **Stage I: Voluntary movement:** The patient will respond to stimuli and can move voluntarily.
- **Stage II: Excitement phase:** As the animal begins to succumb to anesthesia, the patient goes through an excitement phase, which is noted by flailing of its limbs and acting as if it is trying to escape. The patient still sharply responds to stimulus and will blink briskly when the medial nasal border of the eyelid is tapped (**palpebral response**). The pet has tight jaw tone and cannot be intubated with an endotracheal tube at this time. This is a stage of delirium and involuntary movement.
- **Stage III: Surgical anesthesia:** The patient still responds to stimuli but the jaw tone is relaxed so the animal can be intubated. This is the surgical level. The patient may still have a normal heart and respiratory rate and a sharp palpebral response, but can go through a surgical procedure without response to stimuli and have amnesia. This level can progress to a deeper surgical plane in which the animal becomes profoundly depressed. The patient's eyes roll back in its head, there is no jaw or muscle tone, a minimal or absent palpebral response is noted, and there is slowing of heart and respiratory rates. This stage is divided into four planes.
  - **Light:** The light anesthetic plane provides enough central nervous system depression for minor procedures (i.e., skin laceration repair).
  - **Moderate:** The moderate anesthetic plane provides enough central nervous system depression for minor to moderate anesthetic procedures (i.e., castration, subcutaneous lump removal).
  - **Medium:** Medium anesthetic depth produces more profound depression for major procedures such as minor orthopedic care, spays, and declawing.
  - **Deep:** The deep anesthetic plane is the deepest surgical anesthesia used for major surgical procedures that produce significant pain response. Examples of these procedures are major orthopedic surgeries (i.e., tibial plateau leveling osteotomy), or an ear canal ablation.
- **Stage IV:** Deep anesthesia, which is close to death.

Understanding the Anesthetic Machinery

The medical team must have a basic knowledge of the anesthetic equipment. This includes machine maintenance needs and understanding the physical symptoms of the patient that would occur if there is a failure in the machinery. Equipment needs for anesthesia are discussed next.

Endotracheal Tubes

Endotracheal tubes are plastic tubes that range from 2.5 mm to 14 mm and are a connective link between the patient's airway and the anesthetic machine. The tube should be clean prior to intubation and inflated to make sure the balloon cuff does not have any leaks. The balloon cuff expands to fill the tracheal dimensions. The seal prevents air from escaping around the endotracheal tube and food and particulate material from entering the trachea. The endotracheal cuff should always be deflated prior to extubation to prevent tracheal and laryngeal damage.

Laryngoscopes

Laryngoscopes are lighted oral speculums that are used to depress the tongue and adequately visualize the larynx. This enables placing the endotracheal tube into the trachea (**intubation**) with accuracy and limits the possibility of esophageal intubation. There are different sizes of laryngeal blades that allow the intubation of different sizes of animals.

Anesthetic Machines

The purpose of anesthetic machines is to deliver oxygen, control the levels of anesthesia, and assist ventilation. The basic components of the machine are a compressed gas source (oxygen), a pressure regulator that controls pressure leaving the compressed gas canister, a pressure gauge indicating the amount of gas left in the oxygen tank, a flow meter that controls the flow of oxygen, a vaporizer that facilitates delivery of a controlled concentration of anesthesia, and an oxygen flush valve that allows a rapid flush of oxygen directly into the anesthetic circuit, bypassing the vaporizer.

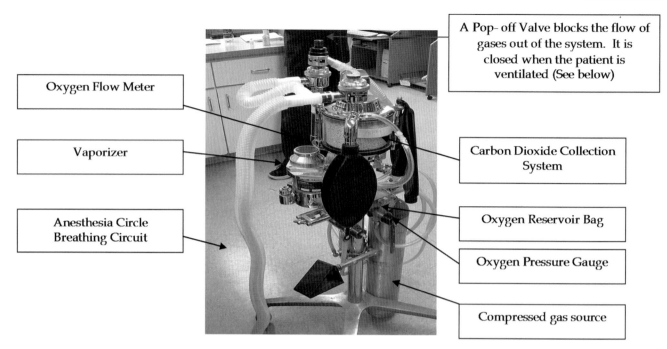

Oxygen Flow Meter

Vaporizer

Anesthesia Circle
Breathing Circuit

A Pop- off Valve blocks the flow of
gases out of the system. It is
closed when the patient is
ventilated (See below)

Carbon Dioxide Collection
System

Oxygen Reservoir Bag

Oxygen Pressure Gauge

Compressed gas source

Figure 29.1.   Image of an anesthetic system.

Equipment Function
Vaporizer
A vaporizer converts a volatile liquid anesthesia into vapor.

Carbon Dioxide Canisters
Canisters containing carbon dioxide-absorbent granules (i.e., Sodasorb) help filter carbon dioxide (toxin) out of the breathing circuit, preventing accumulation of carbon dioxide in the body. If carbon dioxide levels are not controlled, increasing levels can inhibit many physiological processes, such as muscle, brain, and organ system functions. Granules should be changed for every 10 hours of anesthesia. In most cases the granules will show a bluish color change, but not always.

Active Scavenger Systems
Active scavenger systems are venting systems that actively expel anesthetic gases out of the environment. It is important to reduce anesthesia exposure, which can cause fatigue and headache. If using an absorbent canister system, it should be routinely weighed to assess if the canister needs to be changed. These canisters are exhausted when they gain 50 g in weight.

Breathing Circuits
There are two types of breathing circuits: non-rebreather and circle systems. The appropriate type is chosen based on the patient's weight.

• **Circle circuit:** This is the most common type of anesthetic circuit used for patients over 10 pounds (see Figure

29.1). This system allows the animal to rebreathe the mixture of anesthesia and oxygen, reducing the amount of anesthetic liquid and oxygen used during the procedure. Without functional carbon dioxide absorbents, the system can build up an increased amount of carbon dioxide.

• **Non-rebreathing circuit:** Non-rebreathing circuits are used in patients that weigh less than 10 pounds and that can fatigue easily from the increased work of breathing required to move gas through the circle system. The carbon dioxide and waste gases that are expired are eliminated from the patient's next breath by the high oxygen flow into the circuit. This type of circuit increases the amount of liquid anesthesia used because it requires higher oxygen flow to prevent rebreathing of carbon dioxide.

Hospital Team Anesthetic Maintenance Requirements

The hospital team must perform daily, weekly, and monthly maintenance on the anesthetic machinery to make sure that the anesthetic equipment can safely anesthetize the pet. *By far, the most important common cause of anesthetic accidents and death is mismanagement of the anesthetic equipment.* The medical team should maintain the equipment on the following schedule.

Daily
At the beginning of each day, prior to any anesthesia procedures, the medical team must have the equipment evaluated for safety. It must also be set up for the first surgical procedure. An initial checklist follows.

1. **Make sure the oxygen and scavenger systems are on.** Ensure that oxygen levels are sufficient for the day's procedures.
2. **Maintain anesthetic levels in the vaporizer.** The vaporizer should be filled when indicated by the fill lines on the window on the front of the vaporizer.
3. **Evaluate carbon dioxide granules for signs of exhaustion.** If carbon dioxide builds up to toxic levels within an anesthesia circuit, the patient's respiratory center will be inhibited, stopping respiration. The carbon dioxide-absorbent granules should be evaluated for exhaustion after every procedure and at the end of the day.
4. **Assemble the anesthesia machine.** The anesthetic machine should be assembled with the correct circuit based upon the patient's weight. An oxygen reservoir bag should be placed on the machine that best correlates to the patient's weight. The bag should be chosen as follows.

Reservoir Bag Size	Patient's Weight
0.5–l bag (circle or non-rebreather)	<20 lb
1 l	20–40
2 l	40–60
3 l	60–100

5. **Evaluate machinery for gas leaks.**
   - Turn on the oxygen supply to the anesthesia machine. Ensure there is enough oxygen in the oxygen cylinder for the entire procedure.
   - Close off the pop-off valve and cover the Y-piece with the palm or thumb.
   - Turn on the oxygen until the reservoir bag is inflated to 20-cm water pressure.
   - Turn the oxygen off and watch the manometer (pressure gauge) or the reservoir bag, if using a non-rebreathing circuit. If the pressure drops rapidly, or the reservoir bag deflates, gradually turn on the oxygen flow meter until the pressure remains constant. The flow rate of oxygen necessary to maintain a constant pressure indicates the size of the leak, or leaks, in the anesthesia machine.
   - Check the breathing hoses, reservoir bag, vaporizer inlet and outlet, any screw-down fittings, and the seals on the top and bottom of the Sodasorb canister for leaks. When the pressure remains constant with the oxygen turned off, the machine can be considered leak free.
   - **Open the pop-off valve after the leak check.**
6. **Get the endotracheal tube and laryngoscope ready.** Two to three sizes of endotracheal tubes should be readied for the procedure. The size of the endotracheal tube depends on the patient's weight, size, and breed. Certain breeds of dogs (i.e., pugs, shar-peis, English bull dogs) may have a much smaller trachea diameter than their body weight suggests.

A general recommendation for **canine** endotracheal tube size is as follows.

Endotracheal Tube Size	Canine Patient's Weight
5 mm	4–6 lb (1.8–2.7 kg)
5.5 mm	7–8 lb (3.2–3.6 kg)
6 mm	9–11 lb (4–5 kg)
6.5 mm	12–14 lb (5.5–6.4 kg)
7 mm	15–20 lb (6.8–9 kg)
7.5 mm	17–20 lb (7.7–9 kg)
8 mm	21–26 lb (9.5–11.8 kg)
8.5 mm	27–28 lb (12.3–12.7 kg)
9.0 mm	29–31 lb (13–14 kg)
9.5 mm	32–33 lb (14.5–15 kg)
10 mm	31–40 lb (14–18 kg)
11 mm	41–65 lb (18.6–29.5 kg)
12 mm	66–85 lb (30–38.6 kg)
14–16 mm	86–120 lb (39–55 kg)

Recommendations of endotracheal tube size for feline patients are based on weight.

Endotracheal Tube Size	Feline Patient's Weight
3 mm	2–3 lb (0.9–1.4 kg)
3.5 mm	4–6 lb (1.8–2.7 kg)
4 mm	7–10 lb (3.2–4.5 kg)
5 mm	11 lb or more (5 kg +)

7. **Have monitoring devices and warm water heating pads ready.**
8. **Make sure pop-off valve is open.** The pop-off valve is closed for ventilation and to evaluate the anesthetic system for leaks. If the valve is not open while the patient is attached, no gas can escape the system. This creates a buildup of pressure that can damage the lungs and cause potential death. *This cannot be overemphasized as this is the primary cause of anesthetic accident.*

At the end of each day, team members should do the following.

1. Open the pop-off valve all the way and leave it open overnight so that any moisture in the valve can evaporate. If moisture evaporates with the valve closed, it may cause the valve to stick in the closed position.
2. Remove the dome on the expiratory side of the rebreathing circuit, dry the flutter valve, and leave the dome off overnight to allow any moisture that has accumulated in the circuit to dry.
3. Rinse the breathing hoses with mild soap or dilute betadine solution and allow them to air dry overnight.
4. Check the carbon dioxide absorbent. If the absorbent is not discarded when the indicator initially turns color, it

will fade back to white even if the absorbent is exhausted. Baralyme and soda lime are caustic when wet; keep them away from your eyes, nose, and mouth, as well as endotracheal tubes, breathing hoses, and any other means by which it could reach your patients' lungs.

5. Turn all medical gasses off at the tank.
6. Look at the machine, especially the base and wheels. Use a nonvolatile product to clean the machine; Windex works well. *Never* use a petroleum-based product such as WD-40 or Vaseline on your anesthetic machine.

Weekly and Monthly Maintenance Needs

Needed weekly and monthly maintenance can vary from machine to machine. It is recommended that the service manual be reviewed for long-term maintenance needs and that the medical teams implement a schedule of proper weekly and monthly maintenance based on the service manual.

An Overview of the Anesthetic Procedure

Although the veterinarian is responsible for the surgical procedure, the medical team member is responsible for properly monitoring the anesthetized patient and should be able to recognize problems early enough to prevent patient harm. The team member must be able to monitor the patient adequately through a thorough brief physical examination, record their findings, and relate the information to the other team members. The team member responsible for monitoring must be able to perform the following steps.

Step I: Obtain a Thorough Medical History on Admittance

It is recommended that the history be obtained through a written questionnaire that the client signs. Although outlined in Chapter 5, a complete medical history should be discussed with the client to make sure the patient is a good anesthetic candidate. Some key questions should be asked.

When Did the Patient Last Eat?

Patients should not have access to food for 8 hours prior to surgery. A patient may vomit if there is food in its stomach while under anesthesia. The unconscious patient cannot properly swallow, allowing an aspiration of food particles into the trachea and lungs, producing a life-threatening pneumonia (**aspiration pneumonia**). In some situations, surgery may need to be postponed until the animal is properly fasted. However, small amounts of water up to admission should be encouraged to prevent dehydration.

Is There Any History of Previous Disease or Medical Conditions?

A questionnaire with a list of important medical conditions or diseases may help the client focus on primary concerns that could be affected by anesthesia. Conditions such as seizures, heart disease, kidney or liver problems, infectious disease, or hormonal diseases (i.e., diabetes mellitus, hyper-

adrenocorticism, etc.) should be identified prior to administering anesthesia.

Is the Patient on Any Prescribed, Homeopathic, or Over-the-Counter Medication?

Many medications can affect anesthesia or surgery. For example, chronic aspirin therapy can produce slowed platelet function and increased bleeding. Many owners will not realize that drugs such as aspirin are medications. A list of any current medications should be obtained prior to surgery. To prevent improper medication of the patient prior to surgery, place a statement on the surgical release form, such as "*Your pet should not receive any supplements, vitamins, aspirin, or other medications or over-the-counter products 24 hours prior to anesthesia.*"

Has the Pet Ever Shown Allergies to Any Medication, Food or Vaccinations?

It is important to know if a patient is allergic to any medications. If medication is given under anesthesia (i.e., antibiotics) or in recovery, the patient may not show typical symptoms of allergic reaction and may develop a more severe anaphylactic shock. An understanding of any drug allergies may prevent any reaction from occurring while under anesthesia. It is important to evaluate if the patient is sensitive to egg/chicken protein, because propofol anesthesia is egg based.

Has the Patient Ever Had a Problem with Anesthesia?

In some cases owners will report that their pet had a problem with anesthetic during its last procedure, such as a slow recovery, low blood pressure during the procedure, etc. If there has been a concern with a prior procedure, the medical team should be informed immediately and the medical records obtained for the veterinarian to review prior to anesthesia to determine what may have caused the problem.

Step II: Obtaining Presurgery Clinical Diagnostics

Presurgery clinical diagnostics can vary depending on the age, health, history of disease, and the medical concerns by the veterinarian. Each hospital team develops their own list of recommendations/requirements for specific ages, breeds, and species of their patients. An example of possible presurgery clinical diagnostics may be

- Juvenile blood screen (for patients <12 months old):
  — Complete blood count
  — Mini-chemistry (i.e., BUN, creatinine, ALT, glucose, etc.)
- Adult blood screen (for patients 1–6 years):
  — Complete blood count
  — Full chemistry and electrolytes
  — Urinalysis
- Geriatric clinical diagnostic (for patients 7 years +):
  — Complete blood count
  — Full chemistry and electrolytes

— Urinalysis
— Thyroid (felines)
— Electrocardiogram
— Blood pressure

Step III: IV Catheterization and Intravenous Fluid

Placement of an intravenous catheter and administration of fluids during surgery can be very important in maintaining hydration and blood pressure, administering emergency drugs and medications, and ensuring adequate organ and tissue perfusion. Suggest surgical fluid rates are

10–20 ml/kg in the first hour of surgery
5–10 ml/kg/h in each successive hour

Fluid rates should be decreased if the patient is suffering from cardiac disease, acute renal failure, hypoproteinemia, or other diseases that could produce increased risk of fluid overload and pulmonary edema (see Chapter 27). Fluid rates can be increased with concerns of hypotension, blood loss, or disease conditions that require an increased fluid rate. If blood loss is occurring during surgery, it takes three times as much fluid to make up for the amount of blood lost. Furthermore, if the packed cell volume is less than 20%, whole blood should be used immediately. If bleeding is rapid, packed cell volume may not show the actual decrease for 1–2 hours. An estimate of blood loss is

1 blood-soaked 3 × 3 cotton sponge = 10 cc blood
10 Q-tips soaked = 1 ml of blood

Step IV: Evaluating the Anesthetic Patient

This should not be confused with the veterinarian's physical examination of the patient, which should be completed concurrently. Prior to anesthesia and surgery, the monitoring team member should do a thorough precursory physical examination. This allows the team member to appreciate the patient's cardiovascular and other body systems prior to preanesthetic medications or anesthesia. Furthermore, if an abnormality is detected (i.e., pulse deficit) by the team member, the veterinarian can reassess the patient as an anesthetic candidate. The preanesthetic examination (see Chapter 6) should include:

- auscultation of the cardiovascular and respiratory system,
- appreciation of pulse quality,
- temperature,
- appreciation of mucous membrane color and capillary refill time, and
- hydration status.

Step V: Understand the Induction and Maintenance Anesthetics and Their Effect on the Patient

Specific medications can affect mucous membrane color, heart rate, respiratory rate, and other physiological factors of the patient. In order to properly monitor anesthesia, the team member must understand the purpose of each drug used, its physiological effect on the patient, and any possible side effects. A brief overview of the drugs and their purpose in the anesthetic process are discussed next.

Preanesthetic Medication

This category of medication refers to a variety of medications that can be used to sedate the patient, reduce the amount of anesthesia needed, decrease pain, and minimize autonomic reflex activity that slows the heart and respiratory systems. The choices of which medications to use depend on the experience and preference of the veterinarian.

Anticholinergic Drugs
This category of drug blocks the part of the **autonomic nervous system** that reflexively slows the heart, increases production of secretions from the respiratory and gastrointestinal system, produces movement of the intestines, and constricts the iris of the eye. The goal of this medication is to

- increase heart rate,
- increase bronchodilatation, and
- decrease secretions within the gastrointestinal and respiratory system.

Examples
Examples include

- atropine, and
- glycopyrrolate.

Function
Anticholinergic drugs may be included in many anesthetic procedures but are most often used in conjunction with other drugs.

Anesthetics that are most likely to produce bradycardia are

- **Alpha₂ agonists:** xylazine/medetomidine
- **Opioids:** morphine, oxymorphone, hydromorphone
- **Short-term induction anesthetics:** thiamylal (Biotal), propofol (Rapinovet)
- **Gas anesthesia:** isoflurane, sevoflurane
- **Dissociative anesthetics:** for example, ketamine, which can increase salivation.

Side Effects/Contraindications
Due to the pharmacological effects of anticholinergic medications, the following concerns should be noted.

- **Tachycardia:** These drugs can produce a profound tachycardia. Patients with underlying heart disease, especially those prone to arrhythmia, should be treated cautiously with anticholinergic medications. The reflex tachycardia that is produced can stress the cardiovascular system and potentiate shock and collapse.

- **Ileus:** Anticholinergic drugs should also be used with caution with patients with intestinal diseases (i.e., intestinal obstruction, gastric dilatation and volvulus syndrome, etc.) that produce gastrointestinal stasis (**ileus**).

Tranquilizers

These drugs are used to depress the central nervous system, aid in restraint, and reduce struggling of the patient. They also reduce the dose requirement of induction and maintenance drugs and reduce the excitatory signs of early anesthesia.

- **Phenothiazines:** The phenothiazines (i.e., acepromazine) are long-term medications (usually lasting 8–12 hours in duration) used more for sedation. The drug is more effectively used in combination with other sedatives (i.e., butorphanol). Phenothiazines should be used with caution in liver and kidney patients, geriatric and debilitated animals, patients in shock, and animals with seizures. Furthermore, excited or stressed patients may not become sedate when acepromazine is used alone.
- **Benzodinepines:** Drugs such as Diazepam and midozolam can produce mild to moderate sedation more safely in the geriatric patient. These drugs can be used to help control seizures and can be combined with other anesthetics as induction agents (see below). When used alone, benzodinepines can cause unruliness in dogs and cats because the drug can cause loss of inhibition.
- **Alpha$_2$ agonists:** Drugs such as xylazine (Rompun) and medetomidine (Domitor) can produce excellent calming, muscle relaxation, and short-duration analgesia. These drugs are generally combined with opioids or benzodinepines to produce more reliable sedation. These drugs can produce serious hypotension, bradycardia, and arrhythmias and should be used only in healthy cats and dogs. Furthermore, excited or stressed patients may not become sedate when alpha$_2$ agonists are used alone.
- **Opioid agonist/antagonist:** Drugs such as butorphanol (Torbutrol) and buprenorphine (Buprenex) help reduce the patient's response to pain.

Side Effects

Besides the specific side effects listed above, this category of drugs can lead to oversedation, which may be dangerous for the anesthetized animal.

Analgesics

This class of medication helps decrease pain sensitivity prior to, during, and after surgery. By including analgesics in preanesthetic drug combinations, the amount of pain the patient experiences and the amount of subsequent analgesics needed after surgery is reduced.

Example—Opioids

Drugs such as oxymorphone, morphine, and fentanyl are commonly used to produce analgesia and sedation. With the use of transdermal fentanyl, patches need to be applied 12 or more hours before surgery to be effective postoperatively. Caution should be used with patients that have a predisposition to cardiac or respiratory disease. When using a fentanyl patch that does not take affect for 12–18 hours, other analgesics (non-steroidal anti-inflammatory drugs or other opioids) must be given postsurgically to help control acute pain.

Induction Agents

The goal of induction agents is to bypass stage II anesthesia (excitatory phase) so the patient can be intubated, gaining rapid control of the airway, and maintained on gas or injectable anesthesia.

Examples

- **Dissociative agents:** Drugs such as ketamine, in conjunction with benzodiazepines (i.e., Valium), can be used for induction of anesthesia. These combinations have few contraindications and can be used in geriatric and ill patients.
- **Short-acting barbiturates:** Drugs such as thiamylal, propofol, and thiopental can be used for induction to get the animal on anesthesia and then quickly inactivated. These drugs must be used with caution in patients with cardiac disease (especially arrhythmia); they often cause a short-term cessation in respiration (**apnea**).

Side Effects

An anesthetic overdose leads to significant cardiac and respiratory depression, which can result in the death of the patient.

Maintenance Anesthesia Agents

This category refers to inhalant (gas) or injectable anesthesia that produces unconsciousness, muscle relaxation, and analgesia.

Examples

In most hospitals, long-term anesthesia is maintained with gas anesthesia (i.e., isoflurane, sevoflurane) (see Figure 29.2).

Function

Gas anesthesia allows for rapid changes in the depth of anesthesia and more rapid recovery. Inhalant anesthesia, like injectable anesthetics, can produce severe cardiopulmonary effects and requires expense and upkeep of equipment. The most common anesthetics are:

- **Isoflurane:** This newer generation anesthetic has low solubility with 97.4% of the gas exhaled. It produces a variable amount of cardiac and respiratory depression depending on the dose and depth of anesthesia.
- **Sevoflurane:** This is the newest gas anesthesia available. It is the least soluble, producing quick induction and recovery. Patients on sevoflurane must be monitored closely because they can begin to wake up from maintenance at a slightly more rapid rate.

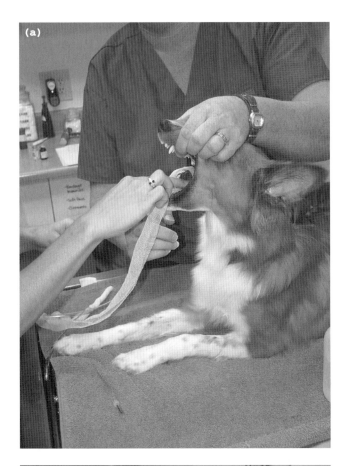

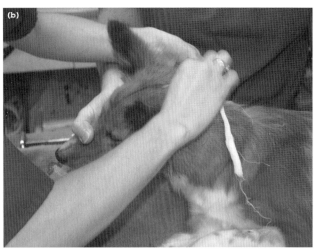

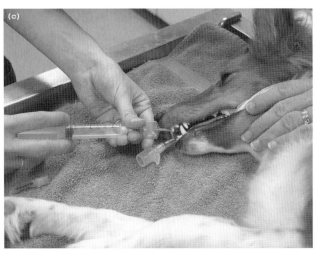

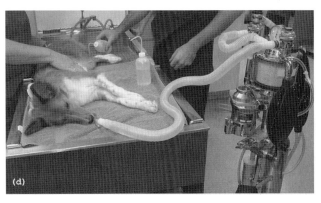

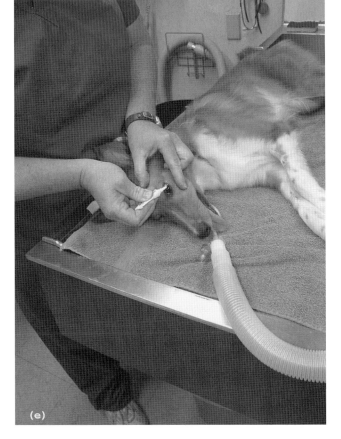

Figure 29.2. Intubation and maintenance. Once the patient is induced, a laryngoscope is positioned to depress the tongue and visualize the larynx, and the endotracheal tube is placed in the trachea (a). The tube is then tied in place (b). The cuff is inflated. Care should be taken not to overinflate the cuff and damage the trachea (c). The animal is placed on a circle circuit (d). A petroleum eye ointment is applied to the eye (e).

Side Effects

Potential side effects depend on the patients and their health status (i.e., heart disease), the length of the procedure, the preanesthetic medication, and the level of gas anesthesia on which a patient is maintained. Specific side effects are listed next.

- **Increased depression of heart and respiratory function:** Slowing of the heart and respiratory rates, **hypoxia**, and decreased cardiac output can be observed as the patient enters deeper anesthesia. In some cases respiratory depression can be so severe that the patient may need assisted ventilation by hand or mechanical ventilation.
- **Cardiac arrhythmias:** With decreased cardiac and respiratory function, tissue can be hypoxic. Decreased oxygenation of cardiac muscle can produce arrhythmias that further decrease cardiac output.
- **Hypotension:** With decreased cardiac output and a depressed central nervous system, the patient's ability to perfuse and maintain blood pressure decreases. In an emergency situation the patient can succumb because the decreased blood pressure cannot maintain adequate perfusion and the body cannot compensate.
- **Hypothermia:** The temperature of the patient must be monitored and maintained to prevent severe hypothermia. Heat is lost to the environment in several ways:
  — Surgical scrub, especially alcohol, increases heat loss through evaporation.
  — An open surgical site can increase heat loss into the environment.
  — A cold surgical table can absorb a great deal of warmth from the patient.
  — Inspired anesthetic can lower core temperature.
  — The patient loses the ability to shiver and vasoconstrict its vessels to produce and maintain heat.
- **Hyperthermia (rare):** Anesthetic reactions producing fever are most common in the following:
  — **Malignant hyperthermia:** In this syndrome patients may have metabolic reactions to the gas itself, producing significant fevers (>105° Fahrenheit) and increasing carbon dioxide to greater then 80–100 mm Hg, producing death.
  — **Nordic breed dogs:** The husky, malamute, etc., have a thicker insulating coat and a higher body temperature, producing higher than normal body temperatures while under anesthesia.
  — **Inhalant anesthesia:** Although more commonly reported in patients undergoing halothane anesthesia, it has been rarely reported in patients anesthetized with isoflurane.
  — **Injectable anesthesia:** Certain drugs (i.e., ketamine and alpha$_2$ agonists) can reset the body's thermoregulatory center for up to 8–12 hours, and as a result fever can be seen.

Step VI: Monitoring Anesthesia

Monitoring anesthesia is the most important technical responsibility associated with surgical procedures. *The anesthetized patient can succumb to anesthesia and die within 5 minutes.* The team member must be able to constantly evaluate the cardiovascular, respiratory, and neurologic systems for changes that could signal a change in status.

Anesthetic Record

Although state requirements for an anesthetic record can vary, the team member is also responsible for maintaining a concise record, which carries physiological data measured throughout the anesthetic period. Team members should record the patient's vital signs every 5 minutes to locate trends that may signal a change in status. This document is a legal record of the anesthetic procedure and should contain documentation of the following.

- Preanesthetic exam and pertinent lab values
- Drugs used for premedication, induction, and maintenance of anesthesia
- Periodic physical examination of the patient's physical attributes, including
  — temperature/pulse/respiration,
  — muscle tone,
  — eye reflexes,
  — capillary refill time, and
  — cardiac and respiratory auscultation (if possible).
- Anesthetic gas level (the vaporizer setting at each evaluation period)

Any clinical data should also be recorded during the periodic physical examinations, depending on the type and length of procedure and the availability of monitoring equipment. These parameters may include

- blood pressure,
- percent oxygenation of blood (SPO$_2$),
- blood gas,
- packed cell volume/total solids, and
- EKG monitoring.

Other data that should be recorded include

- the rate per hour and total amount of fluids administered, and
- how the patient recovers and the time of endotracheal extubation.

Physical Monitoring of the Anesthetic Patient

The monitoring team member must be able to do a quick and thorough physical examination of the patient prior to surgery and then continue monitoring these parameters until the animal is fully recovered. (The triage exami-

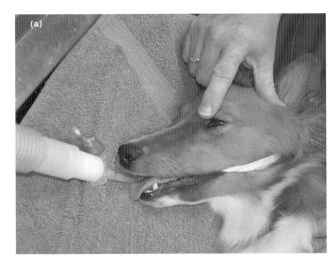
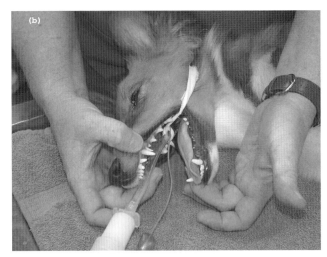
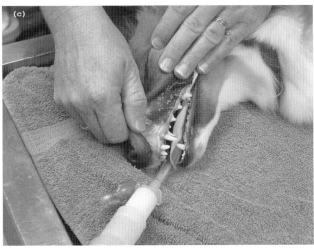
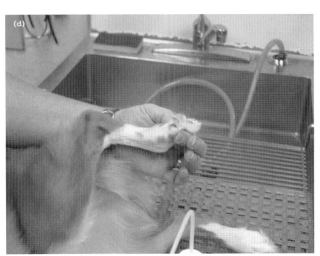

Figure 29.3. Evaluating anesthetic depth. Good monitors of anesthetic depth are palpebral reflex (a), muscular jaw tone (b), mucous membrane color and capillary refill time (c), and the pinch-withdrawal reflex (d).

nation is discussed in Chapter 6.) This process may take a considerable amount of time, even after the endotracheal tube is removed. The following parameters should be carefully monitored during the anesthetic period (see Figure 29.3).

Pulse Quality and Auscultation of the Heart
The team members should both auscultate the heart rhythm and evaluate pulse quality. Any pulse deficits, decreased pulse quality, severe bradycardia, or tachycardia should be reported to the veterinarian immediately.

Respiratory Rate and Auscultation
The patient respiratory rate and character should be observed. Patients that have just been induced can often have decreased or no respiration (apnea). Many patients may need to be ventilated until the animal begins to breathe on its own.

Furthermore, the animal's lungs should be auscultated for crackles suggestive of fluid overload, pulmonary edema secondary to heart disease, or other pathology.

Mucous Membrane Color and Capillary Refill Time
Increases in capillary refill time and paling of the mucous membrane color can suggest decreased cardiac output, bleeding, or early shock. In emergency surgery, spontaneous bruising can suggest bleeding coagulopathy or disseminated intravascular coagulopathy. Any significant changes should be reported to the veterinarian immediately.

Temperature
Hypothermia can challenge the patient and challenge the cardiovascular system. Patients having significant hypothermia (temperature <96° Fahrenheit) should be warmed up with a warm water bottle, surgical warm water heating pads,

or blankets. Rewarming requires that 60% of the patient's body surface area be in contact with an active rewarming device. Covering the legs, tail, and head reduces significant heat loss.

Central Nervous System Evaluation

The patient's anesthetic depth can be evaluated by ocular reflexes, anal and jaw tone, and muscle relaxation.

Ocular Reflexes

Eye Position

As the patient begins light anesthesia, the eyes are generally centered. As the pet begins to enter the surgical anesthetic plane, the eyeballs move downward and medially. If the patient progresses deeper, the eyes can come back to the center position and pupils are usually dilated.

Palpebral Reflex

By placing light pressure on the medial or lateral skin around the eyes, a blink reflex is produced (**palpebral reflex**). In early anesthesia, the reflex is brisk; as the patient progresses deeper, the reflex slows until it disappears completely in deep anesthesia. It should be noted that if done too often, the reflex can exhaust itself.

Corneal Reflex

By placing light pressure on the cornea, the eye should retract and the patient blinks. Care should be taken when evaluating the corneal reflex, since increased digital pressure may produce corneal injury (i.e., corneal ulcer). As the patient enters deeper levels of anesthesia, the corneal reflexes decrease until it disappears completely. This disappears close to death and should always be present unless patient is maintained at a deep plane of anesthesia (i.e., plane 4, deep anesthesia) due to a major orthopedic procedure.

Anal Tone

As the patient enters deeper levels of anesthesia, its normal anal tone relaxes until the anus is fully dilated.

Degree of Muscle Relaxation

As the patient enters a deeper level of anesthesia, muscle tone also decreases. There is absence of voluntary movement, shivering, or withdrawal of the paw when it is pinched (the pinch reflex).

Electronic Anesthetic Monitoring Devices

There are a variety of electronic monitors that aid the medical team in observing body temperature, EKG, pulse oximetry, carbon dioxide levels (**capnography**), respiration, and blood pressure. Each hospital evaluates its needs and decides which monitoring modality best suits its medical team. *However, it is important to understand that no monitoring system can replace the monitoring team member's evaluation of the anesthetized patient.* Examples of monitoring devices are discussed next.

Blood Pressure

Blood pressure is the most important indicator of physiology. Blood pressure monitoring allows the medical team member to evaluate changes in pressure that may indicate a change in status. During anesthesia, the primary concern is decreasing blood pressure, suggesting hypotension, decreased cardiac output, and shock. Decreasing blood pressure may be the first indication of a patient's instability and may need to be aggressively handled by the medical team.

Capnography

The carbon dioxide in expired gas is measured by infra-red spectrophotometry. The measurement of the expired carbon dioxide correlates to the arterial carbon dioxide levels. Increased carbon dioxide levels in the patients can inhibit the respiratory center of the brain and slow or stop respiration.

Temperature

As discussed previously, hypothermia and, rarely, hyperthermia can be side effects of the anesthesia procedure.

Electrocardiogram

The electrocardiogram evaluates the normal EKG rhythm and helps the medical team member detect any cardiac arrhythmias or pathologic changes in the heart rate (see Chapter 24).

Pulse Oximetry

The pulse oximeter evaluates the percentage of oxygenation saturation within the hemoglobin. The sensors are attached to a region of the patient's body where the device can evaluate oxygenation values within the smaller capillaries of the body. Common locations for placement of the probe are the tongue, the interdigital region, the ventral aspect of the tail (with hair shaved, using the rectal probe), or the large muscle masses of the hind legs (tendon probe needed).

Step VII: Recovery

The goal of recovery is to discontinue anesthesia, extubate the patient, return the patient to normal body temperature, and monitor and treat the patient for pain. A suggested protocol for recovery is as follows.

1. **Turn off vaporizer and increase the oxygen flow for 3–4 l/min for 3–5 min:** This will allow the patient to expel any remaining anesthetic gases and increase oxygenation until the patient is fully recovered.
2. **Deflate endotracheal cuff:** This cuff is deflated only when the patient can once again guard its airway (i.e., swallow); **30–50% of patients experience silent regurgitation**. Removal of the tube with the cuff inflated can produce tracheal and laryngeal irritation, causing postoperative coughing, gagging, and possible anorexia.
3. **Change the animal's position and rub the chest:** Changing the patient's position from lateral to sternal re-

cumbency and rubbing the chest gently helps the patient wake.

4. **Reevaluate patient until extubated:** The patient's temperature, pulse, and respiration should be reevaluated periodically and recorded until extubation. If the patient is still hypothermic, warm water blankets, warm towels, and other warming devices covering at least 60% of the patient's surface area should be used until normal body temperature is obtained.

5. **Draw clinical diagnostics:** If postsurgical diagnostics (packed cell volume, blood pressure, etc.) are needed, samples should be obtained at this time.

6. **Monitor for pain:** Depending on the procedure, the patient should be closely monitored for evidence of pain. Tachycardia, increased respiratory effort, or unusual posture or facial expression may suggest that the patient is feeling pain. Any changes within these parameters should be discussed with the veterinarian.

7. **Extubate the patient:** When the patient is sitting sternally and swallowing, the endotracheal tube with the cuff deflated should be carefully removed. Care should be taken to keep the patient sitting sternally when extubating in case the patient begins to vomit. If vomiting is noted, the animal should be immediately positioned with its head lower than its body so that no particles of debris can be aspirated into the trachea or lungs.

Handling Anesthetic Complications

Anesthesia causes stress to the homeostatic processes of the body, causing respiratory and cardiac depression, especially in high-risk patients. Hypotension, cessation of respiration, hypothermia, arrhythmias, and cardiopulmonary arrest can occur in any patient without warning (see Anesthetic Flowchart on p. 432). However, if the team member is observant and monitors vigilantly, certain anesthetic emergencies can be treated in the early phases and the emergency controlled.

Hypotension

This is the most important parameter to monitor in any patient, regardless of health status. It is the only method to assess adequate perfusion, which is necessary to avoid hypoxic tissue damage. Indirect (noninvasive) methods include oscillometric techniques and Doppler ultrasound. Direct (invasive) methods require arterial catheterization.

Normal values for arterial blood pressure in dogs and cats are as follows.

Systolic	110–160 mm Hg
Diastolic	70–90 mm Hg
Mean	70–90 mm Hg

Methods for measuring blood pressure are listed here.

- Oscillometric arterial blood pressure readings are automatically measured by machine. The cuff width must be 40% of the limb circumference for accurate measurements. It may not be reliable in small patients (<5–7 kg). Motion will interfere with measurements and oscillometric readings are inaccurate at low blood pressures. The machines can be relatively expensive.
- Doppler devices used for arterial blood pressure measurement emit an audible noise with every pulse, enabling pulse rate and rhythm to be assessed in addition to arterial blood pressure. Again, cuff width is 40% of the limb circumference for accurate measurement. This method is reliable in all patients, including small patients (<5–7 kg). Doppler is technically more difficult than oscillometry, but can be mastered easily. Devices are relatively inexpensive to acquire.
- Direct arterial blood pressure measurement is the most accurate method. Technically, it is the most difficult method to master, and the monitors are expensive. Risks associated with placing an arterial catheter are small but include infection, arteritis, and hemorrhage. Arterial catheters also provide access for arterial blood sampling and blood gas analysis.

Causes of Hypotension
Causes of hypotension include relative or absolute hypovolemia, shock, sepsis, and drug effects: propofol, inhalant anesthetics, and barbiturates.

Concerns of Hypotension
The most serious adverse effect of hypotension is decreased oxygen delivery to tissues. Anaerobic metabolism is precipitated and acidemia and acidosis will develop. Ischemic organ damage will occur within minutes (less than 20–30) in the kidneys, liver, and brain.

Treatment
Intervention is necessary if the systolic pressure falls below:

Canine: 60 mm Hg (mean blood pressure)
Feline: 100 mm Hg (systolic blood pressure)

Therapies
Therapies for hypotension include the following:

- Decrease the depth of anesthesia.
- Bolus IV fluids in 10 ml/kg intervals (checking pressures between boluses).
- Use colloid fluids (i.e., hetastarch) in a rapid infusion to help increase central perfusion.
- Use medications to help increase blood pressure (i.e., dopamine or dobutamine) by intravenous infusion.

Caution
Hypertension may occasionally be seen in anesthetized patients. Hypertension associated with chronic renal failure

may diminish, or completely resolve, while patients are anesthetized. This is due to the potent vasodilatory actions of the anesthetic drugs. Anesthetic-associated causes of hypertension (systolic >150 mm Hg) include pain, increased carbon dioxide concentration in the body (**hypercarbia**), fever, catecholamine release, and drug effects from ketamine or alpha$_2$ agonists.

Hypoventilation

Hypoventilation is one of the most common anesthesia complications encountered in veterinary practice. A reservoir bag that is the correct volume for the patient will give some indication regarding depth of ventilation (tidal volume). Monitoring blood carbon dioxide levels by arterial blood gas is the most accurate way of monitoring adequacy of ventilation. A second choice is monitoring end-tidal carbon dioxide. The pulse oximeter is actually a very poor way to assess ventilation until a patient is already in a crisis.

Normal Physiologic Response

An appropriately sized reservoir bag empties by one-third if the patient is moving the normal tidal volume of gas (10–15 ml/kg). Normal arterial carbon dioxide measured by blood gas analysis is 35–45 mm Hg. Normal end-tidal carbon dioxide under anesthesia is 35–55 mm Hg. Use the following values to troubleshoot the end-tidal carbon dioxide monitoring:

- Carbon dioxide values **in excess of 55 mm Hg** suggest that assisted or controlled ventilation should be initiated.
- Carbon dioxide values **less than 35 mm Hg** suggest that the patient's breathing should be checked. If the patient is ventilating, rule out hyperventilation.

Cause

If the patient is ventilating normally, or appears to be hypoventilating, and endotracheal tube carbon dioxide is low, then circulation to the lungs must be questioned. At this point, assess APB. If APB is adequate, then there may be a profound ventilation/perfusion mismatch. This occurs when gas is not reaching the alveoli in large areas of the lung that are still receiving normal blood flow, or large areas are receiving a normal amount of gas in the alveoli but have lost their blood supply. In either case, it may be difficult to reestablish a normal ventilation/perfusion pattern.

Concerns

Prolonged hypoventilation produces hypoxia (low tissue oxygen concentration), which can produce cardiac arrhythmias, bradycardia, and cardiorespiratory collapse.

Prevention

Therapy for hypoventilation is very simple: **assisted** or **controlled ventilation**.

- **Long, deep breaths** that are held for 2–3 seconds may help open collapsed alveoli. Assisted ventilation is ac-

complished by squeezing the reservoir bag when the patient starts to inspire. Peak inspiratory pressures (PIP) should be kept to between 20 and 25 cm H_2O in healthy patients. PIP may need to be increased up to 60 cm H_2O for patients with restrictive thoracic disease: pleural effusion, pneumothorax, thoracic mass, etc. Disease of the lung tissue makes it very fragile, and positive pressure ventilation may easily lead to pneumothorax, even at very low PIP.

- **A mechanical ventilator** may also take over the duty of moving gas into and out of the lungs. There are many types of mechanical ventilators; however, the concepts are the same: ensuring an adequate tidal volume (10–15 ml/kg), providing an appropriate number of breaths per minute (8–16), and avoiding pressure trauma to the lungs (**barotraumas**) (PIP less than 30 cm H_2O).
- **Improving circulation** by administering IV fluids and supporting blood pressure will improve circulation to all tissues.

Inadvertent Hypothermia

Of the three most common anesthetic complications (hypothermia, hypotension, hypoventilation), hypothermia is the easiest to document without the aid of expensive equipment. All that is needed is a hand-held thermometer. Rectal temperature is usually 1° to 2° F lower than core temperature due to loss of muscle tone. It may be lower during procedures that expose the perirectal tissues: caudal abdominal, perineal, etc. Tympanic membrane temperatures can be very accurate because the middle ear shares the same vascular supply as the hypothalamus. However, ear thermometers can be technically challenging to use properly in most species. Esophageal readings reflect the temperature of the great vessels. Other methods of monitoring temperature, oral, axillary, and skin surface, are not accurate.

Normal Physiologic Response

The skin surface temperature rises and falls with the environmental temperature. Core body temperature is closely regulated by the hypothalamus.

There are three tissue layers designed to insulate the body and prevent heat loss. These consist of the skin, subcutaneous fat, and hair. These layers are more or less efficient in different patients, depending upon the layers' thickness. Heat transfer through the insulating layers and to the environment occurs in two stages. In stage one, heat is transferred from the core to the skin. In stage two, heat is lost to the environment by radiation, conduction, convection, and evaporation.

In awake animals, there are several reactions to cold. Behavioral reactions include seeking shelter and curling up. Physiologic reactions also occur. These include elevation of the hair (**piloerection**), vasoconstriction, and shivering. Piloerection increases the depth of insulation by forming a stagnant layer of air around the animal. Vasoconstriction of the skin arterioles and arteriovenous anastamoses limits heat loss from the extremities. Shivering increases heat production in all muscle groups. There is also a chemical excitation for heat production. This includes the release of epinephrine, norepinephrine, and thyroxin. The anesthetic drugs affect the thermoregulatory center and all compensatory reactions are abolished during sedation and anesthesia.

Causes

All anesthetics can produce systemic hypothermia. The inhalant gases decrease the thermoregulatory vasoconstriction. The basal metabolic rate is decreased as muscle tone is decreased in the anesthesia. The operating room temperature is often well below body temperature and skin prep solutions at room temperature produce significant heat loss through evaporation. Furthermore, IV fluids at room temperature and prolonged surgical procedures lower core temperatures.

Concerns

Almost all patients that are sedated or anesthetized will lose body temperature. The exceptions are the Nordic breeds of dogs (husky, malamute, Samoyed, etc.) that may actually become hyperthermic under general anesthesia. Some patients develop hypothermia so severe that normal physiology is wrecked. The adverse effects of inadvertent hypothermia include

- **immune system depression**, including impaired leukocyte mobility and phagocytosis, decreased T-cell antibody production, depressed nonspecific host defenses. Postoperative infection rate is increased to three times the normal rate in patients experiencing mild intraoperative hypothermia.
- **coagulopathy**, which is independent of clotting factor levels (more severe in factor deficient patients). Blood viscosity is increased and sludging can occur.
- **systemic vascular resistance** and increased after load. Myocardium is depressed and more prone to arrhythmias and hypoxia.
- **respiratory drive** that is diminished, and physiologic response to hypoxemia and hypercarbia is blunted.
- **central nervous system** that is depressed, with a delayed recovery from anesthesia, confusion, stupor, or coma.
- **hyperglycemia** due to catecholamine release (epinephrine).
- **hypovolemia** due to cold diuresis (may be seen as profound hypotension after rewarming)
- **drug and liver metabolism** significantly decreased, leading to drug toxicity.

Prevention

It is in the best interest of all patients (except those needing deliberate hypothermia) to be kept normothermic preoperatively, during anesthesia, and postoperatively. The prevention of inadvertent hypothermia is more desirable than trying to rewarm patients once they become cold. *Effective*

rewarming cannot happen unless 60% of body surface area is in contact with an external heat source. Desirable methods for preventing inadvertent hypothermia include

- controlling ambient temperature and keeping the OR temperature at least 75° F.
- insulating patients using bubble wrap, plastic wrap, or warm blankets.
- warming skin prep and irrigation solutions.
- warming all intravenous fluids.
- humidifying and heating inspired gasses by using an "artificial nose" such as the HumidVent
- using circulating hot water blankets at 105–107° F
- Using forced air heat-exchange blankets such as the Bair Hugger
- keeping postoperative patients dry or actively drying them using a hand-held blow dryer, taking care to not burn the skin or eyes.

Caution

Using Incorrect Heating Pads

There are other available methods for providing an external heat source, but they are not desirable due to the potential for thermal injury or electrocution. Radiant heaters or heat lamps ("French fry" lamps) cannot be easily regulated and can cause severe thermal injury to the skin. Electric heating pads and electric heating boards can develop hot spots or become wet and shock or electrocute a patient. Hot water bottles can be used provided that they are not above 107° F and are removed when they become cool.

Producing Hyperthermia

It is important to monitor a patient's temperature closely because of the possibility of overshoot; hyperthermia during surgery or rewarming can occur because the blood vessels in the periphery are vasodilated due to the anesthetic drugs. Heat is easily transferred to the core when peripheral vessels are vasodilated. The adverse effects of hyperthermia are also numerous and can be detrimental to a patient's well being.

Cardiac Arrhythmias

Changes in the electrocardiogram can imply derangements in oxygenation (i.e. hypoxia or ischemia) or an electrolyte imbalance (i.e., hyperkalemia) (see Chapter 24). Noted cardiac arrhythmias (premature ventricular contractions, heart block, or other changes) should be reported to the veterinarian immediately. Anesthetic levels should be reduced and oxygen flow should be increased to reduce the effect of hypoxia on the cardiac tissue. Further medication (i.e., lidocaine) may be recommended based on repeated arrhythmic events.

Cardiopulmonary Arrest

If a patient enters cardiopulmonary arrest (see Chapter 31), the veterinarian should be notified immediately, anesthesia

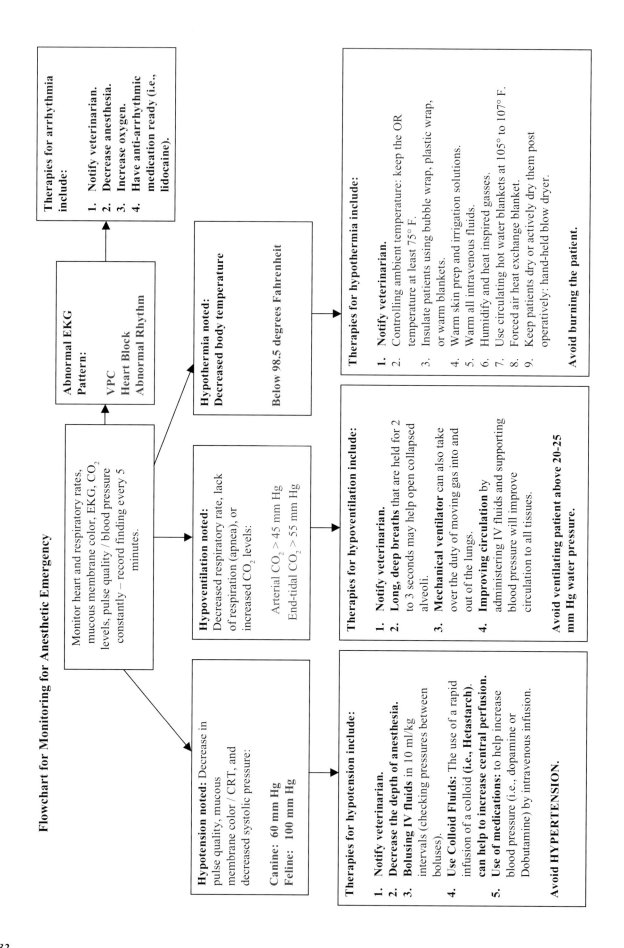

Flowchart for Monitoring for Anesthetic Emergency

Monitor heart and respiratory rates, mucous membrane color, EKG, CO_2 levels, pulse quality / blood pressure constantly – record finding every 5 minutes.

Abnormal EKG Pattern:

VPC
Heart Block
Abnormal Rhythm

Therapies for arrhythmia include:

1. **Notify veterinarian.**
2. **Decrease anesthesia.**
3. **Increase oxygen.**
4. **Have anti-arrhythmic medication ready (i.e., lidocaine).**

Hypothermia noted: Decreased body temperature

Below 98.5 degrees Fahrenheit

Therapies for hypothermia include:

1. **Notify veterinarian.**
2. Controlling ambient temperature: keep the OR temperature at least 75° F.
3. Insulate patients using bubble wrap, plastic wrap, or warm blankets.
4. Warm skin prep and irrigation solutions.
5. Warm all intravenous fluids.
6. Humidify and heat inspired gasses.
7. Use circulating hot water blankets at 105° to 107° F.
8. Forced air heat exchange blanket.
9. Keep patients dry or actively dry them post operatively: hand-held blow dryer.

Avoid burning the patient.

Hypoventilation noted: Decreased respiratory rate, lack of respiration (apnea), or increased CO_2 levels:

Arterial CO_2 > 45 mm Hg
End-tidal CO_2 > 55 mm Hg

Therapies for hypoventilation include:

1. **Notify veterinarian.**
2. **Long, deep breaths** that are held for 2 to 3 seconds may help open collapsed alveoli.
3. **Mechanical ventilator** can also take over the duty of moving gas into and out of the lungs.
4. **Improving circulation** by administering IV fluids and supporting blood pressure will improve circulation to all tissues.

Avoid ventilating patient above 20-25 mm Hg water pressure.

Hypotension noted: Decrease in pulse quality, mucous membrane color / CRT, and decreased systolic pressure:

Canine: 60 mm Hg
Feline: 100 mm Hg

Therapies for hypotension include:

1. **Notify veterinarian.**
2. **Decrease the depth of anesthesia.**
3. **Bolusing IV fluids** in 10 ml/kg intervals (checking pressures between boluses).
4. **Use Colloid Fluids:** The use of a rapid infusion of a colloid **(i.e., Hetastarch) can help to increase central perfusion.**
5. **Use of medications:** to help increase blood pressure (i.e., dopamine or Dobutamine) by intravenous infusion.

Avoid HYPERTENSION.

should be turned off, oxygen flow should be increased, and the patient should be manually ventilated. The medical team should be advised and cardiopulmonary cerebral resuscitation should commence.

Discussing Anesthesia with Clients

The veterinarian is responsible for discussing the overall anesthetic process and concerns with the client; however, the medical team should have a basic understanding of the procedure and be able to discuss basic concerns with the client.

- There is no such thing as a risk-free procedure, but risk is reduced by the veterinarian choosing the appropriate anesthetic drug protocols and vigilant monitoring by the medical team.
- Prior to anesthesia, the patient has a full evaluation to assess their anesthetic risk.
- The patient will be carefully monitored while under anesthesia and during recovery.

CD-ROM 2 will focus on concepts of Understanding the Concepts of Disease and Treatment. The exercises can be done individually or as case rounds as they explore specific topics in veterinary medicine that discuss clinical diagnostics and treatment.

Chapter 30

Shock

The following section outlines the basic concepts of shock and how it affects the physical parameters, diagnostic tests, and treatment options for the patient. This chapter is designed to help the medical team member understand the syndrome of shock, how to identify early signs of the process, how to anticipate diagnostics and treatment options, and how to discuss shock with the client. *Emergency medical treatment is always initiated by the veterinarian.*

Shock is not a disease entity but a syndrome that can arise from many possible disease situations. Simply defined, *shock is the inability of the body to oxygenate blood or perfuse tissue at an acceptable level to keep up with the oxygen demands.* If shock is not reversed quickly and efficiently, the animal can die. There are multiple types of shock, and each syndrome has different treatment components. The forms of shock are as follows.

- Hypovolemic shock
- Cardiovascular shock
- Obstructive shock (obstruction of vessels)
  — Thromboembolism
  — Tumor involving a large vessel
  — Torsion
- Distributive Shock (massive vasodilatation)

Each team member should be able to identify signs of early to moderate shock, obtain a history from the owner to help delineate by which syndrome the patient may be affected, and be ready with diagnostic and treatment components. The key to success in treatment is early detection and effective and efficient treatment.

Obtaining a History with a Patient in Shock

Because shock can result from many possible disease entities, a thorough medical history, as outlined by Chapter 5, should be obtained.

Physical Assessment for an Animal in Shock

Signs of shock can vary depending on the primary cause of the disease and which syndrome of shock is occurring. Furthermore, symptoms can vary in early to severe shock. Some basic changes suggestive of shock (see Table 30.1) are discussed next.

Early Shock
Pulse
- **Rapid, bounding pulse (canine):** Rapid, bounding pulses occur as the body tries to compensate for the acute demands placed upon it. A bounding rapid pulse in a nervous or happy pet does not suggest a shocky state. However, in pets with other changes in mentation, respiration, mucous membrane color, and hydration, this pulse may suggest a serious to life-threatening condition.
- **Bradycardia (feline):** Cats tend to be bradycardic in early shock.
- **Pulse deficit:** In some cases (i.e., cardiovascular shock), the patient may also have **pulse deficits** because the heart cannot produce a pulse for each heart contraction. A team member should always auscult the heart while palpating the pulse in any animal suspected of being in a shocky state. *If there is not a pulse with each heart beat, the patient requires attention immediately.*

Mentation
In early shock, these pets may be dull to depressed because these patients are trying to put all their energy into restoring normal body function. These patients may also show generalized weakness.

Respiration
Pets may have altered respiratory patterns that range from a rapid to a slow rate. There may also be an abdominal component.

Body Temperature
Depending on the type of shock evident, the patients may have extreme aberrations in body temperature. Patients suffering from heatstroke, protracted seizures, or severe infectious disease may have highly elevated body temperature (>105° Fahrenheit). As the animal becomes more shocky, body temperature can become subnormal.

Mucous Membrane Color/Capillary Refill Time
One of the early indicators of shock, mucous membrane color, can become

- **pale** due to blood loss, pain, dehydration, heatstroke, and other causes;
- **injected/red** due to toxin or increased bacterial load; and

Table 30.1.   Physical changes in early/severe shock.

System Examined	Early Shock	Severe Shock
Disposition	Depressed Sternal recumbent Weak	Nonresponsive Comatose Lateral recumbent
Breathing	Increased rate >45 Altered breathing rates Abdominal breathing Open mouth breathing	Abdominal breathing Decreased rate Shallow
Pulses/heart beating	Rapid, bounding pulses Tachycardia (canines) Bradycardia (felines) ± Pulse deficits	Slow weak pulses Bradycardic ± Pulse deficits
Gum color	Pale Purple Yellow	Pale to white Purple/gray Yellow
Capillary refill time	CRT >2–3 seconds	CRT >3 seconds
Body temperature	Normal temp. Temp >106° Hypothermia (felines)	Temp. <98° or >106°
Pupils	Slow to respond to light Anisocoria	Slow to nonresponsive to light Dilated Anisocoria

- **blue/gray/purple (cyanotic)** secondary to heart and lung disease.

Capillary Refill Time
Capillary refill time (CRT) begins to become prolonged (>2–3 seconds) because the body can no longer fill the smallest peripheral capillaries at a regular rate.

Dehydration
Depending on the syndrome, pets can start showing mild to moderate dehydration.

Pupils
Pupils should be even and responsive to light. In some cases, response to a bright light may be slowed. Furthermore, with head trauma, the pupil size may be different sizes (**anisocoria**). *If noted, anisocoria should be brought to the attention of the medical team immediately* (see Figure 30.1).

Severe Shock
As the type of shock worsens, the patient's signs can be more severe. *The time it takes to move from early shock to severe shock can sometimes be within minutes.* A potential critical care patient must be reevaluated constantly until the patient is stabilized. Symptoms of severe shock are discussed next.

Pulses
Because the patient cannot adequately maintain perfusion, the cardiovascular system begins to fail. Pulses become weaker, and the heart rate slows. As the patient deteriorates,

pulses become weak to unapparent and eventually the heartbeat stops.

Mentation
Pets become more depressed, nonresponsive, and even comatose.

Respiration
Respiration becomes shallower and slower.

Mucous Membrane Color/Capillary Refill Time
Mucous membrane color can worsen and CRT can be prolonged. Changes in mucous membrane color depend on the disease entity producing shock (see above).

Dehydration
In specific types of shock, as circulation fails, the patient may become more significantly hypovolemic, decreasing blood flow to the peripheral tissue. This will decrease skin turgor.

Pupils
Pupils become slower to respond to a bright light source. As the patient becomes life threatened, pupils may become fixed and nonresponsive. Anisocoria is still possible.

Clinical Diagnostics of Shock

Because shock can affect the entire body, full diagnostics may be required to both identify the cause of shock and the organs being affected. However, when faced with a patient

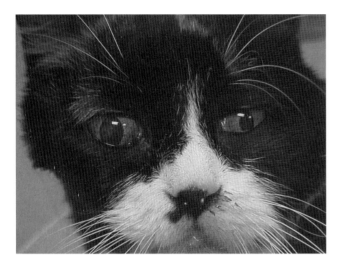

Figure 30.1.   Image of a cat after a trauma. Notice the uneven pupil size suggestive of head trauma or neurologic disease.

in some form of shock, establishing a quick diagnostic baseline (**minimal clinical database**) is very important. Some diagnostic tests (see Table 30.2) may be the following.

- **Packed cell volume (PCV)/total protein (TP):** Changes in packed cell volume and protein in shock situations can help the medical team evaluate significant blood loss, anemia, or dehydration.
- **Glucose:** Glucose is a very important factor to monitor in any shocky patient. The patient must have blood sugar for a normal central nervous system and muscle function. With blood glucose <40–50 mg/dl, patients can become weak, comatose, and have seizures.
- **Electrolytes:** Although not always as easily assessed, aberrant changes in sodium and potassium can produce irregular heart rhythms, weakness, muscle fasciculations, collapse, a slowed heart rate, and death.
- **Clotting times:** Prolonged clotting times producing bleeding can both produce shock and be secondary to the syndrome. If the animal's ability to clot blood is compromised, internal bleeding and severe shock can occur.

Table 30.2.   Changes in clinical diagnostics that could suggest shock.

Parameter	Measurement	Observations

Increased PCV/TP	PCV:
	  Canines >50% +
	  Felines >40% +
	Total protein
	  Canines >8.5 mg/dl
	  Felines >8.5 mg/dl
		Packed cell volume and total proteins above normal are secondary to dehydration.
		
		Elevation of the cell populations and total protein occur as the fluid portion of blood decreases. (See Chapter 21.)

Decreased PCV	PCV:
	  Canines < 25% +
	  Felines < 20 % +
		Decreasing packed cell volume with normal total protein suggests chronic disease or increased red blood cell destruction (hemolysis). In animals with chronic disease, their resources to produce red blood cells and energy may be significantly diminished, lowering the packed cell volume over time.

Normal TP
  Decreased PCV
 	
  Decreased TP
	PCV:
	  Canines <25% +
	  Felines <20% +
	Total protein:
	  Canines <5 mg/dl
	  Felines <5 mg/ dl
		Total protein may be lower, but tends to remain in the normal limits. With acute blood loss, animals can both loose red blood cells and protein.
		
		Protein leaks out of the vessels with the fluid component of blood, hence decreasing as significantly as the packed cell volume.

Glucose	Glucose <40–60 mg/dl	Hypoglycemia can slow the response of the central nervous system and if prolonged can produce severe shock, seizures, coma and death.

Electrolytes	Potassium (K+) >6.0 mg/dl
	Potassium (K+)<3.0 mg/dl
		Potassium is one of three electrolytes of the body to help produce cardiac contraction, muscle movement, nerve firing, and many other basic body functions.
		Significant alterations of this electrolyte can produce
		  • weakness,
		  • abnormal heart rhythms,
		  • muscular tremors,
		  • coma, and
		  • death.

Clotting times	Activated clotting time >120 seconds Activated prothrombin time >120 seconds Prothrombin time >11 seconds	Increases in clotting times can lead to internal bleeding, shock, and death. If increasing clotting times are noted, packed cell volume and total protein should be monitored closely.

Table 30.3. Emergency drug table.

Drug	Indication
50% Dextrose	Significant hypoglycemia (blood glucose <40–60 mg/dl)
Atropine	Bradycardia (heart rate <60 beats/min)
Epinephrine	Cardiac arrest/severe allergic or anaphylactic reaction
Dexamethasone Prednisone	Used to help counteract anaphylactic shock, concerns of spinal injury, or as a general anti-inflammatory medication.
Furosemide	A diuretic that helps increase fluid excretion through the kidneys, removing excess water from the tissues (especially the lungs). Used in the treatment of cardiovascular shock and traumatic brain injury.
Mannitol	A large inert sugar that, when introduced into the bloodstream, helps pull fluids into the vessels. This drug is used primarily to prevent cerebral swelling in the case of a head concussion.
Antihistamines	Antihistamines (i.e., diphenhydramine) are drugs that help slow the allergic response of the body. When the patient is exposed to a foreign allergen, a white blood cell called a mast cell can release histamines, producing signs of an allergic or anaphylactic reaction. Antihistamines help block the process and are used in the treatment of anaphylactic shock.

Emergency Medications for Shock

Although covered in Chapter 26, the team member should have an understanding of what drugs are indicated in an emergency situation. Although this list may not apply to all emergency situations for all medical teams, the drugs listed in Table 30.3 should be available.

Types of Shock

Hypovolemic Shock
Hypovolemic shock occurs when an animal cannot maintain normal blood volume (red blood cells and fluid) or blood pressure.

Etiology
Hypovolemic shock occurs when there is a rapid loss of red blood cells, fluid, or blood pressure. This loss occurs so acutely the patient cannot recover and their body systems begin to fail. Possible causes of hypovolemic shock are

- **acute bleeding:** red blood cell loss, and
- **dehydration:** acute severe loss of fluid from infectious disease, heatstroke, organ failure, and other causes.

Signalment
Hypovolemic shock can occur in any species, sex, and age.

Common Points on Medical History
As discussed previously, a complete medical history should be taken. With concerns of hypovolemic shock, special focus on any possible history of trauma (i.e., hit by car, etc.) or serious underlying disease should be discussed with the client.

Common Points in Initial Assessment
Hypovolemic shock is the inability to perfuse blood to the tissue due to decreased blood volume. As the syndrome progresses, the animal cannot adequately oxygenate tissue and becomes weak, collapsed, and nonresponsive, and the syndrome ends in cardiac failure.

Common initial clinical signs are

- bounding/hyperdynamic pulses (canine),
- bradycardia (feline),
- decreased mentation/depression,
- increased respiration (tachypnea),
- hypothermia (unless heatstroke),
- poor CRT/poor mucous membrane color (pale), and
- generalized weakness.

As the syndrome worsens, signs are

- weak/decreased pulse quality,
- depression progressing to coma (obtund),
- altered respiration (can be bradyneic to tachypnic),
- poor to no mucous membrane color,
- prolonged CRT, and
- severe weakness to borderline coma,

Clinical Diagnostics
As discussed above, a minimal diagnostic database should be obtained to help define the type of shock. In general, hypovolemic shock can demonstrate the changes in clinical diagnostics listed in Table 30.4.

Treatment
The treatment protocol below (see Hypovolemic Shock Flowchart) is a suggestion of how some medical teams would handle a hypovolemic patient. It is meant to give the team member a concept of what steps may need to be taken with a shock patient in order to better anticipate the doctor. This protocol is meant to help the team member assist the veterinarian treat an emergency patient.

The goal of treating hypovolemic shock is to rehydrate the patient and restore normal blood pressure and perfusion. A sample treatment protocol is presented here.

1. **Oxygen therapy:** Have an oxygen environment set up (i.e., cage, mask, nasal oxygen catheter) so that if needed, the pet can be placed on oxygen. *Oxygen is never contraindicated,* and by simply increasing the oxygen concentration in the blood, the patient may become less stressed and shocky.

Table 30.4. Changes noted in clinical diagnostics with hypovolemic shock.

Parameter	Finding
PCV/TP	With dehydration, PCV/TP are elevated.
	With blood loss, PCV/TP are decreased.
Glucose	WNL
Electrolytes	Potassium can be elevated, normal, or low.
Clotting times	If bleeding is occurring, clotting times can be elevated.

2. **Catheter:** Have catheter set up, and if needed set an IV catheter. With a patient in shock, the ability to set a catheter may change within a very small time range. Having a catheter and supplies readily available, and being able to effectively set a catheter, can make the difference in stabilizing the patient.
3. **Fluids:** Be ready to begin fluid administration per the veterinarian recommendations. With life-threatening shock, emergency doses of fluids or bolusing fluids may be requested by the veterinarian.
4. **Minimal clinical database:** Have the supplies ready to run a minimal clinical database. These tests can help the veterinarian begin to determine the type of shock occurring.
5. **Medications:** Have emergency drugs available.
6. **Reevaluation:** Within 5–10 minutes of fluid administration, reevaluate the patient for
   — temperature,
   — pulse quality,
   — respiration, and
   — mucous membrane/CRT.
   If signs do not suggest stabilization, the veterinarian may suggest rechecking the minimal clinical database or other diagnostics to help distinguish other syndromes and disease that may be occurring.
7. **Colloids:** Synthetic colloids are large inert sugar molecules (i.e., hetastarch) that help increase fluid absorption from the tissue into the vessels, producing increased blood pressure.

Septic Shock

A pet with septic shock, a form of distributive shock, has lost its ability to maintain normal tissue perfusion due to massive dilation of all the blood vessels secondary to a massive infection in the body. This causes the blood to pool and not circulate in the normal fashion. In many cases, blood sugar levels are consumed as the body exhausts most of its glucose supplies fighting off the infection. Since the brain and muscle must have blood sugar to function normally, animals in septic shock will show both signs of generalized shock and central nervous system signs.

Signalment

Any patient can develop septic shock. However, very young or old animals can be more predisposed, secondary to a less-responsive immune system.

Etiology

Although any infectious disease can develop into septic shock, the following diseases are more commonly associated with sepsis.

- Canine parvoviral infection
- Canine distemper virus infection
- Bacterial pyometra
- Bacterial pneumonia
- Bacterial hepatitis
- Bacterial kidney disease
- Other bacterial infections especially in the geriatric and neonate pet

Common Points on Medical History

As discussed previously, a complete medical history should be taken. With concerns of septic shock, special focus on any possible history of acute or chronic infectious disease should be discussed with the client.

Common Points in Initial Assessment

Septic shock initially presents with signs of infection, dehydration, and depression. As the disease worsens, shock and neurologic signs occur secondarily as blood sugar and perfusion to the brain decreases.

Common clinical signs of early shock are

- bounding/hyperdynamic pulses,
- decreased mentation/depression,
- increased respiration (tachypnea),
- hyperthermia, secondary to infection,
- poor CRT/poor mucous membranes (pale), and
- generalized weakness.

Clinical signs of severe shock are

- weak/decreased pulse quality,
- depression to coma (obtund),
- unable to see/blind,
- seizures,
- head pressing/circling, and
- dementia.

Diagnostics

As discussed above, a minimal clinical database should be obtained to help define the type of shock the pet presents with. In general, septic shock can show the changes in clinical diagnostics presented in Table 30.5.

Treatment

The treatment protocol below is a suggestion of how some medical teams would handle a septic shock patient (see Septic

Hypovolemic Shock Flowchart

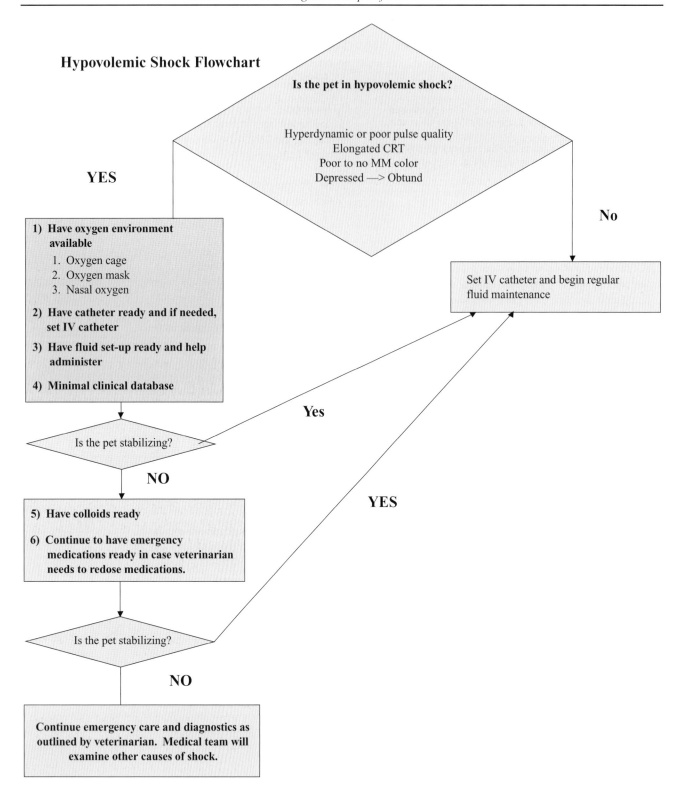

Shock Flowchart). It is meant to give the team member a concept of treatment concerns to better anticipate the doctor.

1. **Treatment:** The most important goal is to identify and treat the underlying disease while restoring and maintaining blood sugar levels and reperfusing the patient.

2. **Oxygen:** Prepare an oxygen environment if needed.
3. **Catheter:** Set up for IV catheter and place in the patient, if needed.
4. **Minimal clinical database:** Get a minimal clinical database. If blood sugar is less than 60 mg/dl administer dextrose infusion.

Table 30.5. Changes noted in clinical diagnostics with septic shock.

Parameter	Finding
PCV/TP	With dehydration, PCV/TP are elevated.
Glucose	Low blood sugar <60 mg/dl, but it can be normal.
Electrolytes	Electrolytes are generally within normal limits.
Clotting times	Clotting times are generally within normal limits.

Table 30.6. Changes noted in clinical diagnostics with anaphylactic shock.

Parameter	Finding
PCV/TP	With dehydration, PCV/TP are elevated
Glucose	Low blood sugar <60 mg/dl can be evident or can be normal
Electrolytes	Electrolytes are generally within normal limits.
Clotting times	Clotting times are generally within normal limits but can be elevated.

Administer Crystalloids

Within 5 minutes of fluid administration, evaluate,

- temperature,
- pulse quality,
- respiration, and
- mucous membrane/CRT

If there is no improvement, have colloids and emergency medication available.

Within 5–10 minutes of fluid administration, reevaluate the pet. If signs do not suggest stabilization, the veterinarian may suggest rechecking the minimal clinical database or other diagnostics to help distinguish other syndromes or disease states that are occurring.

Anaphylactic Shock

Anaphylactic shock (another form of distributive shock) is a massive allergic reaction to a foreign venom, protein, or drug causing massive systemic vasodilatation (hypotension), bronchoconstriction, collapse, and shock.

Signalment

Anaphylactic shock can occur in any species, sex, and age.

Etiology

When the pet encounters a sting, insect bite, or exposure to a drug or medication, a massive allergic reaction can occur produced from the release of histamines from a type of white blood cell called a mast cell. *Unlike an allergic reaction, the pet may not show obvious signs of facial swelling, hives, and redness of the skin (erythema).* The massive release of histamine overwhelms the patient and causes weakness, hypotension and shock.

Common Points on Medical History

As discussed previously, a complete medical history should be taken. With concerns of anaphylactic shock, special focus on any possible history of exposure to insects or reptiles (i.e., snake) and new medication or vaccine should be discussed with the client.

Common Points in Initial Assessment

The pet usually presents with a respiratory wheeze, severe depression, weakness, collapse, low blood pressure, and occasionally a stinger in the tongue region. Common clinical signs of disease are

- weakness, sometimes comatose,
- poor mucous membrane color,
- increased CRT,
- dehydrated,
- poor pulse quality,
- tachypnea,
- facial swelling,
- hives on the body,
- bronchoconstriction, wheezes in respiratory tract,
- stinger on tongue or other body part (occasionally),
- focal swelling and inflammation consistent with insect sting, and
- collapse.

Diagnostics

As discussed above, a minimal clinical database should be obtained to help define the type of shock. In general anaphylactic shock can show the changes in clinical diagnostics listed in Table 30.6.

Treatment

The treatment protocol below (see Anaphylactic Shock Flowchart) is a suggestion of how some medical teams would handle an anaphylactic patient. It is meant to give the team member a concept of what steps may need to be taken with a shock patient to better anticipate the doctor. This protocol is meant to help the team member assist the veterinarian treat an emergency patient. The goal of treatment of anaphylactic shock is to stop the allergic reaction, restore and maintain blood sugar levels if necessary, and rehydrate the patient.

Emergency Medications

1. With anaphylactic shock, the following medications should be available to help stop the allergic process and stabilize the patient.

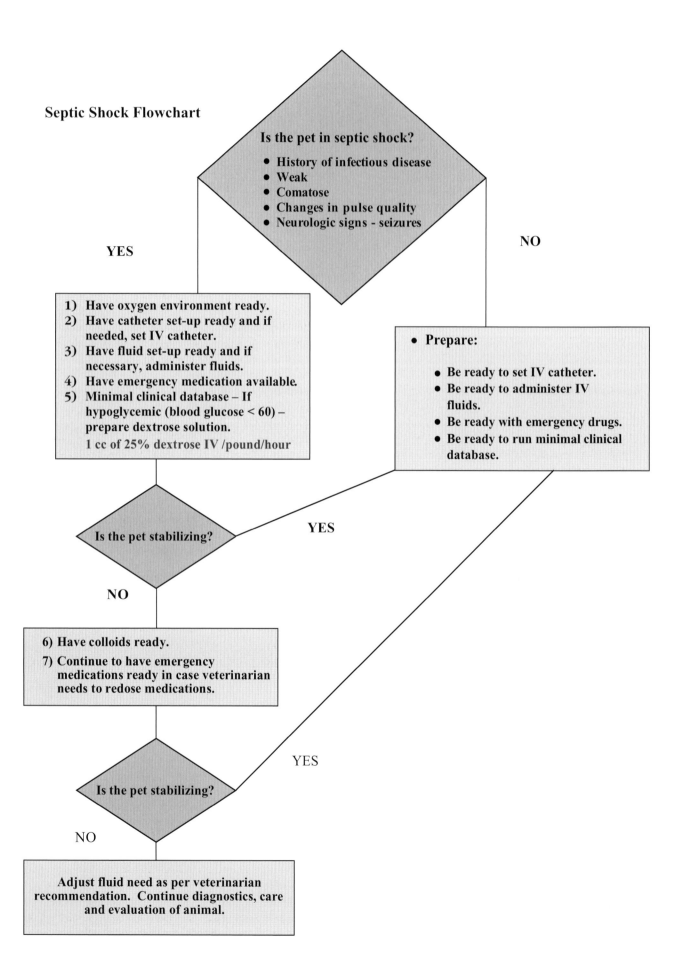

Septic Shock Flowchart

Is the pet in septic shock?

- History of infectious disease
- Weak
- Comatose
- Changes in pulse quality
- Neurologic signs - seizures

YES

NO

1) Have oxygen environment ready.
2) Have catheter set-up ready and if needed, set IV catheter.
3) Have fluid set-up ready and if necessary, administer fluids.
4) Have emergency medication available.
5) Minimal clinical database – If hypoglycemic (blood glucose < 60) – prepare dextrose solution.
1 cc of 25% dextrose IV /pound/hour

- Prepare:
  - Be ready to set IV catheter.
  - Be ready to administer IV fluids.
  - Be ready with emergency drugs.
  - Be ready to run minimal clinical database.

Is the pet stabilizing?

YES

NO

6) Have colloids ready.
7) Continue to have emergency medications ready in case veterinarian needs to redose medications.

Is the pet stabilizing?

YES

NO

Adjust fluid need as per veterinarian recommendation. Continue diagnostics, care and evaluation of animal.

- **Steroid medication:** Steroidal medication (i.e., dexamethasone, prednisone) is focused on reducing the symptoms of the allergic response and stabilizing the patient.
- **Epinephrine:** In extreme anaphylaxis, epinephrine is used to reverse slow heart rate, low blood pressure, bronchoconstriction, and other physical symptoms.
- **Antihistamines:** Antihistamines (i.e., diphenhydramine) may be recommended to stop the histamine's degranulation, which is producing the anaphylactic reaction.

2. **Oxygen:** Prepare oxygen environment if needed
3. **Catheter:** Set up for IV catheter and place if instructed to do so.
4. **Minimal clinical database:** Get a minimal clinical database. If blood sugar is less than 60 mg/dl administer dextrose infusion.

Prepare IV Infusion with Dextrose
In some cases of severe hypoglycemia, the veterinarian may request 25% dextrose solution. To prepare infusion take 50% dextrose and mix it with equal parts sterile fluid in a 1:1 ratio. The general dose is 1 cc/lb 25% dextrose IV.

Prepare IV Fluids with Dextrose
In many cases of persistent hypoglycemia, the veterinarian may request adding 50% dextrose to fluids to help maintain blood glucose levels. The fluids with dextrose component are prepared as follows.

- **2.5% Dextrose solution:** Take a liter of crystalloid fluids (i.e., 0.9% NaCl, lactated Ringer's solution, Normosol, etc.) and remove 50 cc of sterile fluid. Add 50 cc of 50% dextrose to the fluid, which will produce a 2.5% dextrose solution for long-term maintenance.
- **5% Dextrose solution:** Take a liter of crystalloid fluids (i.e., 0.9% NaCl, lactated Ringer's solution, Normosol, etc.) and remove 100 cc of sterile fluid. Add 100 cc of 50% dextrose to the fluid, which will produce a 5% dextrose solution for long-term maintenance.

Within 5 minutes of fluid administration, evaluate

- temperature,
- pulse quality,
- respiration, and
- mucous membranes/CRT.

If there is no improvement, have colloids and emergency medication available. Within 5–10 minutes of fluid administration, reevaluate the pet. If signs do not suggest stabilization, the veterinarian may suggest rechecking the minimal clinical database or other diagnostics to help distinguish other syndromes or diseases that are occurring.

Cardiogenic Shock
Cardiogenic shock occurs when normal blood flow and perfusion is unable to be maintained due to an inability of the heart to properly pump and maintain cardiac output. Pets in cardiogenic shock cannot maintain normal perfusion to the lung fields and oxygenation of tissue.

Signalment
Each type of heart disease has specific breed, sex, and species predispositions (see Chapter 12) for cardiogenic shock.

Etiology
Cardiovascular shock is a syndrome produced by an underlying heart disease, trauma, or congenital defect that challenges the cardiovascular system until the heart is no longer able to maintain normal perfusion and oxygenation of tissues. Once the heart begins to fail, decreased blood perfusion through the lung fields and heart produces an inability to absorb oxygen into the bloodstream and perfuse the body.

Common Points on Medical History
As discussed previously, a complete medical history should be taken. With concerns of cardiovascular shock, special focus should be on any previous history of cardiac disease, current heart medications, and increase in exercise intolerance.

Common Points in Initial Assessment
The pet usually presents with dyspnea (see Figure 30.2), open mouth breathing with an abdominal push, weakness, possible coughing (canines), cyanotic gum color (i.e. purple, blue, or gray), and poor capillary refill time. General common clinical signs of disease are listed in Table 30.7. General common clinical signs of disease are as follows.:

- **Dyspnea:** Pets will present with severe trouble breathing, with increased rate. Their head and neck can be extended upward with their ears pinned back (see Figure 30.2).
- **Color of gums:** Blue or purple coloration suggests poor oxygenation of tissue (cyanosis).
- **Pulses:** Pulse quality can vary depending on the type of cardiac disease (see Chapter 12). Changes in pulse rate and quality can be, in early heart failure (**tachycardia**)
  — **Cat:** >220 beats/min
  — **Dog:** >200 beats/min
  In later failure (**bradycardia**)
  — **Cat:** <80 beats/min
  — **Dog:** <60 beats/min
  Quality for pulses can be
  — weak pulses,
  — paradoxical pulses,
  — pulse deficit, and
  — no pulses.

Auscultation
Changes in heart and lung sounds can also vary depending on disease. Some notable changes can be the following:

- **Cardiac auscultation:** The cardiac sounds can be muffled and decreased with increased respiratory effort, fluid

Anaphylactic Shock Flowchart

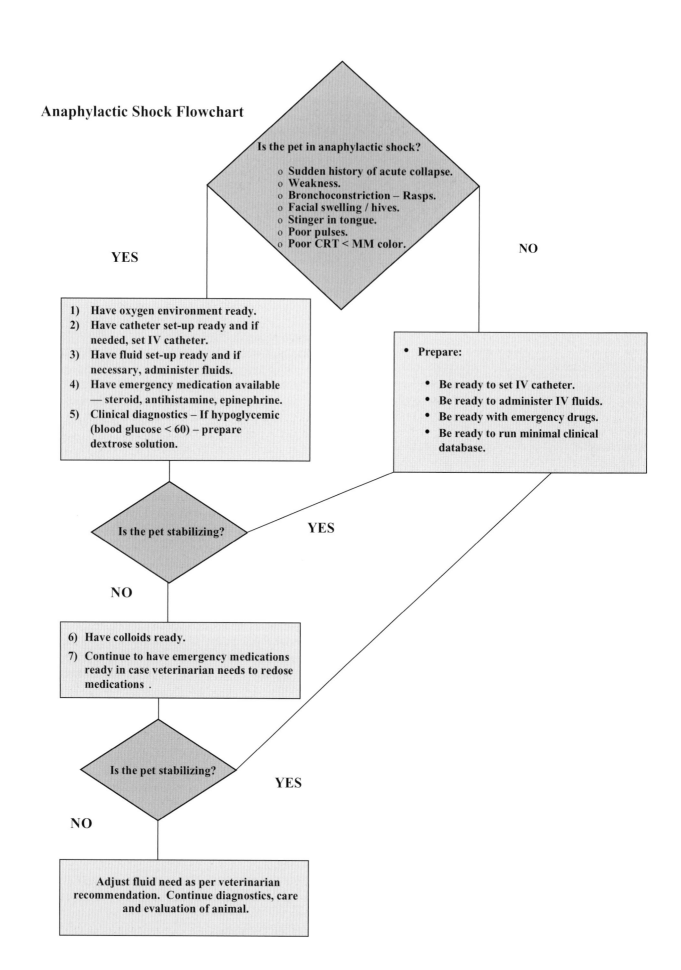

Is the pet in anaphylactic shock?

- o Sudden history of acute collapse.
- o Weakness.
- o Bronchoconstriction – Rasps.
- o Facial swelling / hives.
- o Stinger in tongue.
- o Poor pulses.
- o Poor CRT < MM color.

YES

NO

1) Have oxygen environment ready.
2) Have catheter set-up ready and if needed, set IV catheter.
3) Have fluid set-up ready and if necessary, administer fluids.
4) Have emergency medication available — steroid, antihistamine, epinephrine.
5) Clinical diagnostics – If hypoglycemic (blood glucose < 60) – prepare dextrose solution.

- • Prepare:
  - • Be ready to set IV catheter.
  - • Be ready to administer IV fluids.
  - • Be ready with emergency drugs.
  - • Be ready to run minimal clinical database.

Is the pet stabilizing?

YES

NO

6) Have colloids ready.
7) Continue to have emergency medications ready in case veterinarian needs to redose medications .

Is the pet stabilizing?

YES

NO

Adjust fluid need as per veterinarian recommendation. Continue diagnostics, care and evaluation of animal.

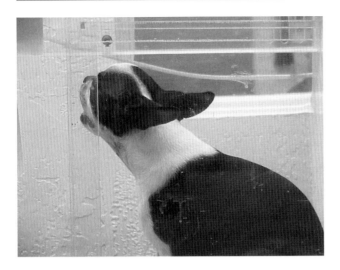

Figure 30.2. An illustration of a patient with severe cardiac distress, note the extension of the neck and placement of the ears. This patient is struggling to bring in every possible breath.

Table 30.7. Changes noted in clinical diagnostics with cardiogenic shock.

Parameter	Finding
PCV/TP	Generally within normal limits.
Glucose	Generally within normal limits.
Electrolytes	Electrolytes are generally within normal limits. However, derangements in the sodium and potassium levels can be affected by cardiac medications. Abnormalities in the electrolytes can produce significant cardiac arrhythmias.
Clotting times	Clotting times are generally within normal limits, but can be elevated.
EKG	Although not discussed with other types of shock, electrocardiograms should be evaluated for abnormal rhythm once the pet is stabilized. Significant arrhythmias must be corrected to stabilize the patient (see Chapter 24).

in the chest or pericardium, or space occupying masses. With valvular disease, heart murmurs may also be noted. Finally if there is an arrhythmia, abnormal extra heartbeats may be heard intermittently with normal beats.

- **Respiratory noise:** With cardiac failure, fluid can accumulate within the lung fields due to pulmonary congestion. As this progress, crackles can be auscultated.

Diagnostics

As discussed above, a minimal clinical database should be obtained to help define the type of shock. In general cardiogenic shock, all test parameters can show the changes in clinical diagnostics presented in Table 30.7.

Treatment

The treatment protocol below (see the Cardiogenic Shock Flowchart) is a suggestion of how some medical teams would handle an cardiogenic patient. It is meant to give the team member a concept of what steps must be taken with a shock patient to better anticipate the doctor. This protocol is meant to help the team member assist the veterinarian treat an emergency patient. *Unlike the other treatments of shock, cardiogenic shock is not usually treated with large amounts of intravenous fluid.* These patients are often symptomatic because of fluid pooling within the lung tissue (**pulmonary edema**) due to poor perfusion and cardiac circulation. In this situation, fluids are contraindicated because intravenous fluids can dramatically increase pulmonary edema. The goals of treatment in these cases are to reduce the stress of the animal, increase oxygen concentration in the body, reduce pulmonary edema, and restore normal cardiac output. Possible treatment protocols may be as follows.

1. **Oxygen:** Placing the pet in an oxygen environment, whether it is a mask, oxygen cage, oxygen E-collar, or

nasal catheter is very important. The only limitation in administering oxygen is not to stress the patient during administration.

2. **Catheter:** Set up for IV catheter and place it if instructed to do so. Setting the catheter may need to occur after the pet is stabilized. If the pet becomes too stressed, it may die; caution should always be practiced in any treatment protocol with this type of patient.

3. **Emergency medications:** With cardiogenic shock, the following medications may be needed to help reduce stress and return to normal cardiac function.
   - **Sedatives:** Sedatives, such as morphine and butorphanol, are used to reduce the amount of stress for the patient and decrease hyperventilation that can worsen pulmonary edema. The goal of these medications is not to anesthetize but to reduce the stress enough to let the animal breathe slower and more deeply.
   - **Furosemide (Lasix):** This diuretic is usually given at high doses hourly to help pull fluid from the tissue (i.e., lungs) into the urine and decrease the amount of pulmonary edema.
   - **Nitroglycerin ointment:** This transdermal paste is usually placed in the ear of the affected patient. It is a potent vasodilator that reduces the amount of pressure the heart must push against to produce a pulse.
   - **Other medications:** Medications such as bronchodilators, atropine, and epinephrine may be recommended by the veterinarian.

4. **Reevaluation:** Completing a physical assessment of the patient depends on how well the patient is responding to initial therapy. If the patient is easily stressed, *visual reevaluation may be the only way to assess the patient.*

   If the patient cannot be stressed, perform a visual evaluation of

- mentation,
- respiration, and
- gum/tongue color.

If the patient can be more fully evaluated, check

- pulse,
- respiration,
- mucous membrane/CRT,
- hydration, and
- temperature.

5. **Evaluation of medications:** Once the patient is initially placed on medication and in an oxygen environment, the pet is then monitored and medication repeated until the pet either stabilizes or succumbs. Often the medical team can only visually monitor the pet as discussed above and medicate at regular intervals. *Some patients will not be able to be stabilized even with all treatment options completed.*

6. **Clinical diagnostics:** Clinical diagnostics should not be collected until the pet is more stable. The increased stress of a blood draw can lead to cardiovascular failure. Clinical diagnostics on the stabilized patient can include the following:
   - Minimal clinical database
     —PCV/TP
     —Electrolytes
     —Kidney function (BUN/creatinine)
   - Electrocardiogram (EKG)
   - Thoracic radiographs
   - Cardiac ultrasound

Heatstroke/Hyperthermia

Heatstroke is defined as a severe elevation in body temperature above 106° Fahrenheit. At this temperature, there can be severe damage to organs and systems.

- **Abdominal organs (liver, kidney, etc.):** Increased temperatures can damage the kidney and liver, producing acute organ failure.
- **Central nervous system:** Increased heat can cause thermal injury that can produce seizures and other neurologic signs.
- **Coagulopathy:** With extreme increases in body temperature, the blood can be stimulated to clot spontaneously in the vessels, exhausting the normal clotting factors. Once the clotting factors are exhausted, the pet can begin to bleed internally. This is called **disseminated intravascular coagulopathy (DIC),** and it is potentially the most life-threatening complication to heatstroke.

Signalment

Heatstroke can affect either dogs or cats of any age but is more common in short-faced breeds that have a harder time panting to regulate body temperature (e.g., bulldogs, pugs, Lhasa apso, etc.) and long, thick-coated breeds (e.g., Arctic breeds such as malamute, American Eskimo, etc.).

Etiology

Heatstroke (hyperthermia) can be caused by many possible conditions.

- **Infection:** High fever can occur in response to overwhelming infection.
- **Heatstroke:** Animals begin to overheat in a humid, hot environment and become overwhelmed and unable to cope with the heat.
- **Seizures:** Animals who have multiple clusters of seizures (**status epilepticus**) can have their body temperature increase due to constant muscular contractions and tetany.
- **Toad poisoning:** Animals exposed to toxins of specific toads can have a severe chemical reaction in which one symptom can be severely high temperatures.
- **Toxin:** Certain types of toxins, such as plant food/pesticides (organophosphates), snail bait (metaldehyde), and poisons (strychnine), can cause severe muscular convulsions that can raise body temperature into dangerous territory (see Chapter 27).

Common Points on Medical History

As discussed previously, a complete medical history should be taken, with a special focus on causes that may produce heatstroke, for example

- environmental exposure,
- history of seizures,
- ingestion of toxin / poison, and
- exposure to poisonous toad.

Common Points in Initial Assessment

Careful attention should be paid to any spontaneous bruising of the gums, skin, or mucous membranes, which could suggest the beginning of internal bleeding (DIC). General common clinical signs of disease are

- panting,
- salivating,
- skin that is hot to the touch,
- dry, red-injected mucous membranes,
- nervous behavior, possibly accelerating to seizure activity,
- weak to collapsed,
- bloody vomiting/diarrhea,
- bruising or small hemorrhages on gums and skin (DIC),
- shock,
- rapid heart rate,
- coma, and
- death.

Diagnostics

As discussed above, a minimal clinical database should be obtained to help define the type of shock the animal has. In general heatstroke shock, all minimal clinical database parameters can show the changes in clinical diagnostics as listed in Table 30.8).

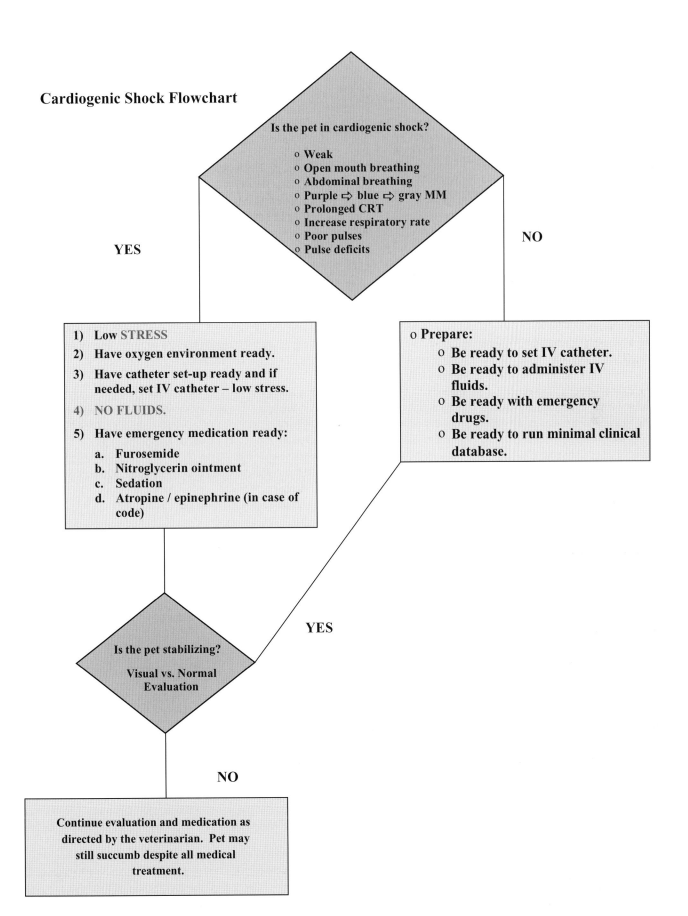

Cardiogenic Shock Flowchart

Is the pet in cardiogenic shock?

- o Weak
- o Open mouth breathing
- o Abdominal breathing
- o Purple ⇨ blue ⇨ gray MM
- o Prolonged CRT
- o Increase respiratory rate
- o Poor pulses
- o Pulse deficits

YES

NO

1) Low STRESS
2) Have oxygen environment ready.
3) Have catheter set-up ready and if needed, set IV catheter – low stress.
4) NO FLUIDS.
5) Have emergency medication ready:
   a. Furosemide
   b. Nitroglycerin ointment
   c. Sedation
   d. Atropine / epinephrine (in case of code)

o Prepare:
   - o Be ready to set IV catheter.
   - o Be ready to administer IV fluids.
   - o Be ready with emergency drugs.
   - o Be ready to run minimal clinical database.

Is the pet stabilizing?

Visual vs. Normal Evaluation

YES

NO

Continue evaluation and medication as directed by the veterinarian. Pet may still succumb despite all medical treatment.

Table 30.8. Changes noted in clinical diagnostics with heatstroke.

Parameter	Finding
PCV/TP	Elevated secondary to dehydration, initially. Can become decreased if pet begins to have internal bleeding problems.
Glucose	Generally within normal limits.
Electrolytes	Electrolytes are generally within normal limits.
Clotting times	Clotting times can be elevated secondary to prolonged hyperthermia. Elevations in clotting time can be severe, suggesting the patient is beginning to bleed internally.

Treatment

The treatment protocol below (see Heatstroke Flowchart) is a suggestion of how some medical teams would handle a heatstroke patient. It is meant to give the team member a concept of what steps may need to be taken with a shock patient to better anticipate the doctor. This protocol is meant to help the team member assist the veterinarian in treating an emergency patient. When treating for heatstroke, the team member may face the challenges of hyperthermia, shock, and DIC all encompassed in one event. Even when stabilized, the patient must be carefully monitored for complications such as organ disease, central nervous system damage, and DIC. *The goal of treatment is to cool the animal down, reestablish perfusion, and monitor for life-threatening side effects.*

1. **Cool down:** If the patient's temperature is more than 106° Fahrenheit, a cool down should be initiated immediately, using
   - cool water bath (*not an ice bath*),
   - fan,
   - alcohol bath on lower limbs, and
   - ice water enema (last resort).
   The animal's temperature should be monitored until temperature falls between 103° and 103.5° Fahrenheit. Then stop the cool down and dry pet off to prevent hypothermia. Temperature should still be monitored for hypothermia.
2. **Catheter:** Be ready to set IV catheter.
3. **Treatment:** Begin treating for shock.
   - Be ready to administer IV fluids.
   - Be ready to collect blood samples and run minimal clinical databases.
   - Be ready with emergency medications, such as
     —dextrose,
     —atropine, and
     —epinephrine.
4. **Evaluation:** If stability is still questionable, have colloids ready.

5. **Monitor:**
   - for ongoing complications of heatstroke.
   - for hypothermia secondary to cool down.
   - diagnostics for complications and be prepared to treat as needed–GET A CLOTTING TIME!
   - oxygen needed.

Traumatic Brain Injury/Head Trauma

Traumatic brain injury is an acute syndrome brought on by a sharp blow to the head or a fall (such as from a moving vehicle) that causes blunt injury to the brain.

Etiology

A sharp blow to the head causes the brain to swell within the cranium bone around it. The swelling can place increasing intracranial pressure on the brain and early central nervous system, impeding normal brain function. If the swelling is severe enough, damage can be permanent. Depending on the pet's presentation and response to treatment, prognosis can be fair to extremely poor.

Signalment

Head trauma can affect any breed, sex, or age of patient.

Common Points on Medical History

As discussed previously, a complete medical history should be taken. With concerns of head trauma, special focus on any history of acute trauma, animal attack, fall, or injury should be discussed with the client.

Common Points in Initial Assessment

These patients can be extremely fragile and could become comatose and die suddenly. Common signs of a traumatic brain injury are

- pupils that are different sizes (anisocoria; see Figure 30.3),
- depression,
- vomiting (usually excessive),
- not aware of surroundings,
- seizures,
- rigidity,
- coma, and
- abnormally low or high body temperature.

Diagnostics

As discussed above, a minimal clinical database should be obtained to help define the type of shock. In general, with head concussions, all test parameters can show the changes listed in Table 30.9.

Practice Tip: If a traumatic brain injury is suspected, a jugular draw should not be attempted because placing pressure on the jugular vein can increase intracerebral pressure.

Heatstroke Flowchart

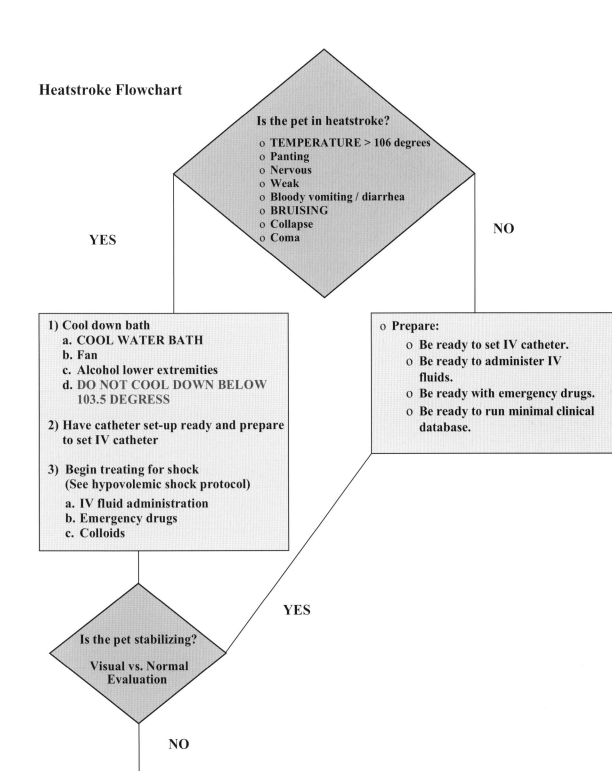

Is the pet in heatstroke?

o **TEMPERATURE > 106 degrees**
o **Panting**
o **Nervous**
o **Weak**
o **Bloody vomiting / diarrhea**
o **BRUISING**
o **Collapse**
o **Coma**

YES

NO

1) **Cool down bath**
   a. **COOL WATER BATH**
   b. **Fan**
   c. **Alcohol lower extremities**
   d. **DO NOT COOL DOWN BELOW 103.5 DEGRESS**

2) **Have catheter set-up ready and prepare to set IV catheter**

3) **Begin treating for shock (See hypovolemic shock protocol)**
   a. **IV fluid administration**
   b. **Emergency drugs**
   c. **Colloids**

o **Prepare:**
   o **Be ready to set IV catheter.**
   o **Be ready to administer IV fluids.**
   o **Be ready with emergency drugs.**
   o **Be ready to run minimal clinical database.**

Is the pet stabilizing?

Visual vs. Normal Evaluation

YES

NO

Continue close evaluation and monitoring of patient. Monitor for concerns of acute organ disease, CNS disease or disseminated intravascular coagulopathy (DIC).

Traumatic Brain Injury Flowchart

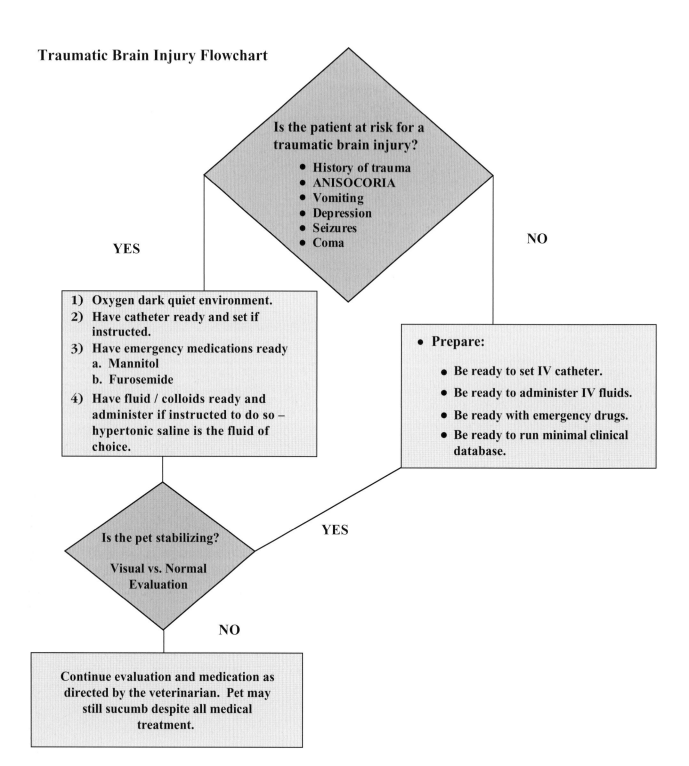

Is the patient at risk for a traumatic brain injury?

- History of trauma
- ANISOCORIA
- Vomiting
- Depression
- Seizures
- Coma

YES

NO

1) Oxygen dark quiet environment.
2) Have catheter ready and set if instructed.
3) Have emergency medications ready
   a. Mannitol
   b. Furosemide
4) Have fluid / colloids ready and administer if instructed to do so – hypertonic saline is the fluid of choice.

- Prepare:
  - Be ready to set IV catheter.
  - Be ready to administer IV fluids.
  - Be ready with emergency drugs.
  - Be ready to run minimal clinical database.

Is the pet stabilizing?

Visual vs. Normal Evaluation

YES

NO

Continue evaluation and medication as directed by the veterinarian. Pet may still sucumb despite all medical treatment.

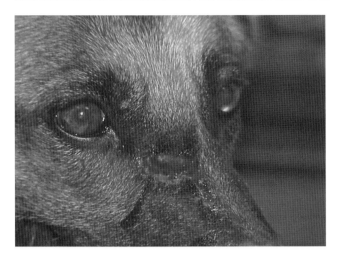

Figure 30.3. Note the different pupil sizes in this pet that was kicked by a horse. With a history of trauma, anisocoria is a strong suggestion of a traumatic brain injury.

Table 30.9. Changes noted in clinical diagnostics with concussion.

Parameter	Finding
PCV/TP	Usually within normal limits unless the trauma has also triggered internal bleeding.
Glucose	With cerebral swelling and edema, these patients may have a hard time regulating blood sugar and may alternate between hyper- and hypoglycemia.
Electrolytes	Electrolytes are generally within normal limits.
Clotting times	Clotting times are generally within normal limits unless the initiating trauma has produced internal bleeding.

Treatment

The goal of treatment is to try to reduce swelling of the brain while supporting the animal through possible shock and coma (see Traumatic Brain Injury Flowchart). The animal must be handled in a quiet, dark, warm environment because traumatic brain injury patients are very sensitive to loud noises and bright stimuli.

1. **Oxygen:** Increasing oxygen concentration in the bloodstream can help maintain normal brain function and aid in tissue perfusion.
2. **Position:** Keep animal immobile and quiet with the patient's head slightly elevated.
3. **Catheter:** Have IV catheter ready and set it if instructed to do so.
4. **Emergency drugs:** Emergency medications are focused on stabilizing the pet and reducing cerebral swelling. Some indicated medications to have ready are as follows.
   - **Mannitol:** Mannitol is a large, inert sugar molecule that is given slowly intravenously over 20–30 minutes to help pull fluid out of the brain tissue and back into the blood vasculature.
   - **Furosemide (Lasix):** Lasix is usually given after the mannitol to help to decrease cerebrospinal fluid production and lower intracranial pressure.
   - **Sedation:** If pet is thrashing, seizuring, or having uncontrolled motor activity, diazepam sedation can be used as needed.
4. **Have intravenous fluids/colloids:** Fluid requirements and types depend on the stability of the patient and its metabolic needs.
5. **Reevaluation/minimal clinical database:** The patient should be monitored closely for overall changes in stability and clinical diagnostics. Many comatose patients may code because the cerebral swelling is too severe to maintain normal cardiac and respiratory function.

Discussing Shock and Emergency Syndromes with the Client
- Shock is a life-threatening syndrome that is caused by a primary trauma, disease, or condition that overwhelms the patient such that its body cannot keep up with demands placed upon it.
- Shock is an emergency condition, and if not reversed and stabilized quickly, the patient can die.
- The initial signs of shock can be weakness, rapid pulses, changes in the breathing patterns, and depression.
- Although signs can be mild at first, the patient can deteriorate rapidly, showing signs of collapse, weak thready pulses, shallow breathing, coma, and death.
- The patient requires critical care treatment and often must be hospitalized for long periods of time.
- Treatment is focused on reestablishing normal blood pressure, heart and breathing rates, and treating the underlying condition producing this syndrome.
- Often patients require intravenous fluids, emergency medications, oxygen therapy, and monitoring of clinical diagnostics.
- If not treated, patients have a poor prognosis and can die.

CD-ROM 2 will focus on concepts of Understanding the Concepts of Disease and Treatment. The exercises can be done individually or as case rounds as they explore specific topics in veterinary medicine that discuss clinical diagnostics and treatment.

Chapter 31

Cardiopulmonary Cerebral Resuscitation (CPCR)

CPCR is the *combined* techniques of chest compressions/defibrillation and mechanical ventilation. The goal of CPCR is to provide adequate circulatory and ventilatory support to the heart and brain until cardiac and pulmonary functions can return. It is used when the patient codes or when the heart and/or respiratory systems fail. Cardiovascular failure can occur in patients undergoing anesthesia, suffering from an acute or chronic systemic disease, after a severe trauma (i.e., hit by car), or any other process that places the pet into a shock syndrome.

This chapter discusses the preparations the veterinary medical team must make in case of cardiovascular failure. CPCR is always initiated and led by the veterinarian, *however, for CPCR to have the highest likelihood of success, it must be handled by the veterinary medical team.* The team approach to managing cardiopulmonary arrest is essential. *Each member* of the hospital staff (including the receptionist and kennel help) should be trained in every aspect of CPCR.

Before CPCR can be initiated, the status of the code must be determined to facilitate the necessary action. In some acutely or chronically ill patients with an overall poor prognosis, the clients may elect not to have any treatment initiated if the animal codes. In other patients, the clients may elect to have full or advanced care initiated. Code statuses are set up by the veterinarian after discussing their concerns with clients whose pets are severely ill and may code. *If a patient codes and their code status is unknown, CPCR should always be initiated.* Table 31.1 outlines the type of code status.

Before faced with a code, the veterinary medical team should assemble a moveable compact **crash kit**. Crash kits can vary from as simple as a tackle box to as elaborate as a mechanic's chest and should allow all necessary supplies to be readily available. Necessary supplies include

- endotracheal tubes,
- laryngoscope ,
- intravenous catheters,
- fluids and administration sets,
- tape and bandage supplies,
- syringes and needles,
- tourniquet,
- drugs and dosage chart for all drugs in the kit
  — atropine,
  — lidocaine,
  — epinephrine,
  — dopram,
  — dopamine/dobutamine, and
  — dextrose (50%), and
- resuscitation (Ambu) bag.

When choosing an area in which to perform CPCR, it should be large enough to allow the medical team and their equipment easy access to all sides of the patient. The lighting should be bright enough for the medical team to intubate and catheterize the patient. If possible, an oxygen source should be available. The table should be flat and hard enough to allow good chest compressions. The height of the table should allow the team member to stand over the patient and effectively compress the chest (see below).

Beginning CPCR

When faced with a patient that has coded, a team member should perform the following steps.

- **Step 1:** Double check.
- **Step 2:** Don't panic: Call for help in no uncertain terms.
- **Step 3:** Begin CPCR!

Once the heart stops, the team has 5 minutes to restore normal circulation before permanent brain damage occurs. If the medical team is not right there to react immediately within the first 30 seconds as cardiopulmonary arrest occurs, overall prognosis is very poor.

Each team member must assume specific responsibilities when first approaching a code (see Table 31.2). In smaller hospitals, where there may be fewer than 2–3 team members available, these responsibilities can be combined. Components of CPCR (i.e., chest compressions) can be physically demanding and exhausting; each team member should be able assume new responsibilities as another team member tires. Practice drills are essential and allow the staff to respond quickly and efficiently.

The primary objective of basic life support is to temporarily support the patient's ventilation, oxygenation, and circulation by administering artificial respiration and chest compressions. The following is a step-by-step discussion of how a medical team could respond to a code. *Overall, the code is always overseen by the veterinarian and can vary*

Table 31.1. Code status.

Code Status	Medical Treatment	Reason
No code—Do not resuscitate (DNR)	No medical treatment is pursued if the patient codes. This does not mean the medical team does not treat the patient aggressively until that point.	Clients may decide that their pet may be a "no code" based on personal reasons or experiences with other animals, the severity and prognosis of the underlying disease, or financial concerns.
Closed chest	Closed chest massage refers to CPCR with respiratory and cardiac support. The cardiac compression occurs by external chest compression	Closed chest massage is the first response when the patient codes.
Open chest	Open chest massage is an advanced treatment option in which the thoracic cavity is opened and the heart is directly massaged.	Open chest massage requires advanced critical care support if the patient is revived. Clients must be aware of the complications and advanced treatment concerns for when a patient goes through an open-chest CPCR.

Table 31.2. CPCR responsibilities.

Responsibility	Tasks
Airway management	Establish airway and ventilate the patient.
Cardiovascular management	Chest compressions.
Venous access	Place IV lines and start fluids as directed.
Monitoring	Check for pulse.
	Check mucous membrane color/CRT.
	Auscultate heart and lungs.
	Attach EKG.
Drug administration	Administer drugs.
	Record time and drugs given.

depending on the patient, the patient's disease, and the hospital's experience and equipment. The steps to take following a code are as follows.

Step I: Determine If the Patient Has Coded
A team member should assess the patient for respiration, heart rate, and pulse (see Figure 31.1). If the patient shows signs of cardiovascular failure, the medical team must be notified immediately.

Step II: Begin Cardiac Compression
While the medical team is beginning to secure an airway and oxygen source, one team member should begin chest compression. This will maintain cardiac output and perfusion while also producing moderate expansion and contraction of the lungs. The effectiveness of cardiac compressions depends entirely upon the force (strength) with which the compressions are administered. *Place the animal in right lateral recumbency.*

Patients Less than 10 Pounds
The thumb and first two fingers can be used to compress the chest (thumb placed on left side of chest and fingers below;

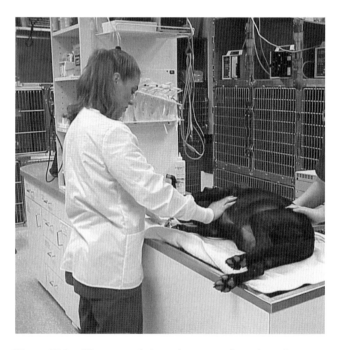

Figure 31.1. If concerned about the status of a patient, the technical team member should evaluate for heart rate, pulse, and respiration. If the patient is in a code status, the veterinarian and team should be notified immediately.

see Figure 31.2]). *Chest compressions should be administered at a rate of 160–200 per minute.*

Patients More than 10 Pounds
Place both hands on the chest over the heart. The heart area can be located by counting four to six rib spaces or use the point of the left elbow against the chest. Keep arms extended and locked. Place the heel of the lower hand over the area of the heart and compress the chest by bending at the waist. Do not bend the elbows because this will not create an appropri-

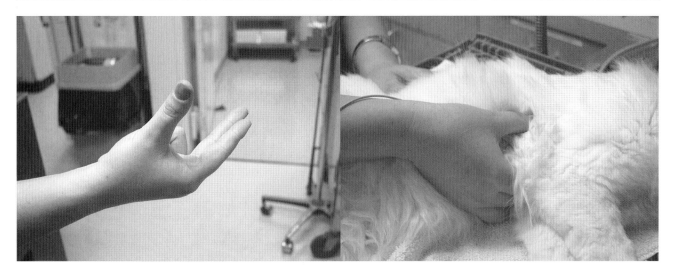

Figure 31.2

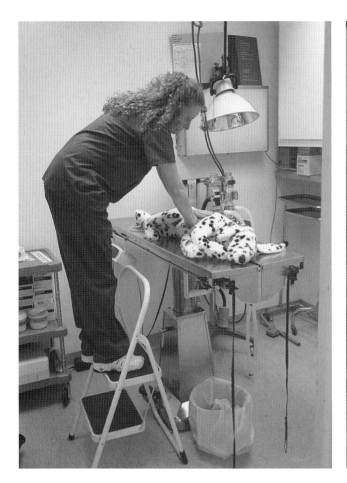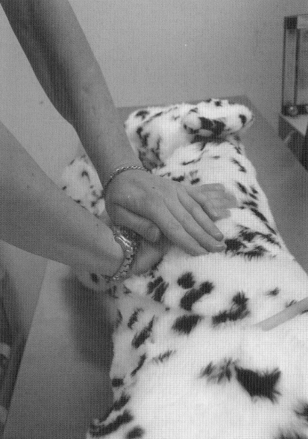

Figure 31.3

ate force to effect circulation. *Chest compressions should be administered at a rate of 80–100 per minute.* The rate of chest compressions suggested above is simply a guide. Although the *number* of compressions is important, main-tain focus on the *effectiveness* of the compression (quality vs. quantity). It may also be necessary to stand on a stool to get the proper height to perform an adequate compression (see Figure 31.3).

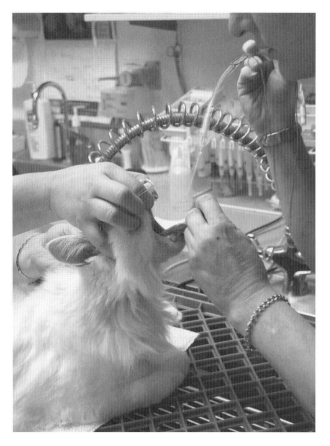

Figure 31.4

Practice Tip: The goal of a good compression is to compress the chest 30–50% of normal volume and produce a palpable pulse.

Administer two quick breaths, initially, then ventilate once every 2–3 seconds.

Step III: Establish an Airway

Establish a patent airway by placing an endotracheal tube. The use of a laryngoscope is recommended because some patients can aspirate food and saliva that can be obstructive if not removed first (see Figure 31.4). Once intubated, the cuff should be inflated and the tube tied in. It is recommended that only new endotracheal tubes be used in the crash kit to prevent using a leaky or damaged cuff that would require a new tube to be placed.

It is important to remember that when cardiopulmonary arrest occurs in anesthetized animals, anesthetic gases should be turned off immediately (see Figure 31.5). Flush the system with 100% oxygen. *Always disconnect hoses attached to endotracheal tubes before flushing.*

Step IV: Breathing

Administer artificial respiration by connecting the endotracheal tube to an Ambu bag (connected to oxygen supply) or anesthesia machine. If there is no Ambu bag or oxygen source, mouth to endotracheal tube can also be attempted.

- If using an anesthetic machine as an oxygen source, the outflow valve should be tightened down and the oxygen reservoir bag compressed to deliver positive pressure ventilation (see Figure 31.6).
- Administer no more than 20 cm of H_2O pressure, and when the breath is completed, open up the outflow valve, flush oxygen into the system, and repeat the procedure for the next breath (see Figure 31.7.)

Step V: Have Drugs Ready and Administer Them as Instructed

Understanding the pharmacology of the drugs used during CPCR is important. The drugs used in CPCR are focused on increasing heart rate and blood pressure, blocking normal control mechanisms of the body to slow heart and respiratory rates, and restoring perfusion. The most common drugs used in CPCR are as follows:

- **Epinephrine:** Epinephrine is a drug of the sympathetic nervous system that elevates heart rate, increases blood

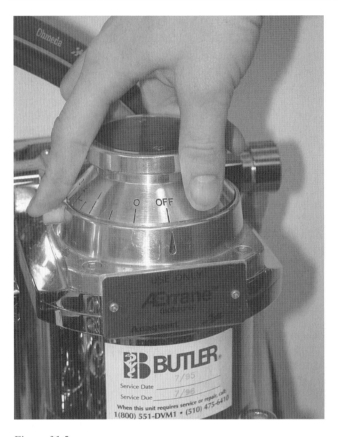

Figure 31.5

pressure, and dilates airways. Epinephrine can be given either intravenously or through the tracheal tube.

- **Atropine:** Atropine blocks the body's normal response to slow the heart rate and respiratory rate when they become too rapid. This drug is mainly used to increase a slowed heart rate. Atropine can be given either intravenously or through the tracheal tube.
- **Doxapram (Dopram):** Doxapram is used to stimulate respiration within the central nervous system. Doxapram is given intravenously. The beneficial effects of the drug are controversial.
- **Dextrose (50%):** Dextrose is used to maintain normal blood sugar levels if the patient is hypoglycemic. The brain and muscle must have sugar to maintain normal function. Without this the patient can become comatose, seizure, and die. Dextrose is mixed 1:1 with sterile water or IV fluids to make a 25% dextrose solution. It is then given intravenously (see Chapter 30).

When handling a code, the medical team should have the drugs available, drawn up, and ready to administer. The two most important drugs to have ready for intratracheal or intravenous administration are *epinephrine* and *atropine*. See Table 30.3 for doses that should be used as the veterinarian recommendations. The amount, route, and time a drug is administered must be recorded for the medical record.

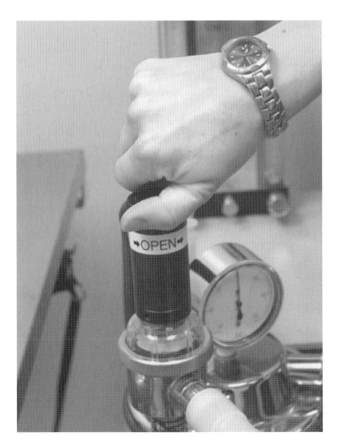

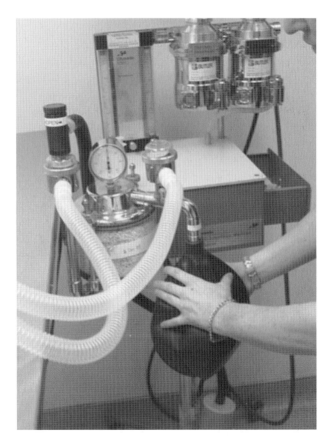

Figure 31.6

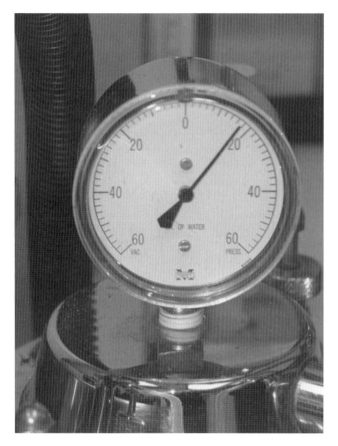

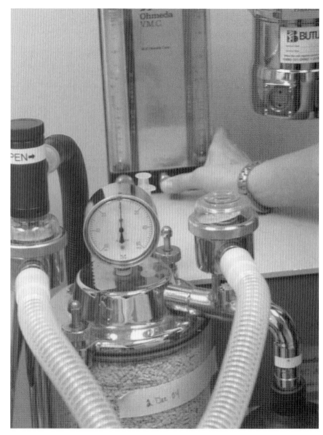

Figure 31.7

Step VI: Have Catheter Ready and Set Catheter

A catheter is extremely important for the administration of drugs and fluids to help maintain circulation. Setting a catheter on a coded patient often is extremely difficult and sometimes impossible. If an animal presents in an emergency situation, it is recommended to set a catheter before the patient's condition worsens. Even if the owner does not want to treat the pet and may opt for euthanasia, a port is extremely helpful in giving any type of medication. The cost factor is minimal for one catheter in comparison with repeated venipuncture. An indwelling catheter can minimize stress, and maximize efficiency. Once a patent catheter is set, begin the fluid and drug administration that the veterinarian outlines. (See Figure 31.8.)

Step VII: Evaluate the Patient

Once CPCR is initiated, the patient should be evaluated every 15–30 seconds for response. Initially, the patient should have its temperature monitored, the heart and lungs should be auscultated, the gum color and capillary refill time evaluated, and the pulse examined. *If chest compressions are being done effectively, there should be a pulse observed with each cardiac compression.* Once initially evaluated, placement of advanced monitoring devices (i.e., EKG, pulse oximeter, esophageal stethoscope) can be useful to detect changes in the patient and the effectiveness of CPCR (see Figure 31.9).

CPCR is then maintained over the next 5–10 minutes. Especially with CPCR in the larger patient, team members will have to switch responsibilities because compressing the chest compression becomes exhausting. Compressions, ventilation, and drug and fluid administration are maintained until the veterinarian calls the code or the animal responds and stabilizes.

Overall, the prognosis once an animal codes is poor to guarded, usually because there is some underlying disease that produced the cardiac arrest. Many animals will never regain consciousness and code again once the emergency medication wears off due to permanent damage to the central nervous system. The owner must be made aware of this from the start so they can begin to prepare in case CPCR is not successful. There can also be permanent brain damage.

In an emergency, every minute counts. Team members recognizing likely problems initially and preparing for anticipated treatments greatly facilitate success of stabilization and outcome for the patient. Practicing cardiac arrest situations with the medical team at regular intervals can make the hospital ready to respond to life-threatening emergencies quickly and more effectively.

Table 31.3.   Emergency dose table—canine.

Weight (pounds)	Epinephrine— Intravenous (1:1000)	Epinephrine— Intertracheal* or Sublingual (1:1000)	Atropine (0.54 mg/ml)	Dopram (20 mg/ml)	Dextrose—50%** (25% /ml)
Common Dose	1 cc/10 pounds	1 cc/20 pounds	1 cc/20 pounds	1 cc/20 pounds	1 cc/pound
1	0.1 ml	0.2 ml	0.05 ml	0.02–0.10 ml	1 cc
2	0.2 ml	0.4 ml	0.1 ml	0.04–0.2 ml	2 cc
3	0.3 ml	0.6 ml	0.15 ml	0.06–0.3 ml	3 cc
4	0.4 ml	0.8 ml	0.20 ml	0.08–0.4 ml	4 cc
5	0.5 ml	1.0 ml	0.25 ml	0.1–00.5 ml	5 cc
6	0.6 ml	1.2 ml	0.30 ml	0.12–0.6 ml	6 cc
7	0.7 ml	1.4 ml	0.35 ml	0.14–0.7ml	7 cc
8	0.8ml	1.6ml	0.40 ml	0.16–0.8 ml	8 cc
9	0.9 ml	1.8 ml	0.45 ml	0.18–0.9 ml	9 cc
10	1.0 ml	2.0 ml	0.5 ml	0.2–1.0 ml	10 cc
15	1.5 ml	3.0 ml	0.75 ml	0.3–10.5 ml	15 cc
20	2.0 ml	4.0ml	1.0 ml	0.4–2.0 ml	20 cc
25	2.5 ml	5.0 ml	1.25 ml	0.5–20.5 ml	25 cc
30	3.0 ml	6.0 ml	1.5 ml	0.6–3.0 ml	30 cc
35	3.5 ml	7.0 ml	1.75 ml	0.7–30.5 ml	35 cc
40	4.0 ml	8.0 ml	2.0 ml	0.8–4.0 ml	40 cc
45	4.5 ml	9.0 ml	2.25 ml	0.9–40.5 ml	45 cc
50	5.0 ml	10.0 ml	2.5 ml	1.0–5.0 ml	50 cc
55	5.5 ml	11.0 ml	2.75 ml	1.1–50.5 ml	55 cc
60	6.0 ml	12.0 ml	3.0 ml	1.2–6.0 ml	60 cc
65	6.5 ml	13.0 ml	3.25 ml	1.3–60.5 ml	65 cc
70	7.0 ml	14.0 ml	3.5 ml	1.4–7.0 ml	70 cc
75	7.5 ml	15.0 ml	3.75 ml	1.5–70.5 ml	75 cc
80	8.0 ml	16.0 ml	4.0 ml	1.6–8.0 ml	80 cc
85	8.5 ml	17.0 ml	4.25 ml	1.7–80.5 ml	85 cc
90	9.0 ml	18.0 ml	4.5 ml	1.8–9.0 ml	90 cc
95	9.5 ml	19.0 ml	4.75 ml	1.9–90.5 ml	95 cc
100	10.0 ml	20.0 ml	5.0 ml	2.0–10.0 ml	100 cc

*For intratracheal treatment dilute with sterile water and administer: 3 ml with a cat or small dog, 5 ml with a medium-sized dog, and 10 ml with a large breed dog.

**Dextrose mixed in equal portions with sterile fluids.

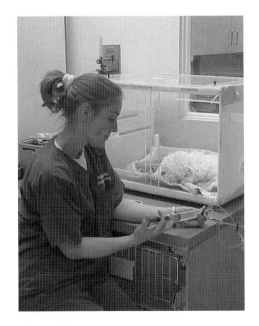
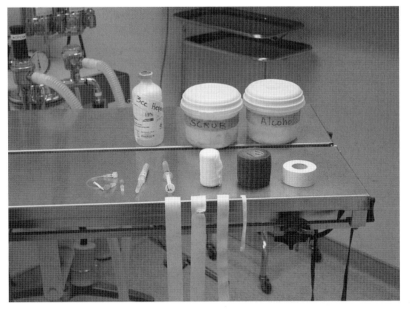

Figure 31.8

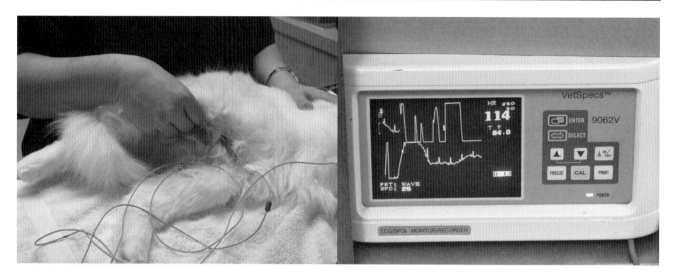

Figure 31.9

Talking to the Client about CPCR

- Cardiopulmonary resuscitation is initiated when a patient's heart and respiratory systems fail.
- Cardiopulmonary resuscitation is a combination of manual chest compressions, emergency drugs, and ventilation for support until the animal's heart and lungs can be restarted.
- The medical team has 5 minutes to successfully stabilize the patient before permanent brain damage occurs.
- If the patient presents in a full code, there is a decreased chance that it will respond and stabilize.
- Some patients that do respond will never gain consciousness and will code again once emergency drugs wear off.
- For the patients that do continue to support themselves, it may take days to weeks to fully evaluate if the pet has suffered permanent brain damage.
- Many patients may have to be maintained for days in a critical care facility to help them fully recover after an arrest episode.

CD-ROM 2 will focus on concepts of Understanding the Concepts of Disease and Treatment. The exercises can be done individually or as case rounds as they explore specific topics in veterinary medicine that discuss clinical diagnostics and treatment.

Appendix

App. A.1   Flowchart for Cardiac Auscultation

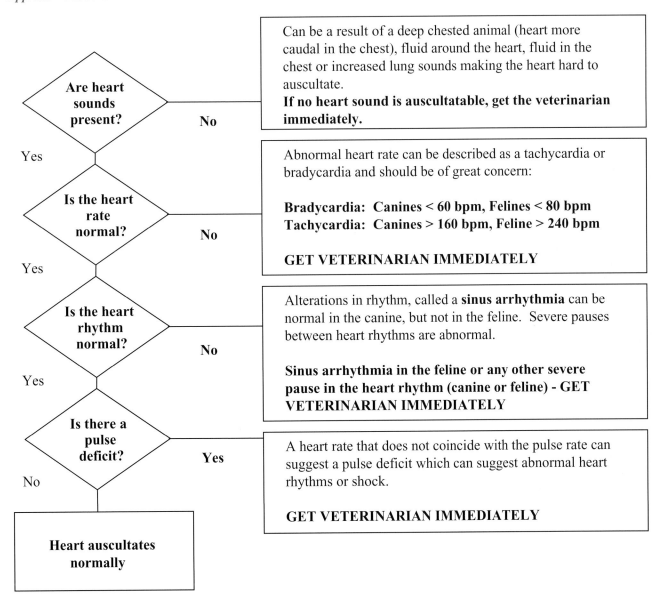

App. A.2 You know you are in trouble based on physical exam when . . .

System Examined	Canine	Feline
Disposition	Nonresponsive Comatose Lateral recumbent	Nonresponsive Comatose Lateral recumbent
Breathing	Increased rate >45 Abdominal breathing	Increase rate >45–60 Abdominal breathing Open mouth breathing (panting)

Pulses/heart
beating
	Increased rate >150
	Pulse quality:
	  None
	  Hyperdynamic
	  Weak
		Increased rate >200
		Pulse quality:
		  None
		  Hyperdynamic
		  Weak

Gum color	White Purple/gray Yellow	White Purple/gray Yellow
Capillary refill time	CRT >2 seconds	CRT >2 seconds
Bruising	Any bruising should be monitored Increased bruising	Any bruising should be monitored Increased bruising
Body temperature	Temp <98° or Temp >106°	Temp <98° or Temp >106°
Body confirmation	Bloated in abdomen Bloated in chest Shift-Sherrington	Bloated in abdomen Bloated in chest Shift-Sherrington

App. A.3 Outline of azotemia.

Type of Azotemia	Urine Specific Gravity	Cause	Prognosis	Other Concerns
Pre-Renal	High	Dehydration	Kidney chemistry values usually return to normal when patient is rehydrated	
Azotemia	Dilute	Primary renal disease	Can be poor due to underlying renal disease	Hypokalemia Proteinuria
Post-renal azotemia	High (but can become dilute with long-term urinary obstruction)	Urinary obstruction (FLUTD)	Can be poor if obstruction is prolonged, which can produce primary renal disease	Hyperkalemia

App. A.4   Diagnostic Tree for Hyperadrenocorticism

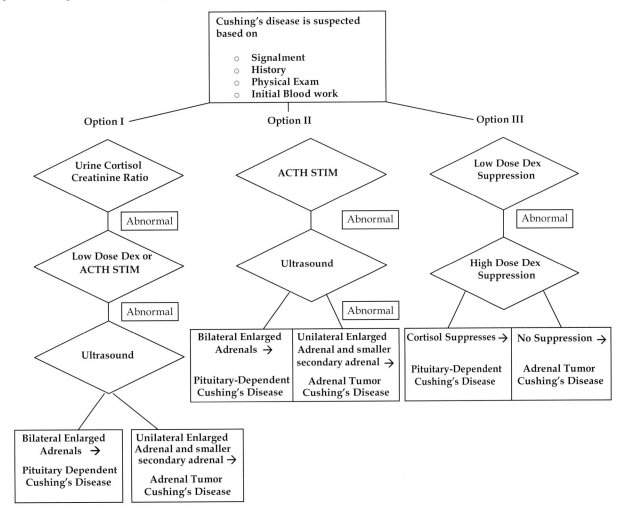

App. A.5 CBC Differential Flowchart: Red Blood Cell Evaluation

White Blood Cell Population: Count 100 Cells

Draw EDTA blood sample and check tube

Is the sample normal?

Blood Clot → Redraw sample and start over

Yes → Make a blood film and evaluate the red blood cells

Agglutination → Check a saline prep for agglutination

Is it agglutination or roleaux?

Roleaux

Agglutination → Concerns of autoimmune-mediated hemolytic anemias **CONSULT DOCTOR**

Is central pallor normal?

NO → Hypochromasia — Decreased hemoglobin production — spleen, liver, kidney disease or iron deficiency **CONSULT DOCTOR**

Yes → Is the cell normal?

Polychromasia — Regenerative anemia **CONSULT DOCTOR**

NO → **CONSULT DOCTOR**

Echinocytes — Altered fat metabolism, tumor, toxin

Schistocytes — Heartworm disease, spleen and liver disease

Spherocytes — AIHA

Intracellular Changes — Parasite, regenerative change, toxic injury

Yes → Go on to WBC evaluation

PCV: _____

TP: _____

App. A.6 Blood film evaluation.

Cell type[1]	Description	Normal Values	Number Seen
Neutrophils	Neutrophils have segmented nuclei with a pink staining cytoplasm.		
Bands	Band neutrophils have unsegmented nuclei (monocyte-like) with a pink-staining cytoplasm. **Increased Bands Suggest Acute Disease**		
Eosinophils	Eosinophils have segmented nuclei with a pink cytoplasm and dark red granules in the cytoplasm. Eosinophils respond to fungal infections or allergic reactions.		
Monocytes	Monocytes have unsegmented nuclei with a purple staining cytoplasm. They are seen with chronic infections.		
Lymphocytes	Lymphocytes are small round cells with round nuclei and purple-staining cytoplasm. They are responsible for producing immunoglobulin.		

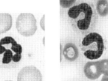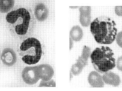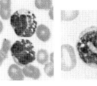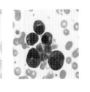

App. A.7 Algorithm for Kidney Disease[i]

Is there an azotemia present?
○ Increased BUN
○ Creatinine

Other elements: Increased phosphorus
Low potassium

Yes → Obtain a urinalysis → Is the USG low?

Yes → Renal Azotemia
Evaluate other functions – i.e., Blood pressure

No → Other cause of azotemia

No → Is there: Low body Albumen
○ PU / PD
○ At risk patient
○ Other signs

Yes → Obtain a urinalysis → Is the USG low?
Is there true proteinuria?
Abnormal Sediment?

Yes → Run advanced diagnostics:
Urine / Protein Quant
Sediment to lab
Hormonal testing

No → At this point there are no concerns of primary renal disease.

No → At this point there are no concerns of primary renal disease.

App. A.8 Algorithm for Liver Disease[ii]

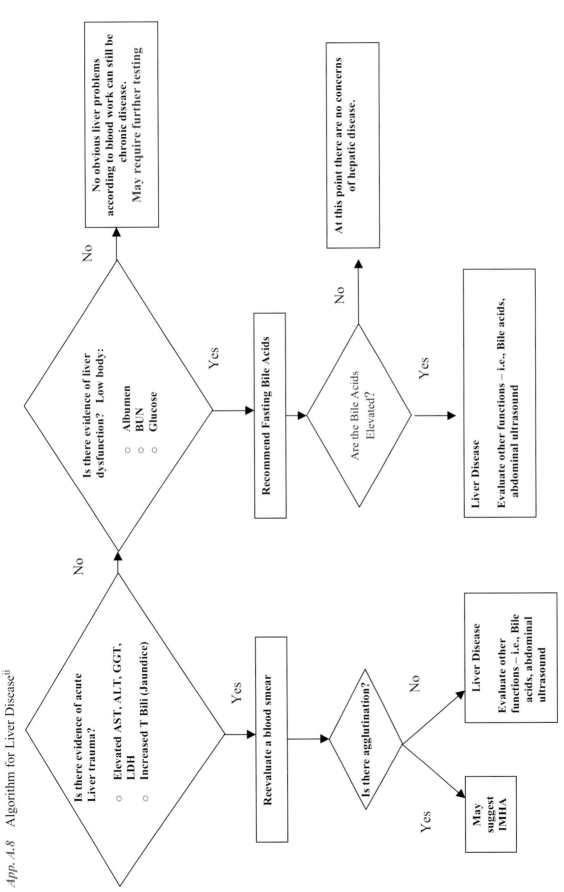

App. A.9   Algorithm for Exocrine Pancreatic Disease (i.e. Pancreatitis)[iii]

App. A.10 Algorithm for Endocrine Pancreatic Disease (Diabetes)[iv]

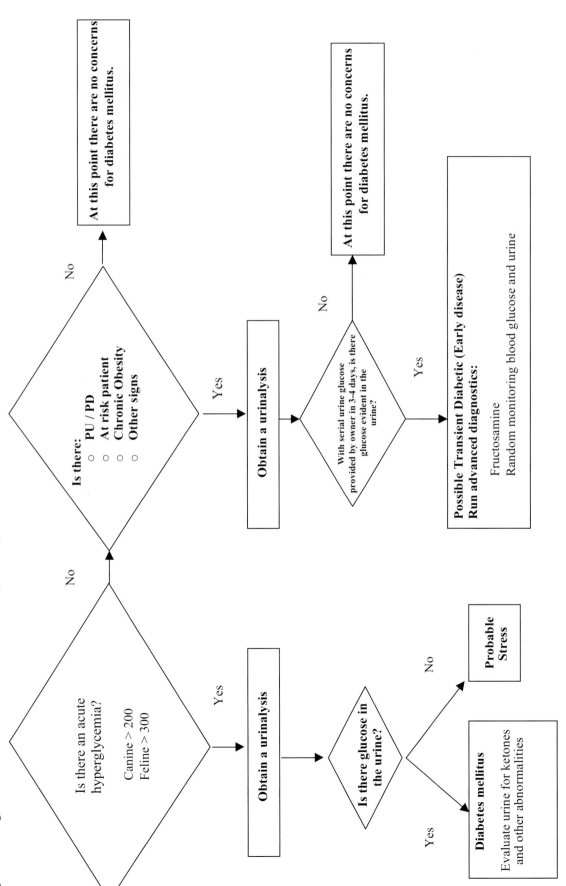

App. 11. Normal values for canine/feline chemistry.

Test	Canine Normal Range	Feline Normal Range
ALP	10–150 U/l	0–62 U/l
ALT (SGPT)	5–60 U/l	27–76 U/l
AST (SGOT)	5–55 U/l	5–55 U/l
GGT	0–14 U/l	0–6 U/l
Albumin	2.5–3.6 g/dl	2.3–3.3 g/l
TP	5.1–7.8 g/dl	5.9–8.5 g/l
Globulin	2.8–4.5 g/dl	3.6–5.6 g/l
Total bilirubin	0–0.4 mg/dl	0–0.4 mg/dl
BUN	7–27 mg/dl	15–34 mg/dl
Creatinine	0.4–1.8 mg/dl	0.8–2.3 mg/dl
Glucose	60–125 mg/dl	70–150 mg/dl
Calcium	8.2–12.4 mg/dl	8.2–11.8 mg/dl
Phosphorus	2.1–6.3 mg/dl	3.0–7.0 mg/dl
Chloride (Cl)	105–115 mEq/l	111–125 mEq/l
Sodium (Na)	141–156 mEq/l	147–156 mEq/l
Potassium (K)	4.0–5.6 mEq/l	3.9–5.3 mEq/l

App. 12. Guidelines for subcutaneous fluid therapy.

Animal's Weight	Approximate Subcutaneous Fluid Amount*
<10 pounds	50–200 ml
11–40 pounds	200–500 ml
41–70 pounds	500–700 ml
>70 pounds +	>700–1000 ml +

*These fluids are suggested fluid ranges based on pet weights. These ranges are meant for animals without primary disease that could produce pulmonary edema and congestion (i.e., congestive heart failure, electric cord injury, etc.).

App. A.13   Flowchart A: Evaluating Urine Color, Turbidity, and Specific Gravity

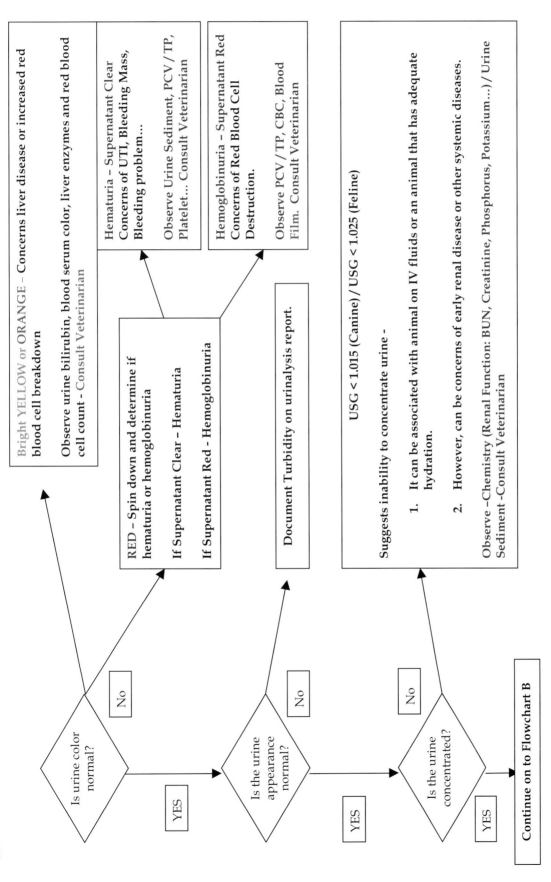

App. A.14 Flowchart B: Evaluating Urine Chemistry

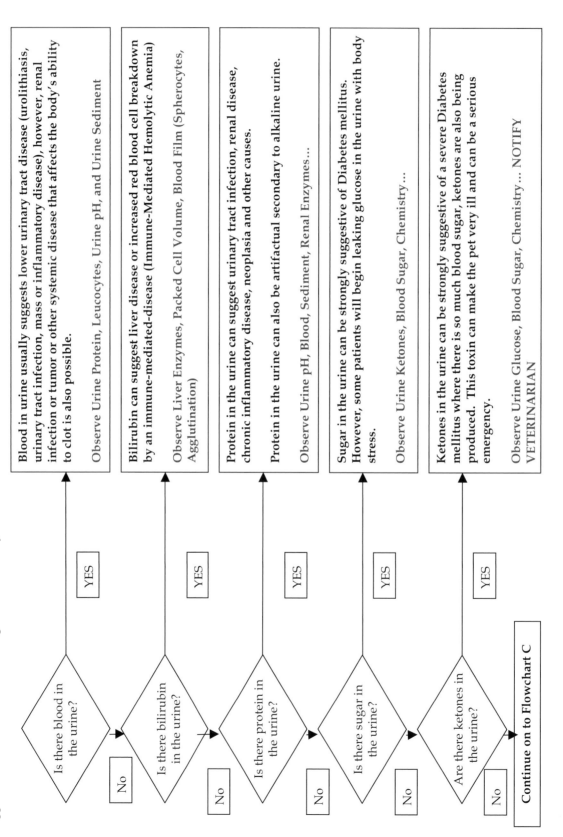

Is there blood in the urine? — YES → Blood in urine usually suggests lower urinary tract disease (urolithiasis, urinary tract infection, mass or inflammatory disease), however, renal infection or tumor or other systemic disease that affects the body's ability to clot is also possible.

Observe Urine Protein, Leucocytes, Urine pH, and Urine Sediment

No ↓

Is there bilirubin in the urine? — YES → Bilirubin can suggest liver disease or increased red blood cell breakdown by an immune-mediated-disease (Immune-Mediated Hemolytic Anemia)

Observe Liver Enzymes, Packed Cell Volume, Blood Film (Spherocytes, Agglutination)

No ↓

Is there protein in the urine? — YES → Protein in the urine can suggest urinary tract infection, renal disease, chronic inflammatory disease, neoplasia and other causes.

Protein in the urine can also be artifactual secondary to alkaline urine.

Observe Urine pH, Blood, Sediment, Renal Enzymes…

No ↓

Is there sugar in the urine? — YES → Sugar in the urine can be strongly suggestive of Diabetes mellitus. However, some patients will begin leaking glucose in the urine with body stress.

Observe Urine Ketones, Blood Sugar, Chemistry…

No ↓

Are there ketones in the urine? — YES → Ketones in the urine can be strongly suggestive of a severe Diabetes mellitus where there is so much blood sugar, ketones are also being produced. This toxin can make the pet very ill and can be a serious emergency.

Observe Urine Glucose, Blood Sugar, Chemistry… NOTIFY VETERINARIAN

No ↓

Continue on to Flowchart C

App. A.15 Flowchart C: Evaluating Urine Sediment

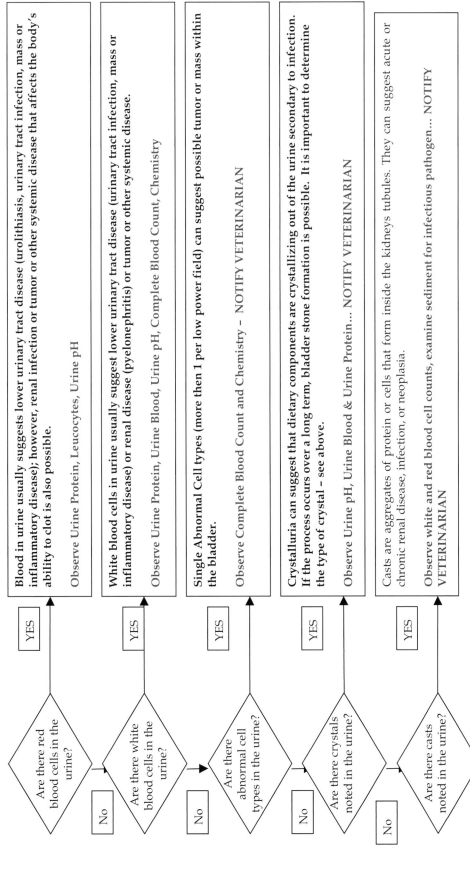

Are there red blood cells in the urine?

YES → Blood in urine usually suggests lower urinary tract disease (urolithiasis, urinary tract infection, mass or inflammatory disease); however, renal infection or tumor or other systemic disease that affects the body's ability to clot is also possible.

Observe Urine Protein, Leucocytes, Urine pH

No ↓

Are there white blood cells in the urine?

YES → White blood cells in urine usually suggest lower urinary tract disease (urinary tract infection, mass or inflammatory disease) or renal disease (pyelonephritis) or tumor or other systemic disease.

Observe Urine Protein, Urine Blood, Urine pH, Complete Blood Count, Chemistry

No ↓

Are there abnormal cell types in the urine?

YES → Single Abnormal Cell types (more then 1 per low power field) can suggest possible tumor or mass within the bladder.

Observe Complete Blood Count and Chemistry – NOTIFY VETERINARIAN

No ↓

Are there crystals noted in the urine?

YES → Crystalluria can suggest that dietary components are crystallizing out of the urine secondary to infection. If the process occurs over a long term, bladder stone formation is possible. It is important to determine the type of crystal – see above.

Observe Urine pH, Urine Blood & Urine Protein…. NOTIFY VETERINARIAN

No ↓

Are there casts noted in the urine?

YES → Casts are aggregates of protein or cells that form inside the kidneys tubules. They can suggest acute or chronic renal disease, infection, or neoplasia.

Observe white and red blood cell counts, examine sediment for infectious pathogen… NOTIFY VETERINARIAN

↓

Finish U/A – Discuss Abnormal with Veterinarian

App. A.16 Algorithm: Evaluating the EKG

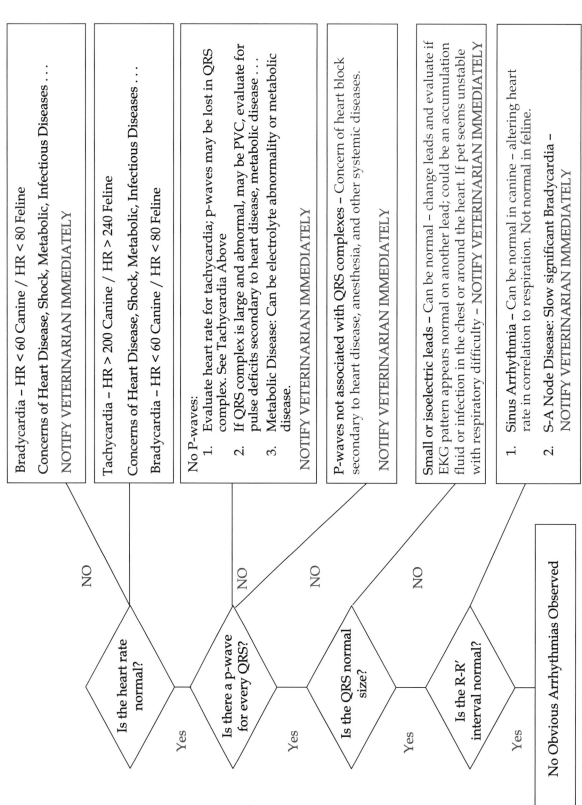

Bradycardia – HR < 60 Canine / HR < 80 Feline

Concerns of Heart Disease, Shock, Metabolic, Infectious Diseases . . .

NOTIFY VETERINARIAN IMMEDIATELY

Tachycardia – HR > 200 Canine / HR > 240 Feline

Concerns of Heart Disease, Shock, Metabolic, Infectious Diseases . . .

Bradycardia – HR < 60 Canine / HR < 80 Feline

No P-waves:
1. Evaluate heart rate for tachycardia; p-waves may be lost in QRS complex. See Tachycardia Above
2. If QRS complex is large and abnormal, may be PVC, evaluate for pulse deficits secondary to heart disease, metabolic disease . . .
3. Metabolic Disease: Can be electrolyte abnormality or metabolic disease.

NOTIFY VETERINARIAN IMMEDIATELY

P-waves not associated with QRS complexes – Concern of heart block secondary to heart disease, anesthesia, and other systemic diseases.

NOTIFY VETERINARIAN IMMEDIATELY

Small or isoelectric leads – Can be normal – change leads and evaluate if EKG pattern appears normal on another lead; could be an accumulation fluid or infection in the chest or around the heart. If pet seems unstable with respiratory difficulty – NOTIFY VETERINARIAN IMMEDIATELY

1. Sinus Arrhythmia – Can be normal in canine – altering heart rate in correlation to respiration. Not normal in feline.
2. S-A Node Disease: Slow significant Bradycardia – NOTIFY VETERINARIAN IMMEDIATELY

NO

NO

NO

NO

Is the heart rate normal?

Yes

Is there a p-wave for every QRS?

Yes

Is the QRS normal size?

Yes

Is the R-R' interval normal?

Yes

No Obvious Arrhythmias Observed

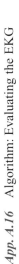

App. A.17 Flowchart of Treating Toxicity—General

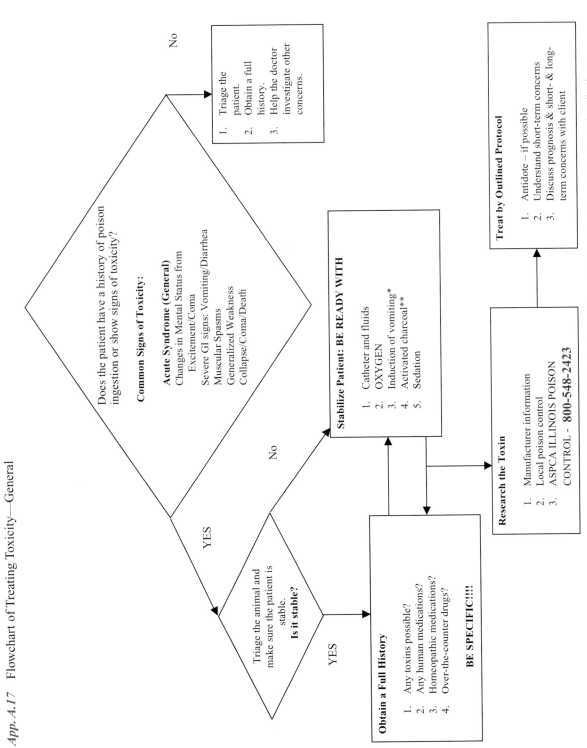

Does the patient have a history of poison ingestion or show signs of toxicity?

Common Signs of Toxicity:

Acute Syndrome (General)
Changes in Mental Status from Excitement/Coma
Severe GI signs: Vomiting/Diarrhea
Muscular Spasms
Generalized Weakness
Collapse/Coma/Death

No

1. Triage the patient.
2. Obtain a full history.
3. Help the doctor investigate other concerns.

YES

Triage the animal and make sure the patient is stable.
Is it stable?

No

YES

Obtain a Full History
1. Any toxins possible?
2. Any human medications?
3. Homeopathic medications?
4. Over-the-counter drugs?

BE SPECIFIC!!!

Stabilize Patient: BE READY WITH
1. Catheter and fluids
2. OXYGEN
3. Induction of vomiting*
4. Activated charcoal**
5. Sedation

Research the Toxin
1. Manufacturer information
2. Local poison control
3. ASPCA ILLINOIS POISON CONTROL - **800-548-2423**

Treat by Outlined Protocol
1. Antidote – if possible
2. Understand short-term concerns
3. Discuss prognosis & short- & long-term concerns with client

* Induction of vomiting should only be done if ingestion is recent. Further induction may be contraindicated with specific toxins and medications. **However, inducing vomiting should never be attempted if the patient is seizing or unable to swallow properly due to the concerns of aspiration.**
** Activated charcoal should never be attempted in comatose or seizuring patients or patients that are unable to swallow.

A.18 IV Fluid Administration Algorithm

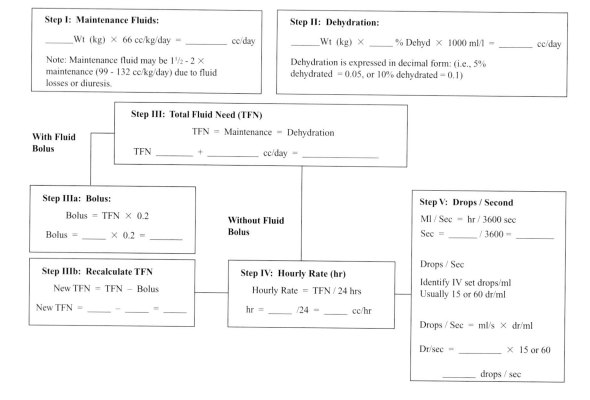

App. A.19 Canine Endotracheal Size Based on Weight

Endotracheal Tube Size	Canine Patient's Weight
5 mm	4–6 lb (1.8–2.7 kg)
5.5 mm	7–8 lb (3.2–3.6 kg)
6 mm	9–11 lb (4–5 kg)
6.5 mm	12–14 lb (5.5–6.4 kg)
7 mm	15–20 lb (6.8–9 kg)
7.5 mm	17–20 lb (7.7–9 kg)
8 mm	21–26 lb (9.5–11.8 kg)
8.5 mm	27–28 lb (12.3–12.7 kg)
9.0 mm	29–31 lb (13–14 kg)
9.5 mm	32–33 lb (14.5–15 kg)
10 mm	31–40 lb (14–18 kg)
11 mm	41–65 lb (18.6–29.5 kg)
12 mm	66–85 lb (30–38.6 kg)
14–16 mm	86–120 lb (39–55 kg)

App. A.20 Endotracheal Size Based on Weight

Endotracheal Tube Size	Feline Patient's Weight
3 mm	2–3 lb (0.9–1.4 kg)
3.5 mm	4–6 lb (1.8–2.7 kg)
4 mm	7–10 lb (3.2–4.5 kg)
5 mm	11 lb or more (5 kg +)14–16

App. A.21 Flowchart for Monitoring Anesthetic Emergency

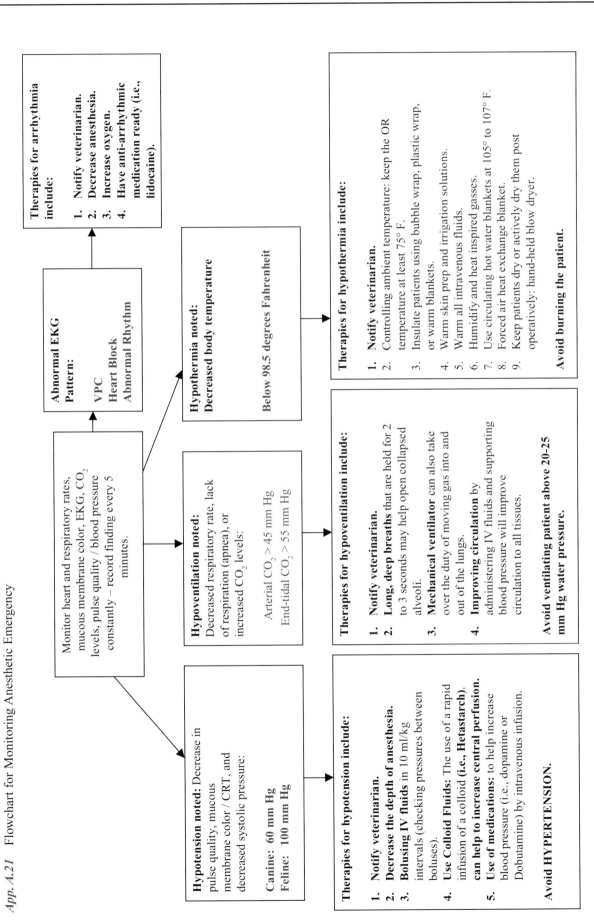

Monitor heart and respiratory rates, mucous membrane color, EKG, CO_2 levels, pulse quality / blood pressure constantly – record finding every 5 minutes.

Abnormal EKG Pattern:

VPC
Heart Block
Abnormal Rhythm

Therapies for arrhythmia include:

1. Notify veterinarian.
2. Decrease anesthesia.
3. Increase oxygen.
4. Have anti-arrhythmic medication ready (i.e., lidocaine).

Hypothermia noted: Decreased body temperature

Below 98.5 degrees Fahrenheit

Therapies for hypothermia include:

1. Notify veterinarian.
2. Controlling ambient temperature: keep the OR temperature at least 75° F.
3. Insulate patients using bubble wrap, plastic wrap, or warm blankets.
4. Warm skin prep and irrigation solutions.
5. Warm all intravenous fluids.
6. Humidify and heat inspired gasses.
7. Use circulating hot water blankets at 105° to 107° F.
8. Forced air heat exchange blanket.
9. Keep patients dry or actively dry them post operatively: hand-held blow dryer.

Avoid burning the patient.

Hypoventilation noted: Decreased respiratory rate, lack of respiration (apnea), or increased CO_2 levels:

Arterial CO_2 > 45 mm Hg
End-tidal CO_2 > 55 mm Hg

Therapies for hypoventilation include:

1. Notify veterinarian.
2. Long, deep breaths that are held for 2 to 3 seconds may help open collapsed alveoli.
3. Mechanical ventilator can also take over the duty of moving gas into and out of the lungs.
4. Improving circulation by administering IV fluids and supporting blood pressure will improve circulation to all tissues.

Avoid ventilating patient above 20-25 mm Hg water pressure.

Hypotension noted: Decrease in pulse quality, mucous membrane color / CRT, and decreased systolic pressure:

Canine: 60 mm Hg
Feline: 100 mm Hg

Therapies for hypotension include:

1. Notify veterinarian.
2. Decrease the depth of anesthesia.
3. Bolusing IV fluids in 10 ml/kg intervals (checking pressures between boluses).
4. Use Colloid Fluids: The use of a rapid infusion of a colloid (i.e., Hetastarch) can help to increase central perfusion.
5. Use of medications: to help increase blood pressure (i.e., dopamine or Dobutamine) by intravenous infusion.

Avoid HYPERTENSION.

App. A.22   Estimate of fluid need based on hydration and fluid loss status.

Species	Condition	Significant V/D	Suggested Fluid Administration Level
Feline & canine	0–5% dehydrated/stable	N	Maintenance→ 1.5 × maintenance
Feline & canine	0–5% dehydrated/stable	Y	Bolus + 1.5–2×/maintenance
Feline & canine	7–9% dehydrated/stable	N	Bolus + maintenance→ 1.5× maintenance
Feline & canine	7–9 % dehydrated/stable	Y	Bolus + 2× maintenance
Feline & canine	9–12 % dehydrated/stable	N	Bolus + 2× maintenance
Feline & canine	9–12% dehydrated/stable	Y	Bolus + 2×/maintenance
Feline	Unstable	Y or N	Shock fluid doses (45 ml/kg/h)
Canine	Unstable	Y or N	Shock fluid doses (90 ml/kg/h)

*This table is a rough estimate of fluid need and should be used only as a reference for the medical team member to ascertain the relative fluid level needed for a sick patient. All fluid administration rates are based solely on the veterinarian recommendations.

App. A.23   Physical changes in early/severe shock.

System Examined	Early Shock	Severe Shock
Disposition	Depressed Sternal recumbent Weak	Nonresponsive Comatose Lateral recumbent
Breathing	Increased rate >45 Altered breathing rates Abdominal breathing Open mouth breathing	Abdominal breathing Decreased rate Shallow
Pulses/heart beating	Rapid, bounding pulses Tachycardia (canines) Bradycardia (felines) ± Pulse deficits	Slow weak pulses Bradycardic ± Pulse deficits
Gum color	Pale Purple Yellow	Pale to white Purple/gray Yellow
Capillary refill time	CRT >2–3 seconds	CRT >3 seconds
Body temperature	Normal temp. Temp >106° Hypothermia (felines)	Temp. <98° or >106°
Pupils	Slow to respond to light Anisocoria	Slow to nonresponsive to light Dilated Anisocoria

App. A.24   Changes in clinical diagnostics that could suggest shock.

Parameter	Measurement	Observations

Increased PCV/TP	PCV:
	  Canines >50% +
	  Felines >40% +
	Total protein
	  Canines >8.5 mg/dl
	  Felines >8.5 mg/dl
		Packed cell volume and total proteins above normal are secondary to dehydration.
		
		Elevation of the cell populations and total protein occur as the fluid portion of blood decreases. (See Chapter 21.)

Decreased PCV	PCV:
	  Canines < 25% +
	  Felines < 20 % +
		Decreasing packed cell volume with normal total protein suggests chronic disease or increased red blood cell destruction (hemolysis). In animals with chronic disease, their resources to produce red blood cells and energy may be significantly diminished, lowering the packed cell volume over time.

Normal TP		Total protein may be lower, but tends to remain in the normal limits.

Decreased PCV	PCV:
	  Canines <25% +
	  Felines <20% +
		With acute blood loss, animals can both loose red blood cells and protein.

Decreased TP	Total protein:
	  Canines <5 mg/dl
	  Felines <5 mg/ dl
		Protein leaks out of the vessels with the fluid component of blood, hence decreasing as significantly as the packed cell volume.

Glucose	Glucose <40–60 mg/dl	Hypoglycemia can slow the response of the central nervous system and if prolonged can produce severe shock, seizures, coma and death.

Electrolytes	Potassium (K+) >6.0 mg/dl
	Potassium (K+)<3.0 mg/dl
		Potassium is one of three electrolytes of the body to help produce cardiac contraction, muscle movement, nerve firing, and many other basic body functions.
		Significant alterations of this electrolyte can produce
		  • weakness,
		  • abnormal heart rhythms,
		  • muscular tremors,
		  • coma, and
		  • death.

Clotting times	Activated clotting time >120 seconds Activated prothrombin time >120 seconds Prothrombin time >11 seconds	Increases in clotting times can lead to internal bleeding, shock, and death. If increasing clotting times are noted, packed cell volume and total protein should be monitored closely.

App. A.25   Emergency drug table.

Drug	Indication
50% Dextrose	Significant hypoglycemia (blood glucose <40–60 mg/dl)
Atropine	Bradycardia (heart rate <60 beats/min)
Epinephrine	Cardiac arrest/severe allergic or anaphylactic reaction
Dexamethasone Prednisone	Used to help counteract anaphylactic shock, concerns of spinal injury, or as a general anti-inflammatory medication.
Furosemide	A diuretic that helps increase fluid excretion through the kidneys, removing excess water from the tissues (especially the lungs). Used in the treatment of cardiovascular shock and traumatic brain injury.
Mannitol	A large inert sugar that, when introduced into the bloodstream, helps pull fluids into the vessels. This drug is used primarily to prevent cerebral swelling in the case of a head concussion.
Antihistamines	Antihistamines (i.e., diphenhydramine) are drugs that help slow the allergic response of the body. When the patient is exposed to a foreign allergen, a white blood cell called a mast cell can release histamines, producing signs allergic or anaphylactic reaction. Antihistamines help block the process and are used in the treatment of anaphylactic shock.

App. A.26   Hypovolemic Shock Flowchart

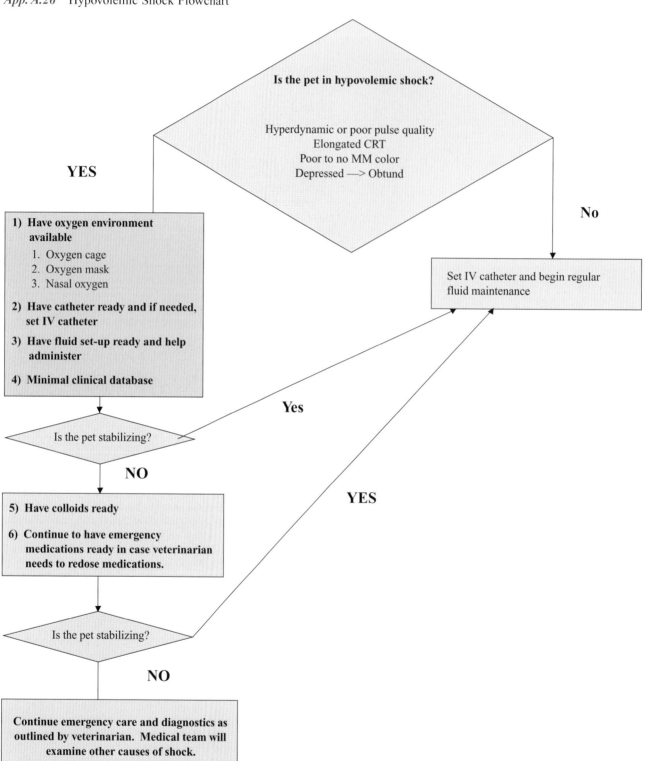

App. A.27   Septic Shock Flowchart

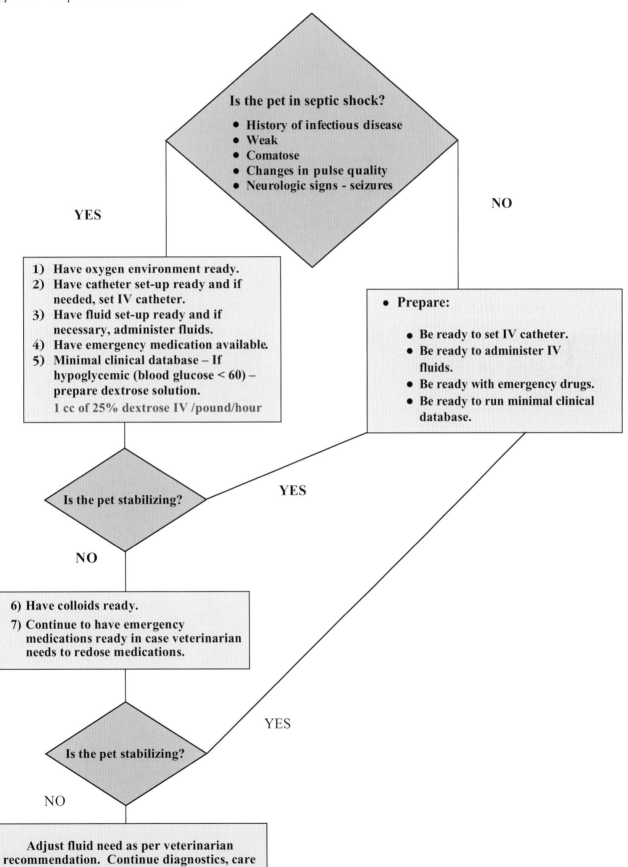

Is the pet in septic shock?

- History of infectious disease
- Weak
- Comatose
- Changes in pulse quality
- Neurologic signs - seizures

YES   **NO**

1) Have oxygen environment ready.
2) Have catheter set-up ready and if needed, set IV catheter.
3) Have fluid set-up ready and if necessary, administer fluids.
4) Have emergency medication available.
5) Minimal clinical database – If hypoglycemic (blood glucose < 60) – prepare dextrose solution.
   1 cc of 25% dextrose IV /pound/hour

- Prepare:

  - Be ready to set IV catheter.
  - Be ready to administer IV fluids.
  - Be ready with emergency drugs.
  - Be ready to run minimal clinical database.

Is the pet stabilizing?   **YES**

NO

6) Have colloids ready.
7) Continue to have emergency medications ready in case veterinarian needs to redose medications.

YES

Is the pet stabilizing?

NO

Adjust fluid need as per veterinarian recommendation. Continue diagnostics, care and evaluation of animal.

App. A.28 Anaphylactic Shock Flowchart

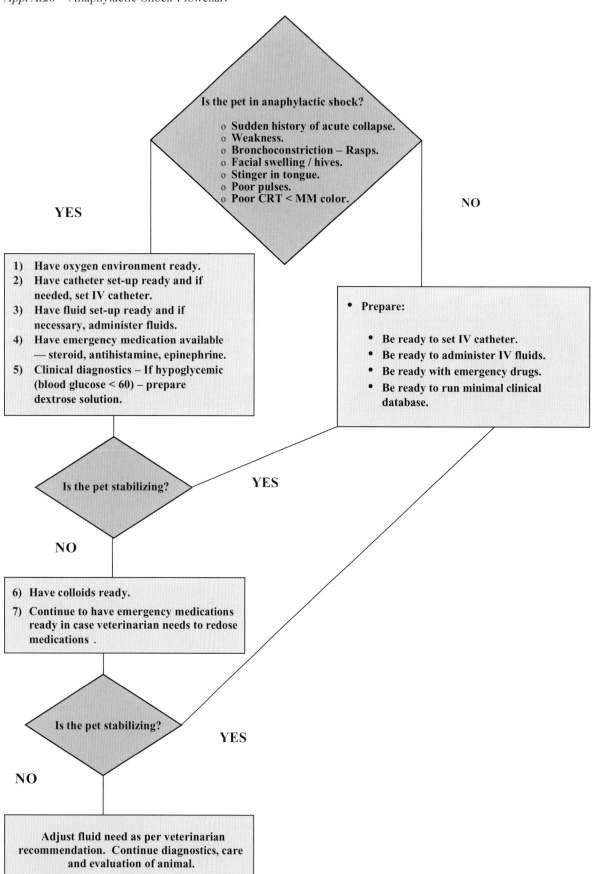

Is the pet in anaphylactic shock?

- o Sudden history of acute collapse.
- o Weakness.
- o Bronchoconstriction – Rasps.
- o Facial swelling / hives.
- o Stinger in tongue.
- o Poor pulses.
- o Poor CRT < MM color.

YES   **NO**

1) Have oxygen environment ready.
2) Have catheter set-up ready and if needed, set IV catheter.
3) Have fluid set-up ready and if necessary, administer fluids.
4) Have emergency medication available — steroid, antihistamine, epinephrine.
5) Clinical diagnostics – If hypoglycemic (blood glucose < 60) – prepare dextrose solution.

- • Prepare:
  - • Be ready to set IV catheter.
  - • Be ready to administer IV fluids.
  - • Be ready with emergency drugs.
  - • Be ready to run minimal clinical database.

Is the pet stabilizing?   **YES**

NO

6) Have colloids ready.
7) Continue to have emergency medications ready in case veterinarian needs to redose medications .

Is the pet stabilizing?   **YES**

NO

Adjust fluid need as per veterinarian recommendation. Continue diagnostics, care and evaluation of animal.

App. A.29   Flowchart for Caridogenic Shock

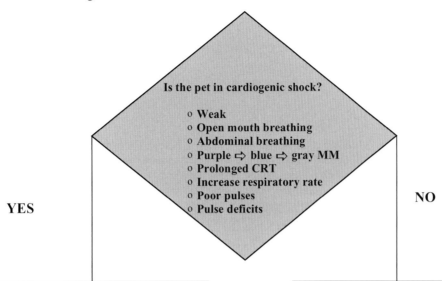

Is the pet in cardiogenic shock?

o **Weak**
o **Open mouth breathing**
o **Abdominal breathing**
o **Purple ⇨ blue ⇨ gray MM**
o **Prolonged CRT**
o **Increase respiratory rate**
o **Poor pulses**
o **Pulse deficits**

YES   **NO**

1) **Low STRESS**
2) **Have oxygen environment ready.**
3) **Have catheter set-up ready and if needed, set IV catheter – low stress.**
4) **NO FLUIDS.**
5) **Have emergency medication ready:**
   a. **Furosemide**
   b. **Nitroglycerin ointment**
   c. **Sedation**
   d. **Atropine / epinephrine (in case of code)**

o **Prepare:**
   o **Be ready to set IV catheter.**
   o **Be ready to administer IV fluids.**
   o **Be ready with emergency drugs.**
   o **Be ready to run minimal clinical database.**

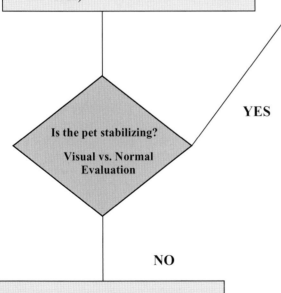

Is the pet stabilizing?

Visual vs. Normal Evaluation

YES

NO

Continue evaluation and medication as directed by the veterinarian. Pet may still succumb despite all medical treatment.

App. A.30 Flowchart for Heatstroke

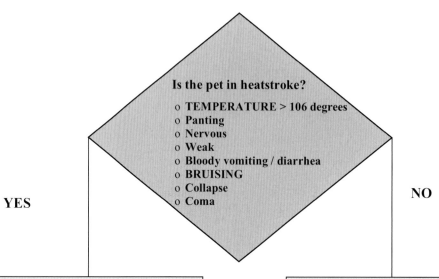

Is the pet in heatstroke?

o **TEMPERATURE > 106 degrees**
o **Panting**
o **Nervous**
o **Weak**
o **Bloody vomiting / diarrhea**
o **BRUISING**
o **Collapse**
o **Coma**

YES

NO

1) Cool down bath
   a. **COOL WATER BATH**
   b. **Fan**
   c. **Alcohol lower extremities**
   d. **DO NOT COOL DOWN BELOW 103.5 DEGRESS**

2) Have catheter set-up ready and prepare to set IV catheter

3) Begin treating for shock (See hypovolemic shock protocol)
   a. **IV fluid administration**
   b. **Emergency drugs**
   c. **Colloids**

o **Prepare:**
   o **Be ready to set IV catheter.**
   o **Be ready to administer IV fluids.**
   o **Be ready with emergency drugs.**
   o **Be ready to run minimal clinical database.**

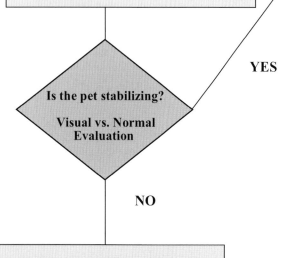

Is the pet stabilizing?

Visual vs. Normal Evaluation

YES

NO

Continue close evaluation and monitoring of patient. Monitor for concerns of acute organ disease, CNS disease or disseminated intravascular coagulopathy (DIC).

App. A.31 Flowchart for Traumatic Brain Injury

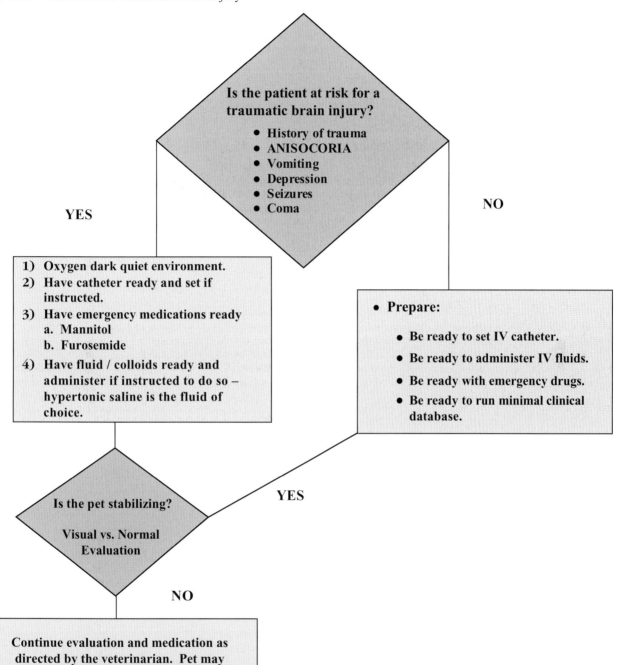

App. A.32 Emergency dose table.

Weight (pounds)	Epinephrine— Intravenous (1:1000)	Epinephrine— Intertracheal* or Sublingual (1:1000)	Atropine (0.54 mg/ml)	Dopram (20 mg/ml)	Dextrose—50%** (25% /ml)
Common Dose	1 cc/10 pounds	1 cc/20 pounds	1 cc/20 pounds	1 cc/20 pounds	1 cc/pound
1	0.1 ml	0.2 ml	0.05 ml	0.02–0.10 ml	1 cc
2	0.2 ml	0.4 ml	0.1 ml	0.04–0.2 ml	2 cc
3	0.3 ml	0.6 ml	0.15 ml	0.06–0.3 ml	3 cc
4	0.4 ml	0.8 ml	0.20 ml	0.08–0.4 ml	4 cc
5	0.5 ml	1.0 ml	0.25 ml	0.1–00.5 ml	5 cc
6	0.6 ml	1.2 ml	0.30 ml	0.12–0.6 ml	6 cc
7	0.7 ml	1.4 ml	0.35 ml	0.14–0.7ml	7 cc
8	0.8ml	1.6ml	0.40 ml	0.16–0.8 ml	8 cc
9	0.9 ml	1.8 ml	0.45 ml	0.18–0.9 ml	9 cc
10	1.0 ml	2.0 ml	0.5 ml	0.2–1.0 ml	10 cc
15	1.5 ml	3.0 ml	0.75 ml	0.3–10.5 ml	15 cc
20	2.0 ml	4.0ml	1.0 ml	0.4–2.0 ml	20 cc
25	2.5 ml	5.0 ml	1.25 ml	0.5–20.5 ml	25 cc
30	3.0 ml	6.0 ml	1.5 ml	0.6–3.0 ml	30 cc
35	3.5 ml	7.0 ml	1.75 ml	0.7–30.5 ml	35 cc
40	4.0 ml	8.0 ml	2.0 ml	0.8–4.0 ml	40 cc
45	4.5 ml	9.0 ml	2.25 ml	0.9–40.5 ml	45 cc
50	5.0 ml	10.0 ml	2.5 ml	1.0–5.0 ml	50 cc
55	5.5 ml	11.0 ml	2.75 ml	1.1–50.5 ml	55 cc
60	6.0 ml	12.0 ml	3.0 ml	1.2–6.0 ml	60 cc
65	6.5 ml	13.0 ml	3.25 ml	1.3–60.5 ml	65 cc
70	7.0 ml	14.0 ml	3.5 ml	1.4–7.0 ml	70 cc
75	7.5 ml	15.0 ml	3.75 ml	1.5–70.5 ml	75 cc
80	8.0 ml	16.0 ml	4.0 ml	1.6–8.0 ml	80 cc
85	8.5 ml	17.0 ml	4.25 ml	1.7–80.5 ml	85 cc
90	9.0 ml	18.0 ml	4.5 ml	1.8–9.0 ml	90 cc
95	9.5 ml	19.0 ml	4.75 ml	1.9–90.5 ml	95 cc
100	10.0 ml	20.0 ml	5.0 ml	2.0–10.0 ml	100 cc

*For intratracheal treatment dilute with sterile water and administer: 3 ml with a cat or small dog, 5 ml with a medium-sized dog, and 10 ml with a large breed dog.

**Dextrose mixed in equal portions with sterile fluids.

Glossary

Term	First Reference	Definition
Accommodation	Chapter 20	The lens is located behind the iris and is supported by fibrous ligaments within the eye. The tension on these ligaments can be changed by muscle activity altering the focal length of the lens, allowing the eye to switch focus from the far field to the near field. This process is called accommodation.
Acetabulum	Chapter 8	A rounded cavity in the hip bone that articulates with the femur as the hip joint.
Acetaminophen	Chapter 27	A non-narcotic analgesic drug with a very small margin of safety in animals: it can cause severe effects on the liver and blood.
Acetone	Chapter 15	A toxin that acidifies the blood, making the pet anorexic, ill, and weak.
Acetylcholine	Chapter 27	In normal muscle activation, an activated neuron releases a chemical called acetylcholine. This chemical diffuses away from the nerve toward the muscle in a space called the neuromuscular junction. The contact of acetylcholine with specific proteins (acetylcholine receptors) on the muscle stimulates muscular contraction.
ACTH	Chapter 17	A hormone produced from the pituitary gland, ACTH stimulates the adrenal gland to produce cortisol.
ACTH stimulation test	Chapter 17	A clinical diagnostic test that evaluates a patient's response to ACTH.
Addisonian crisis	Chapter 27	A disease condition in which a patient cannot respond with normal levels of cortisol and/or aldosterone, and the patient enters a shock-like state.
Adenovirus	Chapter 2	A virus that produces a life-threatening infection of the liver, causing depression, anorexia, icterus, vomiting, and diarrhea.
Adjuvant	Chapter 2	Chemicals or portions of microscopic metal in a vaccine that are attached to weakened or killed pathogenic bacteria or viruses to stimulate an immune response
Adrenal cortex	Chapter 17	The outer layer of the adrenal gland that is responsible for producing cortisol, aldosterone, and some sex hormones.
Agglutination	Chapter 21	A process where the red blood cells precipitate out of the blood like snow in a snow globe due to an immune-mediated process.
Albumin	Chapter 22	Albumin is a small carrier protein that binds to hormones and other components in the bloodstream to maintain and move necessary elements throughout the body.
Aldosterone	Chapter 17	A hormone of the adrenal cortex that regulates re-absorption of sodium and expulsion of potassium in the body.
Alkaline phosphatase (SALP or ALP)	Chapter 22	Alkaline phosphatase refers to a large number of intracellular enzymes that are present within the liver, intestine, bone, kidneys, and placenta.
Alopecia	Chapter 19	Hair loss that can be localized or generalized.
Alpha 2 agonists	Chapter 29	An anesthetic medication that can produce excellent calming effects, muscle relaxation, and short-duration analgesia.
ALT (alanine aminotransferase)	Chapter 22	A hepatic intracellular enzyme that is responsible for the conversion of 2-oxoglutarate to pyruvate and glutamate in the liver cells (hepatocytes).
Alveolar bone	Chapter 9	The bone that forms tooth sockets.
Amylase	Chapter 22	An enzyme that helps break down larger, more complex sugars into small 1-unit sugars for absorption.
Amyloidosis	Chapter 14	A metabolic disease where an inert protein (amyloid) builds up in the tissue and organs.
Anal sac aprocrine gland adenocarcinoma	Chapter 22	A malignant tumor of the anal gland
Analgesics	Chapter 29	This class of medication helps decrease pain sensitivity prior to, during, and after surgery. By including analgesics in pre-anesthetic drug combinations, the amount of pain the patient experiences and the amount of subsequent analgesics needed postsurgically is reduced.
Ancylostoma	Chapter 10	A species of hookworm.
Anemia	Chapter 7	A low red blood cell count.

Term	First Reference	Definition
Anisocoria	Chapter 7, 20	Patients with an uneven pupil size.
Anterior chamber	Chapter 20	Occupies the space cranial to the lens; it is filled with aqueous fluid that helps to maintain the shape and nutrition of the cranial aspect of the eye.
Anterior cruciate ligament (cranial)	Chapter 13	A ligament within the stifle joint (knee) that helps to prevent forward or medial movement of the femur on the tibia.
Anticholinergic drugs	Chapter 29	This category of drug blocks the part of the autonomic nervous system that reflexively slows the heart, increases production of secretions from the respiratory and gastrointestinal systems, produces movement of the intestines, and constricts the iris of the eye.
Antigen	Chapter 10	Specific surface molecules or proteins on pathogenic organisms (i.e., bacteria).
Antigen	Chapter 12	Specific proteins on the surface of the pathogen that stimulate an immune response.
Anuria	Chapter 13	A halting of glomerular filtration, stopping urine production.
Aortic valve	Chapter 12	The valve that separates the left ventricle from the aorta and opens to push oxygenated blood into the entire body.
Apnea	Chapter 27	An absence of breathing.
Aqueous humor	Chapter 20	The eye produces a fluid called aqueous humor, which is produced in a region behind the iris called the ciliary body.
Articular	Chapter 8	A place or union of two or more bones; a joint.
Articular surface	Chapter 8	The region of a joint where bone interdigitates with bone.
Ascariasis	Chapter 10	Roundworm infection.
Ascites	Chapter 12	A clear fluid that begins to collect in the abdominal cavity secondary to liver disease, low blood protein levels, and other metabolic concerns.
Ascites	Chapter 14	The buildup of a low protein–low cellularity abdominal fluid (transudate or a modified transudate) in the abdomen.
Aspartate aminotransferase (AST or SGOT)	Chapter 22	An intracellular enzyme in all cells, but predominantly in muscle and liver cell damage. AST transfers a-amino groups between specific amino acids as a part of normal protein metabolism.
Aspiration	Chapter 27	Vomiting and passing the vomit into the lung field.
Atopy	Chapter 19	Allergies to airborne material, such as pollen, dust, mites, cat dander, and ragweed.
ATP	Chapter 11	A cellular energy source.
Atrial-ventricular node (A-V node)	Chapter 24	A collection of fibers within the heart that focuses the signal from the S-A node to fire a wave of depolarization down to the ventricle.
Atrophy	Chapter 7	A wasting or decrease in size in an organ or tissue.
Aural hematoma	Chapter 20	An aural hematoma is an accumulation of blood between the cartilage of the earflap and the skin causing a firm, enlarging pocket of fluid to build.
Azotemia	Chapter 13	An increase in renal toxins in the blood (i.e., BUN, creatinine).
Babesia	Chapter 21	An intracellular red blood cell parasite.
Bacteruria	Chapter 22	Bacteria in the urine.
Barotraumas	Chapter 29	Pressure trauma to the lungs.
Basal metabolic rate (BMR)	Chapter 16	The rate at which the cells of the body burn energy.
Basophil	Chapter 21	A white blood cell; medium sized cells 1-2 times the size of a red blood cell and having a segmented nucleus, they are thought to function in allergic reactions.
Basophilia	Chapter 21	An increased basophilia level.
Benzodinepines	Chapter 29	Drugs such as Valium and midozolam can produce mild to moderate sedation more safely in the geriatric patient.
Bile acids	Chapter 24	Hepatocytes also produce chemicals called bile acids that help to emulsify fat within the small intestine.
Bilirubin	Chapter 21	A breakdown pigment of hemoglobin from the red blood cell.
Bilirubin	Chapter 22	A potentially toxic metabolite produced from the breakdown of hemoglobin and other pigments in the body.
Bilirubin	Chapter 24	The normal liver de-activates this toxin produced from the breakdown of hemoglobin and other pigments in the body.
Bilirubinuria	Chapter 23	Bilirubin in the urine.
Blastomycosis	Chapter 11	A fungal infection caused by the fungus *Blastomycosis dermatitis*, which can affect the respiratory, skeletal, integumentary (skin), central nervous system, and other systems of the body.
Bloat	Chapter 10	Referring to a disease condition where the canine stomach distends with gas and expands.
Blood dialysis	Chapter 13	This process is the continuous filtering of toxins from the blood using specialized machinery.
Blood urea nitrogen (BUN)	Chapter 13	A form of conjugated ammonia produced within the liver to be excreted by the kidney.

Term	First Reference	Definition
Bone marrow	Chapter 8	The inner aspect of the bone that serves as a location of blood precursor cells responsible for the production of much of the body's red and white blood cells and platelets
Borborgymi	Chapter 15	Increased intestinal sounds.
Brachiocephalic	Chapter 19	Short faced, referring to brachiocephalic breeds (i.e., pug, bull dog, etc).
Bradycardia	Chapter 6	An abnormally slow heart rate.
Bronchoconstriction	Chapter 11	Constriction of the bronchial tissue.
Brucellosis	Chapter 18	A sexually transmitted disease producing infertility in the male and abortion and fetal death in the female.
Buccal mucosa	Chapter 7	The mucosal lining inside the oral cavity lateral to the teeth and tongue.
Calculus	Chapter 9	A mineralized plaque deposit that is often yellow to brown in color.
Calici virus	Chapter 7	An upper respiratory virus in cats causing congestion, ocular discharge, and oral ulcerations.
Cancellous bone	Chapter 8	Soft, spongy bone with a reticular or lattice-like network.
Canine distemper	Chapter 11	A viral infection that attacks the respiratory, gastrointestinal (rare), and central nervous system of canines.
Canine hepatitis virus	Chapter 2	An adenovirus that produces a life-threatening infection of the liver, causing depression, anorexia, icterus, vomiting, and diarrhea.
Canniculi	Chapter 14	Channels running through the layers of hepatocytes that remove de-activated toxins from the liver and pass them into the bile ducts and gall bladder for excretion in the feces.
Cardiac arrhythmia	Chapter 24	An abnormal rhythm of the heart.
Cardiac sphincter	Chapter 10	A thick, circular muscle that separates the esophagus from the stomach, preventing reflux of ingesta back into esophagus.
Cardiovascular shock	Chapter 12	A condition in which there is still an evident heartbeat, but the heart is unable to maintain any cardiac output, producing collapse, weakness, and, potentially, death.
Cardiovascular shock	Chapter 30	Occurs when a pet is unable to maintain normal blood flow and perfusion due to an inability of the heart to properly pump and maintain cardiac output.
Carnassial teeth	Chapter 9	The upper fourth premolars and lower first molars; the largest teeth in an animal's mouth.
Carnivores	Chapter 9	Animals whose diets consist only of meat.
Caudal	Chapter 1	An object or lesion on the body that is behind another object.
Cecum	Chapter 10	The ileum empties into this small vestigial region of the intestines.
Cellular respiration	Chapter 11	A cellular process where cells take 1 unit of sugar molecules and, through a process called cellular respiration, convert sugar into energy (ATP), water, and carbon dioxide.
Chief complaint (CC)	Chapter 7	The client's primary reason for bringing the pet to the hospital.
Cholelithe	Chapter 14	A gall bladder stone.
Cholestasis	Chapter 14	Decreased bile flow through the gall bladder.
Cholestatic disease	Chapter 14	Causes an obstruction of the gall bladder.
Cholinesterase	Chapter 17	A chemical enzyme that inactivates the acetylcholine, giving the muscle time to reset and be stimulated again.
Chronic interstitial nephritis	Chapter 13	An inflammatory disease of the kidneys.
Ciliary body	Chapter 20	A region behind the iris that produces aqueous humor.
Cirrhosis	Chapter 14	An end-stage liver disease where the normal liver tissue is replaced with scar tissue and fibrosis.
Class 2 malocclusion	Chapter 9	In this deformity, the upper jaw is much longer than the lower, causing misalignment of the teeth.
Class 3 malocclusion	Chapter 9	In this deformity, the lower jaw is much longer than the upper, causing misalignment of the teeth.
Class O malocclusion	Chapter 9	This is a normal bite and occlusion of the incisor and canine teeth; also called a scissors bite.
Clotting factors	Chapter 10	Enzymes produced by the liver to begin the clotting cascade when a patient begins to bleed.
Coagulopathy	Chapter 6	An inability of the body to clot blood.
Coagulopathy	Chapter 14	Refers to the body having altered ability to clot blood.
Coccidiomycosis	Chapter 11	A fungal infection that can affect the respiratory, skeletal, abdominal organs, integumentary (skin), central nervous system, and other systems of the body.
Colloids	Chapter 28	This category is made up of fluid types that have an increased density (hypertonic) as compared to blood.
Colon	Chapter 10	The large intestine, which is broken into the ascending loop, the transverse loop, and the descending loop.

Term	First Reference	Definition
Colostrum	Chapter 18	The first maternal milk, which is rich in immunoglobulins and helps produce immunity in the newborn.
Concussion	Chapter 30	An acute syndrome brought on by a sharp blow to the head or a fall (such as from a moving vehicle) that causes blunt injury to the brain.
Cone cells	Chapter 20	Specialized cells that process bright light and colors in the retina.
Congenital patellar disease	Chapter 13	A disease of the young patient where the patella does not sit normally in the patellar grove due to architectural abnormalities in the leg.
Congestion	Chapter 12	As there is decreased flow through major body organs (i.e. lungs, liver . . .) secondary to decreased perfusion, the fluid component of blood begins to move out of the vessels and collect within the organs and/or the body cavity.
Conjunctiva	Chapter 6	Mucus membrane that lines eyelids and is reflected onto the eyeball.
Consensual PLR	Chapter 20	An ocular reflex where a light shines into one iris and the opposite iris constricts as well.
Continuous rate of infusion (CRI)	Chapter 28	A medication added to a fluid to create a continuous rate of infusion (CRI) of the needed drug.
Cornea	Chapter 20	The clear outermost section of the eye.
Corneal reflex	Chapter 29	By placing light pressure on the cornea, the eye should retract and the patient blinks.
Cortical bone	Chapter 8	The densely packed outer column of a long bone.
Cortisol	Chapter 17	A hormone produced from the adrenal cortex that increases blood sugar levels in time of stress or emergency.
Coumadin	Chapter 27	A poison that interferes with the normal clotting agents that stop bleeding.
Cranial	Chapter 1	An object or lesion on the body that is in front of another object.
Cranial draw sign	Chapter 8	An abnormal increased forward movement in the tibia when the bone is pulled cranially while the femur is held in place; suggestive of an anterior cruciate ligament rupture.
Cryptorchid	Chapter 3, 18	Male patients that do not have their testicles descend normally in utero or shortly after birth; the testes may sit within the inguinal canal or anywhere within the abdominal cavity.
Cryptosporidium	Chapter 10	A very small parasite that produces severe diarrhea in young animals.
Crystalloids	Chapter 27	Types of fluid that have a similar concentration (isotonic) density to blood.
Cutaneous larval migrans	Chapter 10	A parasitic infection of humans where the larval form burrows through the skin causing erosive paths usually seen in the feet or legs.
Cyanotic	Chapter 12	A bluish gray hue to the skin due to lack of oxygen within the bloodstream.
Cylinduria	Chapter 23	Increased numbers of casts in the urine.
Cystocentesis	Chapter 13	A needle aspirate of the bladder.
Cystotomy	Chapter 13	A surgical opening of the bladder.
Cytauxoan	Chapter 21	An intracellular red blood cell parasite.
Deciduous teeth	Chapter 9	Baby teeth.
Demodecosis (demodectic mange)	Chapter 19	Demodecosis is a parasitic mite infection of the hair follicle.
Dermatophytes	Chapter 19	Skin fungal agents that produce ringworm infections.
Diabetes mellitus	Chapter 15	A disease process where insulin production is not sufficient to adequately control normal blood sugar levels.
Diaphragm	Chapter 11	The musculoskeletal partition that completely separates the thoracic cavity from the abdomen.
Diaphysis	Chapter 8	Area of dense cortical bone in the middle of the bone shaft, also called the bone shaft.
Diarthrosis	Chapter 8	A synovial joint, these joints are freely movable and are united by a fluid-filled cavity.
Diasystole	Chapter 11	The phase of contraction of the atriums of the heart.
Diplydium	Chapter 10	A species of tapeworms found in dogs and cats.
Direct PLR	Chapter 20	An ocular reflex whereby a light shines into one iris and it constricts.
Dirofilaria immitis	Chapter 12	A bloodborne parasite responsible for heartworm disease.
Disseminated intravascular coagulopathy (DIC)	Chapter 30	A syndrome produced by severe metabolic upset, which stimulates the blood to clot spontaneously in the vessels, exhausting the normal clotting factors. Once the clotting factors are exhausted, the pet can begin to bleed internally.
Distal	Chapter 1	An object or lesion on a limb that is farther from the body than another object.
Distributive shock (massive vasodilatation)	Chapter 30	This syndrome refers to a pet that has lost its ability to maintain normal tissue perfusion due to massive dilation of all the blood vessels.
Diuresis	Chapter 13, 27	Using large amounts of intraveous, subcutaneous, or oral fluids to increase glomerular filtration to help the kidneys push the toxins into the bloodstream.
Dorsal	Chapter 1	An object or region on the body that is closer to the spine than another object.
Draped	Chapter 3	The process by which surgical boundaries are covered with sterile towels.

Term	First Reference	Definition
Ductus venuses	Chapter 14	A small vessel in the embryo that bypasses blood around the animal's liver.
Duodenum	Chapter 10	The first section of the small intestine.
Dypsnea	Chapter 12	Trouble breathing.
Dypsnic	Chapter 11	Labored or difficult breathing.
Dystocia	Chapter 18	Trouble giving birth, an abnormal labor.
Ear pinna	Chapter 7	The ear flap.
Ecchymosis	Chapter 14	Large geographic hemorrhages noted on the skin or mucus membranes.
Echinocytes	Chapter 21	Red blood cells with club-like projections from the cell surface.
Echogenicity	Chapter 25	Refers to the strength or amplitude of the returning echo image on an ultrasound examination.
Eclampsia	Chapter 18	A serious condition affecting the canine shortly after pregnancy. When the female begins to produce milk (lactation), the body's stores of calcium drop quickly. Calcium is needed by almost every cell in the body to control cellular activity, aid in muscular contraction, help heart function, and aid nerve conduction, as well as other body functions. With the demands of lactation, calcium levels fall so rapidly that the patient cannot compensate, and the muscular, cardiac, and neurologic systems are severely affected.
EDTA (ethylene diamine tetra acetic acid)	Chapter 21	A blood-clotting tube that prevents the clotting of blood, used in performing complete blood counts.
Elbow dysplasia	Chapter 8	Congenital misalignment of the elbow joints, potentially producing an arthritic joint.
Emaciated	Chapter 7	To become excessively lean.
Embolism	Chapter 12	Due to abnormal blood flow, small clots can form in the ventricles in cats. These clots can be pushed into the aorta as the ventricle contracts and are then called embolisms or thromboembolisms.
Endemic	Chapter 2	The presence of an infectious disease within a geographic region.
Endocrine glands	Chapter 15	Glands that secrete hormones or other chemicals directly into the bloodstream, which influence metabolism and other body processes (i.e., pituitary, thyroid, sex organs, etc.).
Endometritis	Chapter 18	An infection of the lining of the uterus.
Entropion	Chapter 20	An abnormal turning of the lid with resulting irritation of the cornea by hair and lashes.
Enucleation	Chapter 20	Surgical removal of the eye.
Enzymes	Chapter 9	Chemicals that begin breaking down food.
Eosinopenia	Chapter 21	A decreased eosinophil level.
Eosinophilia	Chapter 21	An increased eosinophil level.
Eosinophils	Chapter 21	White blood cells with segmented nuclei, pink cytoplasm, and dark red granules in the cytoplasm. Eosinophils respond to fungal infections or allergic reactions.
Epinephrine	Chapter 17	A chemical produced by the adrenal medulla that responds to assist the body in times of crisis or life and death concerns (fight or flight system).
Epiphora	Chapter 20	Increased tearing.
Epiphysis	Chapter 8	An active area of bone growth where soft, spongy bone (cancellous bone) is produced.
Epiphysitis	Chapter 8	An inflammation of the growth plate.
Epistaxis	Chapter 2	A nosebleed.
Epithelium	Chapter 11	A layer of skin.
Erythema	Chapter 29	Reddening of the skin.
Erythropoietin	Chapter 13	A hormone produced by the kidney that stimulates red blood cell production in the bone marrow.
Estrogen	Chapter 18	Female hormone produced by the ovary to stimulate the signs of heat.
Ethylene glycol	Chapter 13, 27	Most antifreeze contains ethylene glycol; this toxin begins to crystallize in the bloodstream, especially within the kidneys, and produces acute renal failure.
Etiology	Chapter 8	The study of the causes of the disease.
Euthyroid sick	Chapter 16	A syndrome where chronic organ or infectious disease can suppress thyroid production even though the thyroid gland is not diseased.
Excoriation	Chapter 29	Skin damaged into its deeper layers, producing a red, inflamed, moist lesion.
Exercise intolerance	Chapter 5, 11, 12	Inability to exercise at a normal level; decreasing ability to exercise.
Exocrine glands	Chapter 15	Glands that discharge their secretions outwardly through a duct. Their secretions control many important body functions (i.e., salivary gland, sweat gland, mammary gland, etc.).
External acoustic meatus	Chapter 20	The canal that leads outward from the eardrum.
Favoring	Chapter 7	To avoid bearing weight upon.
Feathered edge	Chapter 21	The feathered edge is a tapering at the end of a blood film where the cells are not touching.

Term	First Reference	Definition
Feline lower urinary tract disease (FLUTD)	Chapter 13	An infectious, nutritional, or inflammatory disease of the lower urinary tract, producing obstruction of the urinary bladder.
Femoral head and neck excision (FHO)	Chapter 8	A surgery for chronic hip arthritis that removes the femoral head from the hip joint out of the acetabulum and then severs the femoral head from the femur.
Fenestration	Chapter 13	Opening.
Fibrosarcoma	Chapter 22	A spindle cell tumor containing increased connective tissue.
Flight or fight response	Chapter 27	A behavior in an animal. The animal will either prepare its body to stand and fight or run.
Fluid overload	Chapter 28	When an animal is receiving too many intravenous fluids or receiving fluids too quickly.
Fossa	Chapter 14	A furrow or shallow depression.
Gastrin	Chapter 13	The hormone that produces stomach acid; it is eliminated in the kidneys.
Gastro-distention volvulus	Chapter 6	A life-threatening condition of large and giant breed dogs where the stomach bloats and rotates on its own axis, cutting off the blood to the stomach and spleen.
Gastropexy	Chapter 10	A permanent surgical attachment of the stomach to the abdominal wall.
Giardia (giardiasis)	Chapter 10	A microscopic protozoal parasite that causes mild to moderate gastrointestinal infection.
Gingiva	Chapter 9	The gums.
Gingivitis	Chapter 3, 9	Swelling and infection of the gums; an inflammation of gums.
Glans penis	Chapter 18	A region of specialization located in the middle of the canine penis. It will swell like a balloon prior to and during sexual contact. It prevents premature separation from the female during coitus and increases the chances of fertilization.
Glaucoma	Chapter 20	A disease of the neural tissue involving the optic nerve and the retina. The major precipitating cause of glaucoma is an increase in intraocular pressure.
Glomerular filtration	Chapter 13	The rate at which the kidneys filter toxins from the blood.
Glucagon	Chapter 25	A hormone produced by the endocrine pancreas that is released in times of hyperglycemia to decrease blood sugar levels.
Gluconeogenesis	Chapter 25	The process whereby the body breaks up fat for the production of sugar.
Glucosuria	Chapter 23	Glucose in the urine.
Granuloma	Chapter 2	Small, nonpainful mass or nodule of chronically inflamed tissue.
Halitosis	Chapter 9	Mild to severe bad breath.
Heart block	Chapter 24	An arrhythmia produced by a blockage of the conduction of the electrical signal through the atrial-ventricular node and the bundle of His. The obstruction prevents the normal transmission of the signal from the S-A node to the ventricle.
Heinz bodies	Chapter 21	Denatured hemoglobin fused to the cell membrane.
Heinz body anemia	Chapter 27	Exposure to onions and garlic (wild onions and store purchased) that produces an oxidative injury to red blood cells, denaturing the hemoglobin in the red blood cell and forming Heinz bodies, which produce a serious to life-threatening anemia.
Hematemesis	Chapter 2	Vomiting frank red blood.
Hematochezia	Chapter 2	Frank red blood in the stool.
Hematocrit	Chapter 21	Many blood cell counters do a calculated hematocrit (HCT), which is an evaluation of red blood cell concentration that is a calculated measurement based on the total red blood cell count and the size of the red blood cells.
Hematuria	Chapter 23	Blood in the urine.
Hemoglobin	Chapter 11	A special iron-based chemical that has the ability to carry oxygen and carbon dioxide throughout the body.
Hemoglobinuria	Chapter 23	Hemoglobin in the urine.
Hemolysis	Chapter 22	Red blood cell breakdown with release of hemoglobin in the serum.
Hepatic artery	Chapter 24	The major arterial blood supply for the liver.
Hepatic congestion	Chapter 22	A pooling of fluid in liver tissue due to decreasing blood flow through the right heart due to heart disease.
Hepatic encephalopathy	Chapter 14	A neurologic syndrome caused by the improper hepatic detoxification of toxins. The toxins build up within the bloodstream and directly affect the central nervous system.
Hepatic lipidosis	Chapter 14	A severe metabolic disease of the liver, mainly affecting cats, in which the liver becomes infiltrated with large amounts of body fat, shutting down the liver and leading to a build up of hepatic toxins in the bloodstream.
Hepatic vein	Chapter 14	The major venous blood supply for the liver.
Hepatocyte	Chapter 14, 22	A liver cell.
Hepatomegally	Chapter 14	Liver enlargement.
High-dose dexamethasone suppression test	Chapter 17	A clinical diagnostic test to differentiate adrenal or pituitary forms of Cushing's disease.

Term	First Reference	Definition
Hip dysplasia	Chapter 8	Congenital misalignment of the hip joints potentially producing an arthritic joint.
Histamine	Chapter 2	A chemical produced by a group of white blood cells in the body (mast cells) to produce an allergic reaction.
Howell-Jowell bodies	Chapter 21	Nuclear remnants seen within the cytoplasm as dark-staining bodies.
Hyperadrenocorticism (Cushing's disease)	Chapter 27	A hormonal imbalance caused by overproduction of a prednisone-like steroid called cortisol in the adrenal glands of the body.
Hyperbilirubinemia	Chapter 22, 23	Increased levels of bilirubin in the blood.
Hypercalcemia	Chapter 22	Increased calcium levels in the bloodstream.
Hypercarbia	Chapter 29	Increased carbon dioxide in the blood.
Hyperdynamic pulse	Chapter 6	A bounding strong pulse that lifts the finger of the skin.
Hyperechoic	Chapter 25	A structure in the ultrasound exam that is brighter than the surrounding tissue.
Hyperglycemia	Chapter 22	Increased blood sugar levels.
Hyperkalemia	Chapter 13	Increased blood levels of potassium.
Hyperpigmentation	Chapter 19	Increased pigment laid down in the skin secondary to chronic inflammation or infection.
Hyperthermia	Chapter 6	Higher than normal body temperature.
Hyperthyroid	Chapter 16	An overproduction of thyroid hormone from the thyroid glands.
Hypertonic	Chapter 28	Fluid types that have an increased density as compared with blood.
Hyphema	Chapter 7	The presence of blood in the eye.
Hypoadrenocorticism (Addison's disease)	Chapter 17	A lack of production of the hormone aldosterone.
Hypoalbuminemia	Chapter 22	Decreased blood albumen levels.
Hypocalcemia	Chapter 18	Low blood calcium level.
Hypochromasia	Chapter 21	An increase in the size of the area of central pallor and most often due to a decrease in the concentration of hemoglobin within the red blood cell.
Hypoechoic	Chapter 25	When performing an ultrasound, hypoechoic structures are those that are less bright than the surrounding tissue.
Hypokalemia	Chapter 13	Decreased blood levels of potassium.
Hyposthenuria	Chapter 27, 28	Urine that is a more dilute specific gravity than plasma or serum. USG < 1.008; the inability to concentrate urine.
Hypothermia	Chapter 6	Lower than normal body temperature.
Hypothyroid	Chapter 26	An underproduction of thyroid gland caused by pituitary or idiopathic/immune-mediated disease of the thyroid.
Hypovolemic shock	Chapter 30	Inability to maintain normal blood volume (red blood cells and fluid) or blood pressure.
Iatrogenic	Chapter 17	A condition or disease produced by effects of treatment.
Icterus	Chapter 2, 14, 22	The yellow coloration of the skin, mucous membranes, and conjunctiva of the eye caused by the buildup of bile pigments in the tissue. Commonly secondary to liver disease, gall bladder obstruction, or immune-mediated hemolytic anemia. *See bilirubin.*
Ileum	Chapter 10	The last section of the small intestine.
Immune-mediated disease	Chapter 8	A disease in which the white blood cells attack other body cells or tissues as if they were foreign invaders or pathogens (i.e., immune mediated hemolytic anemia).
Immune-mediated hemolytic anemia	Chapter 15	Massive destruction of the red blood cells by the patient's white blood cells within the blood vessels of the body.
Immune-mediated hemolytic anemia	Chapter 23	A disease condition whereby red blood cells are lysed by the white blood cells and the immune system as the red blood cells are being attacked as if foreign bacteria.
Immune-mediated thyroiditis	Chapter 16	An inflammatory disease in which the white blood cells of the body attack the thyroid cells as foreign bacteria.
Immunoglobulins	Chapter 21	Specific blood proteins produced by lymphocytes to fight off infection.
Inclusion bodies	Chapter 21	Intracellular remnants from a viral infection.
Induced ovulators	Chapter 18	Induced ovulators will go into heat and become sexually active, but will not ovulate unless sexual contact occurs. The sexual act stimulates a neuroendocrine response that stimulates ovulation.
Induction agents	Chapter 29	The role of an induction agent is to bypass stage II anesthesia (excitatory phase) so the patient can be intubated to gain rapid control of the airway and allow maintenance on gas or injectable anesthesia
Induction chamber	Chapter 4	A large glass or plastic aquarium-like structure with a locking airtight lid used to anesthetize small patients.
Inguinal canal	Chapter 3	A slit in the abdominal muscles that allows the abdomen to communicate with the subcutaneous tissue and scrotum.

Term	First Reference	Definition
Inspiratory/expiratory study	Chapter 11	A specific thoracic radiographic study to evaluate the patient for tracheal collapse.
Insulin	Chapter 15	A hormone produced by the endocrine pancreas that is released in times of hyperglycemia to decrease blood sugar levels.
Insulinoma	Chapter 15	A metabolically active tumor of the endocrine pancreas producing high levels of insulin.
Intercostal muscles	Chapter 11	The muscles between the ribs.
Intussusception	Chapter 10	An invagination of a section of small intestine into another adjoining section causing an obstruction.
Iris	Chapter 20	A color contractile membrane suspended between the lens and the cornea.
Islets of Langerhans	Chapter 15	A region of specialized cells within the pancreas that produce insulin and glucagon.
Isochoic	Chapter 25	Substances of a different medium are isochoic if waves travel through them at the same speed.
Isospora	Chapter 10	A microscopic parasite that causes mild to moderate gastrointestinal infection in the canine and feline.
Isosthenuria	Chapter 23	Refers to urine that has the same specific gravity as plasma or serum. USG 1.010–1.015.
Isotonic	Chapter 28	Fluid types that have the same density as compared to blood.
Jaundice	Chapter 2	The yellow coloration of the skin, mucous membranes, and conjunctiva of the eye from the buildup of bile pigments in the tissue. Commonly secondary to liver disease, gall bladder obstruction, or immune-mediated hemolytic anemia.
Jejunum	Chapter 10	The middle section of the small intestine.
Joint capsule	Chapter 8	A thick connective band of fibrous tissue that surrounds the joint and keeps the bone aligned.
Joint cavity	Chapter 8	Area within the joint capsule filled with the lubricating synovial fluid.
Joint effusion	Chapter 8	When the joint is inflamed from injury or disease, the joint capsule begins to swell outward as joint fluid production increases secondary to inflammation.
Joint mouse	Chapter 8	A small irregular piece of articulate cartilage that has broken off a boney surface.
Joint tap	Chapter 8	With a patient under sedation, a needle is placed into the joint capsule and joint fluid is harvested. The fluid is then prepared for evaluation. Changes in joint fluid can suggest inflammatory joint disease (i.e. arthritis, rheumatoid arthritis), infection (septic joint), or cancer.
Joints	Chapter 8	Joints are the intersections of bones or other articulations that serve to unite the bones firmly or allow free movement.
Juxtomglomerular cells	Chapter 13	Specialized cells present within the arterioles of the glomeruli that aid in the maintenance of blood pressure.
Keratoconjunctivitis sicca	Chapter 16, 20	A disease producing a lack of normal tear production in the eye that leads to irritation of the outer segment of the eye, inflammation of the cornea, and chronic mucoid discharge.
Ketoacidosis	Chapter 25	A condition in response to increased to extremely high blood glucose levels. The body metabolizes excess sugar by converting it to acetone, a ketone. Acetone is a toxin that acidifies the blood, making the pet anorexic, ill, and weak.
Ketonuria	Chapter 23	Ketone in the urine.
Kilovoltage (Kv)	Chapter 25	The amount of energy applied to tungsten filaments to produce a stream of electrons that produces x-ray radiation.
Lateral	Chapter 1	An object or lesion that is farther away from the median plane in respect to another object.
Lavage	Chapter 10	Rinsing the abdomen copiously with sterile fluids.
Left atrioventricular valve (mitral valve)	Chapter 12	The valve that separates the left atrium from the left ventricle.
Lens	Chapter 20	A transparent refracting media.
Lenticular sclerosis	Chapter 20	The normal aging of the lens in animals produces a chronic thickening that is perceived as a bluing of the lens.
Ligated	Chapter 3	The surgical process in which a blood vessel is tied off with sterile suture.
Lipemia	Chapter 15, 22	Increased fat in the bloodstream; a white coloration of serum from the presence of fat.
Loops of Henle	Chapter 13	Specialized structures in the renal medulla that re-absorb the fluid component of the urine.
Low-dose dexamethasone suppression test	Chapter 17	A clinical diagnostic test to evaluate the adrenal gland for overproduction of cortisol (Cushing's disease.).
Lymphocytes	Chapter 21	Small round cells with round nuclei and purple-staining cytoplasm. They are responsible for producing immunoglobulin.

Term	First Reference	Definition
Lymphocytosis	Chapter 21	Increased lymphocyte count.
Lymphoma	Chapter 22	A cancer of the immune system.
Lymphopenia	Chapter 21	A decreased lymphocyte count.
Lysosomes	Chapter 21	Intracellular vacuoles that contain chemicals to help kill bacteria and foreign material.
Macroconidia	Chapter 29	Fungal hyphae and fruiting fungal bodies.
Maldigestion syndrome	Chapter 14	The body is unable to break down nutrients in the small intestine.
Mange	Chapter 7	A cutaneous mite infection. The type of mange is dependent on the infectious mite (i.e., sarcoptes, demodex).
Mastectomy	Chapter 18	A surgical removal of part of or all the mammary chain.
Medial	Chapter 1	An object or lesion that is closest to the median plane in respect to another object.
Median plane	Chapter 1	An invisible plane that splits the pet into two symmetrical halves, used for directional terminology.
Mediastinum	Chapter 11	The region cranial and caudal to the heart and between the lungs.
Medullary canal	Chapter 8	Inside the column of bone. This is where the blood precursor cells (red blood cells, white blood cells, and platelets) develop.
Megacolon	Chapter 10	The loss of nervous control to the large colon, producing a dilation and immotility of the descending colon.
Megaesophagus	Chapter 10	The loss of nervous control to the esophagus, producing a dilation and immotility.
Megakaryocyte	Chapter 21	Large cells within the bone marrow that are the parent cell of platelets.
Melena	Chapter 14	Blood in the stool.
Menisci	Chapter 8	These structures are formed from hyaline cartilage, fibrocartilage, and fibrous tissue. They sit within the joint surface to add stability and absorb shock to the joint.
Mentation	Chapter 6	The mental status or attitude of the pet.
Mesentery	Chapter 10	A sheet of connective tissue that suspends the entire small intestine.
Metaldehyde toxicity	Chapter 27	A key poison in slug and snail bait as well as a fuel used in camp stoves. When ingested, it produces a severe excitatory effect on the central nervous system.
Metaphysis	Chapter 8	Area of primary (trabecular) soft bone located on the farthest ends of the bone. This area of bone flares out to increase the articular surface of the joint, providing a larger surface area to more evenly balance weight distribution.
Metarubricytes	Chapter 21	Large cells within the bone marrow that are precursor cells of the red blood cells.
Metastatic chest protocol	Chapter 11	A specific thoracic radiographic study to evaluate the patient for possible masses in the chest.
Methoxyhemoglobin	Chapter 27	An altered form of hemoglobin that is unable to carry oxygen into the body; thus, the animal slowly begins to suffocate.
Milliamperage seconds (MaS)	Chapter 25	The length of time electrons are exposed to tissue.
Minimal clinical database	Chapter 30	A quick diagnostic baseline usually including a packed cell volume, total protein, blood glucose, and other possible diagnostics.
Mitral insufficiency (cardiac)	Chapter 12	A disease of improper blood flow through the mitral valve (left atrial/ventricular valve).
Monocyte	Chapter 21	Monocytes have unsegmented nuclei with a purple-staining cytoplasm. They are seen with chronic infections.
Monocytosis	Chapter 21	An increased monocyte level.
Mucocutaneous junctions	Chapter 29	Regions where the hair coat meets the skin (i.e., nail bed, lips, around the eye, the nasal planum, and areas around the genitals).
Mucous membranes	Chapter 6	Membrane lining of a passage or cavity that communicates with the air.
Murmur	Chapter 7	A soft blowing or rasping sound heard on auscultation of the heart.
Mycoplasma (formerly hemobartonella)	Chapter 21	An intracellular blood parasite.
Myelogram	Chapter 25	A dye study that uses a water-soluble iodine-based solution, called Iohexol, to check for strictures and pressures in the spinal cord caused by intervertebral disc extrusion or spinal masses.
Myoglobin	Chapter 23	An oxygen-carrying compound within muscle tissue.
Myoglobinuria	Chapter 23	Myoglobin in the urine.
Necrosis	Chapter 24	Death of areas of tissue or bone.
Negative feedback loop	Chapter 27	When the production of a specific chemical inhibits further production of the same compound.
Neoplasia	Chapter 6	An abnormal formation of tissue or growth as in a cancer.
Neoplastic	Chapter 8	Pertaining to the formation of abnormal tissue (cancer).
Nephron	Chapter 8	The glomeruli, the convoluted tubules, and the nephrotic loops are called a nephron and represent the smallest functional unit within the kidney.

Term	First Reference	Definition
Neutropenia	Chapter 21	A decreased neutrophil level.
Neutrophilia	Chapter 21	An increased neutrophil level.
Nonsteroidal anti-inflammatory drugs (NSAIDs)	Chapter 26	A group of drugs that reduces pain and inflammation caused by trauma, fever, wear and tear, and athletic injury.
Nothing per os (NPO)	Chapter 15	A medical term requesting that no food and water be given to a patient.
Nystagmus	Chapter 5	Constant, involuntary, cyclic movement of the eyeball.
Obstructive shock; obstruction of vessels	Chapter 30	A shock syndrome brought on by obstruction of vessels; for example, thrombo-embolism, tumor involving a large vessel, or torsion (GDV).
Omnivores	Chapter 9	Animals whose diets consist of meats and vegetables.
Onchyectomy	Chapter 3	The surgical removal of the fingertip and nail bed of the pet's digits.
Open fracture	Chapter 8	A fracture that has punctured through the skin, increasing the chance of infection in the bone.
Opioid agonist/antagonist	Chapter 29	Drugs such as butorphanol (Torbutrol) and buprenorphine (Buprenex) that help reduce the patient's response to pain.
Opisthotonus	Chapter 7, 27	A spasm or seizure in which the patient becomes lateral recumbent, with the front legs rigid and the head rigid perpendicular to the spine.
Optic nerve	Chapter 20	A cranial nerve that transmits visual images to the brain.
Orchidectomy	Chapter 3	A complete removal of both the testicles of a male animal, rendering the pet unable to reproduce and decreasing their secondary sex characteristics (i.e., aggression, voice change, marking territory, etc.).
Organophosphate/carbamate toxicosis	Chapter 27	Common ingredients in pet flea and tick control, household insecticides, and agriculture products. When the pet is exposed to high levels of these drugs, it interferes with the normal muscle and nervous function.
Os penis	Chapter 28	The male canine penis contains a bone called the os penis.
OSHA	Chapter 4	Occupational Safety and Health Administration; an agency that oversees safety issues within the workplace.
Osteochondritis dissecans (OCD)	Chapter 8	With this disease, there is change in the normal lay down of cartilage lining the joint, which produce areas of thickened, irregular cartilage that is prone to become injured and break loose. When this happens, a nonhealing ulcer occurs, which produces chronic pain upon movement of the joint.
Osteomyelitis	Chapter 25	An infection of the bone.
Osteosarcoma	Chapter 22	A cancer of the bone.
Otitis	Chapter 20	An inflammation or infection of the ear.
Otitis externa	Chapter 20	An inflammation or infection of the external ear canal.
Otitis interna	Chapter 20	An inflammation or infection of the inner ear.
Otitis media	Chapter 20	An inflammation or infection of the middle ear.
Ova	Chapter 18	The female gamete, the egg.
Ovariohysterectomy (spay)	Chapter 3	Complete removal of both ovaries and the uterus to the cervix, rendering the female unable to reproduce or show signs of heat.
Overbite	Chapter 9	A syndrome where the upper jaw is much longer than the lower, causing mis-alignment of the teeth.
Oxidative injury	Chapter 27	*See Heinz body anemia.*
Pacemaker of the heart	Chapter 24	The initiator of the conduction signal is high in the right atrium in a region called the sino-atrial node (S-A node). Because the S-A node has the highest amount of automaticity of the heart fibers, it can stimulate a wave of depolarization on its own without outside stimulation.
Packed cell volume (PCV/total protein)	Chapter 21	The most reliable measurement of red blood cell level in a patient. It is the percentage of red blood cells present in a peripheral blood sample.
Palpebral reflex	Chapter 29	By placing light pressure on the medial or lateral skin around the eyes, a blink reflex is produced.
Pancreatic adenoma/ adenocarcinoma	Chapter 15	Benign and malignant tumors of pancreatic tissue.
Pancreatic duct	Chapter 10	Empties into the duodenum.
Pancreatic lipase immunoreactivity	Chapter 22	A diagnostic test for pancreatitis (especially in the feline).
Pancreatitis	Chapter 15	An acute or chronic inflammatory condition of the pancreas
Panosteitis	Chapter 8	An inflammation of the medullary canal on the long bones in rapidly growing large to giant dog breeds
Panosteitis	Chapter 25	An inflammation of the bone.
Paradoxical pulses	Chapter 12	A syndrome whereby the pulse weakens and strengthens as the patient inhales and exhales. This change suggests a fluid accumulation around the heart, a pericardial effusion.
Parathyroid gland	Chapter 16	Secretes hormones to control the level of calcium within the bloodstream.
Parenteral	Chapter 28	Administration of medication that is other than oral route.
Parotid gland	Chapter 9	A salivary gland.

Term	First Reference	Definition
Pathologic fracture	Chapter 8	A disease process or cancer that produces severe decalcification of the bone so that a bone can break without any trauma.
Perfusion	Chapter 7	Ability to maintain normal blood flow to the tissue.
Pericardial effusion	Chapter 7	Accumulation of fluid around the heart within the pericardial sac.
Pericardium	Chapter 12	A sheet of clear tissue than surrounds the heart.
Perineal urethrostomy	Chapter 13	A surgery to create a new opening above the penis
Periodontal disease	Chapter 9	A process that causes destruction of the supporting structures around the teeth. These supporting structures include the gums (gingiva), the bone that forms the tooth socket (alveolar bone), and the connective tissue that attaches the tooth into the tooth socket (periodontal ligament).
Periodontal ligament	Chapter 9	The connective tissue that attaches the tooth into the tooth socket.
Peripheral edema	Chapter 22	Fluid that pools within the tissue causing swelling of the limbs.
Perisoteum	Chapter 8	A thick connective tissue membrane covering the bone. It is responsible for protection and nutrition of the bone.
Peristalsis	Chapter 10	The normal movement of the intestines to churn food and move it forward through the intestinal tract.
Peritoneal lavage	Chapter 13	Administration of specialized fluids directly into the abdomen; can sometimes help decrease the toxin load.
Peritoneum	Chapter 14	A thin layer of tissue that covers the interior of the abdomen and secretes a clear sterile fluid to prevent attachment of bacteria to help resist infection.
Peritonitis	Chapter 10	A massive infection of the abdomen.
Petechiation	Chapter 14	Small pinpoint hemorrhages noticed in the skin or mucous membranes.
Phagocytosis	Chapter 21	The absorption and digestion of foreign material and bacteria by the white blood cell through the extension of its cell wall around the foreign invader.
Pharynx	Chapter 11	The common region of the nose and mouth.
Phenothiazines	Chapter 29	A long-term medication (usually lasting 8–12 hours in duration) used more for sedation.
Pheochromocytoma	Chapter 17	A metabolically active tumor of the adrenal medulla that secretes epinephrine.
Photophobia	Chapter 20	Sensitivity to light.
Photoreceptors	Chapter 20	The cells of the retina that process light into an electrical signal.
Piloerection	Chapter 29	Elevation of the hair.
Pinna	Chapter 20	The ear flap.
Pituitary-dependent hyperadrenocorticism (PDH)	Chapter 27	A disease syndrome produced by small microscopic pituitary tumors that over-produce ACTH, stimulating the adrenal glands to constantly produce cortisol.
Pituitary gland	Chapter 17	A small gland in the brain, also called the master gland, that secretes many different types of hormones to control other hormone release in the body.
Plantograde gait	Chapter 15	Patients that present walking flat on back legs at the level of the ankle.
Plaque	Chapter 9	The soft "slime" layer of material found on tooth surfaces composed of salivary proteins, decayed food materials, and bacteria.
Platelets	Chapter 21	Small cell components of blood that are several times smaller than normal red blood cells. They function in clot formation.
Pleural effusion	Chapter 11	An accumulation of fluid within the chest, surrounding the lungs and heart.
Pleuritis	Chapter 11	A viral, bacterial, fungal, or rickettsial infection of the lining of the chest (pleura).
Pneumonia	Chapter 11	A bacterial, fungal, or viral infection involving the lung fields, the bronchi, and the trachea.
Pneumothorax	Chapter 11	An injury to the chest or lung fields that allows the introduction of air into the thorax, collapsing the lungs.
Polychromasia	Chapter 21	A bluish coloration in the red blood cells due to remnants of nuclear material.
Polychromatophilic red blood cell	Chapter 21	An immature red blood cell seen on a blood smear that indicates a regenerative response to anemia.
Polydipsia	Chapter 4	Refers to patients with increased consumption of water.
Polyphagic	Chapter 25	With increased appetites.
Polyuria	Chapter 4	With increased urination.
Portal vein	Chapter 14	Large venous system that drains the intestines, taking the absorbed nutrients, microbes, and toxins to the liver for detoxification.
Porto-caval shunt	Chapter 14	A disease process in which the blood supply from the portal system, which carries toxins that are normally metabolized by the liver, bypasses the organ and goes directly into the general circulation and central nervous system, causing severe metabolic and toxic reactions.
Postparturient hypocalcemia	Chapter 18	*See eclampsia.*
Posterior chamber	Chapter 20	The region of the eye that lies between the caudal aspect of the iris and the cranial aspect of the lens.
Postprandial	Chapter 14, 22	After a meal.

Term	First Reference	Definition
Premature ventricular contraction (PVC)	Chapter 24	In this situation a region of ventricular muscle becomes irritated by trauma, disease, or infection. This region is so irritated that it produces a depolarization wave that stimulates a ventricular contraction independent of the S-A node.
Preprandial	Chapter 13	Prior to a meal.
Progesterone	Chapter 18	A female hormone produced by the ovary to sustain pregnancy.
Prophylaxis	Chapter 9	Describes the process of cleaning a patient's teeth under anesthesia in the veterinary hospital.
Prostate gland	Chapter 18	A single gland located around and along the urethra, just behind the excretory ducts of the vesicular gland, producing a small amount of fluids for the ejaculate and producing necessary electrolytes to help sperm motility and fertility.
Prosthesis	Chapter 8	Replacement of a missing part with an artificial substitute.
Protein-losing enteropathy	Chapter 22	A disease affecting the intestine's ability to absorb protein.
Protein-losing nephropathy	Chapter 22	A disease affecting the kidneys, producing an abnormal excretion of protein out of the glomeruli.
Proteins induced by vitamin K antagonism (PIVKA)	Chapter 27	A highly suggestive clinical diagnostic blood test that detects proteins produced when drugs that interfere with vitamin K are present in the body.
Proteinuria	Chapter 23	Protein in the urine.
Protruding third eyelid (cherry eye)	Chapter 20	The swelling and inflammation of the gland on the back side of the third eyelid, producing a protrusion and elevation.
Proximal	Chapter 1	An object or lesion on a limb that is closer to the body than another object.
Proximal convoluted tubules	Chapter 13	A region within the nephron that functions to actively re-absorb all of the necessary nutrients back into the bloodstream.
Pruritic	Chapter 19	Severe itchiness.
Pruritus	Chapter 7	Severe itchiness.
Pseudoarthrosis	Chapter 8	A false joint formation.
Pulmonary edema	Chapter 11	A filling of the airways with fluid.
Pulmonic valve	Chapter 12	The valve that separates the right ventricle from the right outflow tract taking de-oxygenated blood to the lungs.
Pulse deficit	Chapter 7	A lack of pulse associated with a heartbeat. Can be suggestive of a cardiac arrhythmia or shock.
Pulse oximetry	Chapter 12	The percent of oxygen-carrying capacity of the blood.
Pupillary light response (PLR)	Chapter 20	An ocular reflex whereby a light shines into one iris and it constricts.
Purkinje fibers (Bundle of His)	Chapter 24	Specific conductive fibers in the intraventricular septum that carry a wave of depolarization from the atrium to the ventricles.
Purulence	Chapter 7	Containing pus.
Pustules	Chapter 29	Small elevation in the skin filled with lymph or pus.
p-wave	Chapter 24	The electrical wave that spreads over the atrium away from the EKG sensor and then returns to baseline. After the p-wave is produced, both atria contract, producing diasystole.
Pyelonephritis	Chapter 8	Infection or inflammation of the glomeruli.
Pyometra	Chapter 28	A massive infection of the uterus.
Pyuria	Chapter 23	White blood cells in the urine.
QRS wave	Chapter 24	The electrical wave denoted on the EKG after the p-wave, which denotes a wave of depolarization that stimulates ventricular contraction.
Radio-dense	Chapter 10	The ability of a tissue or mass to show up on a radiograph.
Refractometer	Chapter 13, 23	Measures the specific gravity or the measure of concentration of a fluid.
Renal cortex	Chapter 13	The outermost tissue region of the kidney, which houses hundreds of thousands of specialized structures called glomeruli (Bowman's capsules).
Renal glomeruli (Bowman's capsules)	Chapter 13	A set of tubules closely interdigitated with small arterioles, which serves as a filter for the body.
Renal medulla	Chapter 13	The renal medulla houses a section of the nephron called the nephrotic loops (Loops of Henle), which function to re-absorb most of the fluid component of the urine.
Renin–angiotensin system	Chapter 13	A system of enzymes that are released in response to low blood pressure to produce vasoconstriction, producing increased blood pressure.
Renolithiasis	Chapter 13	A kidney stone.
Respiration rate	Chapter 11	The rate at which the animal breathes normally while at rest.
Retina	Chapter 20	The innermost tunic of the eye that receives visual images from the lens and transmits them via the optic nerve to the brain.
Right atrioventricular valve (tricuspid)	Chapter 12	The valve that separates the right atrium from the right ventricle.
Rod cells	Chapter 20	Detect light in dim and dark environments.
Roleaux formation	Chapter 21	Roleaux formation is a stacking of red blood cells, similar to coins, on a saline blood film.

Term	First Reference	Definition
Rubriblast	Chapter 21	An immature red blood cell seen on a blood smear that indicates a regenerative response to anemia.
Rubricyte	Chapter 21	An immature red blood cell seen on a blood smear that indicates a regenerative response to anemia.
Salivary glands	Chapter 9	These glands secrete saliva that helps emulsify food into a liquid solution.
Sanguineous	Chapter 28	Bloody fluid.
Scatter radiation	Chapter 25	Radiation that scatters off in all directions from the x-ray table.
Schirmer tear test	Chapter 20	A test that checks for normal tear production in an eye.
Schistocyte	Chapter 21	Schistocytes are fragmented red blood cells that are produced from colliding with intravascular fibrin strands as the body attempts to form clots within the blood vessels.
Sclera	Chapter 7	A tough, white, fibrous tissue that covers the eye (the white of the eye).
Seborrhea	Chapter 19	A defect in keratinization (skin formation) with increased scaling, with or without excessive greasiness of the skin and coat, and often secondary inflammation.
Seborrhea oleosa	Chapter 19	Oily seborrhea.
Seborrhea sicca	Chapter 19	Dry seborrhea.
Sepsis	Chapter 10	A massive infection of the body.
Serosanguineous	Chapter 18	Bloody/serum fluid.
Sesamoids	Chapter 8	These small bones formed in muscle tendons function to protect tendons at the points of greatest friction.
Shift-Sherrington syndrome	Chapter 6	A syndrome associated with a trauma (usually from being hit by a car) that produces a patient with rigid nonmoveable forelegs and neck, while its hind end is completely relaxed. This syndrome usually suggests that there has been a fracture in the lower back, and the spinal cord may be damaged or severed.
Shiotz tonimetry	Chapter 20	A device that measures pressure within the eye.
Signalment	Chapter 6	A legal description of the patient.
Sino-atrial node (S-A node)	Chapter 24	The initiator of the conduction signal is high in the right atrium in a region called the sino-atrial node (S-A node). Because the S-A node has the highest amount of automaticity of the heart fibers, it can stimulate a wave of depolarization on its own without outside stimulation.
SOAP method	Chapter 6	The SOAP method is a set protocol of recording a physical examination made up of subjective, objective, assessment, and plan components.
Spastic entropion	Chapter 20	Process whereby entropion can occur secondary to chronically inflamed and irritated eyes.
Spherocytes	Chapter 21	Small, dense, red blood cells without the normal central pallor. Usually seen with immune-mediated hemolytic anemia. When serum antibodies adhere to the surface of the red blood cell, the macrophages in the spleen and liver recognize the damaged portion of the red cell membrane and pinch it off. The loss of cell membrane changes the shape of the red blood cell to a sphere. Spherocytes should be suspected when there is large variability in red blood cell size.
Spontaneous ovulators	Chapter 18	Animals that ovulate independently of any neuroendocrine stimulation.
Status epilepticus	Chapter 30	Patients present with constant seizures.
Stenosis	Chapter 12	A narrowing of the area in front, at the valve level, or above the pulmonary or aortic valves of the heart valve that impedes blood flow.
Stridor	Chapter 11	A respiratory noise.
Stump pyometra	Chapter 18	An infection of the uterine stump in a spayed female.
Subcutaneous emphysema	Chapter 11	Air under the skin.
Sublingual gland	Chapter 9	A salivary gland.
Subluxation	Chapter 25	Dislocation of the bones in a joint.
Submandibular gland	Chapter 9	A salivary gland.
Supernatant	Chapter 23	The liquid portion that is poured off after urine has been spun down.
Sutures	Chapter 8	Dense connective tissue that connect bones to form a nonmoveable joint.
Symmetrical flank alopecia	Chapter 19	A bilateral even pattern of hair loss over the lateral abdomen.
Synarthrosis	Chapter 8	A joint formed by bones connected by dense connective tissue sutures.
Synchondrosis	Chapter 8	Cartilaginous joints that contain bones connected by dense cartilage; this includes the joints formed between the epiphysis and diaphysis of young animals' long bones.
Synovial fluid	Chapter 8	Fluid secreted by the synovial membrane of the joint that helps lubricate and aid in the nutrition of the joint.
Synovial joint	Chapter 8	These joints are freely movable and are united by a fluid-filled cavity.
Synovial membrane	Chapter 8	A thin layer of connective tissue that stretches out over the entire articular surface.
Systole	Chapter 12	The phase of contraction of the ventricles of the heart.

Term	First Reference	Definition
Tachycardia	Chapter 6	An abnormally rapid heart rate.
Tachypnea	Chapter 7	Elevated respiratory rate.
Tachypnic	Chapter 11	An increased respiratory rate.
Taenia	Chapter 10	A species of tapeworms found in dogs and cats.
Tartar	Chapter 9	Calculus that is mineralized plaque deposits; often yellow to brown in color.
Tendonectomy	Chapter 3	A surgical procedure that removes a small section of tendon in each toe to prevent the extension of the cat's claws.
The nephrotic loops (Loops of Henle)	Chapter 13	Specialized structures in the renal medulla that function to re-absorb the fluid component of the urine.
Theobromine	Chapter 27	A toxin found in chocolate.
Third phalanx	Chapter 3	Refers to the distal third bone of the finger or toe that produces nail or hoof.
Thoracentesis	Chapter 11	A chest tap.
Thoracotomy	Chapter 10, 25	A surgical opening of the chest.
Thrombocytopenia	Chapter 21	A low platelet count.
Thrombocytosis	Chapter 21	A increased platelet count.
Thromboembolism	Chapter 12	Due to abnormal blood flow, small clots can form in the ventricles of cats; these clots can be pushed into the aorta as the ventricle contracts. They are then called embolisms or thromboembolisms.
Thyroid-stimulating hormone	Chapter 16	A hormone produced by the pituitary to stimulate thyroxine release from the thyroid gland.
Thyroidectomy	Chapter 16	Surgical removal of the thyroid gland.
Thyroxine	Chapter 16	A hormone produced by the adrenal gland that sets the rate the cells of the body burn energy.
Toxocara	Chapter 10	A species of roundworms in the canine and feline.
Trabecular bone	Chapter 8	Soft bone located on the farthest ends of a long bone.
Tracheobronchitis	Chapter 11	A highly infectious upper respiratory and bronchial infection that is a combination of a viral and bacterial or fungal infection; it affects most dogs and cats, especially in a shelter environment.
Tracheoscopy/bronchoscopy	Chapter 11	A noninvasive anesthetic procedure performed by passing a fiber optic camera down the trachea into the lung fields.
Transdermal	Chapter 19	Refers to medication that can be absorbed through the skin.
Transtracheal wash	Chapter 11	A sterile catheter or red rubber feeding tube placed between the tracheal rings of a sedated animal. The catheter is run down the trachea as far as possible, and a small amount of sterile fluid is flushed into the trachea and lower airways. This stimulates the animal to cough and bring up debris. The sterile fluid and debris are then aspirated for culture and cytology.
Transudate	Chapter 14	A low protein–low cellular fluid.
Triage	Chapter 6	The evaluation of an incoming pet for stability, injury, or disease.
Trichuris	Chapter 10	A species of whipworms in the canine and feline.
Trigone	Chapter 13	A region of the caudal bladder where the ureters from the kidneys empty into the bladder.
Triple pelvic osteotomy	Chapter 8	This procedure is done prophylactically in young animals with evidence of early hip dysplasia and poor hip conformation, where the femoral head is not well seated within the hip.
Trypsin-like immunoreactivity (TLI)	Chapter 21	A diagnostic test for pancreatic exocrine insufficiency and chronic pancreatitis (canine).
Tunic	Chapter 20	An investing membrane.
t-wave	Chapter 24	After the full heartbeat occurs, the muscle goes through a wave of repolarization where the electrolytes of the body are rebalanced to make the heart ready for the next beat.
Uncinaria	Chapter 10	A species of hookworm found in the canine and feline.
Underbite	Chapter 9	An abnormal architecture of the jaw where the lower jaw is much longer than the upper, causing misalignment of the teeth.
Upper GI (barium series)	Chapter 25	An upper GI is a radiographic study in which the patient ingests barium, and x-rays are taken at set intervals to evaluate possible obstruction, mass, or ulceration of the esophagus, stomach, and intestines.
Urine cortisol creatinine ratio	Chapter 17	A clinical diagnostic test that evaluates the patient's urine cortisol levels in relation to the urine creatinine levels.
Urine protein/creatinine ratio	Chapter 13	This test is usually run when there is a persistent urine protein presence without evidence of urinary tract disease. Normally, the protein molecules are too large to pass through the glomerular filters. The smaller amino acid creatinine is released in the urine in large amounts. When there is glomerular damage, protein can leak through the filters, increasing the amount of protein in the urine and increasing the protein/creatinine ratio.

Term	First Reference	Definition
Urine specific gravity	Chapter 23	The concentrating ability of urine.
Urolithes	Chapter 13	Bladder stones.
Urolithiasis	Chapter 23	A bladder stone.
Uveal	Chapter 20	The second tunic of the eye, which supplies nutrients and oxygen to the ocular tissue.
Uveitis	Chapter 20	An inflammation of the uveal coat of the eye; the anterior uveal coat is the iris, and the posterior uveal coat is the blood vessels supplying the blood to the retina.
Ventral	Chapter 1	An object or region on the body that is closer to the sternum than another object.
Ventroflexion of the neck	Chapter 13	Patients that are unable to lift their necks into a normal position secondary to severe hypokalemia.
Virulence	Chapter 2	Ability of a pathogenic organism (bacteria, fungus, virus, or protozoa) to cause a disease.
Visceral larval migrans	Chapter 10	A parasitic infection of humans where the larval form burrows through the internal architecture of the body.
Vitreous chamber	Chapter 20	A region in the eye that lies between the caudal aspect of the lens and the retina.
Warfarin	Chapter 27	A poison that interferes with the normal clotting agents that clot blood and stop bleeding.
Zona fasciculata	Chapter 17	Inner regions of the adrenal cortex that produces a prednisone-like steroid called cortisol.
Zona granulosa	Chapter 17	Outermost area of the cortex that is responsible for producing a steroid hormone called aldosterone, also called a mineralocorticoid.
Zona reticularis	Chapter 17	Inner regions of the adrenal cortex that produces a prednisone-like steroid called cortisol.
Zoonotic disease	Chapter 6	Diseases that are communicable from animal to human.
Zygomatic gland	Chapter 9	A salivary gland.

Resources

The following sources are recommended as good referral sources for the veterinary team. They all have strengths in their own field and can be a part of an excellent referral library:

On-Line Sources
- CET University (a Virbac site): www.cetuniversity.com—An online interactive continuing education site on veterinary dentistry.
- Dermatology University (a Virbac site): www.virbac-dermu.com—An online interactive continuing education site on veterinary dermatology.

Textbooks

- Tilley, Larry, and Smith, Francis, *5-Minute Consult: Canine and Feline*, 3rd ed. Blackwell Publishing, Ames, Iowa. 2005.
- Colville, Thomas, and Bassert, Joanna. *Clinical Anatomy and Physiology for Veterinary Technicians*. Mosby, Philadelphia. 2001.

Index

Page references followed by f denote figures. References followed by t denote tables.

Antifungals
kidney toxicity, 184
for pneumonia, 141
Antigens
defined, 108, 488
screening for in heartworm disease, 169
Antihistamines, 140, 168, 384-385, 443
Anti-inflammatory medications. *See also specific medications*
for arthritis, 78
dimethyl sulfoxide (DMSO), 387
glucosamine, 387-388
nonsteroidal anti-inflammatory medications (NSAIDs), 385-386
steroidal medication, 386-387
tramadol, 388
Antiparasitic agents
fendbendazole, 389
ivermectin/avermectin, 388
praziquantel, 389
pyrantel pamoate, 388-389
sulfadimethoxine, 389-390
tylosin tartrate, 390
Anuria, 185, 488
Aortic valve, 147, 148f-151f, 154, 488
Apnea, 406, 424, 488
Appetite
in dental disease, 89
history, 36
in hyperthyroidism, 221
in liver disease, 197
in pancreatic disease, 208
Approaching an animal, 27-28, 27f
cat behavior under stress, 28
dog behavior under stress, 27-28
Aqueous humor, 282, 488
Arrhythmia
causes, 355, 426, 431
defined, 489
in GDV, 126
sinus arrhythmia, 359
Arthritis
age of onset/incubation, 76
breeds commonly affected, 76
complications, 77
defined, 75
diagnosis, 77, 77f
discussing with clients, 79
history points, 76-77
observations on initial assessment, 77
overview, 75, 77f
prevention, 78
signalment, 75-76
treatment, 78
Articular, 63, 488
Articular bone surface, 63
Articular cartilage, 65f, 66, 75
Articular surface, 66, 488
Artificial respiration, 456
AS (left ear), 6

Ascariasis, 488. *See also* Roundworms
Ascites, 162, 195-196, 197, 488
Ascriptin, 78
Aspartate aminotransferase (AST or SGOT)
abnormalities, 314
defined, 488
diagnostic tests to evaluate, 314-315
discussing with clients, 315
function, 314
in liver disease, 199, 314-315
location of production, 314
symptoms associated with elevations, 314
ASPCA-University of Illinois Poison Control, 398
Aspiration, 488
Aspiration pneumonia, 106, 422
Aspirin, 78, 167
Assessment
adrenal disease, 226-227, 227f
cardiac disease, 151-154, 152t, 153f
dental disease, 90-91, 90f, 91f, 92f, 93f
ears, 286, 286f
endocrine pancreas disease, 213, 213f, 214f
exocrine pancreas disease, 209
gastrointestinal system, 107-108, 107t
liver disease, 197-198, 198f, 198t
ocular disease, 275-276, 275f, 276f
orthopedic cases, 70-72, 71f, 72f, 73f
reproductive disease, 241, 241t, 242f
respiratory disease, 132-133, 133f, 133t
skin (integument), 250-252, 250f-252f
in SOAP method, 46
thyroid disease, 218-219, 219f, 220f
urogenital system, 180, 180f, 180t
AST. *See* Aspartate aminotransferase (AST or SGOT)
Asthma. *See* Feline asthma
Atopy, 267, 488
ATP, 129, 488
Atrial septal defect, 155f
Atrial-ventricular node (A-V node), 354, 355f, 488
Atrioventricular block (heart block)
complications, 363
degrees, 363
diagnostics, 363-364, 363f
discussing with clients, 364
etiology, 363
history points, 363
observations on initial assessment, 363
prevention, 364
signalment, 363
treatment, 364
Atrophy
in arthritis, 77
defined, 488
disuse, 77
in OCD, 85

Atropine
drug interactions, 393
emergency dose, 459t, 486t
form of drug, 393
precautions, 393
route of administration, 393
side effects, 393
use in cardiopulmonary cerebral resuscitation (CPCR), 457
AU (each ear), 6
Aural hematoma
complications, 289
defined, 488
diagnosis, 289
discussing with clients, 289
history points, 289
observations on initial assessment, 289, 289f
prevention, 290
signalment, 289
treatment, 289-290
Auscultation
heart, 54-55, 54f, 154, 159, 427, 443, 445, 461
respiratory system, 55, 55f, 133, 134f, 135f, 154, 427, 445
Automaticity, 353
Autonomic nervous system, 423
Avoidance behavior, 27
Axillary artery pulse, 41, 42f
Azotemia
defined, 175, 178, 488
post-renal, 179, 179t, 318, 462t
pre-renal, 178, 178t, 318, 462t
renal, 178-179, 179t, 318, 462t
signs of, 316-317, 319

Babesia, 299, 303f, 488
Bacteria, in urine sediment, 344
Bactericidal antibiotics, 381, 383
Bacteriostatic antibiotics, 381
Bacteriuria, 342, 488
Bad breath. *See* Halitosis
Bands, 301, 304f, 306-307, 465
BAR (bright, alert, and responsive), 4, 51
Barbiturates, 424
Barium
swallow, 117
upper GI series, 109, 110f, 371f
Barotraumas, 430, 488
Basal metabolic rate (BMR)
defined, 488
thyroid hormone regulation of, 217, 220, 222, 330
Basophilia, 307, 488
Basophils, 307, 488
Behavior changes, in hyperthyroidism, 221
Benzodinepines, 424, 488
Beta-blockers, 165
BID (twice per day), 5